A Beginner's Guide
to Targeted Cancer
Treatments and Cancer
Immunotherapy

T0293746

A Beginner's Guide to Targeted Cancer Treatments and Cancer Immunotherapy

SECOND EDITION

Elaine Vickers

WILEY

Registered Offices
John Wiley & Sons, Inc., 111 River Street, Hoboken, NJ 07030, USA
John Wiley & Sons Ltd, The Atrium, Southern Gate, Chichester, West Sussex, PO19 8SQ, UK

For details of our global editorial offices, customer services, and more information about Wiley products visit us at www.wiley.com.

Wiley also publishes its books in a variety of electronic formats and by print-on-demand. Some content that appears in standard print versions of this book may not be available in other formats.

Library of Congress Cataloging-in-Publication Data
Names: Vickers, Elaine (Elaine Ruth), author.
Title: A beginner's guide to targeted cancer treatments and cancer
    immunotherapy / Elaine Vickers.
Description: Second edition. | Hoboken, NJ, USA : Wiley, 2025. | Includes
    bibliographical references and index.
Identifiers: LCCN 2024029662 (print) | LCCN 2024029663 (ebook) | ISBN
    9781119834069 (pb) | ISBN 9781119834076 (adobe pdf) | ISBN 9781119834083
    (epub)
Subjects: MESH: Neoplasms–drug therapy | Molecular Targeted
    Therapy–methods
Classification: LCC RC271.C5 V53 2024 (print) | LCC RC271.C5 (ebook) |
    DDC 616.99/406–dc23/eng/20240708
LC record available at https://lccn.loc.gov/2024029662
LC ebook record available at https://lccn.loc.gov/2024029663

Cover Design: Wiley
Cover Image: © Juan Gaertner/Shutterstock

Set in 9.5/13pt Palatino by Straive, Pondicherry, India
SKY10086953_100424

Contents

Acknowledgments

Firstly, and most importantly, I am enormously indebted to Kathleen Killen, who I met through her work at Cancer Research UK. Kat contacted me at the end of 2022, offering her proofreading skills as a medical writer, and she has contributed enormously to this edition. Not only has Kat scrutinized every word on every page, legend, footnote, and table, but she has also made many valuable contributions to the consistency, accuracy, and inclusivity of the content.

I would also like to thank everyone else who has offered their advice and reviewed and critiqued this edition. They are: Maggie Uzzell, Joanne Bird, Anne Croudass, Karen Turner, Ben Hood, Chloe Beland, Miranda Payne, Nick Duncan, Clayton Wong, and Philip Dean.

As with the first edition, special thanks go to Ruth McLaren. Ruth was the person who first suggested I should teach nurses and other health professionals as my full-time occupation. Without her, my business and my book might never have happened.

Praise for the First Edition

"I wish this book had existed when I began my career in oncology research. It gives an excellent background to proteins within cancer cells and healthy cells as well as microenvironment differences in cancers. Reading this book gave me even deeper insight into some of the studies I had previously worked on. The writing style and presentation of material is very easy to follow and well organized."

–Dr Ben Hood, Cancer Research Consultant Nurse, Sir Bobby Robson Cancer Trials Research Centre

"Well done on such a massive undertaking and a really, really useful book. I've learned a lot as I've read it."

–Dr Sue Brook, Associate Medical Director, Ellipses Pharma

"Very impressive! Supportively written, this will become the "go-to book" for any health care professional wanting information on targeted treatments in cancer."

–Daniel Collins, Deputy Chief Pharmacist, Liverpool Women's NHS Foundation Trust

"As a healthcare professional, I need to know how the drugs I administer to my patients are acting in the body, how they are designed to fight cancer, and to be able to answer the sometimes-difficult questions that patients ask. This book helps me to do this with confidence. It is complicated in parts because the science is complicated, but written in a way that all those working in the field of cancer care will be able to understand, with knowledge that they can apply to practice. Fabulous illustrations throughout the book and a very logical format make this text accessible to all."

–Nikki Hayward, Skin Cancer CNS team lead, Buckinghamshire Healthcare NHS Trust

"What an amazing achievement! Patients and healthcare professionals will be delighted to discover a book that makes incomprehensible concepts accessible, interesting, and logical."

–Heather Phillips, Research Delivery Manager, NIHR

"Really wonderful, so nicely written, exactly what I had been looking for. We are in the very early stages of developing an NIH/NCI grant proposal related to technology that helps clinicians easily align their patients' variants with potential treatment options, and Dr. Vickers' book was absolutely invaluable at opening my eyes to the complexity and the possibilities."

–Bob Dolin, Senior Informaticist, Elimu Informatics

I recommend this book to all of my students who wish to further develop their knowledge of some of the targeted therapies used to treat cancer. The book is well written which strengthens its use as a reference and it is also a book which readers can use to check their understanding of these treatments. It contains excellent illustrations.

–Maggie Uzzell, The Royal Marsden School

About the Author

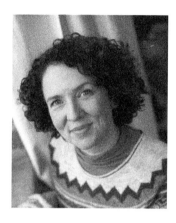

Elaine Vickers has been a cancer educator and writer for over twenty years. Since setting up her company, Science Communicated Ltd (sciencecommunicated.co.uk), Elaine has developed a wide range of study days, courses, and teaching materials that explain cancer biology and the science behind targeted cancer treatments and immunotherapies.

Each year, Elaine teaches hundreds of cancer nurses, doctors, and allied cancer professionals working in the United Kingdom. She also presents a regular program of in-person study days for the Royal Marsden Conference Centre in London and speaks at numerous cancer conferences in the United Kingdom and Europe. In recent years, Elaine has expanded her reach by delivering online courses and creating educational videos and webinars. She has also worked with an animator to create animations that explain cancer and cancer treatments.

Elaine has a degree in Medical Science from the University of Birmingham and a PhD in Molecular Biology from the University of Manchester. Her goal is to unravel the complexities of cancer biology and new cancer treatments and make these topics interesting and accessible to nonscientists.

Elaine considers herself incredibly lucky to live in Manchester with her husband Rowan and her little dog CJ.

How to Use This Book

I wrote the first edition of this book when I couldn't find a resource that would cover all the topics I was teaching on without overwhelming the reader with scientific detail. I felt what was missing was a single book that brought together sufficient information on cancer biology to explain the promise and the limitations of the latest cancer treatments.

Since the first edition was published in 2018, a lot has changed, particularly in the realm of immunotherapy. Thus, in this edition, I have expanded the early chapters to incorporate greater detail on the relationship between cancer and our immune system. I have also vastly expanded the information on immunotherapy. In this edition, immune checkpoint inhibitors have their own chapter. I also devote a second chapter to explanations of the science behind many other immunotherapy approaches.

As with the first edition, although I have called this book "A Beginner's Guide …" I do include a lot of science. I also don't try to hide the complexity of the subjects I am attempting to describe. However, I hope that by providing illustrations and including lots of background information in the first two chapters, you can follow the rest of the book.

You'll also notice that I don't describe any advances in radiotherapy or surgery, and I provide very little information on chemotherapy and hormone therapy. I made this choice because I am a molecular biologist, and I wanted to focus my attention on where I feel I have the most to offer: explaining the science behind targeted therapies and immunotherapies for cancer.

One challenge I had when writing this book was the rapid pace of cancer research and drug development. Although I have done my best to provide up-to-date information, this will no doubt be quickly eroded by the creation of new treatments and new approvals in the months and years to come. I apologize if any drug or bit of science you are interested in – from a professional or personal standpoint – isn't included. I hope that because I have focused on the mechanisms of action of new treatments rather than their stage of development, you will find this book relevant to you.

Another decision I made when writing the book was to provide only passing information on the degree of benefit offered by the treatments mentioned. I made this choice because the difference a treatment makes is context- and disease-specific. For example, a treatment that provides only a modest extension in survival times in people with relapsed, advanced disease may be able to cure people who have early-stage, newly diagnosed disease. As a molecular biologist interested in explaining how treatments work, I decided this level of detail was beyond the scope of this book. For similar reasons, I don't generally provide information about which countries a treatment is licensed in or for which patients.

I have presumed that when you open this book, you will be approaching the subject from one of four perspectives:

1. Because you're interested in **a specific treatment** and want to learn more about it. If that's the case, you might want to start with the index and look it up by name.
2. Because you're involved in caring for people affected by a **certain type of cancer** and want to know about the relevant treatments. If so, you might wish to turn to chapter seven first.
3. Because you'd like to know about treatments that **have a specific target**, such as CDK inhibitors, or that **have a particular mechanism**, such as vaccine-based treatments. If that's you, then chapters 3–6 will likely contain the information you're after.
4. Or, if you're relatively new to the topics covered in this book, I would advise you to begin at the beginning and go from there!

Whatever your reason for reading this book, my sincere hope is that you will find it useful and interesting.

CHAPTER 1	An Introduction to Cancer Cell Biology and Genetics

IN BRIEF

I find it impossible to describe how targeted cancer treatments work without mentioning what it is they target. And when I try to explain what it is they target, I find myself going back to the beginning and explaining where cancers come from, what faults they contain, and why they behave as they do. And, to explain that, I need to explain concepts such as DNA damage, oncogenes, tumor suppressor genes, and the hallmarks of cancer cells.

In recent years, we've also made great progress in using a patient's immune system to treat cancer using immunotherapy. When explaining how immunotherapies work, I find it useful to offer at least a brief description of our immune system and the ways in which cancer cells and white blood cells interact. Armed with this knowledge, various strategies to use the immune system to destroy cancer cells begin to make sense.

In this chapter, my goal is to bring together much of this background knowledge. I hope it will provide you with a useful foundation that enables you to understand individual targeted therapies and immunotherapies that I mention in later chapters.

First, I run through the causes and consequences of DNA mutations in cells. I describe how even just a handful of mutations can force a healthy cell to become a cancer cell.

I also describe the cancer microenvironment – the cells and structures that cancer cells live alongside, including white blood cells of our immune system. Cancer cells have the ability to exploit their local environment and, in many instances, manipulate it. I explain what impact this has when doctors come to treat people with the disease.

In addition, I tackle topics such as genome instability and intratumoral heterogeneity. Perhaps these are topics that right now don't mean anything to you, and you're unsure of why you need to know about them. But it's only through understanding these concepts that you can appreciate the limitations of targeted (and standard) cancer treatments and grasp the potential of immunotherapy. It is also important to understand why cancer spreads and how cancers evolve and change over time.

A Beginner's Guide to Targeted Cancer Treatments and Cancer Immunotherapy, Second Edition. Elaine Vickers.
© 2025 John Wiley & Sons Ltd. Published 2025 by John Wiley & Sons Ltd.

I then turn my attention to the unique properties of hematological cancers. I describe some of the types of mutation that drive their behavior and talk about why these mutations occur. I also explain their greater vulnerability to immunotherapy compared to solid tumors.

Finally, I wrap up the chapter with a brief overview of why cancer is so difficult to treat successfully and why so many people currently cannot be cured.

1.1 INTRODUCTION

This book is about the science that lies behind targeted cancer treatments and cancer immunotherapies. Almost without exception, these treatments work by attaching to, or blocking the actions of, proteins. So, to understand these treatments, it's first of all essential to understand what proteins are, how they work, and how the proteins found inside and on the surface of cancer cells differ from their healthy counterparts.

For this to make sense to you, I need to explain the different types of DNA damage that cancer cells contain, because a cell's DNA is its instruction manual telling it how to make proteins. If we know what DNA damage a cell contains, this will tell us what faulty proteins it's making. And if we know what faulty proteins it's making, we will have a better idea of which treatments might work against it.

So, this chapter contains lots of information about cancer cells, DNA, and proteins. However, even in this chapter, I've made some assumptions about what you do and don't know. For example, I've assumed that you have a rough idea of what DNA is and how cells use their DNA to make proteins. If you're not familiar with these concepts, I would recommend first taking a look at the Appendix, which contains a list of reading materials about cells, DNA, chromosomes, genes, and proteins. When you've had a look at that, you'll be ready to read further.

This chapter doesn't exclusively focus on individual cancer cells and their faults.

Cancer cells don't live alone, nor are tumors a homogenous mass of identical cancer cells. Instead, cancer cells live among other types of cells, such as fibroblasts, fat cells, and numerous types of white blood cells. This composition changes over time and also in response to treatment. In addition, cancer cells themselves evolve and change over time, and this has an enormous impact on the effectiveness, or not, of many treatments.

In this chapter, I'll also provide you with some background information about how cancer cells relate to, and influence, our immune system. Why it is, for example, that in some people their immune system reacts strongly against their cancer cells, while in another person their immune system seems to essentially shrug its shoulders and carry on as normal. I'll also pay special attention to T lymphocytes (T cells), which are at the heart of many different forms of immunotherapy.

Some of the information in this chapter is relevant to all cancers, wherever they occur in the body and whatever type of cell they developed from. However, there are some features of hematological cancers (such as leukemias and lymphomas) that set them apart from solid tumors like breast or bowel cancer. Some of this difference comes down to the mutations that drive hematological cancers, but some of it is due to their accessibility to drugs, and to healthy white blood cells.

Along with the chapter that follows (which is all about the two main groups of cancer treatments in this book: monoclonal antibodies and kinase inhibitors), this chapter hopefully provides you with all the background information you need to make sense of the rest of this book.

1.2 DNA DAMAGE IS THE CAUSE OF EVERY CANCER

Our cells' DNA is essentially a huge instruction manual telling our cells what proteins to make, how to make them, when to make them, what to do with them, and when to destroy them. In turn, the proteins our cells make dictate their behavior. For this reason, if you damage a cell's DNA, it is likely to make the wrong, or damaged, versions of proteins, leading to abnormal behavior (see Figure 1.1).

Cancer starts to develop when a single cell accumulates DNA damage to several important genes. This damage causes the cell to make faulty proteins that force it to behave abnormally. To result in cancer, the cell also needs to overcome whatever hostile forces are exerted by its environment and by neighboring cells. Thankfully, this normally doesn't happen. Instead, a cell that finds its DNA damaged usually tries to repair the damage, or it self-destructs through a process called apoptosis.[1] Or, if the cell doesn't kill itself, it's usually kept in check by its environment or destroyed by white blood cells. But, if a damaged cell survives, and if it avoids or overcomes its hostile neighbors, it might ultimately multiply and cause us to develop cancer.

Over the past 40 years or so, scientists have been gradually uncovering which gene mutations cause cancer. Genes only take up about 1%–2% or so of our cells' total DNA, so it's this DNA they have focused on [1].

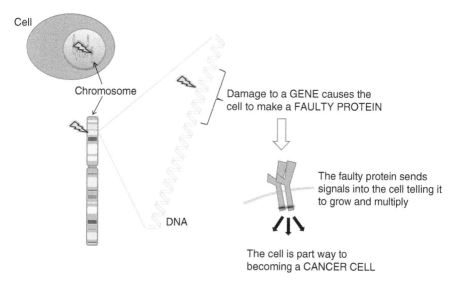

Figure 1.1 Gene mutations cause the production of faulty proteins. Chromosomes are long lengths of DNA found inside the nucleus of each cell. Within our chromosomes are regions of DNA called genes. These are stretches of DNA that contain the instructions to make proteins. If a gene is affected by a mutation (represented by a lightning bolt), the cell might then make a faulty protein. In this example, the faulty protein is a cell surface receptor that gives the cell a continuous signal to grow and multiply.

---

[1] Apoptosis is also referred to as "programmed cell death."

Box 1.1   The names of genes and their proteins

As you read this book, you might notice that protein names are written normally but that gene names are written in italics. For example, the *HER2* gene contains the instructions for making HER2 protein. You might also notice that sometimes the gene and the protein have different names. An example of this is the *TP53* gene, which contains the instructions for making a protein called p53. It's also possible for a gene to contain the instructions for making more than one protein. For instance, the *CDKN2A* gene (sometimes referred to as the *CDKN2A* locus) contains the instructions for making several proteins, two of which are called p16^{INK4a} and p14^{ARF}.

To add to the confusion, some genes and proteins have more than one name. For example, the *HER2* gene is also called *ERBB2* and *NEU*. The reasons behind the various names often have a lot to do with what organism or group of cells the gene/protein was discovered in; if it's similar to another gene/protein that has already been discovered; what role the gene/protein is thought to play in the cells or organism it was found in; and whether or not abnormalities in the gene/protein cause disease. For example, HER2 stands for "human epidermal growth factor receptor-2," because it's similar in structure to HER1 (although we usually refer to HER1 as the EGF receptor or EGFR). *HER2* is also called *ERBB2* because a very similar gene, called *ERBB*, was discovered in a disease-causing virus called the avian erythroblastosis virus. *HER2* is also called *NEU* because a faulty version of it can cause a cancer called neuroblastoma in rodents.

A final point to note is that gene names are often written in capital letters, whereas protein names aren't. But this convention isn't always adhered to.

(What exactly the rest of our cells' DNA is for is a matter of continued debate among scientists.)

Through initiatives such as The Cancer Genome Atlas [2] and the International Cancer Genome Consortium [3], hundreds of scientists have amassed an incredible catalog of information about the thousands of different DNA mutations cancer cells contain [4, 5]. They've also discovered that different types of cancer differ from one another in terms of the mutations they contain and the treatments they respond to. In addition to these differences, we know that important similarities can exist between cancers that arise in different organs. For example, the cancer cells of some breast

cancers overproduce[2] a protein called HER2, and the same is true of the cancer cells in some stomach cancers and other cancer types [6].

Because there's lots I want to say about the DNA mutations found in cancer cells, I'm going to split it up into different topics. First, I'll talk about what causes the DNA mutations found in cancer cells (Section 1.2.1). Then I'll describe what types of mutation occur (see Section 1.2.2), how the number and pattern of mutations in cancer cells varies (see Section 1.2.3), and which mutations have the greatest effect on cell behavior (see Section 1.2.4). Then I'll talk about some of the most common gene mutations in cancer cells and what impact they have (Section 1.2.5).

---

[2] Scientists generally talk about proteins being "overexpressed" rather than "overproduced," but they essentially mean the same thing.

All this information is gradually helping scientists create the new, more targeted cancer treatments described in this book.

1.2.1 Causes of DNA Mutations

There are many different reasons why our cells' DNA gets damaged. Much of this damage is natural and unavoidable, whereas some of it is down to our lifestyle, behaviors, exposures, geographical location, and even local customs.[3] We can also inherit damaged DNA from our parents. Depending on what sort of data scientists look at (e.g., whether they examine individual cells or whole organs or tissues, or look at populations of people in different countries), they end up drawing very different conclusions about what proportion of cancers could be avoided [7–10]. So, although I've listed some of the causes of DNA damage later, and in Figure 1.2, I haven't

tried to pin down exactly how many cancers are caused by each one.[4]

Unavoidable Causes of DNA Damage

1. The byproducts of chemical reactions. Unfortunately for us (and for all living things), our cells' DNA gets damaged every second of every day. Scientists think that even without the influence of external factors, each of our cells sustains damage to its DNA roughly 20,000 times each day [15].

   Much of this damage is caused by the products of chemical reactions that are essential to keep us alive. For example, many of our cells' important chemical reactions produce oxygen free radicals[5] – high-energy oxygen atoms that essentially bash into and break DNA [16]. Our cells contain well over 100 different DNA repair proteins to fix this damage [17]. But sometimes they

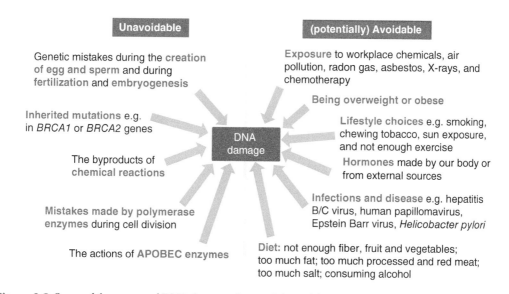

| Unavoidable | (potentially) Avoidable |

Genetic mistakes during the **creation of egg and sperm** and during **fertilization** and **embryogenesis**

Exposure to workplace chemicals, air pollution, radon gas, asbestos, X-rays, and chemotherapy

Inherited mutations e.g. in *BRCA1* or *BRCA2* genes

Being overweight or obese

The byproducts of chemical reactions

Lifestyle choices e.g. smoking, chewing tobacco, sun exposure, and not enough exercise

DNA damage

Hormones made by our body or from external sources

Mistakes made by **polymerase enzymes** during cell division

Infections and disease e.g. hepatitis B/C virus, human papillomavirus, Epstein Barr virus, *Helicobacter pylori*

The actions of **APOBEC enzymes**

Diet: not enough fiber, fruit and vegetables; too much fat; too much processed and red meat; too much salt; consuming alcohol

Figure 1.2 Some of the causes of DNA damage. *Source:* Adapted from Ref. [11–14].

---

[3] For example, in countries like Iran, people are used to drinking much hotter tea than people do in the United Kingdom, and this has been linked to a higher incidence of esophageal cancer.
[4] If you do want to learn more about what you can do to reduce your risk, I would recommend looking at the Cancer Research UK website: http://www.cancerresearchuk.org/about-cancer/causes-of-cancer/can-cancer-be-prevented.
[5] These are also called reactive oxygen species – ROS.

fail to spot all the damage, or they simply can't keep up.

2. Cells make mistakes as they multiply. Tissues that need to renew and replenish their cells often (such as the lining of our bowel, our skin, and those that comprise our immune system) are at the highest risk of cancer[6] [9, 18–20]. This is because for a cell to multiply, it has to make a complete copy of all of its DNA – all 3000 million base pairs of it. The enzyme that copies DNA, called DNA polymerase, although spectacularly fast and accurate, does occasionally make mistakes [18]. Therefore, cells that need to multiply often are at a greater risk of becoming cancer cells than cells that rarely, if ever, multiply.

3. The actions of APOBEC enzymes. APOBEC[7] enzymes are a family of proteins that our cells use to help protect them from viruses. APOBEC enzymes attack viruses by introducing mutations into their DNA. However, if an uninfected cell accidentally makes APOBEC enzymes, the enzymes will attack the cell's own DNA and introduce lots of mutations that could cause cancer [19]. Also, after a cell has become a cancer cell, APOBEC enzymes continue to add more and more damage to the cell's genes [20].

4. Inherited mutations. Some people are born with DNA faults that put them at a higher risk of cancer. Sometimes the fault has been passed down from generation to generation, with many family members affected. For example, actress and film director Angelina Jolie has inherited a fault in one copy of her *BRCA1* gene (we inherit two copies of each gene). Because this fault is shared by many of her relatives, she lost her mother, grandmother, and aunt to cancer [21]. Faults in high-risk genes such as *BRCA* genes are relatively rare, but they can have an enormous impact on a person's cancer risk. More commonly, subtle variations in many genes will combine to affect our risk.

Faults can also arise in an egg or sperm; if the faulty egg or sperm goes on to create an embryo, this fault will be present in every cell. Or, the fault might occur later, as the growing embryo is developing. For example, faults that occur in an embryo's white blood cells as its immune system forms can cause infant or childhood leukemia [11].

Potentially Avoidable Causes of DNA Damage

1. Lifestyle and exposures. Cells that are exposed to high levels of carcinogens (anything that causes cancer is called a carcinogen) are particularly vulnerable to becoming cancer cells. This includes cells that line our lungs, skin, bowel, and stomach. Carcinogens include various constituents of cigarette smoke, alcohol, UV light from the sun or from sunbeds, radiation from X-rays, some viruses, asbestos, and food toxins [13].

Our cancer risk is also linked to our diet (including our consumption of fruit and vegetables, red and processed meat, salt, and fiber), our level of physical activity, and our weight. This is a huge topic. If you would like to learn more, I suggest looking at the Cancer Research UK [22] and American Cancer Society [23] websites.

---

[6] If this seems like a simple and straightforward association, don't be fooled. There is huge controversy around the exact relationship between cancer risk and tissue renewal, number of stem cells, and DNA damage by environmental versus natural mechanisms. I've supplied a handful of references if you want to explore further.

[7] In case you're curious, APOBEC stands for apolipoprotein B mRNA editing enzyme, catalytic polypeptide-like.

2. The influence of sex hormones. When discussing the causes of cancer, we shouldn't ignore the influence of sex hormones such as estrogen, progesterone, and testosterone. These tiny, fat-soluble chemicals encourage cells that contain receptors for them to survive, grow, and multiply (estrogen can also cause DNA damage [24]). Cancers that develop from hormone-sensitive tissues in the breast and prostate often retain their sensitivity to hormones. These cancers often respond to treatments that block the production of hormones in the body or that block the impact of hormones on cancer cells.

    The risk of various cancers, including breast, ovarian, and endometrial cancer, is linked to a person's exposure to sex hormones such as estrogen. Reproductive factors (such as age of menarche[8] and menopause, along with the number of pregnancies and length of time they breastfed) and bodyweight affect a person's lifetime exposure to estrogen and thus also influence their cancer risk [25].

3. The influence of inflammation. For many people, their cancer diagnosis was preceded by years of inflammation, infection, or irritation [26]. For example, people with a chronic hepatitis B or hepatitis C virus infection are at high risk of liver cancer, whereas people with inflammatory bowel disease are at an increased risk of bowel cancer [27, 28]. It seems that the presence of white blood cells in a tissue can increase the DNA mutation rate in the tissue's cells and encourage the cells to multiply, raising the risk of cancer [28].

4. Cancer treatments. Most chemotherapies and radiotherapy work by causing so much DNA damage that cancer cells die. However, not every cell is killed. Cells that

sustain damage to their DNA and yet survive may later become cancer cells. Because of this, people treated for cancer sometimes develop second cancers months or even many years later [29, 30].

Causes of DNA Mutations – Summary
Our risk of cancer in any particular place in our body is therefore a combination of the following [8–10]:

- The natural rate that the cells multiply in that tissue.
- The extent to which DNA polymerase, oxygen free radicals, and APOBEC enzymes have caused mutations in the tissue's cells (the amount of damage will gradually increase as we age).
- Our biological sex and our inherited genetic makeup.
- Our lifestyle and behaviors (which will be hugely impacted by our cultural background, physical location, personal choices, and opportunities).
- Our cells' exposure to carcinogens, hormones, and factors that cause inflammation.

    Cancer Research UK estimates that around 4 in every 10 cases of cancer diagnosed in the United Kingdom are potentially preventable through changes to lifestyle, behaviors, exposures, and weight [31, 32]. However, we cannot influence factors such as the activity of APOBEC enzymes or the accuracy of DNA polymerase. As I said before, estimating what proportion of cancers can be prevented is an incredibly contentious topic, and estimates vary widely depending on how the research was done [7].

1.2.2 Types of DNA Mutations

DNA mutations come in many forms. For the sake of simplicity, I'm going to split them into two groups: (1) mutations affecting long

---

[8] The age at which a girl has her first period.

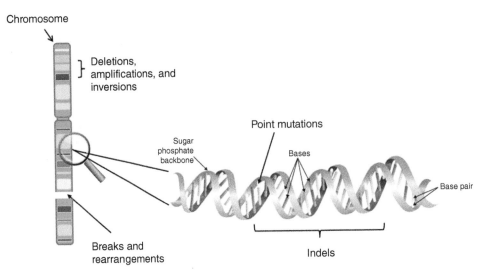

Figure 1.3 DNA damage can come in many forms. Deletions, amplifications, and inversions can affect tens of thousands of DNA bases at a time. Breaks and rearrangements affect whole chromosomes. Smaller-scale mutations include point mutations (insertions, deletions, or substitutions) affecting a single DNA base. Insertions and deletions that involve up to 1000 DNA bases are called indels. *Source:* Adapted from Ref. [33], the image of DNA double helix was created by the Genomics Education Programme and licensed under the Creative Commons Attribution 2.0 Generic license. https://www.flickr.com/photos/genomicseducation/13081113544/Image of magnifying glass from pixabay.com.

stretches of DNA and whole chromosomes and (2) mutations affecting under 1000 DNA base pairs (see Figure 1.3).

Mutations Affecting Long Stretches of DNA and Whole Chromosomes

For a start, many cancers are aneuploid – that is, the cells contain the wrong number (i.e., not the normal 23 pairs) of chromosomes [34]. Often, there is evidence that at an early point in the cancer's development, its entire genome – all 46 chromosomes – have been duplicated (called whole-genome doubling [35]). In addition, chromosomes often show signs of having shattered into small pieces and then been stitched back together in a haphazard fashion – called chromothripsis [36, 37]. These types of DNA damage are no doubt important. However, it's not always clear what impact they have on cancer cells, nor what we could do about them in terms of offering better treatments. Because detecting

these types of DNA damage doesn't generally help doctors decide what treatment to give to their patients, I'm not going to talk about them further.

What can be more helpful is detecting chromosome faults such as translocations, inversions, insertions, deletions, and amplifications.

Chromosome Translocations and Rearrangements

A chromosome translocation is when two chromosomes break, and the cell accidentally sticks them back together incorrectly (see Figure 1.4). Chromosomal rearrangements are similar, but both breaks occur in a single chromosome. More often than not, the chromosomes break in regions that don't contain any genes (remember that the information to make proteins only takes up 1% or so of our chromosomes). However, sometimes translocations and rearrangements do affect genes, and this can have dire consequences.

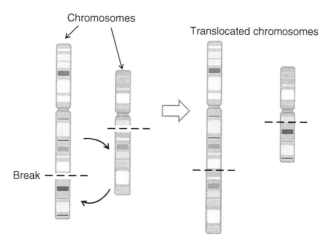

Figure 1.4 A chromosome translocation. Two chromosomes (colored turquoise and orange) break. The cell attaches them back together incorrectly. If the chromosomes have broken where genes are located, this may result in two genes from different chromosomes becoming fused together on the same chromosome (a gene fusion).

For example, the cancer cells of chronic myeloid leukemia (CML) almost always contain a translocation in which chromosome 9 and chromosome 22 have broken and been stitched back together incorrectly. This causes the *BCR* gene on chromosome 22 to become fused together with the *ABL* gene on chromosome 9. The fusion of these two genes causes the cell to make a Bcr-Abl fusion protein (a protein made using the information in the fusion gene), which forces the cells to grow and multiply [38, 39].

In some other cancers, you find translocations and gene rearrangements in which a control region from one gene (a promoter or enhancer[9]) has become fused to the protein-coding region[10] of a second gene. This has often happened during the development of prostate cancer and some forms of blood cancer such as non-Hodgkin lymphomas and myeloma (sometimes called multiple myeloma).

In prostate cancer, the rearrangement often involves the *ERG* and *TMPRSS2* genes on chromosome 21. The rearrangement places the promoter from the *TMPRSS2* gene (a gene that is always active in prostate cells) next to the protein-coding region from a powerful, pro-growth protein called *ERG* [40] (see Figure 1.5). The consequence of this mutation is the massive overproduction of ERG protein, which forces the prostate cell to multiply.

Chromosome Insertions

An insertion is when part of one chromosome is inserted into another chromosome (Figure 1.6). It can also occur when part of a chromosome is reinserted back into the chromosome it came from, but in the wrong place. An example is the "internal tandem duplications" affecting the *FLT3* gene, which are found in the cancer cells of around a third of people with acute myeloid leukemia (AML) [41].

---

[9] The Khan Academy website has a nice description of gene regulation: https://www.khanacademy.org/science/ap-biology/gene-expression-and-regulation/regulation-of-gene-expression-and-cell-specialization/a/overview-of-eukaryotic-gene-regulation.
[10] That is, the part of the gene that contains the instructions to make a protein.

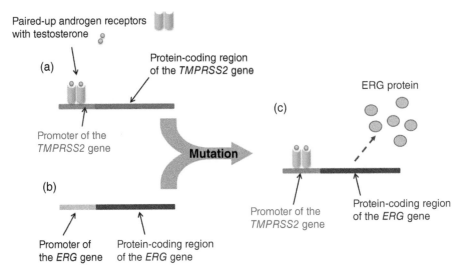

Figure 1.5 The TMPRSS2-ERG gene fusion often found in prostate cancer cells. (a) In healthy prostate cells, androgen receptors pair up due to the presence of testosterone. Paired-up receptors then attach to the *TMPRSS2* gene promoter and cause the cell to produce TMPRSS2 protein. **(b)** Prostate cells only rarely produce ERG because the *ERG* gene does not contain attachment sites for androgen receptors. **(c)** 50% of prostate cancers contain a mutation that puts the protein-coding region of the *ERG* gene under the control of the promoter from the *TMPRSS2* gene. This mutation causes the cell to overproduce ERG protein, which in turn forces the cell to multiply. *Source:* Adapted from Ref. [40].

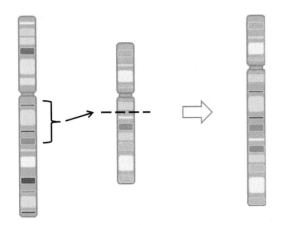

Figure 1.6 A chromosome insertion – part of one chromosome is inserted into another chromosome (as shown) or back into the chromosome it came from.

The insertion involves part of the *FLT3* gene, which is copied and reinserted back into the original gene. This causes the cell to make an extra-large, overactive version of FLT3 protein, which can be blocked with FLT3 inhibitors (see Section 3.6.8 for more on this).

Chromosome Deletions

Not surprisingly, a chromosome deletion is when part of a chromosome gets deleted (Figure 1.7a). An example is the deletion of the part of chromosome 17 that contains the *TP53* gene – this is often referred to as del(17p). *TP53* is a vital tumor suppressor gene that prevents faulty cells from becoming cancer cells (there is more about *TP53* in Sections 1.2.5 and 4.7). The loss of *TP53* means that part of the cell's protection against cancer has gone.

Chromosome Inversions

Inversions (Figure 1.7b), in which part of a chromosome is cut out, flipped over, and then reinserted, can also disrupt genes. For example, an inversion of part of chromosome 2 is found in about 4%–7% of non-small cell lung cancers (NSCLCs; this is the most common type of lung cancer). The inversion joins together the *ALK* gene with part of the *EML4* gene, creating an uncontrollable ALK fusion

(a)   (b)

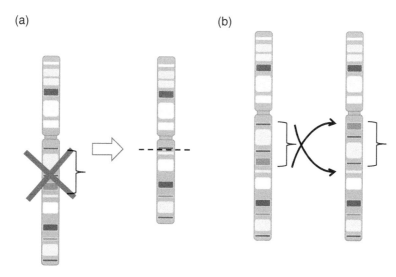

Figure 1.7 Chromosome deletions and inversions. (a) In a chromosome deletion, part of a chromosome is (not surprisingly) deleted. **(b)** Chromosome inversion – a segment of the chromosome is cut out, flipped over, and inserted back into the chromosome.

protein that forces the cells to multiply [42]. (For more about *ALK* mutations in lung cancer, and ALK inhibitors, see Section 3.6.5.)

Gene Amplification

Gene amplifications occur when a cell's DNA replication machinery accidentally makes extra copies of a region of a chromosome that contains one or more genes (see Figure 1.8). As a consequence, the cell overexpresses[11] the proteins made from the amplified genes. A common amplification is that of the *HER2* gene (also referred to as *NEU* or *ERBB2*), which is amplified in about 15%–20% of breast cancers [43].

Point Mutations and Indels

A point mutation is when one DNA base is accidentally added, deleted, or swapped for a different one. The term "indel" is used to refer to small insertions and deletions affecting fewer than 1000 DNA base pairs. Most point

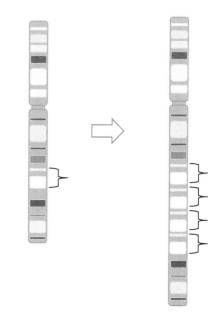

Figure 1.8 Gene amplification. The cell accidentally makes extra copies of a section of a chromosome. The duplicate segments are inserted into other chromosomes or back into the same chromosome.

---

[11] When a cell uses the information in a gene to make the corresponding protein, that gene is "expressed." So, if a gene is said to be overexpressed, that means that more of the corresponding protein is being made than is normal.

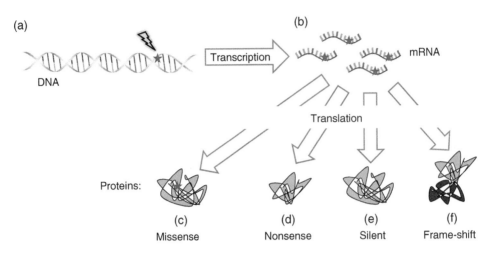

(a)

DNA

Transcription

(b)

mRNA

Translation

Proteins:

(c)
Missense

(d)
Nonsense

(e)
Silent

(f)
Frame-shift

Figure 1.9 Point mutations. A point mutation (shown by a red star) is when one DNA base is added, deleted, or swapped for a different one in the cell's DNA. **(a)** If the mutation is in a gene, the mutation will be copied into the mRNA **(b)** and it may alter the resulting protein. The consequence might be that **(c)** due to a missense mutation, the protein made by the cell differs from the normal version of the protein by one amino acid, **(d)** a nonsense mutation in the DNA introduces a stop signal into the mRNA, and the cell makes an extra-short (truncated) protein, **(e)** a silent mutation has no impact on the protein produced, and **(f)** a frameshift mutation causes the cell to make a very different protein compared to the normal protein, which is only partly the same as the original. *Source:* DNA image from Pixabay. mRNA image by Christine I Miller, licensed under the Creative Commons Attribution-Share Alike 4.0 International license.

mutations and indels have no impact on the cell, as they occur outside of genes. However, if a mutation (such as a base substitution, addition, or deletion) occurs within a gene, it can have various consequences (see Figure 1.9).[12] Point mutations are classed as missense, nonsense, or silent, depending on what consequence the mutation has on protein production. They are also classified as "in-frame" or "frameshift" mutations [44]. All of these terms are explained in greater detail later.

Just one extra piece of information before I move on: The unmutated, normal version of any gene is often referred to as the "wild-type" version of that gene.

Missense and Nonsense Mutations

If one DNA base is substituted for a different one, this might change a single codon. As you might already know, proteins are constructed from long chains of 20 different amino acids. Each set of three bases (called a codon) in the mRNA strand tells the ribosome what amino acid to add next to the protein it's making.[13]

In a missense mutation, the change in a codon means that the protein made from that gene differs by one amino acid from the normal protein (Figure 1.9c) [44]. Two examples are the faulty version of the B-Raf protein (called V600E), which is often found in the

---

[12] If you need a refresher on gene transcription and translation at this point, I suggest taking a look at some of the resources suggested in the Appendix.

[13] If you're struggling to make sense of this, I would suggest looking at the Appendix and learning a bit about gene transcription and translocation.

cancer cells of people with malignant melanoma [45], and some of the faulty versions of EGFR, which are found in the cancer cells of some people with lung cancer [46]. In both cases, the faulty, cancer-causing versions of these proteins (both of which contain hundreds of amino acids) are just one amino acid different from the normal version of the protein. However, even changing that one amino acid is sufficient to create a massively overactive version of B-Raf or EGFR.

In contrast, nonsense mutations are those that cause the cell to make a shortened (truncated) version of the protein (Figure 1.9d). This happens because the original codon has now become a "stop codon." There are three codons (UAA, UAG, and UGA) that tell the ribosome to stop adding any more amino acids to a protein. If a DNA point mutation creates one of these stop codons part way through the mRNA, then the ribosome will stop part way through making the protein. For example, some of the inherited *BRCA* gene mutations that increase the risk of breast and ovarian cancer cause cells to produce a shortened version of a BRCA protein [47].

Silent Mutations

These point mutations don't have any impact on the protein the cell makes even if they occur within a gene (Figure 1.9e). For example, if a ribosome comes across the mRNA sequence CCC, this tells it to add a proline amino acid to the protein it's making. If a point mutation changes the mRNA from CCC to CCA, this has no impact because the sequence CCA also tells the ribosome to add a proline.

In-Frame and Frameshift Mutations

If one or two DNA bases are added to or deleted from a gene's sequence (or any number that isn't a multiple of three), this creates a frameshift mutation that is likely to have an enormous impact on what protein is

produced (Figure 1.9f). An example is if one DNA base (a C) is added to a gene so that the mRNA goes from ….CGACGACGA…. to … CCGACGACGA…. Now, instead of adding three arginine amino acids to the protein (as directed by CGA-CGA-CGA), the ribosome adds a proline followed by two threonines (CCG-ACG-ACG). The ribosome carries on going from there, adding a completely different selection of amino acids from the normal sequence. As a result, the protein the cell makes may bear very little resemblance to the normal protein. Frameshift mutations also commonly introduce stop codons that create truncated proteins.

An "in-frame" mutation is opposite to a frameshift mutation in that it doesn't affect the rest of the protein. For example, if three bases are added to ….CGACGACGA…. so that it becomes ….CGACCCCGACGA…, the ribosome will insert an extra proline in between the arginines, but it has no further impact.

1.2.3 Numbers and Patterns of DNA Mutations in Cancer Cells

In recent years, technologies have been developed that allow scientists to pinpoint the location and identity of thousands of DNA mutations inside cancer cells. They have discovered that different cancers contain different numbers, types, and patterns of mutations that arise due to different mutational processes. For example, lung cancers that develop in people with a history of smoking usually contain lots of point mutations in which a C DNA base has been changed to an A. A different pattern of mutations – where there are lots of insertions and deletions of more than three DNA bases at a time – is common in people with cancers associated with inherited *BRCA* gene mutations. Other patterns are linked to overactive APOBEC enzymes.

Scientists have discovered well over 100 different patterns of mutations in cancer cells, which they call "mutation signatures" [48–51]. It's possible for one cancer cell to contain multiple patterns of mutations because the cancer has arisen due to a combination of causes. This means that the various patterns of mutations found in a person's cancer cells are a bit like an archeological record showing what has happened inside the cell during the person's lifetime [48–52]. Some of the patterns will be due to natural aging processes, while others might reflect the person's choices through life, such as whether they took up smoking (Figure 1.10). The amount of damage in cancer cells' DNA varies greatly from cancer type to cancer type, and from one person to another [5, 53]. Cancers that have come about because of the effects of

powerful carcinogens often contain a vast amount of DNA damage. For example, lung cancers in people who are current smokers or have smoked in the past contain roughly ten times the amount of damage as lung cancers in people who have never smoked [54]. Melanoma skin cancers, which are almost always caused by UV light from the sun (or from sunbeds), also contain a vast number of mutations [5]. In general, cancers in older people contain more mutations than those in children and young adults simply because their cells have had more years in which to accumulate mutations.

Although cancer cells often contain hundreds or even thousands of mutations, most of these mutations have no discernible impact on the cell's behavior. They have occurred because the cancer cell is damaged and unstable and is

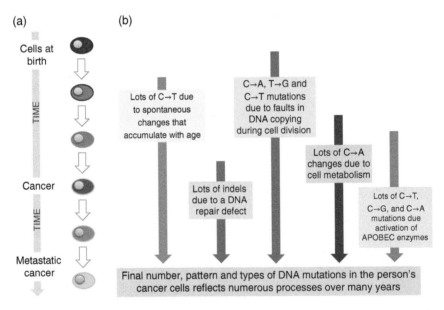

Figure 1.10 **The mutations found in a person's cancer cells are a record of all the mutations that the cells have sustained throughout their lifetime. (a)** At birth, the person's cells only contain the *germline* mutations they were born with. However, as they go through life, their cells accumulate additional *sporadic* mutations due to a variety of processes. Distinct patterns caused by different processes are called *mutational signatures*. The mutations in one cell may eventually cause it to become a cancer cell. The cancer cells later accumulate further mutations that cause metastasis. **(b)** Various mutational signatures are caused by different processes (e.g., aging and metabolism) and defects (e.g., faults in DNA repair processes and overactive APOBEC enzymes). *Source:* Adapted from Ref. [49].

picking up new mutations all the time. The mutations that are important in driving the cancer cells' abnormal behavior are referred to by scientists as driver mutations. Mutations that add little or nothing to the cells' behavior are called passenger mutations.

Perhaps not surprisingly, scientists are much more interested in finding a cancer's driver mutations than its passenger mutations. They want to know what's driving the cells' behavior so that they can do something about it.

1.2.4 Driver Mutations – Those that Affect Cancer Cell Behavior

For DNA damage to cause cancer, some of it must affect genes that control the cell's behavior. These "driver mutations" affect cell processes and behaviors such as:

- How fast the cell grows
- How frequently it multiplies
- The way it communicates with neighboring cells
- How often and how thoroughly it checks its own health and monitors and repairs DNA mutations
- Its ability to survive in adverse conditions such as low oxygen levels
- Its ability to extract itself from its normal environment and move elsewhere
- Whether it goes through all the normal checks and balances during the cell cycle[14]
- Whether it still has the ability to self-destruct by a process called apoptosis
- The way it produces energy
- Whether it can hide from or suppress the person's immune system.

The genes that control these behaviors are classed as oncogenes, tumor suppressor genes, and DNA repair genes.

Oncogenes

Many of the proteins made from oncogenes encourage our cells to survive, grow, and multiply.[15] Others can make cells more mobile and invasive or help them to hide from the immune system. All these genes need to be tightly controlled to avoid cancer. In cancer cells, the proteins that are made by oncogenes are often overproduced and/or overactive due to mutations. Examples of oncogenes include *EGFR, RAS,*[16] *BRAF, MYC, HER2,* and *SRC.*

Tumor Suppressor Genes

The proteins made from these genes slow down or stop cell growth and proliferation and trigger apoptosis. In cancer cells, they're damaged in a way that causes their protection to be lost. Examples include *TP53, PTEN, RB1,* and *APC.*

DNA Repair Genes

The proteins made from these genes sense and repair DNA damage. In cancer cells, they're damaged in such a way that they can no longer do their job properly. Because of this, cancer cells pick up more and more DNA damage as time goes on. Examples of DNA repair genes include *BRCA1, BRCA2, ATM, ATR, RAD51,* and *ERCC1.*

In healthy cells, the proteins made from DNA repair genes keep the cell's DNA free from faults. There is also a balancing act between the oncogenes and the tumor suppressor genes. For example, a protein called Bcl-2 protects cells from death, whereas a protein called p53 triggers death. The gene for making Bcl-2 (called *BCL2*) is an oncogene; the gene for making p53 (called *TP53*) is a tumor suppressor gene. Healthy cells contain

---

[14] The cell cycle is the normal, step-by-step process our cells go through when they multiply.
[15] For an explanation of oncogenes vs. proto-oncogenes, look in the Glossary.
[16] There are three main *RAS* genes: *KRAS, NRAS,* and *HRAS.*

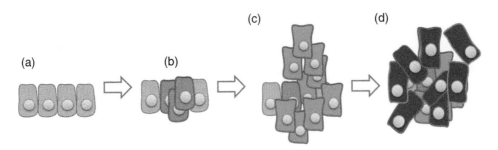

Figure 1.11 **A series of mutations leads to bowel cancer** [5]. **(a)** Orderly, well-connected cells in the lining of the bowel. **(b)** A random mutation in a bowel cell leads to loss of APC protein activity; this cell starts to multiply slightly faster than its neighbors, forming a little lump – an adenoma. The faulty cells are not cancer cells but, because they are multiplying more quickly than normal, they are prone to collecting more mutations. **(c)** Weeks, months, or years later, a mutation in the *KRAS* gene causes the K-Ras protein to become overactive; the cells now multiply rapidly and in a disorderly fashion. **(d)** Finally, genes like *TP53*, *PIK3CA*, and *SMAD4* are mutated. The faulty cells are now full-blown cancer cells, able to invade through local tissues, disrupt their function, and spread to other parts of the body.
Abbreviations: *APC* – adenomatous polyposis coli; *KRAS* – Kirsten rat sarcoma virus; *PIK3CA* – phosphatidylinositol-4,5-bisphosphate 3-kinase catalytic subunit alpha; *SMAD4* – SMAD family member 4; *TP53* – tumor protein 53.

strict amounts of both proteins that balance each other out. But cancer cells often contain too much Bcl-2 and too little, or faulty, p53.

Multiple Driver Mutations Are Necessary for a Cell to Become a Cancer Cell

The gradual accumulation of mutations in several oncogenes, tumor suppressor genes, and DNA repair genes can ultimately cause someone to develop cancer. A sequence of events that frequently leads to bowel cancer is often given as an example (Figure 1.11).

Our bowel is lined by orderly layers of cells known as epithelial cells. Because bowel cells are constantly getting scraped off by food passing through, our bowel cells have to multiply pretty often in order to keep the number of cells constant. Cells that multiply are prone to picking up mutations. So, our bowel cells tend to contain more and more mutations as we get older. If a mutation affects a gene called *APC*, this is bad news as *APC* is an important tumor suppressor gene. But the situation isn't desperate as it's only one mutation, which isn't enough to cause

bowel cancer. However, if it's followed by a mutation in *KRAS*, then the situation becomes worse; *KRAS* is a powerful growth-promoting oncogene that forces the cell to multiply more rapidly. As the cells multiply, they pick up yet more mutations. The cell still isn't a cancer cell because other protective proteins are still doing their job. But if genes such as *PIK3CA* (an oncogene), *SMAD4* (a tumor suppressor gene), and *TP53* (a tumor suppressor gene) become faulty, then the cell will become a full-blown cancer cell [5].

In other cancers, a similar combination of mutations in a handful of important genes is thought to drive their behavior [55].

1.2.5 The "Usual Suspects" – Genes Commonly Mutated in Many Cancers

Some gene mutations are common only in one or two types of cancer. These include the *VHL* mutations that are very common in kidney cancer and some of the translocations that are very common in hematological cancers (such as leukemias, lymphomas, and myeloma). But other gene mutations crop up time and time again in many different cancer types. I'll be mentioning some of these gene mutations at various points in this book, so I've listed some of them in Table 1.1.

One thing that might (or might not!) jump out at you from the table is that many of the most commonly mutated genes in cancer cells are involved in cell communication pathways.

These pathways are used by all our body's cells to sense and respond to changes in their environment, signals sent out by neighboring cells, the presence or absence of hormones, and signals sent out by white blood cells.

A wide variety of communication pathways exist in our cells, and they involve many different proteins. These pathways are often overactive in cancer cells, and they are the

Table 1.1   A selection of some of the most commonly mutated oncogenes, tumor suppressor genes, and DNA repair genes in human cancers.

Gene name (protein name)	What protein is made from this gene?	What is the consequence for the cell if the gene is mutated?
Oncogenes		
RAS (Ras)	There are three main versions of the gene (*KRAS*, *NRAS*, and *HRAS*), which contain the instructions for making three Ras proteins (K-Ras, N-Ras, and H-Ras). They are enzymes that play a central role in cell communication [56].	All the proteins made from these genes are involved in cell communication pathways – the sequences of events triggered inside a cell when it receives a signal to grow and multiply from its neighbors. Therefore, all these proteins cause cells to grow and multiply. Overactive communication pathways also force cells to survive (even when damaged) and to become more mobile and invasive. For more on cell communication pathways and how they work, see Chapter 3, Section 3.2.
PIK3CA (p110alpha)	The PI3K protein is an enzyme involved in cell communication. It comes in many different forms and is made up of two component parts: an enzyme part and a regulatory part. The *PIK3CA* gene encodes an enzyme part called p110alpha (p110α) [57].	
HER2/NEU/ErbB2 (HER2)	A receptor found on the cell surface, which activates cell communication pathways inside the cell [58].	
MYC (MYC)	A transcription factor – it attaches to the promoters of various genes and triggers gene transcription. Many of the genes it controls are involved in cell growth and proliferation [59].	
BRAF (B-Raf)	An enzyme involved in cell communication, activated by Ras proteins [60].	
EGFR (EGFR)	A receptor found on the cell surface, which activates cell communication pathways inside the cell [58].	
Tumor suppressor genes		
TP53 (p53)	A transcription factor activated by DNA damage and other triggers – it attaches to various gene promoters and triggers gene transcription. The proteins produced as a result of p53 activity block cell proliferation and cause cell death [61].	If p53 is not working properly or is missing from a cell, the cell loses the ability to stop multiplying or die in response to DNA damage.
PTEN (PTEN)	An enzyme involved in cell communication that blocks the activity of PI3K. PTEN also helps cells avoid DNA damage [62].	If PTEN is not working properly or is missing from a cell, the PI3K-controlled communication pathway becomes overactive.

(Continued)

Table 1.1   (Continued)

Gene name (protein name)	What protein is made from this gene?	What is the consequence for the cell if the gene is mutated?
RB (RB)	RB has a pocket in its surface that fits E2F proteins, which control entry into the cell cycle[a]. RB holds onto and blocks E2F proteins, and this prevents cells from multiplying [63].	If RB is not working properly or is missing from a cell, E2F can force the cell into the cell cycle (for more about RB and E2F, see Chapter 4, Section 4.5).
CDKN2A (p16 INK4a)	p16^{INK4a} is a protein that blocks a set of enzymes called the cyclin-dependent kinases (CDKs). CDKs force RB to let go of E2F proteins (see the description of RB mentioned earlier). By blocking CDKs, p16^{INK4a} prevents cells from entering the cell cycle (see Chapter 4, Figures 4.18 and 4.19) [64].	If p16^{INK4a} is not working properly or is missing from a cell, E2F proteins force the cell into the cell cycle.
NF1 (neurofibromin)	A large protein that inactivates Ras proteins (see the description of Ras earlier in this table) [65].	If neurofibromin is not working properly or is missing from a cell, Ras proteins become overactive.
APC (APC)	The surface of the APC protein has various different regions through which it interacts with many different proteins involved in cell communication, mobility, adhesion to neighboring cells, and other processes [66].	If APC is not working properly or is missing from a cell, then levels of another protein, beta-catenin (β-catenin), rise. Beta-catenin causes cells to multiply.
DNA repair genes		
BRCA1 (BRCA1) and BRCA2 (BRCA2)	BRCA1 and BRCA2 proteins are both necessary for a DNA repair process called homologous recombination (HR). Our cells use HR to accurately repair double-strand breaks in their DNA [67] (see Chapter 4, Section 4.3 for more information on BRCA proteins).	If either BRCA1 or BRCA2 is not working properly or is missing from a cell, the cell can no longer perform HR. The cell then has to rely on less accurate repair mechanisms and is liable to pick up further DNA mutations.
ATM and ATR	Cells trigger the activity of ATM and ATR proteins when they detect damage to their DNA. Together, these enzymes coordinate the cell's response to the damage [68].	If either ATM or ATR is damaged or missing from a cell, its ability to respond to DNA damage is compromised.

Abbreviations: APC – adenomatous polyposis coli; ATM – ataxia-telangiectasia mutated; ATR – ATM and Rad3 related; BRCA – breast cancer susceptibility gene; EGFR – epidermal growth factor receptor; HER2 – human epidermal growth factor receptor-2; NF1 – neurofibromatosis type 1; *PIK3CA* – phosphatidylinositol-4,5-bisphosphate 3-kinase catalytic subunit alpha; PTEN – phosphatase and tensin homolog; Ras – rat sarcoma virus; RB – retinoblastoma protein; TP53 – tumor protein p53.
[a] The cell cycle is the very orderly and precise sequence of events that a cell goes through in order to multiply.

target of various cancer drugs. The whole of Chapter 3 is dedicated to cell communication pathways and the drugs that block them.

1.3 THE DEFINING FEATURES (HALLMARKS) OF CANCER CELLS

All cancers are presumed to begin with a single cell that has sustained damage to its DNA and has multiplied out of control. As an adult, it's true that every cell in our body contains some sort of damage to its DNA [69, 70]. However, what sets a cancer cell apart from a non-cancer cell is the following:

- The amount and type of DNA damage the cells contain
- Damage in oncogenes, tumor suppressor genes, and DNA repair genes
- The changes in behavior that the damage causes
- The ability of the damaged cell to overcome suppression by neighboring cells and avoid destruction by the person's immune system.

The behavioral changes that set a cancer cell apart from a healthy cell are collectively known as "the hallmarks of cancer." These hallmarks are the brainchild of two scientists called Professor Douglas Hanahan and Professor Robert Weinberg, who came up with a list of six back in 2000 [71]. They added two more in 2011 and another two in 2022 [72, 73]. They also described four "enabling characteristics" – features of cancers and their environment that allow them to develop and that sustain their growth.

1.3.1 Ten Hallmarks of Cancer (Plus Four Enabling Characteristics)

The hallmarks can be summarised as: [71, 72, 74]

1. They can tell themselves to multiply. A normal cell only multiplies when it receives an instruction[17] to do so. A cancer cell can generate those instructions itself

2. They are insensitive to negative feedback, because proteins that would normally tell them to stop multiplying and die (like p53) have been lost or don't work properly.

3. They resist death. Every day, millions of cells in our body self-destruct because they have worn out or become damaged. Cancer cells have defects that make it almost impossible for them to do this.

4. Cancer cells can multiply forever because they contain a protein called telomerase. Healthy cells lack this protein and eventually stop multiplying.

5. They develop a blood supply to gain access to oxygen and nutrients. Cancer cells release a tiny protein called VEGF that tells nearby blood vessels to sprout and grow (a process called angiogenesis – see Section 1.6.3 for more on this process). They also take advantage of existing blood vessels.

6. They can invade and spread. Most of our body's cells are connected to each other in orderly arrangements. Cancer cells have lost connective proteins from their surface, and they are independent and mobile.

7. They have changed the way they produce energy. Healthy cells use sugars from our food to make energy using a highly efficient, oxygen-dependent process. Cancer cells use an inefficient process that requires less oxygen but helps them multiply more quickly.

8. They can avoid destruction by the immune system. White blood cells constantly patrol our body, looking for defective cells. Cancer cells hide from white blood cells, suppress cancer-fighting white blood cells and co-opt white blood cells for their own purposes (there is lots more about this in Section 1.5).

9. They are more changeable than healthy cells. Normal cells mature and specialize until they are perfectly adapted for a specific function. Cancer cells are more plastic – they adapt and change depending on their circumstances.

10. Tumors contain senescent cells. Senescent cells (those that have stopped multiplying and that have shut down many internal systems) appear to send signals that encourage cancer cells to multiply and protect them from the effects of treatments.

Enabling Characteristics

1. Cancer cells are genetically unstable. Cancer cells gain new DNA mutations all the time, and they evolve and diversify as time goes by. (I'll come back to this topic and its importance in Sections 1.4 and 1.9.4.)

2. Cancer cells are also epigenetically unstable. When a scientist talks about epigenetics, they're referring to chemical changes that influence how tightly packed DNA is. This influences whether the genes in that region

---

[17] This instruction is usually in the form of small proteins known as "growth factors" released by the cells' near neighbors – see Chapter 3, Section 3.2.1 for more on this.

of DNA are active and used to make pro-teins or not. Inside tumors, low levels of oxygen and nutrients and other cues cause cancer cells to alter their epigenetics. This is another cause of variation among cancer cells and their ability to adapt to changing circumstances.

3. Cancer cells live in an inflammatory environment. Normal inflammation occurs in response to tissue damage – it encourages repair and acts as a magnet for white blood cells that clear up any infection. This same mechanism is hijacked by cancer cells. Inflammatory white blood cells found inside tumors help cancer cells avoid destruction and support their growth and spread (for more on this, see Section 1.5.3).

4. Cancer cells and cancer treatments are influenced by bacteria and other microbes. The range and types of bacteria, fungi, and other microbes found inside a tumor differ from person to person and affect cancer

cell behavior. The effectiveness of some cancer treatments is also influenced by the microbes living in the person's digestive tract (the gut microbiome). This is a new and complicated area of cancer research and biology, and we have a lot still to learn. I'll return to it in Chapter 5 when I discuss biomarkers of response to checkpoint inhibitor immunotherapy.

1.4 VARIATION AMONG CANCER CELLS IN A SINGLE TUMOR

A major reason why many tumors fail to respond to treatment or become resistant later is intratumoral heterogeneity – the fact that inside a tumor there are various populations of cancer cells that are different from each other. This variation is often genetic, with different populations of cells containing different combinations of DNA mutations (Figure 1.12).

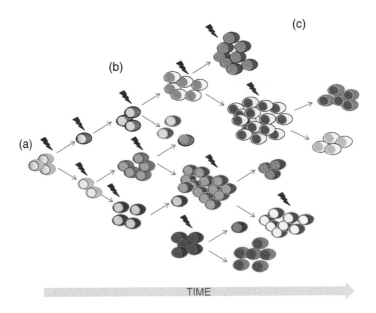

Figure 1.12 Genome instability causes intratumoral heterogeneity. (a) In a newly emerged cluster of cancer cells, all the cells are likely to contain the same genetic faults. However, each cell is genomically unstable and likely to pick up more mutations over time. (b) The cells start to evolve and become different from one another. (c) As time goes on, the cells diverge from each other more and more, creating distinct populations of cells driven by different sets of mutations.

For example, scientists analyzing multiple biopsies from a single tumor have found huge variations in the number, type, and chromosome location of genetic mutations in the person's cancer cells. One of the first and most comprehensive analyses of this phenomenon was conducted by a group of British scientists who studied tumor biopsy samples from people with kidney cancer [73]. When investigating 12 samples taken from one patient, they found that only a third of the 128 DNA mutations they discovered were present in all 12 samples. Similar studies investigating tumor samples from people with other cancer types have revealed similar stories [75–77].

1.4.1 Causes of Genetic Heterogeneity

It seems that as a cancer grows, the cells within it evolve and change. This is because cancer cells are genomically unstable – they accumulate DNA damage at a faster rate than healthy cells. There are various reasons for this instability, some of the most important of which are the following [78, 79]:

- Cancer cells contain faults in DNA repair genes and this compromises their ability to detect and repair DNA damage.
- Cancer cells' apoptosis machinery is faulty, which means they stay alive despite containing lots of DNA damage.
- The normal mechanisms that ensure each cell has the correct number of chromosomes and that help to avoid chromosome breakages and fusions are lost.
- The cells' ability to replicate their DNA accurately is compromised.
- Some cancer cells are continually exposed to mutagens such as tobacco smoke or UV light.

- Cancer cells contain mutations in powerful oncogenes that destabilize the cell and lead to further mutations.

Because of genomic instability, over the weeks, months, and years that go by before a cancer is diagnosed (and in the weeks, months, and years afterward), cancer cells emerge that have different combinations of mutations compared to their predecessors. And, as time goes on, the cancer cells within a tumor become more diverse.

1.4.2 Other Types of Heterogeneity

In addition to the cancer cells in a tumor (and any metastases[18]) being genetically diverse, they are also epigenetically diverse. In some parts of a tumor, certain genes might be suppressed because their DNA is too tightly coiled to allow gene transcription. In other parts of a tumor, or perhaps in a metastasis, those same genes might be relaxed and used to make protein.

Epigenetic gene regulation is influenced by a cell's environment (such as oxygen levels, nutrient availability, acidity, and the presence of chemical signals released by other cells). Many mutations found in cancer cells also affect epigenetic enzymes. As a result, epigenetic diversity can arise from both environmental and genetic influences on the cells' DNA [80].

Other causes of diversity include metabolic differences, with groups of cells performing all the chemical reactions they need to sustain life using distinct combinations of enzymes and chemicals. Cells can also differ in other ways, such as in terms of their appearance and what proteins they secrete into their surroundings [81].

---

[18] Metastases are tumors found in new locations of the body, in contrast to the primary tumor, which is where the cancer started. Metastases are also referred to as "secondaries."

The amount of variation among cancer cells in a person's body has a profound impact on the effectiveness of treatment, so I shall return to this topic in Section 1.9.

1.5 CANCER'S RELATIONSHIP WITH OUR IMMUNE SYSTEM

The fact that someone has cancer indicates that at least two important things have happened:

1. One of their cells has sustained damage in the form of DNA mutations that have caused it to become a cancer cell. This cell has then multiplied many times to become a detectable tumor or blood cancer.
2. For some reason, their immune system has failed to recognize and destroy their cancer cells.

So far in this book I have focused on the DNA mutations inside cancer cells. But now I want to shift my attention away from DNA mutations and look at the interaction between cancer cells and our immune system.

If you'd like to learn a bit about the immune system before we start, then you might want to get hold of an immunology textbook such as *How the Immune System Works* by Lauren Sompayrac [82] or, for more detail, the classic undergraduate textbook is Janeway's *Immunobiology* [83]. Or you could look on YouTube for immunology lectures. For example, a doctor in Australia called Armando Hasudungan has created a series of illustrated videos that introduce you to many immunology concepts (http://armandoh.org/subjects/immunology). As he says himself, his videos don't cover everything, but they're a great starting point if you've not learned any immunology before.

For the rest of this section, I'll focus on how cancer cells avoid getting destroyed by white blood cells, but also how they eventually use white blood cells for their own purposes.

I'll begin by describing how our immune system monitors our cells for signs of damage, and I'll introduce you to T cells. Then I'll look at the "cancer-immunity cycle" – the name given to the process through which our body generates a cancer-fighting immune response. From there, I'll describe the sorts of white blood cells you commonly find inside tumors, and their role in helping cancer cells thrive and survive. Lastly, I'll explain how cancer cells are ultimately able to hide from, suppress, and escape the immune system's control.

1.5.1 How Our Immune System Monitors for Signs of Damage and Destroys Faulty Cells

Probably the first thing to say is that one of the roles of our immune system is to protect us from cancer by detecting and destroying cancer cells.

We'll probably never know how often cancer cells pop up in our body. But immunologists reckon that our immune system is *"recognizing and destroying little cancers as they develop all the time. If we didn't have an immune system, then we would be developing cancer a lot more often"* [84].

Various types of white blood cells participate in destroying any cancer cells that emerge, but the most important are our T cells (aided by dendritic cells) and natural killer (NK) cells (see Box 1.2 for a description of various types of white blood cells).

At the heart of our immune system's ability to detect cancer cells is the fact that all our cells are constantly showing our immune system what's going on inside them. This means that passing white blood cells can instantly see which cells are healthy and identify any that have become faulty.

Box 1.2   Descriptions of some of the white blood cells mentioned in this book listed in alphabetical order

Antigen-presenting cells (APCs). These include dendritic cells and macrophages. These cells display tiny protein fragments (called **peptide antigens**[19]) to T cells. The peptides can have many different sources, such as being a fragment of a mutated protein from a cancer cell (sometimes called a neoantigen) or being part of a virus that is causing an infection. APCs "present" antigens to T cells using tiny cup-like structures on their surface called MHC proteins.

B cells (B lymphocytes). These lymphocytes have B cell receptors (BCRs) on their surface. Once they have matured in the bone marrow, they move to lymph nodes and other lymphoid organs (like the spleen) in search of infections. If their BCRs connect with an antigen (such as a protein fragment from a bacterium or virus), the B cell may become fully active. When fully active, some of these B cells become long-lived, antibody-producing B cells called **plasma cells**. These plasma cells move back to the bone marrow, from where they release millions of copies of their antibody into the blood.

Dendritic cells. Starfish-shaped APCs that shuttle between tissues and lymphoid organs (such as lymph nodes, spleen, and tonsils). A different set of dendritic cells – the follicular dendritic cells – spend their whole life in lymph nodes and other lymph tissues. They capture antigens delivered to them by the flow of lymph fluid and display them to B cells.

Leukocytes. A collective term for all white blood cells.

Lymphocytes. A collective term for B cells and T cells.

Macrophages. The most versatile, "jack-of-all-trades" cells of the immune system. They have the capacity to ingest and destroy invaders, act as APCs, activate T cells, and rid the body of cell debris. However, whereas dendritic cells can shuttle to lymph nodes and other lymphoid organs, macrophages generally stay put in our organs and tissues. Macrophages found in particular locations often look distinctive and have different names, such as Kupffer cells in the liver, Langerhans cells in the skin, and microglia in the brain.

Mast cells. Myeloid cells with histamine-containing granules inside them. The release of their histamine granules helps fight infections but also causes allergic reactions and inflammation.

Myeloid cells. A collective term for white blood cells that develop from myeloblasts. They include macrophages, basophils, neutrophils, eosinophils, and dendritic cells.

Myeloid-derived suppressor cells. Scientists don't really understand these cells, but large numbers of them are found inside tumors and in the blood of people with cancer. They can suppress cytotoxic T cells and also seem to be involved in angiogenesis.

---

[19] Any peptide (or other molecule) that triggers an immune response is called an antigen. If the source of the antigen is a mutated protein found inside a person's cancer cells, then it's often referred to as a **neoantigen**.

Neutrophils. Short-lived myeloid cells that enter tissues and destroy infections. They are the most numerous white blood cells in our body.

T cells (T lymphocytes):

Helper T cells. T cells that respond via their T cell receptor (TCR) to antigens presented to them by APCs via MHC class 2 proteins. They require further activation signals (called "costimulatory signals") from APCs to become fully active. Once active, they then activate B cells and enhance the activity of other white blood cells.

Cytotoxic T cells (CTLs). T cells that respond via their TCR to antigens presented to them by APCs via MHC class 1 proteins. Once they have received the necessary co-stimulatory signals from the APC, they directly destroy virus-infected cells and cancer cells in the affected tissue by releasing cell-killing enzymes.

Regulatory T cells (Tregs). T cells whose job it is to suppress any T cells that might otherwise attack the body's tissues and cause autoimmune diseases; they also prevent the overactivity of T cells that would otherwise cause tissue damage.

Natural killer (NK) cells. Short-lived T cells that enter tissues, release cytokines, and directly destroy virus-infected cells and cancer cells.

Source: Adapted from Ref. [85].

None of this would be possible without special proteins found on our cells' surface called major histocompatibility complex (MHC) class 1 proteins (see Box 1.3 for more about them). These proteins are like little cups sticking out from the cells' surface. Inside each of these cups is a tiny fragment from one of the proteins the cell is making. The fragments (called peptides or peptide antigens)[20] are usually just 8–11 amino acids long [86]. All our cells should be decorated with thousands of cups, which they use to show passing white blood cells tens of thousands of different peptides (Figure 1.13).

Specialized T cells (called cytotoxic T cells) that are passing by take a look at the peptide antigens presented to them by each cell. If the peptides displayed by a cell indicate that it is infected by a virus or has become faulty, the passing T cells immediately release toxic, cell-killing enzymes that destroy the faulty cell. However, T cells are only able to do this if they have already been activated by a dendritic cell.

Another type of white blood cell that can detect and destroy cancer cells is the NK cells. These cells destroy cells that have lost MHC class 1 proteins from their surface altogether and that have avoided destruction by cytotoxic T cells.

I apologize if this is already starting to feel very complicated. Immunology is one of those subjects that triggers long sighs and tired brains, and yet, once you get into it, it's

---

[20] Proteins are made from tiny chemical building blocks called amino acids, which are linked together in long chains to form proteins. There are about 20 or so different amino acids, and some proteins contain many thousands of them. A peptide is a short piece of protein – the term is usually used to describe a piece of protein containing anywhere from 2 up to 50 amino acids. "Peptide antigen" is the name given to any peptide that can trigger a response from the immune system.

Box 1.3 MHC proteins

MHC (major histocompatibility complex) proteins come in two main types: MHC class 1 and MHC class 2. Whereas all our cells have MHC class 1 proteins on their surface, only specialized cells called antigen-presenting cells (APCs) have MHC class 2 proteins on their surface. MHC proteins allow our cells to present small protein fragments (peptides) to one another.

MHC class 1 proteins are used by our cells to display peptides from proteins that they have manufactured themselves.

MHC class 2 proteins are found on APCs such as dendritic cells, which use them to display peptides that they have picked up from their environment.

Source: Adapted from Ref. [86,87].

hard not to be captivated by its beauty and complexity [88]. If you feel like you've already had enough for now, then I suggest moving on to the next section and coming back to this later, maybe once you start reading the chapters on immunotherapy. Or, if you're happy to prepare yourself with a cup of tea (I am from the United Kingdom after all), then do take a deep breath and prepare to continue!

T cell activation is a rather complicated process. But I do want to describe it to you as I think it will help you in a couple of ways: (1) It will help you to make sense of the sentence in which I said that only T cells that have been activated by dendritic cells can kill faulty cells, and (2) it will help you to understand how diverse forms of immunotherapy can all activate T cells (such as peptide and DNA vaccines, dendritic cell vaccines, oncolytic viruses, and checkpoint inhibitors).

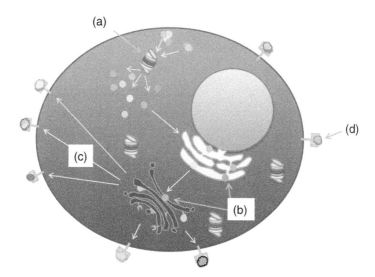

Figure 1.13 Cells use MHC class 1 proteins to display their inner workings to the immune system.
(a) The cell breaks up a representative sample of its proteins into short peptides using its proteasomes.
(b) These peptides are processed further in the endoplasmic reticulum and Golgi apparatus and assembled with MHC class 1 proteins. **(c)** Peptide-MHC class 1 complexes are transported to the cell's outer membrane. **(d)** Peptides are "presented" to passing T cells and then recycled and replaced with new ones.
Source: Adapted from Ref. [86].

Let's start with the fact that dendritic cells activate T cells. Dendritic cells are starfish-shaped cells that act as our body's patrolmen. They are found throughout our body, taking position wherever we're most likely to be exposed to infections, e.g., in our digestive tract, skin, and airways. A key feature of dendritic cells is that they're constantly hoovering up stuff (like bacteria, viruses, and cell debris) from their surroundings. If they detect signs of an infection or another problem, they journey to nearby lymph nodes.[21] As they move, they become fully mature. They also transfer the debris to their surface in the form of short peptide antigens, which they assemble into their MHC proteins and display on their surface. During their journey, which typically takes a day or so, they also increase their production of B7 proteins [86].

When they reach a lymph node, fully mature dendritic cells search for T cells whose T cell receptors (TCRs) match the shape of the peptide antigens displayed by the dendritic cells' MHC proteins. (Apparently, each dendritic cell can scan the surface of about 1000 T cells per hour.) If such a match occurs, the T cell might become active. But to do so, it also needs to receive further activation signals, such as connecting with a B7 protein and receiving suitable signals in the form of cytokines from other white blood cells (Figure 1.14). Activated

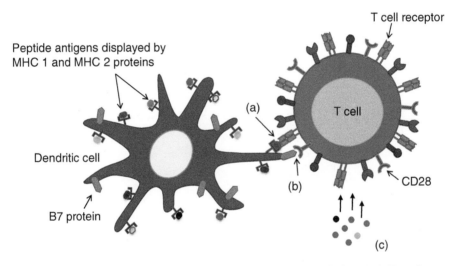

Figure 1.14 T cells are activated by dendritic cells. There are three signals that a T cell needs to receive to become fully active. **(a)** The first activation signal comes from a dendritic cell that displays a peptide antigen on its surface that matches the shape of the T cell's T cell receptor. **(b)** The second signal also comes from the dendritic cell in the form of a B7 protein on the dendritic cell's surface, which connects with CD28, found on the T cell. **(c)** The third signal comes from cytokines – a family of small proteins that act as signals sent out by white blood cells. They include interleukins (e.g., IL-6, IL-2, and IL-4). Interleukins connect with more receptors on the surface of the T cell, telling the T cell what sort of T cell to become (there are many subtypes of T cells) and encouraging it to multiply and survive. *Source:* Adapted from Ref. [89].

---

[21] Lymph nodes are small, bean-shaped patches of tissue, and we have hundreds of them scattered throughout our body. They are places where white blood cells congregate, and where bacteria and viruses get carried by the flow of lymph fluid. They are also where dendritic cells take everything they've picked up while out on patrol.

T cells now multiply rapidly. If they're cyto-toxic T cells, they'll leave the lymph node and start hunting down and destroying cells that display on their surface the same pep-tide antigen shown to them by the dendritic cell [89].

You might have already noticed from Box 1.2 that there are various T cell types (and many subtypes) in our body. Out of all of them, it's the cytotoxic T cells[22] that can directly interact with and destroy other cells. They do this by getting close to the target cell and then releasing cell-killing enzymes called perforin and granzymes. These enzymes do things like drilling holes in the target cell's surface, causing it to become leaky and die – a process that takes about half an hour [90].

1.5.2 The Cancer-Immunity Cycle

Hopefully, by now, you're beginning to under-stand how our immune system can detect and destroy cancer cells. Perhaps the most famous journal article describing this process is the review written by two American scientists, Daniel Chen and Ira Mellman. They published their article in 2013 in the prestigious scientific journal "Cell" and coined the phrase, The Cancer-Immunity Cycle [91] (Figure 1.15).[23]

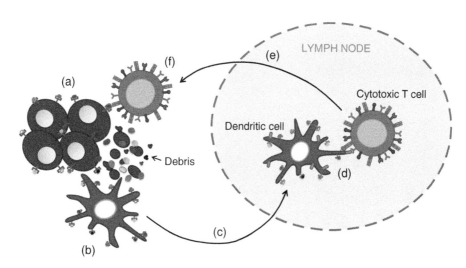

Figure 1.15 The Cancer-Immunity Cycle. (a) Tumors contain living cancer cells and a lot of debris from dead and dying cells. **(b)** Dendritic cells that find their way into a tumor may be activated by this debris, so long as it is accompanied by "danger" signals released by the dying cells and other cells in the tumor, such as various white blood cells. If the right signals are present, the dendritic cell hoovers up some debris. **(c)** The dendritic cell breaks up the debris to create short peptides that it displays on its surface using both class 1 and class 2 MHC proteins. It travels to a nearby lymph node. **(d)** In the lymph node, the dendritic cell presents the peptides on its surface to T cells, trying to find a match. T cells with T cell receptors that match the shape of peptides on the dendritic cell are activated and multiply. **(e)** Some of these activated T cells find their way into the tumor. **(f)** In the tumor, activated T cells destroy cancer cells with the same peptides displayed on their surface as those presented to the T cells by dendritic cells.

---

[22] Cytotoxic T cells are also referred to as "CD8-positive" T cells, or as "killer" T cells.
[23] You can find out how their famous article came about in this profile piece on the Genentech website: https://www.gene.com/stories/behind-the-cycle.

I hope you've noticed that this process has lots of "ifs, buts, and maybes" about it.

For example, IF a dendritic cell gets into a tumor, it MIGHT become active, but ONLY if it also receives other signals. Also, if an activated dendritic cell reaches a lymph node, and IF it finds suitable T cells to activate, those T cells MIGHT know where the cancer cells are located, and they MIGHT get into the tumor environment. In that new environment, they MIGHT manage to stay active long enough to kill some cancer cells. But there are no guarantees that any of this will happen. This brings us to the next Section: How cancer cells avoid detection and destruction by the immune system.

1.5.3 How Cancer Cells Avoid Destruction by the Immune System

There are many reasons why a person's cancer cells might not be destroyed by their immune system. Some of these reasons are important to understand as they can help us make sense of various forms of immunotherapy, such as the immune checkpoint inhibitors I describe in Chapter 5 like nivolumab, pembrolizumab, and ipilimumab.

These reasons can be categorized depending on whether they're directly to do with the person's cancer cells, their T cells, or a different mechanism. I've listed some of these reasons later, but this is by no means an exhaustive list.

Reasons Why the Person's Cancer Cells Aren't Detected by Their Immune System

- The person's cancer cells might not contain the types of DNA mutations that lend themselves to recognition by the immune system. For example, cancer cells with a handful of large-scale chromosome defects are much less visible to the immune system than those with thousands of small-scale mutations caused by powerful mutators

such as components of tobacco smoke, UV light, defects in DNA repair processes, or overactive APOBEC enzymes [92].

- If there's too much diversity in terms of the mutations the cancer cells contain, this can bamboozle the immune system. The immune system has a better chance of detecting cancer if there are lots of mutations that are the same in every cancer cell in the tumor and in any metastases (called *clonal mutations*), rather than when there are diverse cancer cells with different mutations inside them [92, 93].
- If the person's cancer cells have lost much of their ability to process peptides and display them via MHC class 1 proteins, they will be invisible to the immune system [94].
- Some of the gene mutations found in cancer cells seem to go hand-in-hand with a lack of immune response. Examples include amplification of the *CCND1* gene, and mutations affecting *RAS* genes, *MYC*, *EGFR*, *HER2*, *PTEN*, and *TP53* [92, 95].

Sometimes Their Dendritic Cells Don't Present Peptide Antigens to T Cells
Reasons for this could be: [94]
- In some people, their cancer cells seem able to prevent dendritic cells from becoming mature and active, so they never pick up any tumor debris.
- Some cancer cells limit the ability of activated dendritic cells to internalize and process cancer peptides, reducing their ability to present peptide antigens to T cells.
- The continued presence of cancer cells in a tissue can gradually lead to a phenomenon called immune tolerance (see Box 1.4). This is a situation in which dendritic cells (and other white blood cells) start believing that the presence of cancer cells is normal and nothing to be concerned about, so they don't raise the alarm.

Box 1.4 Immune tolerance

Immune tolerance is essential to life. It describes the fact that our immune system ignores (and therefore doesn't attack) the normal proteins and other molecules that make up our body. If our immune system can't ignore our own healthy proteins, then we develop autoimmune diseases. However, cancers often hide from the immune system by inducing immune tolerance. If the immune system is tolerant to cancer cells and believes that they're normal, it will no longer try to attack them.

Box 1.5 Why do we have immune-suppressing white blood cells?

Our immune system fights off infections, destroys faulty cells, and keeps us healthy. However, it's important that immune responses don't outlive their usefulness. If immune responses last too long, the activated white blood cells will start doing damage to otherwise healthy tissues and organs. Hence, we have white blood cells such as **regulatory T cells** that exist to suppress and restrain other white blood cells. In addition, these restraining white blood cells prevent our immune system from destroying helpful bacteria in our gut, and they help prevent the growing embryo from being destroyed in the womb during pregnancy.

Sometimes the Person's Immune System Creates Cancer-fighting T Cells, But They Can't Get to Where They're Needed

Reasons for this could be: [93, 94]

- Tumor blood vessels are strange and chaotic. They can act as a barrier that prevents T cells from leaving the blood and getting in among the cancer cells (I come back to the strangeness of tumor blood vessels in Section 1.6.3) [93, 94].
- Cytotoxic T cells that recognize peptide antigens displayed by cancer cells don't necessarily know where the tumor is and may end up elsewhere in the body rather than inside the tumor.

Sometimes Cancer-Fighting T Cells Get into a Tumor But then Become Suppressed or Exhausted

Reasons for this could be: [96–99]

- In many tumors, cancer cells produce signaling molecules that attract and activate immune-suppressing white blood cells such as regulatory T cells (Tregs), myeloid-derived suppressor cells (MDSCs), and certain types of B cells. These white blood cells suppress any cancer-fighting cytotoxic T cells or NK cells in their vicinity

(see Box 1.5 for more about immune-suppressing white blood cells) [96–99].

- Activated T cells that enter tumors and start killing cancer cells eventually become overworked, overstimulated, and exhausted.
- Various types of cell in a tumor, including cancer cells and white blood cells, produce a range of small proteins called *growth factors* and other signaling molecules (e.g., prostaglandin E2, transforming growth factor-β, and interleukin-10) that directly suppress cytotoxic T cells.
- Cancer cells (and white blood cells) sometimes manufacture and release an enzyme called indoleamine 2,3-dioxygenase (IDO), which suppresses the activity of T cells.
- Cancer cells sometimes display proteins on their surface that suppress the actions of T cells. These proteins, which are often found on the surface of other white blood cells in the tumor too, are known as inhibitory checkpoint proteins. They include PD-L1 and PD-L2 (I'll be coming back to this in Chapter 5).

- T cells become suppressed and inactive due to the toxic tumor environment, which is often acidic, low in oxygen, and lacking nutrients.

All or some of the mechanisms mentioned earlier are likely to be at play in someone with cancer. They explain why someone's cancer might not be controlled or destroyed by their immune system. But they don't explain how cancer cells use white blood cells to help them thrive, which is what we'll turn to next.

1.5.4 How Cancer Cells Ultimately Survive, and Thrive, Among White Blood Cells

Cancer cells in a tumor are often outnumbered by their non-cancer neighbors. Some of these neighbors are white blood cells that I've already mentioned, such as T cells and NK cells. But many of them are white blood cells we commonly think of as being involved in inflammation, such as macrophages and neutrophils. Instead of killing cancer cells, these inflammatory white blood cells often help cancer cells to survive and thrive [28, 96, 100]. They do this by producing:

- Small proteins known as growth factors that cause cancer cells to multiply[24]
- Small proteins and chemicals collectively called "survival factors" that help cancer cells stay alive despite being in a hostile and toxic environment[25]
- Small proteins and chemicals that promote cancer cell migration, invasion, and metastasis.

On top of this, as I mentioned earlier, cancer cells and other cells in the tumor environment actively recruit white blood cells that suppress T cells and prevent them from attacking and destroying cancer cells such as Tregs and MDSCs.

1.5.5 Elimination, Equilibrium, and Escape

So far, I have described how cancer cells interact with white blood cells and explained the role played by different white blood cell types. But what's true for a small cluster of cancer cells isn't necessarily going to be true for a large tumor that has developed over several decades. The relationship between cancer cells and the person's immune system changes over time as the cancer grows. Scientists often refer to this as a process of elimination, equilibrium, and escape (Figure 1.16).

These three phases may take days, weeks, months, years, or even decades. But by the time a person is diagnosed with cancer, generally because it is causing symptoms, their cancer will have reached the escape phase. In this phase, their cancer is no longer being controlled by their immune system.

Together, whether a person's cancer is hidden from T cells, whether T cells have been generated but then suppressed, and what other white blood cells are present in the person's tumor (and what they're doing there) will all influence a person's prognosis and whether they benefit from immunotherapy; something we turn to again in Chapter 5.

1.6 THE CANCER MICROENVIRONMENT

As I've already mentioned, tumors are not lumps of tissue made from millions of identical cancer cells. Instead, they contain a variety

---

[24] We return to the topic of growth factors in Chapter 3, as many cancer treatments work by blocking growth factor receptors.

[25] This might not seem obvious, but because cancer cells grow in a haphazard manner and there aren't enough decent blood vessels around to supply them with everything they want and to take toxins away, their environment is toxic.

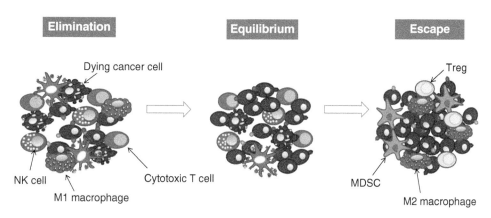

Figure 1.16 Elimination, equilibrium, and escape. In the initial *elimination phase*, cancer cells are successfully spotted and destroyed by both cytotoxic T cells and natural killer (NK) cells. However, any cancer cells that are hidden from the immune system will survive, such as those that present very few antigens on their surface via their MHC proteins. The tumor may then reach an *equilibrium phase*, where some cancer cells are destroyed but other, less visible, or more protected cancer cells are able to multiply. Finally, due to the accumulation of further mutations or changes in the tumor's microenvironment, the tumor reaches the *escape phase*. In this phase, cancer cells multiply at a faster pace than they are destroyed. In addition, immune-suppressing white blood cells such as MDSCs and Tregs accumulate, along with other cells that support, nurture, and protect cancer cells and aid tumor growth and metastasis. *Source:* Ref. [98, 99, 101, 102].

of non-cancer cells (collectively known as stromal cells) such as various types of white blood cells, fibroblasts (these are common, structural cells found in many locations around the body), cells that make up the blood vessels (endothelial cells and pericytes), fat cells (also called adipocytes), nerve cells, and other cell types (see Figure 1.17) [103].

The cells in a tumor are also embedded in a network of proteins and complicated sugar molecules known as the ECM – the extracellular matrix.[26] This intricate web surrounds the cells in all our tissues and organs, and its makeup and role differ from place to place around the body. When a cancer develops, cancer cells and non-cancer cells (which are now under the cancer cells' influence) cause the makeup and density of the ECM to change.

For example, in breast cancer, the ECM becomes stiffer, and this seems to help cancer cells move and escape into the lymph vessels and bloodstream [104].

1.6.1 The Role of White Blood Cells

As I described in Section 1.5, each person's tumor will have a different collection of white blood cells inside it and at its outer fringes. The type of cells present, their number, and their behavior have a huge impact on how quickly or slowly the tumor grows and whether the person can be cured [28, 100, 105]. Some of these are "friends" to cancer cells; they protect cancer cells or encourage their growth. Others are "foes" that attack and destroy cancer cells (Figure 1.18).

---

[26] Examples of ECM proteins include collagen, fibronectin, laminin, and elastin. The ECM also contains long, complicated sugar molecules (called glycosaminoglycans) that are generally chemically linked to proteins to form protein-sugar hybrids called proteoglycans. These proteoglycans form a jelly-like substance in which the fibrous proteins like collagen are embedded.

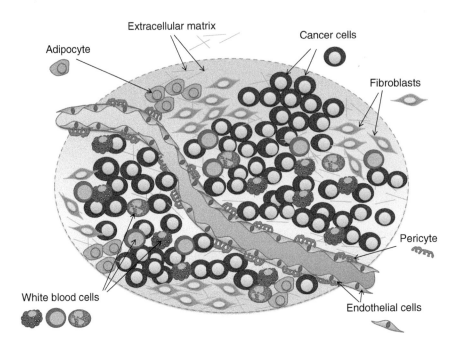

Figure 1.17 The cancer microenvironment contains many different types of cells. Tumors contain cancer cells, many different types of white blood cells, fibroblasts, fat cells (adipocytes), and other cell types (not shown). Winding their way through them are blood vessels, which are made up of endothelial cells and pericytes. Lymph vessels might also be present (not shown). All of these proteins are embedded in a complex network of structural proteins called the extracellular matrix.

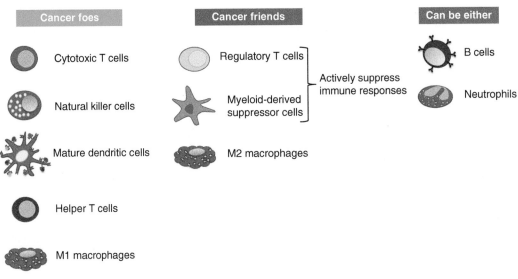

Figure 1.18 The influence of various infiltrating white blood cells on patient prognosis and response to treatment. The presence of some types of white blood cells (Cancer Foes) is generally a good sign for the patient as these create a cancer-fighting immune response and are linked to longer survival times. Whereas the presence of "Cancer Friends" is generally a bad sign and linked to shortened survival. Depending on cues from other cells, macrophages can become "M1" macrophages that produce molecules that kill cancer cells, or they can become "M2" macrophages that suppress immune responses and encourage angiogenesis. The presence of some other types of white blood cell can be a good or a bad sign depending on the cancer type and other influences. *Source:* Ref. [27, 101, 106, 107].

However, as with all things immunology-related there is a lot of subtlety and variation to this. For example, white blood cells that are located among lots of cancer cells will exert a different influence compared to white blood cells that are located around the tumor's fringes or trapped inside blood vessels [101].

1.6.2 The Role of Other Cell Types

Fibroblasts sit in our tissues, and they normally produce structural proteins that form the ECM [108]. In tumors, fibroblasts change in response to chemicals and other signals sent out by cancer cells. They become perpetually activated and behave as though they are in a damaged tissue. For example, they release vast quantities of ECM proteins – much more than normal – and they produce growth factors and chemicals that encourage cancer cells to multiply [103]. These same proteins can be an enormous obstacle to successful treatment [104].

Also found in some tumors are fat cells called adipocytes. Again, the adipocytes found within tumors aren't normal; they've been altered by signals sent out by cancer cells. And, like the fibroblasts in tumors, the adipocytes also encourage and help cancer cells to grow and multiply [103].

1.6.3 Angiogenesis

Angiogenesis (the formation of new blood vessels) is almost always necessary for a cancer to become life threatening. By the time a cancer has reached a few millimeters in size, the cells will be experiencing a drop in oxygen levels (hypoxia). Cancer cells then trigger angiogenesis to gain a blood supply and get access to oxygen and nutrients.

The most important trigger for angiogenesis is a tiny protein called vascular endothelial growth factor (VEGF)[27], which is released by cancer cells (and other cells) when oxygen levels drop. VEGF attaches to receptor proteins on the surface of endothelial cells – the cells that line our blood vessels. Once VEGF has attached to its receptors, the endothelial cells multiply and move into place to form a new blood vessel, which is supported by other cells called pericytes [107, 108]. VEGF isn't the only thing that triggers angiogenesis. Other triggers include angiopoietins, fibroblast growth factor, and ephrins. The fact that VEGF isn't in sole control will become important when we look at the class of cancer drugs called angiogenesis inhibitors (Section 4.1).

When properly controlled, angiogenesis is an important and entirely healthy process. It happens normally during the healing of cuts and wounds, during the menstrual cycle, during the formation of the placenta in pregnancy, and in a growing embryo [109]. The blood vessels that form during these healthy processes are evenly distributed and well supported by pericytes.

However, when angiogenesis happens in a tumor, it helps the cancer to grow and spread by supplying cancer cells with oxygen and nutrients and providing access to the bloodstream. In addition, tumor blood vessels tend to be lumpy, leaky, and disorderly [110]. Endothelial cells are no longer tightly connected to each other and are poorly supported by pericytes, which normally feed, protect, and physically support them [111]. On top of this, the supply of blood (and therefore oxygen) through tumor blood vessels is patchy and some areas in the tumor are constantly deprived of oxygen, changing the behavior of cancer cells nearby (Figure 1.19).

---

[27] There is in fact a whole family of VEGF proteins, called VEGF-A, VEGF-B, VEGF-C, VEGF-D, and placental growth factor.

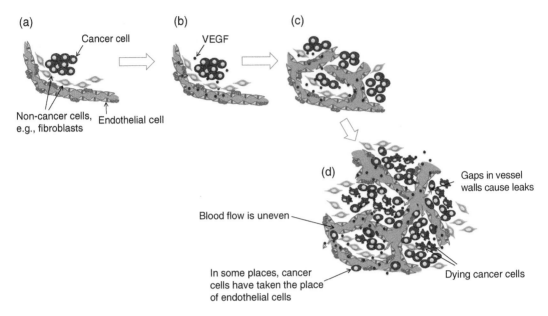

Figure 1.19 Cancer angiogenesis. (a) A cluster of cancer cells is too far away from the nearest blood vessel to receive an adequate blood supply. **(b)** Low oxygen levels trigger the cancer cells to release VEGF and other angiogenesis factors into their surroundings. **(c)** VEGF attaches to VEGF receptors on the surface endothelial cells, causing the blood vessel to sprout side branches and grow. **(d)** The tumor contains a convoluted, lumpy, leaky network of blood vessels; many cancer cells now have sufficient blood supply, but many others do not. **Abbreviations:** VEGF – vascular endothelial growth factor.

1.6.4 Two Examples of the Importance of the Tumor Microenvironment

Perhaps the best way to illustrate the importance of the makeup of the tumor microenvironment in determining how cancers behave and respond to treatment is to give a couple of examples. The two I've chosen are NSCLC and pancreatic cancer. The microenvironment of these two cancers is organized very differently. Each one has a distinctive set of non-cancer cells arranged in a particular way. As you'll hopefully see, this has a powerful impact on how these cancers respond to various treatments.

Non-Small Cell Lung Cancer

NSCLCs contain some of the highest numbers of infiltrating white blood cells, particularly T cells, of any cancer (Figure 1.20).

But perhaps equally important is the presence of tertiay lymphoid structures (TLSs). These are small patches of tissue within tumors that contain many white blood cells arranged in the same way as you normally find in lymph nodes (such as cytotoxic T cells, helper T cells, mature dendritic cells, and B cells). Our lymph nodes are where T cells are activated, and TLSs are the same. This means that cancer-fighting cytotoxic T cells are being generated within the tumor, and then they don't have far to go to find some cancer cells to destroy. The presence of TLSs in NSCLC and other tumors correlates with a better prognosis for the patient, and with a greater benefit from immunotherapy [27, 112–114].

Pancreatic Cancer

The cancer microenvironment of the most common sort of pancreatic cancer (pancreatic ductal adenocarcinoma) is very different from that of NSCLC (Figure 1.21).

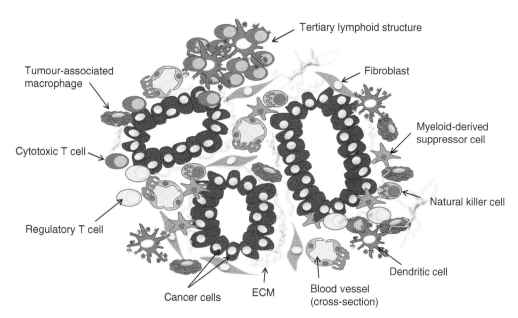

Figure 1.20 The microenvironment of non-small cell lung cancer (NSCLC). Inside the tumor are cancer cells and various non-cancer cell types, including various types of white blood cells. Dotted throughout the tumor are tertiary lymphoid structures (TLSs), and there is a profusion of cytotoxic T cells inside TLSs and elsewhere. There are relatively few macrophages compared to other tumor types.
Abbreviation: ECM – extracellular matrix; TLS – tertiary lymphoid structure.

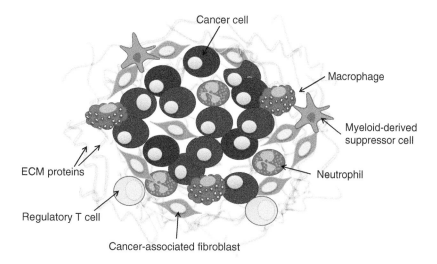

Figure 1.21 The pancreatic cancer microenvironment can protect cancer cells from the effects of treatment. Pancreatic cancers usually contain a fibrous network of ECM proteins that compress blood vessels and prevent cancer drugs from penetrating the tumor. Cancer-associated fibroblasts produce fibrous proteins and release pro-survival proteins such as growth factors. White blood cells such as macrophages secrete many small proteins and chemicals that protect cancer cells from treatments. Cytotoxic T cells are rare.
Abbreviation: ECM – extracellular matrix.

One important difference is the presence of desmoplasia. This refers to the dense accumulation of lots of tightly packed fibrous ECM proteins that have been created by cancer-associated fibroblasts (these are fibroblasts whose behavior is being controlled by cancer cells). Desmoplasia creates a physical barrier that prevents angiogenesis and that limits the number and types of white blood cells that can enter the tumor. Pancreatic tumors tend to contain lots of cancer-assisting macrophages, lots of immune-suppressing Tregs and MDSCs, and very few cytotoxic T cells [115]. As a result, pancreatic cancer is one of the most aggressive and difficult to treat types of cancer. In addition, immunotherapy has so far shown little sign of being an effective treatment approach.

1.7 CANCER SPREAD/ METASTASIS

As soon as a cancer spreads (metastasizes) to another part of the body, treatment becomes more complicated, and the person's likelihood of being cured of their disease drops dramatically [111, 112]. Scientists estimate that metastasis is responsible for around 90% of cancer deaths [116]. Sadly, once a cancer has metastasized, surgery is often no longer helpful and other treatments are likely to have limited impact. The various new cancer growths go on to disrupt and destroy vital tissues and organs.

Also, even when a cancer doesn't *appear* to have spread, there can be individual cancer cells, or microscopic clumps of cells that are circulating in the person's blood or lodged in distant organs or tissues [117]. These initially dormant cells can later cause metastasis and relapse.

There are numerous reasons why cancers metastasize. For example:
- Some cancer cells contain DNA mutations that force them into behaviors that cause metastasis.
- Cancer cells that are on the move might enter a blood or lymph vessel and get carried along by the blood/lymph to distant sites.
- The cells, proteins, and structures in the cancer cells' environment, and the cancer cells' limited access to oxygen, can encourage cancer cells to become more mobile or to move in specific directions.

One important thing to realize is that cancer cells that metastasize might contain lots of mutations and display behaviors that aren't present in cancer cells that stay put. As a result, a patient's metastases might behave differently and respond to different treatments than the primary tumor.

1.7.1 Routes Through Which Cancers Spread

There are five main routes through which a cancer can spread: [118]
- Local invasion
- Lymph vessels
- Blood vessels
- Nerves
- Fluid in the abdomen.

Routes of Cancer Spread – Via Local Invasion

"Local invasion" describes the process whereby cancer cells digest ECM proteins in their surroundings and gradually move into, infiltrate, and destroy nearby tissues. Local invasion is often the first step toward metastasis to distant organs.

Routes of Cancer Spread – Via Lymph Vessels (Lymphatic)

The fluid around our cells drains into lymphatic vessels and from there into lymph nodes (also called lymph glands), and finally back into the bloodstream.[28] Cancer cells that have become detached from the cells around them are often caught up in this flow and carried to nearby lymph nodes.

Routes of Cancer Spread – Via Blood Vessels (Vascular)

Individual cancer cells (and small clusters) are sometimes able to squeeze their way into small blood vessels. The red and white blood cells in the vessel then sweep the cancer cells along until they get stuck somewhere else. Cancer cells that have found their way into the bloodstream are called circulating cancer cells or circulating tumor cells (CTCs).

Routes of Cancer Spread – Via Nerves (Perineural)

This is a relatively rare but dangerous route of cancer spread in which cancer cells spread along the course of nerve bundles. This type of spread is often very painful because cancer cells produce chemicals that trigger nerve activity.

Via Fluid in the Abdomen or (Transcoelomic)

Cancers that arise in the abdomen, particularly ovarian cancers, are liable to spread via the fluid that circulates within the abdomen. Cancer cells on the surface of the tumor break away and float in the abdominal fluid that bathes our internal organs. Cancer cells are carried along in the fluid and then adhere to tissues and organs in the abdomen such as the omentum[29] or bowel.

Once a cancer cell has reached a new location in the body, it won't necessarily cause a new cancer to grow. In fact, the vast majority of breakaway cancer cells die in the lymph or blood, are killed by white blood cells, or simply remain dormant (see Figure 1.22). In order for the cell to cause metastasis, it must survive and thrive in its new environment. And only a tiny proportion of breakaway cancer cells are ultimately able to go through this process.

1.7.2 Locations to Which Cancers Spread

Some cancers have particular routes of spread that are more likely than others (e.g., breast cancer commonly spreads via the lymph system). And each type of cancer is also more likely to spread to some locations than others [119]. For example:

- Breast cancers often spread to the bones, brain, liver, and lungs
- Prostate cancers often spread to bones
- Bowel cancers often spread to the liver, lungs, and the lining of the abdominal cavity (peritoneum)
- Lung cancers often spread to the adrenal glands, bone, brain, liver, and/or into the other lung
- Melanoma skin cancers often spread to the lungs, brain, other parts of the skin, and liver.

The preference that cancers have for spreading to some locations rather than others is often due to the anatomical layout of lymph and blood vessels. For example, the blood supply to the bowel goes from there to the liver, hence the liver is where bowel cancers often spread to first [120].

1.7.3 Reasons Why Cancers Spread

Many of the cells in a tumor seem to be relatively inert and dormant, perhaps because of low oxygen levels or due to signals sent out by their cancer and non-cancer neighbors.

---

[28] For a colorful illustration of the lymph system, see the Cancer Research UK website: http://www.cancerresearchuk.org/what-is-cancer/body-systems-and-cancer/the-lymphatic-system-and-cancer [Accessed January 11, 2022].
[29] The omentum is a fold of fatty tissue that hangs down from the stomach and covers our intestines and other organs.

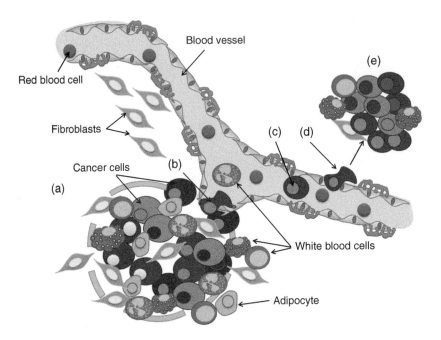

Figure 1.22 The path to metastasis. (a) A primary tumor containing many different cell types.
(b) A cancer cell that is particularly mobile might invade locally and squeeze its way into blood vessels.
(c) A cancer cell circulating in the blood. **(d)** The cancer cell squeezes out of the blood vessel into a new
environment. **(e)** In its new location, the cancer cell may die or remain dormant for weeks or even years,
kept in check by its new environment. However, eventually a change in its environment or the impact of
new mutations might enable it to multiply and create a metastasis.

However, other cancer cells can be highly
mobile and be much more likely to cause
metastasis. Scientists believe that these mobile
cells have gone through a change in appearance and behavior called the epithelial-to-
mesenchymal transition (EMT) [117, 119]
(Figure 1.23).

The EMT is a change that some healthy cells
undergo in a developing embryo or in an
adult when a tissue is damaged. It's when
a stationary, well-connected epithelial cell[30]
becomes more like a mobile, independent
mesenchymal cell. During the EMT, the cell
produces more ECM proteins, becomes more
resilient, and changes shape [121].

The EMT is thus a natural process that is
hijacked and reactivated by cancer cells.
Understandably, if a cancer cell goes through
this change, it's more likely to cause metastasis than other cancer cells.

Triggers that encourage cancer cells to go
through the EMT include growth factors and
other chemicals released by neighboring cells,
low oxygen levels, and contact with various
ECM proteins [122].

The EMT appears to be very important
and it poses huge problems for doctors. For
example, cancers that contain a high proportion of mesenchymal cells are more likely to
resist treatment and spread quickly [123].

---

[30] Cancers that develop from epithelial cells are called carcinomas. These are the most common type of cancer
diagnosed in the United Kingdom, accounting for about 85% of cancers [*Source:* Cancer Research UK].

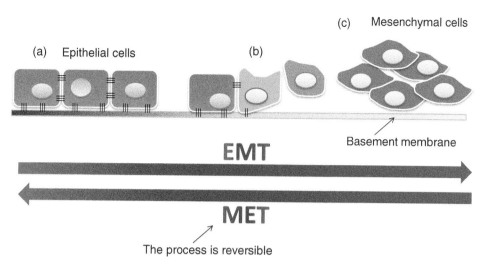

Figure 1.23 The epithelial-to-mesenchymal transition (EMT). (a) All our body's organs and tissues are lined with epithelial cells. Epithelial cells tend to be lined up and well connected to one another. They are also physically attached to the basement membrane (The basement membrane is a thin, dense sheet of ECM. It sits underneath layers of epithelial cells and anchors them to the tissue beneath. It also acts as a barrier separating different types of tissue. In addition, it wraps around blood vessels and provides structural support for endothelial cells.). **(b)** During the EMT, cells gradually stop making epithelial cell proteins and start making lots of proteins common in mesenchymal cells. **(c)** Mesenchymal cells are mobile and resilient and less well connected to one another and the basement membrane.
Abbreviations: EMT – epithelial-to-mesenchymal transition; MET – mesenchymal to epithelial transition.

Also, some treatments seem to cause cancer cells to go through the EMT, helping the cells survive the effects of treatment and causing metastasis [124, 125].

1.8 CANCER STEM CELLS

Over the past 20 years or so, scientists have increasingly become convinced that a proportion of cancer cells behave somewhat like our body's stem cells[31] and can be classed as cancer stem cells [126]. That is, they not only have the ability to multiply to generate further cancer stem cells, but they can also produce cancer cells with various other properties. Therefore, if you kill all the other cells in a tumor but leave the stem cells behind, they will cause the cancer to return. Evidence suggests that cancer stem cells are relatively rare, slow-growing, drug-resistant cancer cells that can survive many cancer treatments [126, 127]. The strength of evidence for their existence varies from cancer type to cancer type.

The precise properties of cancer stem cells and where they come from are hotly debated by scientists [128–130]. Some scientists suggest that they could start out life as healthy adult stem cells that, due to DNA mutations, start behaving like cancer cells. Other scientists

---

[31] Adult stem cells are slow-growing, versatile cells found in small numbers in our organs and tissues. When they multiply, they create mature, specialized cells that replenish, repair, and renew the tissue and keep it healthy. The number of stem cells differs from organ to organ and tissue to tissue around the body, depending on the turnover of cells in that tissue. For example, there are many stem cells in the lining of the bowel because cells are continually being scraped off as food passes through, and these cells need to be replaced.

point to the similarities between cancer stem cells and cancer cells that have gone through the EMT. They suggest that cancer stem cells are derived from cancer cells that have gone through the EMT and that have later undergone further changes [127, 130–132].

Two of the problems scientists face when trying to study cancer stem cells are that (1) these cells are highly changeable and adaptable and (2) what constitutes a cancer stem cell varies from cancer to cancer and even from patient to patient [127]. So, it's best not to get too worked up about the label "cancer stem cell." Instead, we will simply acknowledge that there are often cells in a cancer that are not easily destroyed by treatments and that can cause a cancer to return weeks, months, or years later.

1.9 UNIQUE PROPERTIES OF HEMATOLOGICAL CANCERS

Much of the information I've provided so far has been more relevant to solid tumors than to hematological cancers – those that develop from faulty white blood cells. Hematological cancers have unique features that set them apart from solid tumors, and I'll describe them here.

1.9.1 Introducing Hematological Cancers

Hematological cancers all develop from faulty white blood cells or hematopoietic stem cells (see Figure 1.24). The type of cancer the person develops, and how it behaves and responds to treatment, depends on factors like:

- What type of white blood cell went wrong and caused the person's cancer.
- How mature or immature the cell was when it went wrong.
- What combination of mutations or other faults the cell contains.
- Where it was when it went wrong (e.g., the bone marrow, a lymph node, or lymphoid tissue in the gastrointestinal tract).

- Whether it was in the process of responding to an infection when it went wrong.
- Whether it had responded to an infection in the past.
- Whether the infection the cell had responded to is still around (e.g., most MALT (mucosa-associated lymphoid tissue) lymphomas are linked to an ongoing *H. pylori* infection [133]).

For example, a very immature white blood cell that has just begun to specialize to become some sort of myeloid cell might give rise to acute myeloid leukemia, whereas a fully mature B cell in a lymph node might cause a non-Hodgkin lymphoma.

In addition to being derived from white blood cells or hematopoietic stem cells, hematological cancers have other important characteristics. I've listed a few of these later, as they will hopefully help you make sense of the treatments I mention in later chapters.

1.9.2 Most of Them Develop from Faulty B Cells

Most hematological cancers develop from faulty B cells. Only a minority are T cell cancers or cancers that develop from faulty myeloid cells or stem cells (see Table 1.2).

B cells seem to be more prone to going wrong than other white blood cells for a couple of reasons: First, because of the processes they go through as they mature in the bone marrow. Second, because of the activation steps involved in responding to an infection.

Both processes (maturation and activation) involve the B cell deliberately cutting up, mutating, and rejoining sections of its DNA (see Figure 1.25). The crucial thing here is that unlike most of our cells, which take great pains to prevent their DNA from changing, B cells alter their DNA deliberately. They do this during V(D)J recombination in the bone marrow. They also do it during class switching and somatic hypermutation as they become active in response to an infection.

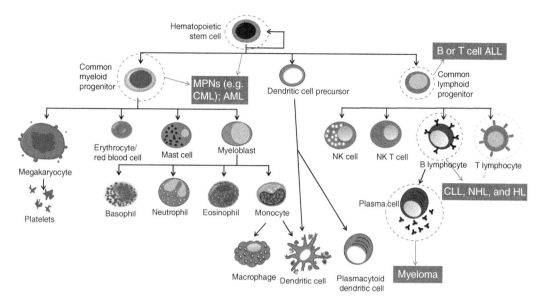

Figure 1.24 Diagram of hematopoiesis showing the cell of origin of common hematological cancers.
Stem cells (top) create progenitor cells that gradually specialize and become mature myeloid or lymphoid
white blood cells. If a stem cell or immature myeloid progenitor cell goes wrong, this may cause a
myeloproliferative neoplasm (MPN) such as chronic myeloid leukemia (CML), or it could cause acute
myeloid leukemia (AML). If an immature lymphocyte goes wrong, this may lead to a B cell or T cell acute
lymphoblastic leukemia (B cell or T cell ALL). Mature T cells rarely lead to cancer; in the rare cases when
this happens, they may cause one of various types of T cell non-Hodgkin lymphoma (T cell NHL). Mature
B cells are the cell of origin of the vast majority of chronic lymphocytic leukemias (CLLs); they also cause
B cell non-Hodgkin lymphomas (NHLs) and Hodgkin lymphoma (HL). B cells that are releasing
antibodies to fight an infection are known as plasma cells. Myeloma is a cancer that develops from faulty
plasma cells. There are many rare hematological cancers and disorders that are not shown in this diagram.
Abbreviation: NK – natural killer. *Source:* Original figure taken from Wikipedia: https://en.wikipedia.
org/wiki/Haematopoiesis#/media/ File:Hematopoiesis_simple.svg.

In addition, during B cell activation, B cells
multiply rapidly and receive protection from
death from their environment. This combination, rapid proliferation, protection, and delib-
erate DNA mutation, makes them vulnerable
to cutting/mutating their DNA in the wrong
places. It also makes them prone to aneuploidy (when a cell ends up with the wrong
number of chromosomes) [134, 135]. Perhaps
it's not so surprising that B cell cancers like
chronic lymphocytic leukemia (CLL) and B
cell non-Hodgkin lymphoma (NHL) are quite
so common.

The last thing to mention about B cell cancers is that many of them rely on the BCRs on
their surface for survival. I'll come back to this
in Section 4.8 when I discuss treatments that
target BCR-controlled signaling pathways.

1.9.3 Certain Translocations Are Common to Each Type and Subtype

Chromosome translocations (where two chromosomes break and end up stuck together
incorrectly) are a common feature of hematological cancers.

Many types, and subtypes, of hematological
cancers have characteristic translocations that
exist alongside other mutations and abnormalities. Table 1.3 lists a few of the most common

Table 1.2   The expected incidence of various hematological cancers in the United Kingdom.

Type of cancer	Expected number of cases each year in the United Kingdom
Cancers that develop from stem cells or myeloid white blood cells:	**9010**
Acute myeloid leukemia	2890
Chronic myeloid leukemia[a]	720
Myeloproliferative neoplasms (MPNs): myelofibrosis, polycythemia vera, essential thrombocythemia, or MPN – unclassifiable	4530
Myelodysplastic syndromes	870
Cancers that develop from B cells:	**23,140**
B cell acute lymphoblastic leukemia	630
Chronic lymphocytic leukemia	4720
B cell non-Hodgkin lymphomas (marginal zone, follicular, mantle cell, large B cell, and Burkitt's)	11,260
Hodgkin lymphoma	1870
Myeloma	4660
Cancers that develop from T cells and NK cells:	**1140**
T cell acute lymphoblastic leukemia	150
T cell non-Hodgkin lymphomas	990
Proportion of cancers in this table that are of:	
Myeloid/stem cell origin	27%
B cell origin	70%
T cell origin	3%

[a] Chronic myeloid leukemia is often classified as a form of MPN.
Source: Data are from hmrn.org.

translocations [134, 135]. It seems that for some hematological cancers, a translocation between two chromosomes was the first mutation that occurred in an otherwise normal cell that put it on the path to becoming a cancer cell. However, all of us will have some white blood cells in our body that contain the same chromosome translocations found in cancer cells. So, the translocation itself is generally insufficient to cause cancer [135, 143].

Knowing what translocations have taken place in a patient's cancer can provide important information as to the likely future course of their cancer, how aggressive it's going to be, and whether it will respond to certain treatments. The discovery of translocations has also led to the discovery of important genes and proteins that have since led scientists to create new treatments. Sometimes, such as in CML, mantle cell lymphoma, and follicular lymphoma, there's just one specific translocation found in the cancer cells of virtually every person. In other cancers, you find a range of different translocations.

The Three Main Types of Translocations
As I outlined in Section 1.2.2, translocations can have a variety of consequences for a cell. In hematological cancer cells, you find three main types of translocations:
1. Translocations (such as the t(9;22) translocation found in CML) that create a fusion protein that is a faulty version of a kinase. Examples include Bcr-Abl and NPM-ALK, which force cells to grow and multiply.

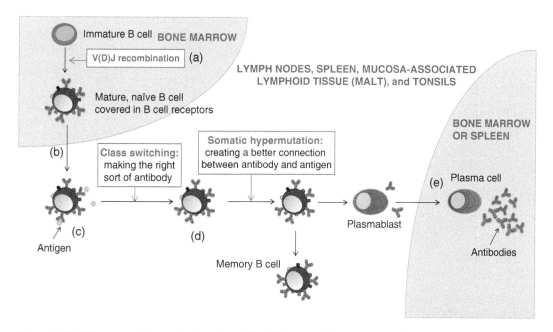

Figure 1.25 The maturation and activation of B cells is a multistep process. (a) As a B cell matures, it creates a unique B cell receptor (BCR) gene by a process called V(D)J recombination. A fully mature B cell has thousands of copies of the unique BCR protein made from this gene on its surface. (b) Mature B cells leave the bone marrow and travel to lymph nodes and other immune tissues. (c) Mature B cells are constantly meeting bacteria, viruses, and other pathogens, all of which have potential antigens on their surface that the B cell's BCRs might be able to recognize. (d) If a B cell does recognize an antigen, it might enter a multistep activation process involving somatic hypermutation and class switching. (e) Finally, the B cell might become a fully fledged plasma cell capable of releasing thousands of copies of a soluble version of its BCR protein (now called an antibody) into the blood. Plasma cells are mostly found in bone marrow and spleen. Activated B cells can also become long-lived memory B cells, ready to react if they encounter the same antigen again in the future. **Abbreviation:** BCR – B cell receptor.

2. Translocations that create a fusion protein that is a faulty version of a transcription factor. The faulty transcription factor suppresses genes and prevents the cell from making proteins that would help it mature properly. Examples include TEL-AML1, AML1-ETO, and PML-RARA.
3. Translocations that put together the control region of one gene with the protein-coding region of an oncogene, causing overproduction of an oncogenic (cancer-causing) protein. Examples include the t(14;18) translocation in follicular lymphoma (a form of B cell NHL), which causes overproduction of Bcl-2.

However, do remember that translocations aren't the only mutations found in hematological cancer cells. For example, in the cancer cells of CLL, the region of chromosome 17 that contains the *TP53* gene is commonly deleted or mutated. Lack of functional p53 protein in CLL cells causes the disease to be aggressive and resistant to chemotherapy [144].

1.9.4 They Have CD Antigens on Their Surface

All the proteins (and other large, complex molecules) found on the surface of our white blood cells have been allocated a number

Table 1.3 Some of the common translocations found in hematological cancer cells.

Translocation	Genes affected	Type of cell	Name of cancer
t(**14**;18)	*BCL2* (Bcl-2)	B cell	Follicular lymphoma
t(8;**14**)	*MYC*	B cell	Burkitt's lymphoma
t(3;**14**)	*BCL-6*	B cell	Diffuse large B-cell lymphoma
t(9;22)	*BCR-ABL* fusion	Myeloid cell	Chronic myeloid leukemia
t(11;**14**)	*CCND1* (Cyclin D1)	B cell	Mantle cell lymphoma
t(10;**14**)	*HOX11* (TLX1)	T cell	T cell ALL
t(2;5)	*NPM-ALK* fusion	B cell	Anaplastic large cell lymphoma
t(12;21)(p12;q22)	*TEL-AML1*[a] fusion	B cell	B cell ALL
t(1;19)(q23;p13)	*E2A-PBX1* fusion	B cell	B cell ALL
t(8;**14**)(q24;q32)	*MYC*	B cell	B cell ALL
t(15;17)(q21;q21)	*PML-RARA* fusion	Myeloid cell	Acute promyelocytic leukemia[b]
t(8;21)(q22;q22)	*AML1-ETO* fusion	Myeloid cell	Acute myeloid leukemia

Abbreviation: ALL – acute lymphoblastic leukemia.
Translocations that create an overactive kinase are in orange; those that create a faulty transcription factor are in purple; those that cause the overexpression of an oncogenic protein are in turquoise.
[a] This fusion protein created is also called ETV6-RUNX1.
[b] Acute promyelocytic leukemia is a rare subtype of acute myeloid leukemia.
Source: Ref. [135–142].

known as a "CD antigen" number.[32] (CD stands for "cluster of differentiation," but it doesn't mean anything very much.)

CD numbers correspond to the order in which the proteins were discovered (CD1 came first, then CD2 was discovered, then CD3 …). Scientists have now discovered and numbered over 370 CD antigens; regular workshops are held to discuss CD antigens found since the previous meeting.

So, the number assigned to a CD antigen doesn't tell you anything about that antigen itself (other than give you a rough idea of when it was discovered). But the range of CD antigens on the surface of a white blood cell can tell you things like:

- What type of white blood cell it is (e.g., only B cells have CD20 on their surface).
- Whether it's a mature, fully functioning white blood cell, or an immature one, or somewhere in between.
- What its job is.
- Whether, if it's a B or T cell, it has recognized and responded to an antigen.[33]

Each type of white blood cell has a wide variety of different CD antigens on its surface. Many of these proteins help our white blood cells communicate with one another. Other CD antigens transport things in and out of the cell, help the cell move through the bloodstream and into tissues, or help it destroy invaders.

[32] Numbering and naming of CD antigens are the responsibility of the participants of workshops run by the Human Cell Differentiation Molecules (HCDM) organization. Details of every CD antigen are available on the HCDM.org website.
[33] Although "antigen" and "CD antigen" sound like they're very similar to one another, it's probably easiest to think of them as two entirely different things: "antigens" being things that can trigger an immune response, and "CD antigens" being proteins and other large molecules found on the surface of white blood cells.

Box 1.6   The conventions of writing down translocations

When someone writes **t(9;22)(q34;q11)**, they are giving you detailed information about the translocation that has taken place. First, **t** stands for translocation. Second, the translocation involves chromosomes 9 and 22. The term **q34** tells you that it was the long arm (rather than **p** – the short arm) of chromosome 9 that broke, specifically at position 34. And **q11** tells you that it was the long arm of chromosome 22 that broke, at position 11. All chromosomes have a long arm and a short arm, which are separated by a narrow region of the chromosome called the centromere.

It's worth noting a couple more things about CD antigens at this point:

- They're found on the surface of white blood cells, and they are therefore accessible to monoclonal antibody treatments.
- Many of them are not necessary for the survival of the white blood cells that they are found on; therefore, blocking them with an antibody won't necessarily kill the cell.

Each type of white blood cell has a very particular set of CD antigens on its surface. If a cell goes wrong and becomes a cancer cell, the cancer cell often has (more or less) the same CD antigens on its surface as its healthy counterpart. Knowing what CD antigens a person's cancer cells have on their surface can therefore tell you things like what sort of white blood cell their cancer developed from and which antibody-based treatments might be helpful for them.

1.9.5 They Live in Close Proximity to Other White Blood Cells

As with cancer cells in solid tumors, hematological cancer cells live in an environment that contains lots of other white blood cells. And, like solid tumors, hematological cancer cells influence and reshape their environment to suit their purposes and to avoid destruction. For example:

- In CLL, the person's cancer cells are generally found in protected environments within the bone marrow, lymph nodes, and spleen (as well as accumulating in the blood). The cancer cells are surrounded by T cells, NK cells, macrophages (called nurse-like cells), endothelial cells, and other cell types. These cells provide support, protection, and encouragement to CLL cells [145, 146].
- In ALL, AML, and other leukemia types, leukemic cells hijack and destroy the normal bone marrow environment. Normal bone marrow supports and guides the development of hematopoietic stem cells. In leukemia, the normal balance between white blood cell creation and death changes, and the microenvironment supports the rapid multiplication of cancer cells and protects them from the effects of treatment [147].
- Different types of B cell NHL, such as follicular lymphoma and diffuse large B cell lymphoma (DLBCL), contain different types of non-cancer white blood cells. For example, follicular lymphomas tend to contain lots of helper T cells, but these are virtually absent from the DLBCL environment. Follicular lymphoma cells are also very dependent on signals from their environment for their survival. In contrast, the cancer cells of DLBCL are more resilient and independent [148].
- In Hodgkin lymphoma, only 1%–10% of the cells in the person's tumor are cancer-causing (these are known as Reed-Sternberg cells). The rest are T cells, B cells, plasma cells, and other white blood cells that cluster around the cancer cells and provide support and protection [149].

The consequences of all of this are twofold:

1. To cure someone with a hematological cancer, you need to give them treatments that destroy their cancer cells and that overcome the protection provided by other white blood cells in their environment.

2. There are possibilities for immunotherapy for hematological cancers that don't exist with solid tumors. Although the microenvironment of hematological cancers does contain lots of altered white blood cells, fresh white blood cells are coming and going all the time. After all, the bone marrow, lymph nodes, and other lymph tissues (like the spleen, and Peyers patches in the intestines) are places where white blood cells are constantly congregating and being refreshed. As a result, there is a wider range of successful immunotherapy strategies for people with hematological cancers compared to those for people with solid tumors.

1.10 OBSTACLES THAT PREVENT US FROM CURING CANCER

In this chapter, I've explained some of what we now know about how cancers come about and why cancer cells behave as they do. I've also described some of the behaviors that cancer cells exhibit. In addition, I've tried to portray the diversity that often exists within tumors in terms of the types of cells found in them and the genetic diversity among cancer cells. Armed with all this knowledge about cancer, it's tempting to believe that we might know enough to cure everyone affected by the disease. However, as I'm sure you are fully aware, this sadly isn't the case.

So, what is it that still thwarts us? What features of cancer cells and cancer behavior are responsible for our inability to cure it, particularly when it has metastasized?

As a conclusion to this introductory chapter, I'm going to go through some of the chief obstacles to curing more cancer patients:

1. The similarities between cancer cells and healthy cells
2. The great dissimilarities between different types of cancer
3. The fact that cancer spreads
4. Intratumoral heterogeneity
5. The tumor microenvironment

There are, of course, other obstacles to successfully curing a patient of cancer. Not least are the issues of late diagnosis, the impact of racial, sex, and socioeconomic disparities, and the fact that many people who develop cancer are relatively elderly and frail and have other medical complaints that often preclude the use of aggressive treatments. However, these issues are beyond the scope of this book, so I'll stick to describing the five obstacles I listed above. If you are interested in age and other disparities, I would suggest taking a look at the following references [150–158].

1.10.1 The Similarity Between Healthy Cells and Cancer Cells

All our cells, cancer cells and non-cancer cells alike, have the same repertoire of roughly 21,000 genes. These genes contain the instructions for making all the proteins our cells will ever need. As you might have already gathered from the rest of this chapter, cancer cells never do anything completely new. Instead, they overproduce or produce faulty, overactive versions of proteins that help them grow, multiply, and stay alive. They also underproduce or produce dysfunctional versions of proteins that would normally limit their growth or encourage them to die.

The result of this is that although we might think that cancer is an unnatural aberration that needs destroying, a patient's body doesn't necessarily think the same. So, although it's true that our immune system is powerful

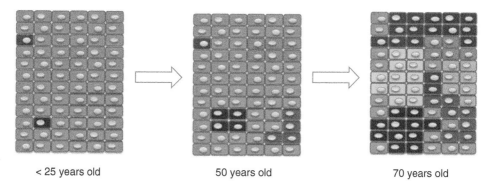

< 25 years old   50 years old   70 years old

Figure 1.26 As we age, our tissues become a patchwork of colonies of mutated cells. In our youth, our cells contain relatively few mutations. However, as we enter middle age and beyond, mutated cells have outcompeted and outgrown their near neighbors, creating colonies of mutated cells. These cells might never become cancer cells, but they often contain many of the same faults. *Source:* Ref. [159–165].

enough to rid the body of cancer, it often doesn't do so (although it's impossible to say exactly how many of us have avoided cancer thanks to the vigilance of our immune system).

Because cancer cells are very similar to healthy cells, it's very difficult to create drugs that can kill one without the other. Newspapers and websites are often littered with stories about chemicals from many different sources that can kill cancer cells grown in a lab. But that isn't difficult. The difficulty is finding chemicals that can kill the cancer cells in a person while leaving their healthy cells alone. And this is virtually impossible. So, every treatment, no matter how targeted we might think it is, will kill some healthy cells alongside killing cancer cells. That means that every cancer treatment causes side effects. The severity of a treatment's side effects often limits how much of the treatment can be given to a patient safely, and that ultimately compromises the treatment's ability to cure them.

Another aspect to this is that our so-called "healthy" cells often aren't all that healthy [159–162]. Every cell in our body sustains DNA damage every day we're alive, and not all of it gets repaired. This damage might not be enough to cause a cell to become a fully fledged cancer cell, but it might be enough

to make the cell a bit weird and cause it to multiply faster than normal, creating a group of mutated cells. The consequence of this is that as we get older our tissues and organs gradually become a patchwork of groups of mutated cells (Figure 1.26) [163]. These cells might never cause cancer, but they often contain some of the mutations that we typically find inside cancer cells and that might be the target of some cancer treatments [164–167]. This adds to the difficulty in selectively targeting and destroying cancer cells while leaving our "healthy" cells unharmed.

1.10.2 Differences Between Different Cancer Types

I'm often asked whether there will ever be "a cure for cancer." And if all cancers shared the same DNA mutations and behaviors, my answer might perhaps be "yes." But as it is, there are many, many different types of cancer, and each cancer has its own unique vulnerability to different treatments. Additionally, not only is it possible to develop liver cancer, stomach cancer, bowel cancer, skin cancer, and so on, but there are also many different types of cancer that can occur in each location. For example, there are adenocarcinoma and squamous cell carcinoma versions of NSCLC, estrogen receptor-positive and estrogen receptor-negative breast cancer, and various types of skin cancer.

In recent years, scientists have uncovered more and more information about the various forms of cancer, what drives them, and what impacts their behavior. Thankfully, this knowledge is gradually improving our ability to treat people more effectively. However, the complexity is mind-blowing. Even when two cancers appear to be driven by the same mutations, it's not necessarily the case that they will respond to the same treatments. It depends on precisely how the cells' internal proteins interact with one another, and how the cancer cells interact with the cells around them. For example, in 50% of people with melanoma skin cancer, the cancer cells contain a mutation in a gene called *BRAF*. Treatment with a B-Raf inhibitor shrinks 50%–80% of these cancers (described in Section 3.7.4) [168]. The same *BRAF* mutation is also found in the cancer cells of 8%–10% of people with bowel cancer. But, in bowel cancer, a B-Raf inhibitor does not work, at least not unless it's combined with a treatment that targets the EGF receptor [169–171].

So, for every cancer, and for every subset of every cancer, we have to discover exactly how the cells are wired up – what's driving them and what's protecting them – before we can uncover how best to treat them. As a result, there will never be "one cure" for all cancers.

1.10.3 Cancer Spread

Scientists have made lots of progress in identifying the gene mutations that cause cancer and that drive its growth. They've also created many treatments that target the consequences of these mutations. However, a lot less progress has been made in identifying the mutations that drive metastasis. Very few treatments that specifically target metastatic cancer cells have been developed [117]. So, once a cancer has metastasized and become resistant to treatment, doctors currently have very little to offer their patients.

Also, there is often a lag between the cancer cells' arrival in a new location and their growth into a metastasis. During the lag period, the cancer cells are dormant and unlikely to be killed by chemotherapy or other cancer treatments [172, 173]. The length of time the cancer cells remain dormant, and the likelihood that they will cause metastasis, varies from cancer to cancer. For example, relapses several years after surgery are common in people with breast, prostate, kidney, or melanoma skin cancer.

In addition, cancer cells that have traveled to locations like the brain or bone marrow receive protection and support from their new environment [172–175]. The brain in particular is difficult for drugs to penetrate, has a large nutrient supply, and is relatively protected from the immune system [172, 174]. Likewise, the bone marrow is full of white blood cells and other cells that churn out substances like various cytokines that can help cancer cells survive and multiply [175].

Lastly, cancer cells in distant organs might contain different mutations compared to those in the original (primary) tumor. Consequently, they might not be destroyed by a cancer treatment chosen by a doctor for its ability to target the person's primary tumor [117].

1.10.4 Intratumoral Heterogeneity

Intratumoral heterogeneity[34] is a huge obstacle to curing people of cancer. As I described in Section 1.4, heterogeneity comes in many

---

[34] As you might remember from Section 1.4, intratumoral heterogeneity is the phrase scientists use to describe the fact that most cancers contain multiple populations of cancer cells driven by different combinations of gene mutations. Cancer cells in a single patient can also differ in terms of the proteins they make, their epigenetics, their metabolism, and their ability to change and adapt in response to changing circumstances.

different forms. It can be genetic, with different pockets of cancer cells containing different combinations of DNA mutations. Cancers can also vary internally in terms of their epigenetics or in their metabolism. And of course, cancer cells don't live alone. Various parts of a person's tumor, and any metastases, are going to have variations in their blood supply, in the number and behavior of fibroblasts and adipocytes, and in what white blood cells are present and what they're doing there. These variations make it impossible for cancer treatments to have a uniform effect on every part of a tumor and any metastases.

The Impact of Heterogeneity on the Effectiveness of Targeted Cancer Treatments

As we create treatments that precisely target cancer cells, it becomes more and more likely that our treatments will kill some cells in a tumor while leaving others unharmed [79, 81, 176–179].

If someone has millions upon millions of cancer cells in their body, it is inevitable that among the different populations of cells there will be some that contain mutations that make them resistant to treatment (see Figure 1.27a & b).

Thus, the precise targeting that is a feature of many of the treatments mentioned in this book is also the treatments' greatest weakness. The more precisely targeted a treatment is, the less likely it is to kill every cancer cell in a person's body [79, 178, 180].

In fact, there are often multiple treatment-resistant clones of cancer cells in the person's tumor and in any metastases. Each clone may have a different resistance-causing mutation [181, 182]. Following treatment, if the cancer reemerges, it's likely to be these resistant cancer cells that are the cause. In addition,

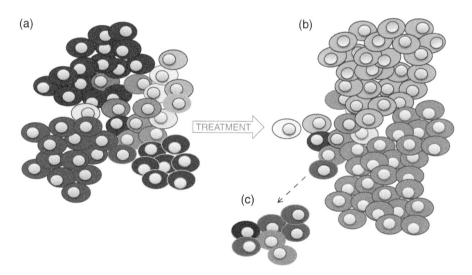

Figure 1.27 Intratumoral heterogeneity is an obstacle to effectiveness of targeted cancer treatments. (a) Due to the genomic instability of cancer cells, cancers generally contain multiple populations of cancer cells driven by unique combinations of mutations (represented by the different colors). Each population exhibits a different level of sensitivity to any particular cancer treatment. (b) Some populations of cancer cells have been killed by the treatment the person was given. However, some cells contained mutations that made them resistant and able to survive. Some of these resistant cells have multiplied and caused the person's disease to return. (c) Cancer cells that leave the original tumor and create a metastasis elsewhere in the body may have different properties from the original tumor.

because the reemergent clones contain different combinations of mutations, a single treatment approach is unlikely to help [181].

Another problem that intratumoral heterogeneity causes is that a biopsy sample from a patient's cancer might not give an accurate picture as to the presence or absence of a particular mutation [176]. It might be that the targetable mutation picked up in the biopsy analysis is only present in a proportion of the cancer cells and absent in others. This would mean that targeting the mutation in question is doomed to fail.

The opposite situation is when a biopsy sample contains such a small proportion of cells with a particular mutation that the testing doesn't pick it up. For example, a colorectal cancer sample might appear to be free of *KRAS* mutations, suggesting that an antibody treatment targeted against the EGF receptor will work [183]. But even a tiny number of *KRAS*-mutant cells that survive treatment might cause recurrence later.

Another problem caused by intratumoral heterogeneity is the way it enables cancers to change over time. Therefore, the cancer cells that drive recurrence and metastasis might contain different gene mutations and have different survival mechanisms than the cancer cells that were first present (Figure 1.27c) [81]. So, when a cancer starts growing again, it's likely to be impervious to the treatments used previously (any cancer cell that was vulnerable to that treatment is already dead); hence, the cancer gets harder and harder to treat

The Impact of Heterogeneity on the Effectiveness of Immunotherapy

The degree of heterogeneity in a tumor also influences whether immunotherapy is likely to work [182]. Because different pockets of cancer cells contain different combinations of mutations, they also differ in their visibility to the person's immune system. As time goes by,

visible cancer cells will be destroyed, leaving less visible cells behind – a process called immuno-editing.

In addition, different parts of a tumor will vary in terms of their accessibility and hostility to different types of white blood cells. Thus, one part of a tumor might be full of cancer-fighting T cells, while another part is full of MDSCs and Tregs (both of which actively suppress T cells) [184].

The degree and pattern of genetic heterogeneity in a tumor appear to influence how likely it is that immunotherapy will work.

If a person's cancer cells all developed from a single cancer cell with many mutations (Figure 1.28a), every cancer cell in their body will also have all these mutations inside them (called clonal mutations). T cells that recognize any of these clonal mutations have the potential to seek out and destroy cancer cells wherever they might be in the body [93, 185]. Excitingly, they can even cure someone with metastatic disease.

In contrast, if the person's cancer cells diversified very early on, and most mutations are only present in a few subsets of cells (called subclonal mutations), then their immune system has a much harder job (Figure 1.28d). Some mutations might fail to elicit an immune response at all; others are so rare that, even if suitable T cells are activated, they have virtually no impact on the tumor as a whole. Pockets of cells with unique mutations might go undetected. Cancers with a high proportion of subclonal mutations are therefore less likely to respond to immunotherapy than those with lots of clonal mutations [186, 187].

Strategies to Overcome the Problem of Intratumoral Heterogeneity

Thus, intratumoral heterogeneity is a huge barrier to the successful treatment of patients with cancer. Efforts to overcome this problem center on the following: [82, 148], [155, 156]

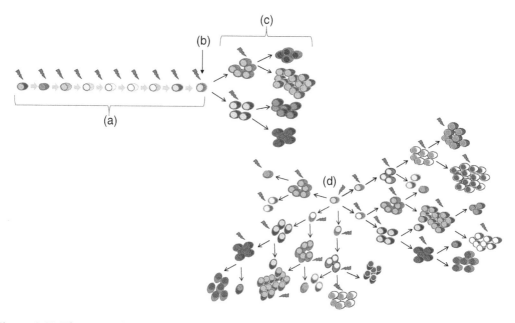

Figure 1.28 The proportion of clonal vs. subclonal mutations influences the effectiveness of immunotherapies that boost T cells. (a) A cell may accumulate many mutations before it finally becomes a cancer cell. **(b)** The first, fully fledged cancer cell. **(c)** Cancer cells are unstable and pick up new mutations, causing heterogeneity. However, all the mutations present in the first cancer cell **(b)** are still present in every cell descended from it – the cancer cells in the person's body contain many clonal mutations. T cells activated in response to clonal mutations can destroy any cancer cell in the person's body, and an immunotherapy that boosts T cell activity is likely to work. **(d)** If a person's cancer cells evolve and diversify right from the start, there will be very few clonal mutations. Most mutations will be subclonal. T cells activated in response to subclonal mutations will only be able to destroy pockets of cancer cells, making it less likely that the person's cancer will be controlled with a treatment that boosts T cell activity.

- Using logical combinations of drugs that target different faulty proteins and pathways and that synergize with one another to kill a more diverse range of cancer cells than any individual treatment used on its own.
- Innovations in the analysis of cancer cells or cancer cell DNA (often called ctDNA – circulating tumor DNA) in a patient's bloodstream, and using these cells/DNA to track the cancer cells' evolution and predict drug resistance-causing mechanisms.
- Taking multiple biopsies from a tumor and its metastases to gain a fuller picture of the mutations driving the cancer.
- Developing treatments such as immunotherapies that are less selective and may be able to kill a broad range of cancer cells driven by different mutations (see Chapters 5 and 6).
- Using mathematical methods to model the outcome of different treatment approaches. The timing, dose, and combination of drugs given to each patient are then chosen to kill the highest proportion of cancer cells over the longest possible period of time – called adaptive therapy.
- Implementing a broad range of tests looking for potentially hundreds of DNA mutations, proteins, and other possible

biomarkers, to match a patient's treatment to the features of their cancer as closely as possible.

1.10.5 The Cancer Microenvironment

The environment in which cancer cells live can have an enormous impact on whether a treatment given to a patient is effective. Even if a drug is theoretically highly effective against a patient's cancer, it still might have no impact if the cancer cells' microenvironment is protecting them. Two main issues that affect a drug's effectiveness are (1) the physical environment in which the cancer cells live and whether the treatment can reach them and (2) the behavior of the non-cancer cells that live alongside the cancer cells. For example [95]:

- Growth factors and other proteins released by non-cancer cells such as fibroblasts, white blood cells, endothelial cells, and adipocytes (fat cells) can protect cancer cells from the effects of various treatments.
- In some cancers, the cancer cells' microenvironment contains a dense network of structural proteins (called desmoplasia) that compresses blood vessels and prevents cancer drugs from reaching the cancer cells.

As I mentioned in Section 1.6.4, a classic example of the problems posed by the cancer microenvironment is pancreatic cancer. Many scientists have found combinations of chemotherapy and other treatments that can successfully kill pancreatic cancer cells cultured in a lab or grown in mice (called xenografts). However, these same treatments have failed to improve the survival times of most patients with pancreatic cancer [158]. One of the chief obstacles that stop treatments from working against pancreatic cancer is its microenvironment (Figure 1.21). It's not unusual for non-cancer cells to outnumber the cancer cells in these tumors, and the microenvironment is awash with a diverse array of cells and densely packed structural proteins that

together prevent drugs from penetrating and protect cancer cells from death. Treatments that remodel the microenvironment might be our best chance at improving the situation, but many have already been tried and have failed [114].

1.11 FINAL THOUGHTS

In this chapter, I have tried to give you a good idea of why cancers come about, what drives them, how they behave, and why we can't yet cure everyone who develops this disease.

Do be aware, though, that this chapter covers just a small percentage of all the knowledge that scientists have accumulated about cancer. There are some big areas of science that I have missed out, such as most of the research on epigenetics; micro-RNAs; exosomes; the role of metabolic pathways and of viruses and infections; the similarities and differences between cancers in different organs; the difference between a benign tumor, a precancerous lesion, and an invasive cancer, etc.

Therefore, this chapter is just a selection of information that I have chosen because I think it might come in handy when you read later chapters.

Throughout the rest of this book, I'll be focusing much of my attention on cancer treatments. Most of these treatments target just one protein, or one cell process that is faulty in cancer cells or that controls their relationship with the immune system. However, the proteins and processes that are targeted by these treatments represent just a small proportion of all the faulty proteins and processes that drive cancer cells and are responsible for the way they behave. I hope that in this chapter I have given you a sense of this complexity.

Even so, the treatments described in the rest of this book target a range of different features of cancer cells. These include treatments that target aspects of cell communication, the cell cycle, DNA repair, angiogenesis, and the interaction between cancer cells and the immune system. Despite mentioning them briefly in this introductory chapter, I will explain these processes in more detail when I come to describe the various treatments in later chapters.

REFERENCES

1 Pray L (2008). Eukaryotic genome complexity. *Nat Educ* **1**(1): 96–96.

2 National Cancer Institute. The cancer genome atlas program. https://www.cancer.gov/ccg/research/genome-sequencing/tcga [Accessed March 18, 2024].

3 Zhang J *et al.* (2019). The international cancer genome consortium data portal. *Nat Biotechnol* **37**(4). doi: 10.1038/s41587-019-0055-9.

4 Stratton MR, Campbell PJ, Futreal PA (2009). The cancer genome. *Nature* **458**(7239). doi: 10.1038/nature07943.

5 Vogelstein B *et al.* (2013). Cancer genome landscapes. *Science (1979)* **339**(6127). doi: 10.1126/science.1235122.

6 Meric-Bernstam F *et al.* (2019). Advances in HER2-targeted therapy: Novel agents and opportunities beyond breast and gastric cancer. *Clin Cancer Res* **25**(7). doi: 10.1158/1078-0432. CCR-18-2275.

7 Yong E (2017). No, we can't say whether cancer is mostly bad luck. *The Atlantic.* [Online] Available: https://www.theatlantic.com/science/archive/2017/03/no-cancer-isnt-mostly-bad-luck/521049/ [Accessed March 18, 2024].

8 Wodarz D (2009). Dynamics of cancer: Incidence, inheritance, and evolution . Princeton Series in Evolutionary Biology. By Steven A. Frank. Princeton (New Jersey): Princeton University Press. $99.50 (hardcover); $39.50 (paper). xiii + 378 p.; ill.; author and subject indexes. 978-0-691-13365-2 (hc); 978-0-691-13366-9 (pb). 2007. *Q Rev Biol* **84**(1). doi: 10.1086/598317.

9 Tomasetti C, Vogelstein B (2015). Variation in cancer risk among tissues can be explained by the number of stem cell divisions. *Science (1979)* **347**(6217). doi: 10.1126/science.1260825.

10 Thomas F, Roche B, Ujvari B (2016). Intrinsic versus extrinsic cancer risks: The debate continues. *Trends Cancer* **2**(2). doi: 10.1016/j.trecan.2016.01.004.

11 Greaves M (2018). A causal mechanism for childhood acute lymphoblastic leukaemia. *Nat Rev Cancer* **18**(8). doi: 10.1038/s41568-018-0015-6.

12 Laconi E, Marongiu F, DeGregori J (2020). Cancer as a disease of old age: Changing mutational and microenvironmental landscapes. *Br J Cancer* **122**(7). doi: 10.1038/s41416-019-0721-1.

13 Bernstein C et al. (2013). DNA damage, DNA repair and cancer. *New Research Directions in DNA Repair.* doi: 10.5772/53919.

14 Włodarczyk M, Nowicka G (2019). Obesity, DNA damage, and development of obesity-related diseases. *Int J Mol Sci* **20**(5). doi: 10.3390/ijms20051146.

15 de Bont R, van Larebeke N (2004). Endogenous DNA damage in humans: A review of quantitative data. *Mutagenesis* **19**(3). doi: 10.1093/mutage/geh025.

16 Valko M *et al.* (2004). Role of oxygen radicals in DNA damage and cancer incidence. *Mol Cell Biochem* **266**(1–2). doi: 10.1023/B:MCBI.0000049134.69131.89.

17 Wood RD *et al.* (2001). Human DNA repair genes. *Science (1979)* **291**(5507). doi: 10.1126/science.1056154.

18 Lange SS, Takata KI, Wood RD (2011). DNA polymerases and cancer. *Nat Rev Cancer* **11**(2). doi: 10.1038/nrc2998.

19 Roberts SA *et al.* (2013). An APOBEC cytidine deaminase mutagenesis pattern is widespread in human cancers. *Nat Genet* **45**(9). doi: 10.1038/ng.2702.

20 Swanton C *et al.* (2015). APOBEC enzymes: Mutagenic fuel for cancer evolution and heterogeneity. *Cancer Discov* **5**(7). doi: 10.1158/2159-8290.CD-15-0344.

21 Jolie Pitt A (2015). Angelina Jolie Pitt: Diary of a surgery. *The New York Times*, March 24, 2015.

22 Cancer Research UK. Causes of cancer and reducing your risk. https://www.cancerresearchuk.org/about-cancer/causes-of-cancer [Accessed March 19, 2024].

23 American Cancer Society. Diet and physical activity: What's the cancer connection? https://www.cancer.org/cancer/cancer-causes/diet-physical-activity/diet-and-physical-activity.html [Accessed March 19, 2024].

24 Miller K (2003). Estrogen and DNA damage: The silent source of breast cancer? *J Natl Cancer Inst* **95**(2). doi: 10.1093/jnci/95.2.100.

25 Travis RC, Key TJ (2003). Oestrogen exposure and breast cancer risk. *Breast Cancer Res* **5**(5). doi: 10.1186/bcr628.

26 Shacter E, Weitzman SA (2002). Chronic inflammation and cancer. *Oncology (Williston Park, NY)* **16**(2): 217.

27 Fridman WH *et al.* (2017). The immune contexture in cancer prognosis and treatment. *Nat Rev Clin Oncol.* doi: 10.1038/nrclinonc.2017.101.

28 Hussain SP, Hofseth LJ, Harris CC (2003). Radical causes of cancer. *Nat Rev Cancer* **3**(4). doi: 10.1038/nrc1046.

29 Kruseova J *et al.* (2021). Possible mechanisms of subsequent neoplasia development in childhood cancer survivors: A review. *Cancers* **13**(20). doi: 10.3390/cancers13205064.

30 Dracham CB, Shankar A, Madan R (2018). Radiation induced secondary malignancies: A review article. *Radiat Oncol J* **36**(2): 85–94. doi: 10.3857/roj.2018.00290.

31 Cancer Research UK. Statistics on preventable cancers. https://www.cancerresearchuk.org/health-professional/cancer-statistics/risk/preventable-cancers#heading-Zero [Accessed March 19, 2024].

32 Parkin DM, Boyd L, Walker LC (2011). The fraction of cancer attributable to lifestyle and environmental factors in the UK in 2010. *Br J Cancer* **105**. doi: 10.1038/bjc.2011.489.

33 Yi K, Ju YS (2018). Patterns and mechanisms of structural variations in human cancer. *Exp Mol Med* **50**(8). doi: 10.1038/s12276-018-0112-3.

34 Gordon DJ, Resio B, Pellman D (2012). Causes and consequences of aneuploidy in cancer. *Nat Rev Genet* **13**(3). doi: 10.1038/nrg3123.

35 López S *et al.* (2020). Interplay between whole-genome doubling and the accumulation of deleterious alterations in cancer evolution. *Nat Genet* **52**(3). doi: 10.1038/s41588-020-0584-7.

36 Forment J v, Kaidi A, Jackson SP (2012). Chromothripsis and cancer: Causes and consequences of chromosome shattering. *Nat Rev Cancer* **12**(10). doi: 10.1038/nrc3352.

37 Voronina N *et al.* (2020). The landscape of chromothripsis across adult cancer types. *Nat Commun* **11**(1). doi: 10.1038/s41467-020-16134-7.

38 Quintás-Cardama A, Cortes JE (2006). Chronic myeloid leukemia: Diagnosis and treatment. *Mayo Clin Proc.* doi: 10.4065/81.7.973.

39 Dorfman LE *et al.* (2018). The role of cytogenetics and molecular biology in the diagnosis, treatment and monitoring of patients with chronic myeloid leukemia. *J Bras Pat Med Lab* **54**(2). doi: 10.5935/1676-2444.20180015.

40 Tandefelt DG *et al.* (2014). ETS fusion genes in prostate cancer. *Endocr Relat Cancer* **21**(3). doi: 10.1530/ERC-13-0390.

41 Grafone T *et al.* (2012). An overview on the role of FLT3-tyrosine kinase receptor in acute myeloid leukemia: Biology and treatment. *Oncol Rev* **6**(1). doi: 10.4081/oncol.2012.e8.

42 Shaw AT, Solomon B (2011). Targeting anaplastic lymphoma kinase in lung cancer. *Clin Cancer Res* **17**(8). doi: 10.1158/1078-0432.CCR-10-1591.

43 Krishnamurti U, Silverman JF (2014). HER2 in breast cancer: A review and update. *Adv Anat Pathol* **21**(2). doi:10.1097/PAP.0000000000000015.

44 Scitable. DNA is constantly changing through the process of mutation. *Nature Education.* [Online]. Available: https://www.nature.com/scitable/topicpage/dna-is-constantly-changing-through-the-process-6524898/ [Accessed March 1, 2022].

45 Davies H *et al.* (2002). Mutations of the BRAF gene in human cancer. *Nature* **417**(6892). doi: 10.1038/nature00766.

46 Rosell R *et al.* (2010). Non-small-cell lung cancer harbouring mutations in the EGFR kinase domain. *Clin Transl Oncol* **12**(2). doi: 10.1007/S12094-010-0473-0.

47 Bergman A *et al.* (2005). A high frequency of germline BRCA1/2 mutations in western Sweden detected with complementary screening techniques. *Fam Cancer* **4**(2). doi: 10.1007/s10689-004-5812-2.

48 Alexandrov LB *et al.* (2020). The repertoire of mutational signatures in human cancer. *Nature* **578**(7793). doi: 10.1038/s41586-020-1943-3.

49 COSMIC (2023). Mutational signatures. https://cancer.sanger.ac.uk/signatures/ [Accessed March 19, 2024].

50 Koh G *et al.* (2021). Mutational signatures: Emerging concepts, caveats and clinical applications. *Nat Rev Cancer* **21**(10). doi: 10.1038/s41568-021-00377-7.

51 Degasperi A *et al.* (2022). Substitution mutational signatures in whole-genome–sequenced cancers in the UK population. *Science (1979)* **376**(6591). doi: 10.1126/science.abl9283.

52 Helleday T, Eshtad S, Nik-Zainal S (2014). Mechanisms underlying mutational signatures in human cancers. *Nat Rev Genet* **15**(9). doi: 10.1038/nrg3729.

53 Chalmers ZR *et al.* (2017). Analysis of 100,000 human cancer genomes reveals the landscape of tumor mutational burden. *Genome Med* **9**(1). doi: 10.1186/s13073-017-0424-2.

54 Swanton C, Govindan R (2016). Clinical implications of genomic discoveries in lung cancer. *N Engl J Med* **374**(19). doi: 10.1056/nejmra1504688.

55 Kandoth C *et al.* (2013). Mutational landscape and significance across 12 major cancer types. *Nature* **502**(7471). doi: 10.1038/nature12634.

56 Prior IA, Lewis PD, Mattos C (2012). A comprehensive survey of ras mutations in cancer. *Cancer Res* **72**(10). doi: 10.1158/0008-5472.CAN-11-2612.

57 Karakas B, Bachman KE, Park BH (2006). Mutation of the PIK3CA oncogene in human cancers. *Br J Cancer* **94**(4). doi: 10.1038/sj.bjc.6602970.

58 Wieduwilt MJ, Moasser MM (2008). The epidermal growth factor receptor family: Biology driving targeted therapeutics. *Cell Mol Life Sci* **65**(10). doi: 10.1007/s00018-008-7440-8.

59 Dang CV (2012). MYC on the path to cancer. *Cell* **149**(1). doi: 10.1016/j.cell.2012.03.003.

60 Leicht DT *et al.* (2007). Raf kinases: Function, regulation and role in human cancer. *Biochim. Biophys. Acta Mol. Cell. Res.* **1773**(8). doi: 10.1016/j.bbamcr.2007.05.001.

61 Bieging KT, Mello SS, Attardi LD (2014). Unravelling mechanisms of p53-mediated tumour suppression. *Nat Rev Cancer* **14**(5). doi: 10.1038/nrc3711.

62 Milella M *et al.* (2015). PTEN: Multiple functions in human malignant tumors. *Front Oncol* **5**(FEB). doi: 10.3389/fonc.2015.00024.

63 Giacinti C, Giordano A (2006). RB and cell cycle progression. *Oncogene* **25**(38). doi: 10.1038/sj.onc.1209615.

64 Zhao R *et al.* (2016). Implications of genetic and epigenetic alterations of CDKN2A (p16INK4a) in cancer. *EBioMedicine* **8**. doi: 10.1016/j.ebiom.2016.04.017.

65 Yap YS *et al.* (2014). The NF1 gene revisited – from bench to bedside. *Oncotarget* **5**(15). doi: 10.18632/oncotarget.2194.

66 Aoki K, Taketo MM (2007). Adenomatous polyposis coli (APC): A multi-functional tumor suppressor gene. *J Cell Sci* **120**(19). doi: 10.1242/jcs.03485.

67 Prakash R *et al.* (2015). Homologous recombination and human health: The roles of BRCA1, BRCA2, and associated proteins. *Cold Spring Harb Perspect Biol* **7**(4). doi: 10.1101/cshperspect.a016600.

68 Maréchal A, Zou L (2013). DNA damage sensing by the ATM and ATR kinases. *Cold Spring Harb Perspect Biol* **5**(9). doi: 10.1101/cshperspect.a012716.

69 Fiala C, Diamandis EP (2020). Mutations in normal tissues – some diagnostic and clinical implications. *BMC Med* **18**(1). doi: 10.1186/s12916-020-01763-y.

70 Martincorena I *et al.* High burden and pervasive positive selection of somatic mutations in normal human skin. *Science (1979)* **348**(6237): 2015. doi: 10.1126/science.aaa6806.

71 Hanahan D, Weinberg RA (2000). The hallmarks of cancer. *Cell* **100**(1). doi: 10.1016/S0092-8674(00)81683-9.

72 Hanahan D, Weinberg RA (2011). Hallmarks of cancer: The next generation. *Cell* **144**(5). doi: 10.1016/j.cell.2011.02.013.

73 Gerlinger M *et al.* (2012). Intratumor heterogeneity and branched evolution revealed by multiregion sequencing. *N Engl J Med* **366**(10). doi: 10.1056/nejmoa1113205.

74 Hanahan D (2022). Hallmarks of cancer: New dimensions. *Cancer Discov* **12**(1): 31–46. doi: 10.1158/2159-8290.CD-21-1059.

75 Murugaesu N *et al.* (2015). Tracking the genomic evolution of esophageal adenocarcinoma through neoadjuvant chemotherapy. *Cancer Discov* **5**(8). doi: 10.1158/2159-8290.CD-15-0412.

76 Losic B *et al.* (2020). Intratumoral heterogeneity and clonal evolution in liver cancer. *Nat Commun* **11**(1). doi: 10.1038/s41467-019-14050-z.

77 le Pennec S *et al.* (2015). Intratumor heterogeneity and clonal evolution in an aggressive papillary thyroid cancer and matched metastases. *Endocr Relat Cancer* **22**(2). doi: 10.1530/ERC-14-0351.

78 Burrell RA *et al.* (2013). The causes and consequences of genetic heterogeneity in cancer evolution. *Nature* **501**(7467). doi: 10.1038/nature12625.

79 Turner NC, Reis-Filho JS (2012). Genetic heterogeneity and cancer drug resistance. *Lancet Oncol* **13**(4). doi: 10.1016/S1470-2045(11)70335-7.

80 Guo M *et al.* (2019). Epigenetic heterogeneity in cancer. *Biomark Res* **7**(1). doi: 10.1186/s40364-019-0174-y.

81 Allison KH, Sledge GW (2014). Heterogeneity and cancer. *Oncology (Williston Park)* **28**(9): 772–778. [Online]. Available: https://pubmed.ncbi.nlm.nih.gov/25224475/ [Accessed January 14, 2022].

82 Sompayrac L (2019). Lecture 3 B Cells and Antibodies. In *How the Immune System Works*. 6th ed. Wiley-Blackwell. pp. 27–41.

83 Murphy KM, Weaver C (2016). *Janeway's Immunobiology*, 9th ed. WW Norton & Co.

84 Beer G (2019) Science surgery: 'Why doesn't the immune system attack cancer cells? https://news.cancerresearchuk.org/2019/02/28/science-surgery-why-doesnt-the-immune-system-attack-cancer-cells/ [Accessed March 19, 2024].

85 British Society for Immunology. BiteSized immunology. *BiteSized Immunology*. [Online] Available: https://www.immunology.org/public-information/bitesized-immunology [Accessed April 3, 2023].

86 Lauren S (2019). Lecture 4 The Magic of Antigen Presentation. In *How the Immune System Works*. 6th ed. Wiley-Blackwell. pp. 42–54.

87 Trombetta ES, Mellman I (2005). Cell biology of antigen processing in vitro and in vivo. *Annu Rev Immunol* **23**. doi: 10.1146/annurev.immunol.22.012703.104538.

88 Yong E (2020). Immunology is where intuition goes to die. https://www.theatlantic.com/health/archive/2020/08/covid-19-immunity-is-the-pandemics-central-mystery/614956/ [Accessed March 19, 2024].

89 Sompayrac L (2019). Lecture 5 T Cell Activation. In *How the Immune System Works*. 6th ed. Wiley-Blackwell. pp. 55–61.

90 Sompayrac L (2019). Lecture 6 T Cells at Work. In *How the Immune System Works*. 6th ed. Wiley-Blackwell. pp. 62–70.

91 Chen DS, Mellman I (2013). Oncology meets immunology: The cancer-immunity cycle. *Immunity* **39**(1). doi: 10.1016/j.immuni.2013.07.012.

92 Litchfield K *et al.* (2021). Meta-analysis of tumor- and T cell-intrinsic mechanisms of sensitization to checkpoint inhibition. *Cell* **184**(3). doi: 10.1016/j.cell.2021.01.002.

93 McGranahan N, Swanton C (2019). Neoantigen quality, not quantity. *Sci Transl Med* **11**(506). doi: 10.1126/scitranslmed.aax7918.

94 Jhunjhunwala S, Hammer C, Delamarre L (2021). Antigen presentation in cancer: Insights into tumour immunogenicity and immune evasion. *Nat Rev Cancer* **21**(5). doi: 10.1038/s41568-021-00339-z.

95 van Weverwijk A, de Visser KE (2023). Mechanisms driving the immunoregulatory function of cancer cells. *Nat Rev Cancer* **23**(4): 193–215. doi: 10.1038/s41568-022-00544-4.

96 Rabinovich GA, Gabrilovich D, Sotomayor EM (2007). Immunosuppressive strategies that are mediated by tumor cells. *Annu Rev Immunol* **25**. doi: 10.1146/annurev.immunol.25.022106.141609.

97 Labani-Motlagh A, Ashja-Mahdavi M, Loskog A (2020). The tumor microenvironment: A milieu hindering and obstructing antitumor immune responses. *Front Immunol* **11**. doi: 10.3389/fimmu.2020.00940.

98 Hossain MA *et al.* (2021). Reinvigorating exhausted CD8+ cytotoxic T lymphocytes in the tumor microenvironment and current strategies in cancer immunotherapy. *Med Res Rev* **41**(1). doi: 10.1002/med.21727.

99 Chow A *et al.* (2022). Clinical implications of T cell exhaustion for cancer immunotherapy. *Nat Rev Clin Oncol* **19**(12): 775–790. doi: 10.1038/s41571-022-00689-z.

100 Slaney CY, Kershaw MH, Darcy PK (2014). Trafficking of T cells into tumors. *Cancer Res* **74**(24). doi: 10.1158/0008-5472.CAN-14-2458.

101 Barnes TA, Amir E (2017). HYPE or HOPE: The prognostic value of infiltrating immune cells in cancer. *Br J Cancer* **117**. doi: 10.1038/ bjc.2017.220.

102 Zhang Y, Zhang Z (2020). The history and advances in cancer immunotherapy: Understanding the characteristics of tumor-infiltrating immune cells and their therapeutic implications. *Cell Mol Immunol* **17**: 807–821. doi: 10.1038/s41423-020-0488-6.

103 Balkwill FR, Capasso M, Hagemann T. The tumor microenvironment at a glance. *J Cell Sci* **125**: 5591–5596. doi: 10.1242/jcs.116392.

104 Cox TR, Erler JT (2011). Remodeling and homeostasis of the extracellular matrix: Implications for fibrotic diseases and cancer. *Dis Model Mech* **4**(2). doi: 10.1242/dmm.004077.

105 Anderson KG, Stromnes IM, Greenberg PD (2017). Obstacles posed by the tumor microenvironment to T cell activity: A case for synergistic therapies. *Cancer Cell* **31**(3). doi: 10.1016/j.ccell.2017.02.008.

106 Gajewski TF, Schreiber H, Fu Y-X (2013). Innate and adaptive immune cells in the tumor microenvironment. *Nat Immunol* **14**: 1014–1022. doi: 10.1038/ni.2703.

107 Chen Z, You J, Liu X (2017). Dynamic interplay between tumour, stroma and immune system can drive or prevent tumour progression. *Converg Sci Phys Oncol* **3**: 34002. doi: 10.1088/ 2057-1739/aa7e86.

108 Cho W *et al.* (2020). Extracellular matrix in the tumor microenvironment and its impact on cancer therapy. *Front Mol Biosci | www. frontiersin.org* **1**: 160. doi: 10.3389/fmolb.2019. 00160.

109 Lugano R, Ramachandran M, Dimberg A (2020). Tumor angiogenesis: Causes, consequences, challenges and opportunities. *Cell Mol Life Sci* **77**: 1745–1770. doi: 10.1007/s00018-019-03351-7.

110 Nagy JA *et al.* (2009). Why are tumour blood vessels abnormal and why is it important to know? *Br J Cancer* **100**: 865–869. doi: 10.1038/ sj.bjc.6604929.

111 Bergers G, Song S (2005). The role of pericytes in blood-vessel formation and maintenance. *Neuro-Oncology* **7**(4): 452–464. doi: 10.1215/ S1152851705000232.

112 Salmon H *et al.* (2019). Host tissue determinants of tumour immunity. *Nat Rev Cancer* **19**: 215–227. doi: 10.1038/s41568-019-0125-9.

113 Federico L *et al.* (2022). Distinct tumor-infiltrating lymphocyte landscapes are associated with clinical outcomes in localized non-small-cell lung cancer. *Ann Oncol* **33**(1). doi: 10.1016/j.annonc.2021.09.021.

114 Vanhersecke L *et al.* (2021). Mature tertiary lymphoid structures predict immune checkpoint inhibitor efficacy in solid tumors independently of PD-L1 expression. *Nat Cancer* **2**(8): 794–802. doi: 10.1038/s43018-021-00232-6.

115 Jin Ho W, Jaffee EM, Zheng L. The tumour microenvironment in pancreatic cancer – clinical challenges and opportunities. *Nat Rev Clin Oncol*. doi: 10.1038/s41571-020-0363-5.

116 Chaffer CL, Weinberg RA (2011). A perspective on cancer cell metastasis. *Science* **331**(6024). doi: 10.1126/science.1203543.

117 Steeg PS (2016). Targeting metastasis. *Nat Rev Cancer* **16**(4): 201–218. doi: 10.1038/nrc.2016.25.

118 CancerQuest. How cancer spreads (metastasis). https://www.cancerquest.org/cancer-biology/ metastasis [Accessed March 18, 2024].

119 National Cancer Institute (2020). Metastatic cancer: When cancer spreads. https://www. cancer.gov/types/metastatic-cancer [Accessed March 18, 2024].

120 Wan L, Pantel K, Kang Y (2013). Tumor metastasis: Moving new biological insights into the clinic. *Nat Med* **19**(11). doi: 10.1038/nm.3391.

121 Kalluri R, Weinberg RA (2009). The basics of epithelial-mesenchymal transition. *J Clin Invest* **119**(6). doi: 10.1172/JCI39104.

122 Jung H-Y, Fattet L, Yang J (2015). Molecular pathways molecular pathways: Linking tumor microenvironment to epithelial-mesenchymal transition in metastasis. *Clin Cancer Res* **21**(5). doi: 10.1158/1078-0432. CCR-13-3173.

123 Chang JT, Mani SA (2013). Sheep, wolf, or werewolf: Cancer stem cells and the epithelial-to-mesenchymal transition. *Cancer Lett* **341**: 16–23. doi: 10.1016/j.canlet.2013.03.004.

124 Yeon Lee S *et al.* (2017). Induction of metastasis, cancer stem cell phenotype, and oncogenic metabolism in cancer cells by ionizing

radiation. *Mol Cancer* **16**(1): 10. doi: 10.1186/s12943-016-0577-4.

125 Shah PP *et al*. (2017). Common cytotoxic chemotherapeutics induce epithelial-mesenchymal transition (EMT) downstream of ER stress. *Oncotarget* **8**(14): 22625. doi: 10.18632/ONCOTARGET.15150.

126 Galassi C *et al*. (2021). The immune privilege of cancer stem cells: A key to understanding tumor immune escape and therapy failure. *Cells* **10**(9). doi: 10.3390/cells10092361.

127 Pattabiraman DR, Weinberg RA (2014). Tackling the cancer stem cells-what challenges do they pose? *Nat Rev Drug Discov* **13**(7). doi: 10.1038/nrd4253.

128 Clevers H (2011). The cancer stem cell: Premises, promises and challenges. *Nat Med* **17**(3). doi: 10.1038/nm.2304.

129 Wang T *et al*. (2015). Cancer stem cell targeted therapy: Progress amid controversies. *Oncotarget* **6**(42). doi: 10.18632/oncotarget.6176.

130 Rossi F *et al*. (2020). Differences and similarities between cancer and somatic stem cells: Therapeutic implications. *Stem Cell Res Ther* **11**(1). doi: 10.1186/s13287-020-02018-6.

131 Singh A, Settleman J (2010). EMT, cancer stem cells and drug resistance: An emerging axis of evil in the war on cancer. *Oncogene* **29**(34). doi: 10.1038/onc.2010.215.

132 Zheng X *et al*. (2021). Communication between epithelial–mesenchymal plasticity and cancer stem cells: New insights into cancer progression. *Front Oncol* **11**. doi: 10.3389/fonc.2021.617597.

133 Du M-Q, Isaccson PG (2002). Gastric MALT lymphoma: From aetiology to treatment. *Lancet Oncol* **3**(2): 97–104. doi: 10.1016/S1470-2045(02)00651-4.

134 Aplan PD (2006). Causes of oncogenic chromosomal translocation. *Trends Genet* **22**(1): 46–55. doi: 10.1016/j.tig.2005.10.002.

135 Küppers R (2005). Mechanisms of B-cell lymphoma pathogenesis. *Nat Rev Cancer* **5**(4): 251–262. doi: 10.1038/nrc1589.

136 Molyneux EM *et al*. (2012). Burkitt's lymphoma. *Lancet* **379**(9822): 1234–1244. doi: 10.1016/S0140-6736(11)61177-X.

137 Jares P, Colomer D, Campo E (2007). Genetic and molecular pathogenesis of mantle cell lymphoma: Perspectives for new targeted therapeutics. *Nat Rev Cancer* **7**(10): 750–762. doi: 10.1038/nrc2230.

138 Troppan K *et al*. (2015). Molecular pathogenesis of MALT lymphoma. *Gastroenterol Res Pract* **2015**: 1–10. doi: 10.1155/2015/102656.

139 Baliakas P *et al*. (2014). Chromosomal translocations and karyotype complexity in chronic lymphocytic leukemia: A systematic reappraisal of classic cytogenetic data. *Am J Hematol* **89**(3): 249–255. doi: 10.1002/ajh.23618.

140 Moorman AV (2016). New and emerging prognostic and predictive genetic biomarkers in B-cell precursor acute lymphoblastic leukemia. *Haematologica* **101**(4): 407–416. doi: 10.3324/haematol.2015.141101.

141 Rowley JD (2008). Chromosomal translocations: Revisited yet again. *Blood* **112**(6): 2183–2189. doi: 10.1182/blood-2008-04-097931.

142 De Kouchkovsky I, Abdul-Hay M (2016). Acute myeloid leukemia: A comprehensive review and 2016 update. *Blood Cancer J* **6**(7): e441. doi: 10.1038/bcj.2016.50.

143 Seifert M, Scholtysik R, Küppers R (2019). Origin and pathogenesis of B Cell lymphomas. *Methods Mol Biol*: 1–33. doi: 10.1007/978-1-4939-9151-8_1.

144 Campo E *et al*. (2018). TP53 aberrations in chronic lymphocytic leukemia: An overview of the clinical implications of improved diagnostics. *Haematologica* **103**(12): 1956–1968. doi: 10.3324/haematol.2018.187583.

145 Svanberg R *et al*. (2021). Targeting the tumor microenvironment in chronic lymphocytic leukemia. *Haematologica* **106**(9): 2312–2324. doi: 10.3324/haematol.2020.268037.

146 Kipps TJ *et al*. (2017). Chronic lymphocytic leukaemia. *Nat Rev Dis Primers* **3**(1): 16096. doi: 10.1038/nrdp.2016.96.

147 Duarte D, Hawkins ED, Lo Celso C (2018). The interplay of leukemia cells and the bone marrow microenvironment. *Blood* **131**(14):1507–1511. doi:10.1182/blood-2017-12-784132.

148 Tarte K (2017). Role of the microenvironment across histological subtypes of NHL. *Hematology* **2017**(1): 610–617. doi: 10.1182/asheducation-2017.1.610.

149 Opinto G *et al.* (2021). Hodgkin lymphoma: A special microenvironment. *J Clin Med* **10**(20): 4665. doi: 10.3390/jcm10204665.

150 Singer S *et al.* (2017). Socio-economic disparities in long-term cancer survival – 10 year follow-up with individual patient data. *Support Care Cancer* **25**(5): 1391–1399. doi: 10.1007/s00520-016-3528-0.

151 Vaccarella S *et al.* (2023). Socioeconomic inequalities in cancer mortality between and within countries in Europe: A population-based study. *The Lancet Regional Health – Europe* **25**: 100551. doi: 10.1016/j.lanepe.2022.100551.

152 Ludmir EB *et al.* (2019). Factors associated with age disparities among cancer clinical trial participants. *JAMA Oncol* **5**(12): 1769. doi: 10.1001/jamaoncol.2019.2055.

153 Craigs CL *et al.* (2018). Older age is associated with less cancer treatment: A longitudinal study of English cancer patients. *Age Ageing* **47**(6): 833–840. doi: 10.1093/ageing/afy094.

154 Esnaola NF, Ford ME (2012). Racial differences and disparities in cancer care and outcomes. *Surg Oncol Clin N Am* **21**(3): 417–437. doi: 10.1016/j.soc.2012.03.012.

155 Vera R *et al.* (2023). Sex differences in the diagnosis, treatment and prognosis of cancer: The rationale for an individualised approach. *Clin Transl Oncol* **25**(7): 2069–2076. doi: 10.1007/s12094-023-03112-w.

156 Hirko KA *et al.* (2022). The impact of race and ethnicity in breast cancer – disparities and implications for precision oncology. *BMC Med* **20**(1): 72. doi: 10.1186/s12916-022-02260-0.

157 Kadambi S *et al.* (2020). Older adults with cancer and their caregivers – current landscape and future directions for clinical care. *Nat Rev Clin Oncol* **17**(12): 742–755. doi: 10.1038/s41571-020-0421-z.

158 Dharmarajan KV, Presley CJ, Wyld L (2021). Care disparities across the health care continuum for older adults: Lessons from multidisciplinary perspectives. *Am Soc Clin Oncol Educ Book* **41**: 1–10. doi: 10.1200/EDBK_319841.

159 Colom B *et al.* (2020). Spatial competition shapes the dynamic mutational landscape of normal esophageal epithelium. *Nat Genet* **52**(6). doi: 10.1038/s41588-020-0624-3.

160 Colom B *et al.* (2021). Mutant clones in normal epithelium outcompete and eliminate emerging tumours. *Nature* **598**(7881). doi: 10.1038/s41586-021-03965-7.

161 Yizhak K *et al.* (2019). RNA sequence analysis reveals macroscopic somatic clonal expansion across normal tissues. *Science (1979)* **364**(6444). doi: 10.1126/science.aaw0726.

162 Martincorena I *et al.* (2018). Somatic mutant clones colonize the human esophagus with age. *Science (1979)* **362**(6417). doi: 10.1126/science.aau3879.

163 Hesman Saey T Almost all healthy people harbor patches of mutated cells. Science News.

164 Kato S *et al.* (2016). The conundrum of genetic 'drivers' in benign conditions. *J Natl Cancer Inst* **108**(8): djw036. doi: 10.1093/jnci/djw036.

165 Adashek JJ *et al.* (2020). The paradox of cancer genes in non-malignant conditions: Implications for precision medicine. *Genome Med* **12**(1): 16. doi: 10.1186/s13073-020-0714-y.

166 Yamanishi Y *et al.* (2002). Regional analysis of p53 mutations in rheumatoid arthritis synovium. *Proc Natl Acad Sci* **99**(15): 10025–10030. doi: 10.1073/pnas.152333199.

167 Anglesio MS *et al.* (2017). Cancer-associated mutations in endometriosis without cancer. *N Engl J Med* **376**(19): 1835–1848. doi: 10.1056/NEJMoa1614814.

168 Holderfield M *et al.* (2014). Targeting RAF kinases for cancer therapy: BRAF-mutated melanoma and beyond. *Nat Rev Cancer* **14**(7). doi: 10.1038/nrc3760.

169 Gong J, Cho M, Fakih M (2016). RAS and BRAF in metastatic colorectal cancer management. *J Gastrointest Oncol* **7**(5). doi: 10.21037/jgo.2016.06.12.

170 Cohen R *et al.* (2020). Molecular targets for the treatment of metastatic colorectal cancer. *Cancers* **12**(9). doi: 10.3390/cancers12092350.

171 Grothey A, Fakih M, Tabernero J (2021). Management of BRAF-mutant metastatic colorectal cancer: A review of treatment options and evidence-based guidelines. *Ann Oncol* **32**(8). doi: 10.1016/j.annonc.2021.03.206.

172 Giancotti FG (2013). Mechanisms governing metastatic dormancy and reactivation. *Cell* **155**(4): 750–764. doi: 10.1016/j.cell.2013.10.029.

173 Dittmer J (2017). Mechanisms governing metastatic dormancy in breast cancer. *Semin Cancer Biol* **44**. doi: 10.1016/j.semcancer.2017.03.006.

174 Neophytou CM, Kyriakou TC, Papageorgis P (2019). Mechanisms of metastatic tumor dormancy and implications for cancer therapy. *Int J Mol Sci* **20**(24). doi: 10.3390/ijms20246158.

175 Byrne NM, Summers MA, McDonald MM (2019). Tumor cell dormancy and reactivation in bone: Skeletal biology and therapeutic opportunities. *JBMR Plus* **3**(3). doi: 10.1002/jbm4.10125.

176 Dentro SC *et al.* (2021). Characterizing genetic intra-tumor heterogeneity across 2,658 human cancer genomes. *Cell* **184**(8). doi: 10.1016/j.cell.2021.03.009.

177 Bedard PL *et al.* (2013). Tumour heterogeneity in the clinic. *Nature* **501**(7467). doi: 10.1038/nature12627.

178 Lim ZF, Ma PC (2019). Emerging insights of tumor heterogeneity and drug resistance mechanisms in lung cancer targeted therapy. *J Hematol Oncol* **12**(1). doi: 10.1186/s13045-019-0818-2.

179 Gatenby RA, Brown JS (2020). Integrating evolutionary dynamics into cancer therapy. *Nat Rev Clin Oncol* **17**(11). doi: 10.1038/s41571-020-0411-1.

180 Tangella LP, Clark ME, Gray ES (2021). Resistance mechanisms to targeted therapy in BRAF-mutant melanoma – a mini review.

Biochim Biophys Acta Gen Subj **1865**(1). doi: 10.1016/j.bbagen.2020.129736.

181 Romano E *et al.* (2013). Identification of multiple mechanisms of resistance to vemurafenib in a patient with BRAF V600E-mutated cutaneous melanoma successfully rechallenged after progression. *Clin Cancer Res* **19**(20). doi: 10.1158/1078-0432.CCR-13-0661.

182 Dagogo-Jack I, Shaw AT (2017). Tumour heterogeneity and resistance to cancer therapies. *Nat Publ Group* **15**. doi: 10.1038/nrclinonc.2017.166.

183 Knickelbein K, Zhang L (2015). Mutant KRAS as a critical determinant of the therapeutic response of colorectal cancer. *Genes Dis* **2**(1). doi: 10.1016/j.gendis.2014.10.002.

184 Vitale I *et al.* (2021). Intratumoral heterogeneity in cancer progression and response to immunotherapy. *Nat Med* **27**(2). doi: 10.1038/s41591-021-01233-9.

185 McGranahan N *et al.* Clonal neoantigens elicit T cell immunoreactivity and sensitivity to immune checkpoint blockade. *Science (1979)* **351**(6280): 2016. doi: 10.1126/science.aaf1490.

186 Jamal-Hanjani M *et al.* (2015). Translational implications of tumor heterogeneity. *Clin Cancer Res* **21**(6). doi: 10.1158/1078-0432.CCR-14-1429.

187 Fisher R, Pusztai L, Swanton C (2013). Cancer heterogeneity: Implications for targeted therapeutics. *Br J Cancer*. doi: 10.1038/bjc.2012.581.

CHAPTER 2

Monoclonal Antibodies and Small Molecules as Cancer Treatments

IN BRIEF

Targeted cancer treatments are those that target specific proteins, processes, and pathways known to have gone awry in cancer cells, whereas immunotherapies aim to create or boost cancer-fighting immune responses.

Most (but not all) of these treatments fall into one of two categories: They are either antibody-based treatments or they are small molecule drugs. Hence, before we look at individual treatments and their targets in the chapters that follow, I'm first going to pause and explore what antibodies and small molecule drugs are, and what they can and cannot do.

Some antibody-based treatments are very similar to the natural antibodies made by B lymphocytes (B cells) of our immune system. They therefore retain many of the properties of antibodies, namely their ability to attach to a target and trigger a reaction from the person's immune system. There are also antibody treatments that affect checkpoint proteins on T cells and boost their activity. These are the checkpoint inhibitors.

In addition, we now have treatments that involve modifying an antibody's structure. In fact, some are made from more than one antibody, or they're part-antibody, part-something else. We can even deliver the gene for a modified antibody to the patient's own T cells – a form of gene therapy. As antibody-based treatments get more complicated, and more diverse, their range of mechanisms of action also increases. Perhaps some of the most interesting and exciting antibody-based treatments are the antibody-conjugates, where the antibody has been chemically linked to a chemotherapy or a radioactive isotope. These antibodies combine the natural functions of an antibody with a cell-killing dose of chemotherapy or radiotherapy.

Another thing to note about antibody-based treatments is their size. These are large, complex proteins. Scientists use clones[1] of living cells as "factories" to manufacture them in large

---

[1] A clone of cells is a population of genetically identical cells. They have been modified so that they all produce the exact same antibody protein. Thus, when this antibody is purified and given to patients, it is referred to as a "monoclonal antibody therapy."

A Beginner's Guide to Targeted Cancer Treatments and Cancer Immunotherapy, Second Edition. Elaine Vickers.
© 2025 John Wiley & Sons Ltd. Published 2025 by John Wiley & Sons Ltd.

quantities. Antibody-based treatments are therefore a type of biological therapy – treatments that are manufactured using living cells.

Small molecules, in contrast, are tiny chemical compounds, similar in size to chemotherapies. They are manufactured by chemists from their constituent atoms (generally lots of carbon, hydrogen, nitrogen, and oxygen and maybe one or two other atoms such as chlorine, fluorine, or platinum). What sets them apart from standard chemotherapies is their target. Instead of attacking any cell that is multiplying (the mechanism of most chemotherapies), they block enzymes and other proteins that cancer cells use to survive and multiply. Often the enzymes they block are part of the kinase family of enzymes. Over 500 kinase enzymes exist in our cells, and they control many of our cells' functions and behaviors. Various kinases are overactive in cancer cells, forcing them to grow, multiply, and survive.

Lastly in this chapter, I also briefly outline a few small molecule cancer treatments that have non-kinase targets. These include drugs that target a survival protein (Bcl-2), DNA repair enzymes, the cell's proteasomes, epigenetic enzymes, and the Hedgehog signaling pathway – all of which I will return to in Chapter 4.

2.1 INTRODUCTION

Over the past 30 years or so, scientists and doctors have used their growing scientific knowledge to create cancer treatments that target cancer cells in a more precise way than chemotherapy. These are often referred to as "targeted cancer treatments" (see Figure 2.1 for their place in the history of cancer treatments).

Even more recently, we have seen an explosion in the number of people treated with immunotherapy. This began with the licensing of the first checkpoint inhibitor in the United States in March 2011.

However, there are no uniformly agreed definitions as to what constitutes either a "targeted cancer treatment" or an "immunotherapy." This creates confusion about how and when to use these terms, and you can't always presume that what you mean by them is the same as someone else. There is also a lot of overlap between the two treatment approaches (Figure 2.2).

For the purposes of this book, I will use the term "targeted therapy" to refer to treatments that target a specific protein, process, or pathway known to play a role in cancer.

The targeted treatments I describe in this book include those that:
1. Target cell surface proteins known as growth factor receptors. These are found on almost every cell in the human body, and too much of them, or faulty, overactive versions of them, are found on the cell surface of many cancer types (Figure 2.3a).
2. Get inside cancer cells and block kinases[2] or other enzymes that are normally controlled by growth factor receptors (kinases are depicted in Figure 2.3b and described further in Section 2.3).
3. Block kinases involved in the cell cycle (Figure 2.3d).

---

[2] You'll be finding out a lot about kinases in this chapter. For now, I'll just say that kinases are a family of specialized enzymes (catalysts) that cause important chemical reactions to take place in our cells and that are often overactive in cancer cells.

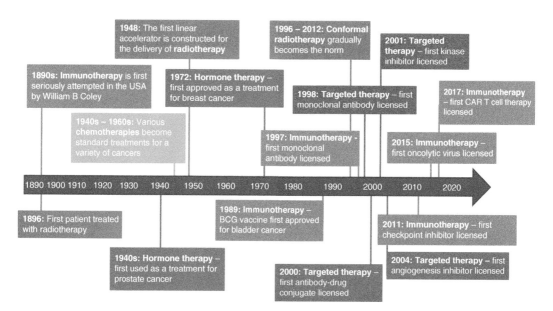

Figure 2.1 Some important milestones in the development of non-surgical cancer treatments. The timeline includes milestones in radiotherapy, chemotherapy, hormone therapy for prostate cancer and breast cancer, targeted therapies such as monoclonal antibodies and kinase inhibitors, and immunotherapies.
Abbreviations: BCG – Bacillus Calmette-Guérin; CAR – chimeric antigen receptor. *Source:* Adapted from Ref. [1–9].

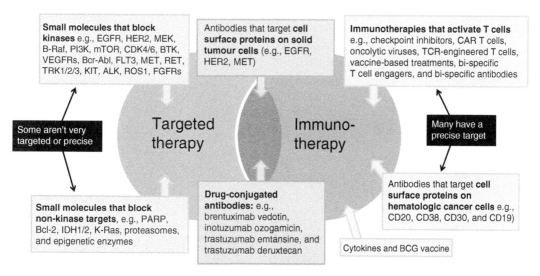

Figure 2.2 Overlap between targeted therapies and immunotherapies. Some treatments fit neatly into just one category, such as small molecules that block overactive kinases in cancer cells (targeted therapy), or treatments that hinge on their ability to activate white blood cells (immunotherapy). But some treatments do more than one thing. For example, antibody treatments given to people with some solid tumors. These antibodies block the actions of overactive receptor proteins found on cancer cells, and this kills cancer cells outright. But these antibodies also recruit and activate white blood cells such as macrophages, which then destroy some cancer cells. So, you can argue that they are both targeted therapies and immunotherapies. To add to the confusion, many immunotherapies work by attaching tightly to a specific target (although that target might be on white blood cells rather than cancer cells). And, to make matters worse, some treatments described by many as "targeted therapies" have very little selectivity for cancer cells and/or block multiple targets.
Abbreviations: BCG – Bacillus Calmette-Guérin; CAR – chimeric antigen receptor; TCR – T cell receptor. For protein names, direct people to the Human Protein Atlas website: https://www.proteinatlas.org/.

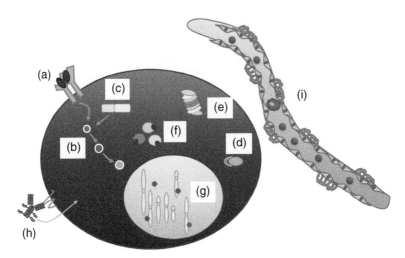

Figure 2.3 Some of the targets of the targeted cancer treatments covered in this book. (a) Cancer cells often overproduce proteins called growth factor receptors. Sometimes these growth factor receptors are faulty and overactive. **(b)** Growth factor receptors trigger the activity of other proteins inside the cell, many of which are kinase enzymes that can be blocked with kinase inhibitors. **(c)** Some cancers contain fusion proteins. Fusion proteins often trigger the same signaling pathways as growth factor receptors. **(d)** Cyclin-dependent kinases (CDKs) control the cell cycle and are the target of CDK inhibitors. **(e)** Our cells use proteasomes to recycle broken, misfolded, and unwanted proteins. Some cancer cells are dependent on proteasomes for their survival and respond to proteasome inhibitors. **(f)** Cancer cells often contain high levels of proteins such as Bcl-2 that prevent cell death. Drugs that target Bcl-2 or another of these proteins can force cancer cells to die. **(g)** Many cancers have difficulty repairing DNA damage; this vulnerability can be exploited with treatments that target DNA repair enzymes such as PARP proteins. **(h)** Some antibody-based treatments attach to cell surface proteins and deliver chemotherapy or another toxic substance. **(i)** When cancer cells experience low oxygen levels, they produce proteins that trigger the growth of blood vessels by a process called angiogenesis. This process is the target of angiogenesis inhibitors. **Abbreviation:** PARP – poly(ADP-ribose)polymerase.

4. Block angiogenesis – tumor angiogenesis is the name given to the process through which small blood vessels sprout new side branches that grow to form new blood vessels, enabling blood to reach the tumor's cells and fuel its growth (Figure 2.3i).
5. Block fusion proteins[3] such as Bcr-Abl or ALK fusion proteins; fusion proteins are created by some chromosome rearrangements and translocations (described in Section 1.2) (Figure 2.3c).
6. Block the proteasome – proteasomes are our cells' protein-recycling units. Myeloma cells seem particularly dependent on them; therefore, proteasome inhibitors are mostly given to people with this type of cancer (Figure 2.3e).

[3] Fusion proteins are proteins made from two separate proteins (or bits of proteins) that have been fused together by the cell to create a single protein that should not normally exist. They are often the result of a chromosome translocation or other chromosome rearrangement.

7. Take advantage of cancer cells' inability to accurately repair DNA damage by blocking DNA repair proteins such as poly(ADP-ribose)polymerase (PARP) and overwhelming the cells with DNA damage (Figure 2.3g).
8. Attach to a cell surface protein and deliver chemotherapy, radiotherapy, or a toxin directly to cancer cells (these are called antibody-drug conjugates) (Figure 2.3h).
9. Overcome cancer cells' resistance to apoptosis[4] and thereby trigger them to self-destruct (Figure 2.3f).
10. Block a range of different enzymes involved in the transport of proteins around the cell, in cell metabolism, and in the epigenetic regulation of genes.

Immunotherapies are treatments that aim to create or boost a cancer-fighting immune response. This can be done using a variety of different treatment approaches.

The immunotherapies I describe in this book include those that:

1. Attach to proteins on the surface of cancer cells and kill them by recruiting and activating white blood cells (such as macrophages and natural killer (NK) cells) and complement proteins.
2. Modulate various aspects of a cancer's behavior and microenvironment by altering the behavior of a protein called cereblon. These are known as the immunomodulators (IMiDs) or cereblon modulators (CELMoDs),[5] and they include thalidomide.
3. Boost the activities of cancer-fighting T cells by preventing checkpoint proteins

on their surface from being triggered (these are known as immune checkpoint inhibitors).
4. Involve genetically modifying some of the patients' own white blood cells (usually T cells) so that they track down and destroy their cancer cells. These are known as adoptive cell therapies or effector T cell therapies, and they include CAR (chimeric antigen receptor) T cell therapy and TCR (T cell receptor) engineered T cell therapy.
5. Attach to a protein on the surface of cancer cells and to a protein found on the surface of T cells (usually CD3). This tethers together a cancer cell with a T cell, causing the T cell to kill the cancer cell. These treatments are called T cell engagers.
6. Trigger an immune response by alerting the patient's immune system to the presence of cancer. These are known as vaccine-based treatments, and they include oncolytic viruses, antigen vaccines, dendritic cell vaccines, and mRNA vaccines.

Before I move on to talk about the physical nature of these treatments, I want to point out a couple of anomalies:

• There are some immunotherapies for cancer that aren't covered by this list. Some, I've chosen to miss out because they're too new and experimental and they might fail long before they reach the late-phase clinical trials that would be needed for their approval. For others, I've chosen not to include them because they boost the person's immune system in a very general way, and they don't really belong in a book

[4] I mentioned apoptosis in Chapter 1. It is the orderly process that damaged cells use to self-destruct.
[5] If you're looking for logic in the inclusion of various letters and their capitalization (or not) in the terms IMiD and CELMoD, I would suggest giving up now.

that is all about targeting and precision. These include cytokines such as interferon-alpha and interleukin-2.

- There are many treatments that either target the production of a sex hormone (estrogen or testosterone) or that block the receptors for these hormones (estrogen or androgen receptors). Because these treatments aren't usually thought of as targeted therapies, I'm not going to say very much about them. If you'd like more detail on them, I did describe them in the first edition of this book [10].

Most (but by no means all) of the treatments covered in this book fall into one of two categories: they are either antibody based or they are small molecules.

For the rest of this chapter, I am going to explore antibodies and small molecules in more detail. However, each individual treatment will really only make sense once we have also looked at its target, which we will do in later chapters.

2.2 ANTIBODY-BASED CANCER TREATMENTS

Many targeted cancer treatments and immunotherapies are based on the structure of the natural antibody proteins that our body makes as it fights off infections (Figure 2.4).

It's worth knowing that anything that a B cell might react to is called an antigen. Antigens are often proteins on the surface of pathogens such as bacteria or viruses (it's worth noting that antigens that activate T cells are different; they are small fragments of proteins called peptide antigens). The precise bit of an antigen an antibody attaches to is called its epitope. Only the very tips of an antibody attach to its target. They are known as the antigen-binding sites (Figure 2.5), and they are part of a larger section of the antibody known as the variable region (Fv). The back portion of the antibody, the part that attracts and activates white blood cells, is known as the constant region (Fc). Another

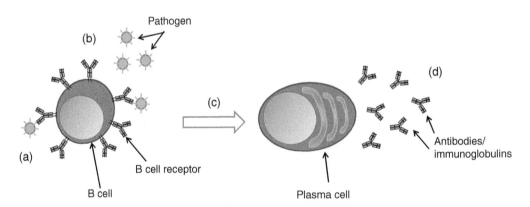

Figure 2.4 Antibodies are made by specialized B cells called plasma cells. (a) Our bodies contain many millions of white blood cells known as B cells (also called B lymphocytes), each of which has around one hundred thousand (100,000) copies of a unique B cell receptor (BCR) on its surface. **(b)** B cells use their BCRs to recognize and connect with one particular protein or other complex molecule, which is often something found on the surface of an invading pathogen such as a bacterium or virus. **(c)** When a B cell's BCRs connect with their target, the BCRs cluster together and become active. After numerous further activation steps, the B cell might become a plasma cell and release millions of copies of its BCR into the blood. **(d)** BCRs that have been released into the blood are known as antibodies or immunoglobulins. *Source:* Adapted from Ref. [11].

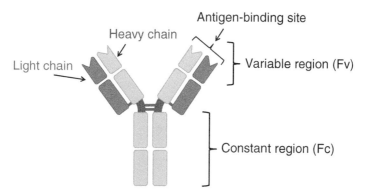

Figure 2.5 Antibodies are large proteins constructed from four separate pieces. Each antibody is made from two larger, heavy chain proteins (turquoise) and two smaller, light chain proteins (blue). These four proteins are held together by chemical bonds (red). Each B cell makes an antibody with a unique antigen-binding site, which is formed by the ends of the heavy and light chains wrapping around one another. Because the antigen-binding regions vary, they are called the "variable region" of the antibody. *Source:* Adapted from Ref. [11].

thing worth remembering is that the terms antibody and immunoglobulin can be used interchangeably.

Using various technologies, scientists can create antibodies that attach to a specific protein found on the surface of cancer cells. They then make it into a treatment that contains millions upon millions of copies of that one particular antibody. This is called a monoclonal antibody therapy as every copy of the antibody in the treatment is the same.

One thing that is important to know is that, because of their size, an antibody's target must be something on the surface of cells. Antibodies cannot simply diffuse across cell membranes in the same way that many small molecules can, so their target can't be hidden away in the cell's cytoplasm or nucleus.

Another thing to note is that antibodies must be given to patients in a way that avoids their digestive system. After all, antibodies are proteins, and our digestive system has evolved many ways to digest, destroy, and release amino acids and energy from the proteins we eat. Because of this, antibodies are given straight into a vein or injected underneath the skin or into muscle.

Lastly, our B cells have the capacity to make different types of antibodies depending on what type of infection or other problem they're reacting to. Different types of antibodies include immunoglobulin-A (IgA), IgG, IgE, IgD, and IgM. All the cancer treatments I've ever come across are made from IgG antibodies.

2.2.1 Why Antibodies Make Good Cancer Treatments

Antibodies have a number of properties that make them an ideal starting point for use as cancer treatments [12–14]. I've listed some of these properties below:

1. They are incredibly precise; an antibody designed to attach to one antigen on the surface of cancer cells will almost never attach to anything else.
2. Many millions of identical copies of an antibody can be reliably made using living cells (this makes them a type of biological therapy or biologic – a treatment manufactured using living cells).
3. Antibodies are very stable and last in the body a long time (usually two to four weeks, if not longer). They can therefore be given to patients as weekly or even monthly treatments.

4. They can be used to block or interfere with cell surface receptors such as growth factor receptors or checkpoint proteins and their ligands.[6]

5. They can also be used to activate receptors (receptor agonists).

6. They can be used to attract and activate white blood cells and thereby trigger an immune response against cells they attach to.

7. They can be tweaked and changed in a variety of nuanced ways to enhance useful features; for example, by altering the sequence of amino acids they're made from or by altering the complex sugar molecules attached to them by the cells they're manufactured by.

8. The genetic instructions (the gene) for making an antibody can be cut into pieces and combined in new ways to create entirely new antibody-based proteins with tailor-made functions that would never normally exist in the natural world.

9. They can be used as transportation devices to deliver toxic drugs, radioactivity, or toxins to cancer cells – these are the antibody conjugates.

2.2.2 How Antibody Therapies Have Changed Over the Years

The idea of using monoclonal antibodies as treatments first became popular in the 1970s. But it was in the 1990s that the first antibody, called rituximab, was approved for use as a cancer treatment [15, 16]. Rituximab is still an important, effective, and widely used treatment for people with some types of leukemia and lymphoma (as well as having some uses outside of cancer such as rheumatoid arthritis).

Since the creation of rituximab, many other antibodies have become important treatments for people with a variety of cancer types – both people with solid tumors and those with hematological cancers like leukemia or lymphoma. As the years have progressed, scientists have also played around with antibodies to enhance various features. I've described some of these alterations below.

Removing Mouse Protein from Antibodies

When scientists first started to make antibody treatments for patients with cancer, they were very limited as to how these antibodies could be made. The most common method was to put the target protein (generally something found on the surface of human cancer cells) into a mouse and then wait for the mouse's immune system to respond. By isolating B cells from the treated mouse, they could create manufacturing cells that churned out millions of copies of an antibody that attached to the chosen target [17]. However, the antibodies they created were mouse antibodies. This meant that the person's immune system would often recognize the antibody as being foreign and mount an immune reaction against it, and this severely restricted their usefulness.

Since the 1980s, scientists have been using newer technologies to create a variety of antibodies that contain less and less mouse protein. These include part-human part-mouse antibodies (known as chimeric antibodies), humanized antibodies, and fully human antibodies (Figure 2.6). In general, as the

---

[6] A ligand is something that binds to a receptor. For example, epidermal growth factor (EGF) is a ligand for the EGF receptor (EGFR). EGF and other growth factors are small proteins that float around freely. But sometimes the ligand for a receptor is something attached to the surface of another cell. This is the case with the ligands for checkpoint proteins.

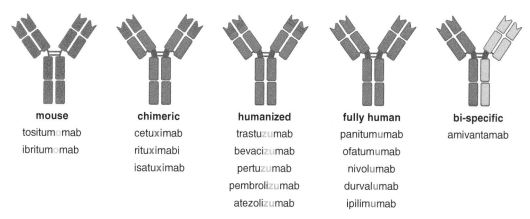

Figure 2.6 Different types of antibodies used as cancer treatments. The scientific name (i.e., not the marketing name) of monoclonal antibodies always ends in mab to denote it as a monoclonal antibody. Letters within the name tell you whether it's a mouse antibody (o), a chimeric (part-mouse, part-human) antibody (xi), a humanized (almost completely human) antibody (zu), or a fully human antibody (u). The letters "li" or simply "l" in pembrolizumab, atezolizumab, nivolumab, and durvalumab tell you that these are immunotherapies. Bi-specific antibodies attach to two different targets.

amount of mouse protein is reduced, the antibody becomes less likely to trigger immune reactions. However, even a fully human antibody is still foreign to the patient's immune system – it's not one made by their own B cells. Thus, fully human antibodies can still cause dangerous infusion reactions [18].

Swapping and Recombining Pieces of Antibody Protein

For several decades, scientists have been able to chop up genes, switch them around, and put them back into living cells (called recombinant DNA technology). The modified cells then use the engineered gene to manufacture the corresponding protein.

Using recombinant technologies, scientists can create proteins that contain segments of two or more different antibodies or that are made from part of an antibody fused to part of a completely unrelated protein. One way of applying this technology is to create back-to-back fusions of antibodies. However, if you took two complete antibodies and fused them back-to-back, the resulting protein would be enormous and would (1) be difficult to

manufacture and (2) probably get stuck in blood vessels and never make it into a tumor. For these reasons, scientists tend to use smaller sections to make a much more manageable-sized protein (Figure 2.7).

I shall be covering these mix-and-match protein structures in greater detail in Section 6.9.

Another example where an antibody has been completely reconstructed is in CAR-modified T cell therapy. In this therapy, the variable region of an antibody has been fused to protein segments taken from a variety of other proteins that activate and enhance the longevity of T cells (this is called a CAR protein). There is lots more information about CAR T cell therapy in Section 6.6.

Other Tweaks and Changes

Even subtle modifications to an antibody can have an enormous impact on its effectiveness. For example, slight changes to the antigen-binding region can hugely improve the antibody's ability to attach to its target. Also, as cells make antibodies, they naturally attach chains of sugar molecules to the protein's

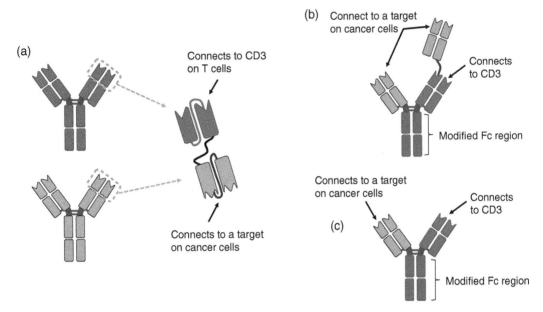

Figure 2.7 Antibody segments can be rearranged to create new structures. **(a)** T cell engagers are constructed from the variable regions of two different antibodies. One end of structure attaches to a protein found on T cells (invariably the chosen protein is CD3), and the other end attaches to a protein found on the surface of cancer cells. The two antibody pieces are connected by a flexible linker. The goal is for the T cell engager to connect together cancer cells with T cells, directing the T cells to destroy the cancer cells. **(b)** Many different antibody-derived T cell engagers have been developed. For example, the structure shown includes the constant region (Fc) of an antibody. The inclusion of a modified Fc region extends the protein's survival time in the body. **(c)** Another T cell engager design that includes an Fc region. *Source:* Adapted from Ref. [19].

structure (this is called glycosylation). Just by making small changes to these sugar molecules, you can increase the antibody's ability to attract and activate white blood cells. Small changes to the order of amino acids in the Fc portion of an antibody can also alter the way it attracts white blood cells and complement proteins [20] (Figure 2.8).

2.2.3 Mechanisms of Action of Antibody-Based Cancer Treatments

As you might have already gathered, antibody-based cancer treatments have a variety of different mechanisms of action. This variety has led to confusion as to which antibody-based cancer treatments should be classed as targeted cancer treatments, and which as immunotherapies (see Box 2.1).

The precise mechanism (or mechanisms) of action of any particular antibody-based treatment will depend on the following: (summarized in Figure 2.9)

- The antibody's target (or targets)
- Exactly where on the target the antibody attaches to – this might dictate whether the target protein is activated or blocked
- What type of antibody has been used (e.g., IgG or IgM)
- Whether anything has been added or subtracted from the antibody's structure.

I have split antibodies into two main groups that are detailed in the following sections: those that can directly kill cancer cells and

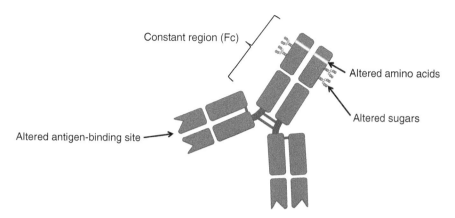

Figure 2.8 An antibody's effectiveness can be improved by tweaking its structure. Some antibodies have been improved upon by making slight changes to the antibody's antigen-binding site. Other modifications include altering the Fc region of the antibody (either by changing the amino acid sequence or adding sugar molecules) to improve the antibody's ability to attract white blood cells and complement proteins.

those that trigger an immune response against the person's cancer cells. (Of course, as you can see from Figure 2.9, many antibodies do both.)

2.2.4 Antibodies that Kill Cancer Cells Directly

Antibodies that kill cancer cells outright either (1) block a target that cancer cells need to stay alive or (2) deliver something toxic to cancer cells.

Antibodies that Block a Target

These antibodies are summarized in Figure 2.10. Many of these antibodies attach to a growth factor receptor (or occasionally they attach to a ligand of a growth factor receptor). Growth factor receptors are common targets of antibody-based cancer treatments because: [12, 13, 22, 23]

- They are found on the cell surface and are therefore accessible to antibodies.
- They are often overproduced by cancer cells, which end up with much higher levels of them on their surface than their healthy cell equivalents.

- Growth factor receptors control many internal proteins that force cancer cells to grow, multiply, and survive. When an antibody attaches to one of these receptors, this is sometimes sufficient to block the signaling pathways under the receptor's control and trigger the cell's death.
- Targeting growth factor receptors found on endothelial cells (the cells that line blood vessels) can alter the properties of tumor blood vessels. In some instances, this disrupts a cancer's blood supply or aids the distribution of chemotherapy (see Chapter 4 for much more on these "angiogenesis inhibitors").

Because growth factor receptors are such an important target of antibody-based cancer treatments, I will revisit them at length in Chapter 3, which is all about treatments that target cell communication pathways.

Antibodies that Deliver Toxic Substances

Another way of using an antibody to kill cancer cells outright is to use the antibody to deliver chemotherapy (Figures 2.11a & 2.12), a

Box 2.1   Should all antibody-based cancer treatments be classed as immunotherapies?

This is a perpetual area of confusion, with different people (and organizations) coming to different conclusions. Let us take a look at four antibody-based cancer treatments and their mechanisms of action as examples:

- **Trastuzumab.** This antibody attaches to a protein called HER2, which is overproduced by some cancer cells due to amplification of the *HER2* gene (this is most commonly found in breast cancer and stomach cancer). HER2 generates signals telling cancer cells to grow, multiply, and survive (there's lots more on this in Chapter 3). When trastuzumab attaches to HER2, this prevents the internal signals from being generated. In addition, trastuzumab also has the ability to attract and activate white blood cells, which destroy cancer cells [21]. *Despite this, I would still class trastuzumab as a* **targeted therapy** *because of its ability to directly kill cancer cells.*
- **Trastuzumab deruxtecan.** This treatment is made from the same trastuzumab antibody, but several copies of a chemotherapy drug have been chemically attached to the antibody. The treatment can therefore do everything the original trastuzumab antibody can do, but now with an extra dimension: The antibody delivers chemotherapy directly to the person's cancer cells (see Figure 2.12) *As with trastuzumab, I would classify this as a* **targeted therapy**.
- **Rituximab.** This antibody attaches to a protein called CD20, which is found on the cancer cells of some leukemias and lymphomas. When rituximab attaches to CD20, this is unlikely to kill the cell. Instead, rituximab attracts and activates white blood cells and complement proteins, and it's these that kill the cancer cells (you can learn about this in Figure 2.13). *I would class this an* **immunotherapy**, *as it primarily works by using the patient's immune cells.*
- **Nivolumab.** This antibody attaches to a protein called PD-1, which is found on activated T cells. PD-1 is a **checkpoint protein** used by our body to prevent T cells from being overactive, or from staying active too long. When its PD-1 proteins are triggered, the T cell becomes inactive and suppressed. Nivolumab prevents this from happening and **boosts the activity of T cells**. Some of these active T cells hopefully then recognize and destroy the person's cancer cells (see Chapter 5 for lots more on nivolumab and the other checkpoint inhibitors). *I would classify nivolumab as an* **immunotherapy** *as its primary mechanism of action is to activate the person's T cells.*

You can see that although these four antibodies share the same basic structure, that of an antibody, they have different (but overlapping) mechanisms of action. I have told you how I would classify each one, but other people have different opinions. For example, some people would say that all antibody-based treatments should be classed as immunotherapies. They would argue that they all have the potential to trigger an immune response, even if that's not their primary mechanism of action, and I can understand their point of view.

radioactive isotope (Figure 2.11b), or a toxin (Figure 2.11c). These are called conjugated antibodies (as opposed to antibodies that don't have anything attached to them, which are often referred to as naked antibodies).

Although all three conjugated antibody approaches have proven successful [24–26], it's the antibody-drug conjugates (ADCs) that have really taken off (see Section 4.2 for more details). There are several approved for use as

- Conjugated antibodies

- Antibodies that target growth factor receptors on solid tumour cells
- Angiogenesis inhibitors

- Antibodies that attach to proteins such as CD20 and CD38 on hemato-logical cancer cells

- Checkpoint inhibitors
- Bi-specific antibodies and bi-specific T cell engagers
- CAR T cells

Work independently of the patient's immune system

Need the patient's immune system for their effects

Figure 2.9 An antibody-based treatment's overall impact is a combination of immune system-dependent and immune system-independent effects. Some antibody-based treatments completely rely on the patient's immune system for their effects. For example, T cell engagers attach to cancer cells and recruit the patient's own T cells to kill them, whereas antibodies that attach to cell surface proteins such as CD20 often have some ability to kill cancer cells directly, without needing to recruit and activate white blood cells. The balance of immune system-dependent and immune system-independent effects of antibodies that target growth factor receptors is more complicated. These antibodies are likely to kill many cancer cells outright, although they do have the potential to attract and activate white blood cells, if suitable cells exist. Antibodies that target angiogenesis target the tumor's blood vessels but are also thought to assist T cells. Conjugated antibodies deliver a potent, toxic entity to cancer cells, such as a form of chemotherapy or a radioactive isotope, which presumably kills the cells outright. *Source:* Adapted from Ref. [19–23].

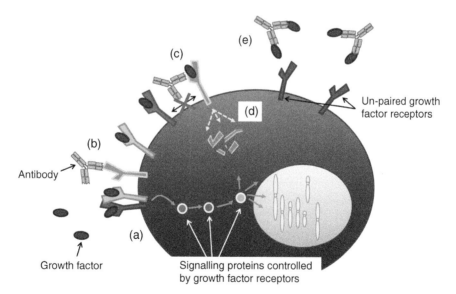

Figure 2.10 Antibodies can block growth factor receptors and the pathways under their control. **(a)** When suitable growth factors attach to growth factor receptors, this triggers the receptors to pair up and activate proteins within the cell. **(b)** Some antibody therapies attach to growth factor receptors and prevent growth factors from attaching to their receptors. **(c)** Some antibodies physically prevent receptors from pairing up (growth factor receptors are only active when in pairs). **(d)** Some antibodies cause their target to be drawn inside the cell and destroyed. **(e)** Some attach to a growth factor and prevent it from binding to its receptor. Blocking the growth factor receptors on the surface of cancer cells is sometimes sufficient to kill them.

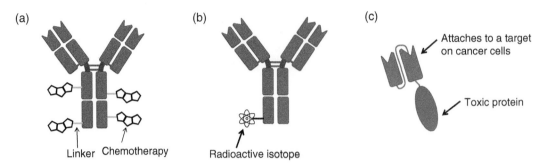

Figure 2.11 Conjugated antibodies can deliver chemotherapy, radioactivity, or a toxin. (a) Antibody-drug conjugates are made from an antibody, a linker, and one or more molecules of a chemotherapy. Two commonly used chemotherapies are calicheamicin and auristatins. **(b)** Antibodies can be used to deliver a radioactive isotope to cancer cells. **(c)** An "immunotoxin" is made from the tip (Fv portion) of an antibody, linked to the cell-killing portion of a toxic protein such as exotoxin A from the *Pseudomonas* bacterium.

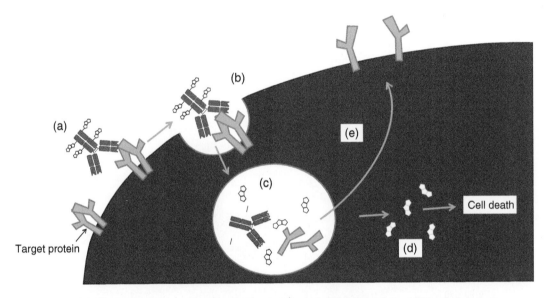

Figure 2.12 Mechanism of action of antibody-drug conjugates (ADCs). (a) An ADC attaches to its target protein on the surface of a cell. **(b)** The cell's membrane folds inward to create a compartment (an endosome) containing the ADC. **(c)** The ADC's linker is broken, releasing toxic chemotherapy. **(d)** The chemotherapy is released into the cell cytoplasm, where it kills the cell by destroying its microtubules or by causing DNA breaks. **(e)** The antibody's target protein may be destroyed or recycled back to the cell surface.

cancer treatments, and more are coming through trials all the time. One of the exciting properties of these antibodies is that they do everything the parent antibody can do (such as blocking a growth factor receptor and/or attracting white blood cells) plus they also deliver chemotherapy.

However, it's worth bearing in mind that only roughly 0.1% (one in every thousand) of an antibody-drug conjugate actually reaches the person's cancer cells inside a solid tumor. The rest gradually gets degraded, causing side effects that reflect the toxicity profile of the conjugated chemotherapy [27].

2.2.5 Antibodies that Create a Cancer-fighting Immune Response

Again, I'll split these treatments into two groups depending on what sort of immune response they create:

- Naked antibodies that attract white blood cells and complement proteins
- Antibody-based treatments that create a T cell response

Naked Antibodies that Attract White Blood Cells and Complement Proteins

The antibody therapies I've depicted in Figure 2.13 are those that attach to a cell surface protein on cancer cells and attract white blood cells and complement proteins. Antibodies that work through this mechanism have been around for decades and the classic example is rituximab, which targets a cell surface protein called CD20.

The CD20 protein is found on B lymphocytes (B cells), including the faulty B cells that cause B cell non-Hodgkin lymphoma (NHL) or chronic lymphocytic leukemia (CLL). It's these cancers that rituximab and other CD20-targeted antibodies are used to treat.

Daratumumab and isatuximab work in a similar way. They both target a protein called CD38 and are given to some people with myeloma [29]. You can find out more about all these antibodies in Section 6.2.

Antibodies that recruit the immune system like this are mostly given to people with hematological cancers. However, some of the antibodies that target growth factor receptors and that are given to people with solid tumors can, in theory at least, do the same thing. But,

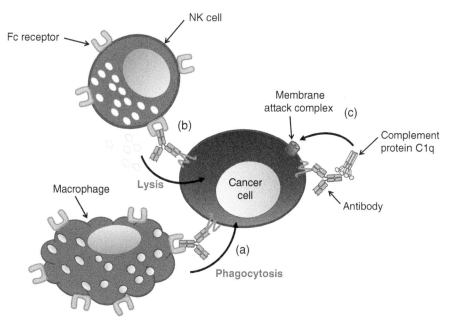

Figure 2.13 Antibodies can kill cancer cells by attracting white blood cells and complement proteins. When an antibody attaches to a protein on a cancer cell, it can attract white blood cells with Fc receptors on their surface such as macrophages and natural killer (NK) cells. **(a)** Macrophages engulf and digest cancer cells with antibodies attached to them through a process called phagocytosis. **(b)** NK cells release cell-killing enzymes that lyse (destroy) the cell. **(c)** Antibodies attached to cancer cells also attract complement proteins that come together to form a membrane attack complex (MAC) that punches holes through the cell's membrane and kills the cell. *Source:* Adapted from Ref. [22, 23, 28].

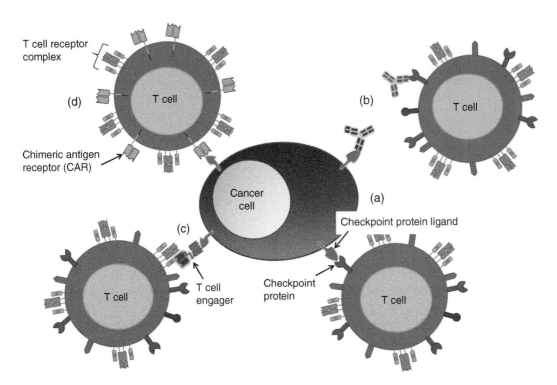

Figure 2.14 **Antibody-based cancer treatments can create a T cell-mediated response to cancer.**
(a) T cells have on their surface a range of inhibitory checkpoint proteins. If one of these is triggered (e.g., by a ligand on the surface of a cancer cell), the T cell is suppressed. **(b)** An antibody that attaches to a checkpoint protein, or to a checkpoint protein ligand, can prevent and reverse the suppression of T cells. The active T cell might then destroy cancer cells. **(c)** A T cell engager binds to proteins on the surface of a cancer cell and a T cell. The physical connection created activates the T cell and causes it to destroy the cancer cell. **(d)** A CAR-modified T cell (CAR T cell) attaches to a cell surface protein on a cancer cell and then destroys it. *Source:* Adapted from Ref. [12, 14, 22, 23].

as I said back in Chapter 1, cancer cells in solid tumors tend to live in a very protected and immune-suppressing environment. So, the antibodies' ability to create an immune response is probably limited [30].

Antibody-based Treatments that Create a T Cell Response

In Figure 2.14, I've illustrated some of the other ways that an antibody-based treatment can create an immune response, this time by triggering the activity of T cells. Some of these antibodies, like the other antibodies I've already described, are made from a complete, intact antibody, with nothing added or removed from the antibody's structure. For example, we have the immune checkpoint

inhibitors (Figure 2.14a & b). These antibodies attach either to a checkpoint protein on the surface of a T cell (such as PD-1) or to a checkpoint protein's ligand (PD-L1), which might be on a cancer cell. There's so much to say about immune checkpoint inhibitors in terms of how they work and who they help that I've given them their own chapter – Chapter 5.

A much less well-known and, so far, unproven approach (in that there aren't any licensed treatments that work like this) is to use an antibody that blocks a checkpoint protein on a white blood cell *other than a T cell*. For example, one possible target is a protein called CD47. Cancer cells (like all our cells) use CD47 to send "don't eat me" signals to macrophages. However, unlike healthy cells, cancer cells are damaged and also give out a range of "eat me" signals. Antibodies that attach to CD47 block the "don't eat me" signal, allowing macrophages to respond to the "eat me" signals on cancer cells [31–33]. I've written more about these antibodies in Section 5.8.

More well-known are T cell engagers and CAR T cells (Figure 2.14c & d). These strategies both involve cutting and stitching back together pieces of the antibody gene. When this gene is inserted into living cells, the cells are forced to create the corresponding protein from this gene – a protein that wouldn't normally exist in the natural world.

In the case of T cell engagers, the engineered gene is inserted into manufacturing cells grown in a lab.[7] These cells create billions of copies of the corresponding protein, which are purified and given to patients [17]. In contrast, CAR T cell therapy involves introducing an engineered gene into the patient's own T cells. Scientists modify the person's T cells in a lab and encourage them to multiply there too. But the modified T cells are then infused back into the patient's blood as living cells [34]. I cover both T cell engagers and CAR T cells in far greater detail in Chapter 6.

2.2.6 Limitations of Antibody Treatments and Reasons for Side Effects

As with all treatments, antibody-based treatments aren't perfect. I've described just some of their limitations below.

Reasons why they might not work at all or only work for a limited amount of time: [35, 36]
- Because of antibodies' size, they can have difficulty getting into all the body's tissues and organs and penetrating the blood-brain barrier.[8] An additional problem arises if

there are regions within a tumor that contain few blood vessels – antibodies are often unable to penetrate these parts of a tumor.
- If an antibody's main mechanism of action is to attract and/or activate white blood cells, its ability to do this will depend on the types of white blood cells present in the cancer, and whether or not they can be provoked into action. The environment in solid tumors is often hostile to cancer-fighting white blood cells, making it difficult to provoke this sort of response.
- Often, an antibody elicits its effects by first of all attaching to a target on the surface of the person's cancer cells (e.g., HER2, EGFR, and CD20). However, if this target is only present on some (but not all) cancer cells, then it's only these cells that will be destroyed and the treatment will be only partially effective.
- Some antibodies work by attaching to a growth factor receptor on the cell surface and preventing the activation of internal proteins under the receptor's control. If the internal proteins under the receptor's control are overactive (perhaps because of a mutation or the presence of a different receptor on the cell surface), then blocking the receptor won't help (see Figure 3.10).
- A mutation might cause cancer cells to create an altered version of the target protein, one that lacks the antibody's binding site. The antibody is then unable to attach.

Reasons why they cause side effects: [37–39]
- Antibodies used as cancer treatments are foreign to the patient's body; the person's immune system therefore sometimes reacts to them, causing allergy-type reactions, such as fever, chills, headaches, and red and itchy skin.

---

[7] Any treatment that is manufactured using living cells is a "biological therapy" or "biologic."
[8] In our brain, the cells lining the blood vessels are slightly different and closer together than in the rest of the body. This makes it harder for things to get through the blood vessel wall and into the brain. This less permeable lining to our brain's blood vessels (known as the blood-brain barrier) protects our brain from many infections and toxins, but it also makes it difficult for cancer treatments to get into our brain and can prevent them from reaching any cancer cells that are hiding there.

- If the antibody's target is found on healthy cells as well as on cancer cells, then it's likely that healthy cells will be destroyed too. For example, epidermal growth factor receptor (EGFR), the target of cetuximab and panitumumab, is found in the skin, digestive tract, and elsewhere. Therefore, these antibodies often cause skin and digestive problems.
- Antibodies that work by boosting the activity of T cells, such as checkpoint inhibitors (e.g., nivolumab and pembrolizumab), can inadvertently activate T cells that attack the body's healthy tissues. These are called immune-related adverse events, and I'll come back to them in Chapter 5.
- Antibody-drug conjugates, which carry chemotherapy to cancer cells, generally cause side effects that relate to the release of their chemotherapy payload into the blood [27].

Reasons why we don't have an antibody-based treatment available for every patient:
- Antibodies are large proteins and cannot cross the cell membrane in the way that small drugs can; therefore, their target must be on the cell's surface. This severely limits the range of proteins in cancer cells that can be targeted with these treatments. There are many cancer types for which it hasn't yet been possible to identify a suitable cell surface target.
- The proteins found on the surface of cancer cells are often very similar to, or the same as, the proteins found on the healthy cells that they developed from. For example, a breast cancer cell often has the same proteins on its surface as a normal breast cell. It can therefore be incredibly difficult to find something on the surface of a person's cancer cells that it is safe to target and that won't lead to the destruction of healthy cells.
- If you want a naked antibody treatment to kill cancer cells outright (i.e., without activating white blood cells or delivering

chemotherapy), then its target needs to be something the cancer cells are depending on for their survival. Again, it's difficult to find such a target for every cancer and every patient.

2.2.7 Uses of Monoclonal Antibody Treatments for Cancer

The first monoclonal antibody given to patients with cancer was rituximab, which targets the CD20 protein found on B cells. Other common targets of monoclonal antibody treatments for cancer are listed in Table 2.1, along with the antibody treatments that target them.
In general:
- Antibodies that target CD antigens on the surface of white blood cells (e.g., CD19, CD20, CD38, CD22, and CD33) are used in the treatment of leukemias, lymphomas, and myeloma. They primarily kill cancer cells by recruiting and activating healthy white blood cells (via the mechanisms shown in Figure 2.13) unless they are an ADC, in which case they also deliver chemotherapy. However, these treatments also cause the death of many healthy white blood cells, and, as a consequence, they are likely to suppress the patient's immune system. (These treatments are described in greater detail in Chapter 6.)
- Antibodies that attach to growth factor receptors (such as EGFR and HER2) are given to people with solid tumors such as bowel or breast cancer. These antibodies probably primarily kill cancer cells outright (as shown in Figure 2.10) as opposed to activating white blood cells [36].
- Antibodies that deliver chemotherapy have a range of different targets. Current targets include proteins found on the surface of cancer cells in solid tumors, such as human epidermal growth factor receptor-2 (HER2) or nectin-4, or proteins found on hematological cancer cells, such as CD33 or CD79b (Section 4.2).

Table 2.1 Examples of targets and uses of antibody-based cancer treatments.

Target protein	Where is it found? [40]	Treatment examples	Indications
Targeted against proteins on hematological cancer cells (leukemias, lymphomas, and myeloma)			
CD19	On cancer cells from B cell leukemias and lymphomas; on the majority of the body's healthy B cells [41]	Blinatumomab, tafasitamab, tisagenlecleucel, lisocabtagene maraleucel, brexucabtagene autoleucel, and axicabtagene ciloleucel	Acute lymphoblastic leukemia (ALL), B cell non-Hodgkin lymphoma (NHL), and chronic lymphocytic leukemia (CLL)
CD20	On cancer cells from B cell leukemias and lymphomas; on the majority of the body's healthy B cells [42]	Rituximab, ofatumumab, obinutuzumab, veltuzumab, ocrelizumab, ibritumomab tiuxetan, mosunetuzumab, epcoritamab, and glofitamab	CLL and B cell NHL
CD22	On cancer cells of ALL and on healthy immature B cells [43]	Inotuzumab ozogamicin and moxetumomab pasudotox	ALL and hairy cell leukemia
CD30	On cancer cells from Hodgkin lymphoma and anaplastic large cell lymphoma; also found on healthy, activated B and T cells [44]	Brentuximab vedotin	Hodgkin lymphoma and anaplastic large cell lymphoma
CD33	On cancer cells of acute myeloid leukemia (AML); found on a variety of immature myeloid white blood cells [45]	Gemtuzumab ozogamicin	AML
CD38	On a variety of white blood cells, including the cancer cells of myeloma [46]	Daratumumab, isatuximab, and talquetamab	Myeloma
CD79b	Found on all healthy B cells and on cancer cells derived from B cells [47]	Polatuzumab vedotin	B cell non-Hodgkin lymphoma
CS1 (SLAMF7)	A receptor protein found on the surface of plasma cells (these are antibody-releasing B cells), on NK cells, and a subgroup of other white blood cells [48]	Elotuzumab	Myeloma
BCMA	Essential for the survival of healthy plasma cells and of myeloma cells [49]	Belantamab mafodotin, idecabtagene vicleucel, ciltacabtagene autoleucel, teclistamab, and elranatamab	Myeloma

(Continued)

Table 2.1 (Continued)

Target protein	Where is it found? [40]	Treatment examples	Indications
Targeted against proteins found on cancer cells in solid tumors			
EGF receptor (EGFR)	On cells of many cancers, including those of the bowel, ovaries, lungs, head and neck, esophagus, and brain; found on healthy cells of many tissues and organs [50, 51]	**Cetuximab, panitumumab, and necitumumab**	Bowel cancer and head and neck cancer
HER2[a]	On about 20% of breast cancers and stomach cancers; also a proportion of lung, bladder, bowel, biliary, ovarian, pancreatic, and prostate cancers [52]; found in lower levels than EGF receptor on a variety of healthy cells and tissues [53, 54]	**Trastuzumab, pertuzumab, margetuximab, trastuzumab emtansine, and trastuzumab deruxtecan**	HER2-positive breast cancer, stomach cancer, and gastroesophageal junction cancer
GD2	On neurons, skin melanocytes, and peripheral pain fibers; also on the cancer cells of neuroblastoma, melanoma skin cancer, some soft tissue sarcomas, osteosarcomas, and small cell lung cancer [55]	**Dinutuximab and naxitamab**	Neuroblastoma
Gp-100	On normal melanocytes and melanoma cells [56]	Tebentafusp (targets Gp-100 and CD3)	Uveal melanoma
MET	On the cells of many healthy tissues; also found on the cancer cells of various tumors [57]	Amivantamab (targets both EGFR and MET)	Non-small cell lung cancer
Nectin-4	Not found on healthy adult tissues; present on cancer cells of breast, lung, urothelial, colorectal, pancreatic, and ovarian cancer	**Enfortumab vedotin**	Bladder cancer
Tissue factor	On cells found in the lining of blood vessels, also found in the brain, heart, kidney, and placenta; found in all types of cancers, particularly adenocarcinomas [58, 59]	**Tisotumab vedotin**	Cervical cancer
TROP2	On the cells of a variety of tissues, particularly skin, esophagus, and tonsils; also found in most cancers of epithelial origin, such as lung, breast, pancreas, liver, colorectal, and ovarian cancer [60]	**Sacituzumab govitecan**	Triple-negative breast cancer
Claudin 18.2	On the cells in healthy stomach lining, and in stomach (gastric), pancreatic, and esophageal cancer. [137]	Zolbetuximab	Stomach cancer, gastroesophageal cancer

Targeted against tumor blood vessels/angiogenesis

VEGF receptor-2 (VEGFR2)	Found on endothelial cells engaged in angiogenesis, such as healthy cells involved in wound healing and the formation of the placenta; also found on endothelial cells that form tumor blood vessels [61]	Ramucirumab	Stomach cancer, non-small cell lung cancer, bowel cancer, and liver cancer
VEGF-A	Released by cells that require a blood supply; produced by the cells of many cancer types [61, 62]	Bevacizumab and aflibercept[b]	Bowel cancer, ovarian cancer, kidney cancer, cervical cancer, breast cancer, non-small cell lung cancer, liver cancer, and glioblastoma

Targeted against T cell checkpoint proteins or their ligands

CTLA-4	Found on T cells and on some other white blood cells [63, 64]	Ipilimumab and tremelimumab	Melanoma
PD-1	On T cells, B cells, NK cells, and myeloid white blood cells [64]	Nivolumab, pembrolizumab, cemiplimab, dostarlimab, tislelizumab, retifanlimab, and toripalimab	Melanoma, non-small cell lung cancer, kidney cancer, bladder cancer, head and neck cancer, Hodgkin lymphoma, breast cancer, cervical cancer, endometrial cancer, squamous cell skin cancer, esophageal cancer, stomach cancer, liver cancer, Merkel cell carcinoma, and bowel cancer
PD-L1	Found on T cells, dendritic cells, and macrophages; also found on the surface of cancer cells in many solid tumors [64, 65]	Atezolizumab, durvalumab, and avelumab	Bladder cancer, non-small cell lung cancer, liver cancer, melanoma, small cell lung cancer, Merkel cell carcinoma, and kidney cancer

[a] Human epidermal growth factor receptor-2 (HER2) is also known as Neu and ErbB2.

[b] Aflibercept is an engineered protein: part-VEGF receptor, part-antibody.

Color key: **black – other conjugated antibody; blue – a naked antibody; orange – drug-conjugated antibody; red – CAR T cell therapy;** turquoise – T cell engager or bi-specific antibody

- Antibodies that block the activity of VEGF receptors (either by attaching to vascular endothelial growth factor (VEGF) or to one of its receptors) are used to target a tumor's blood supply, and they are referred to as angiogenesis inhibitors. These antibodies are given to people with a range of solid tumors [62]. (These treatments are described in greater detail in Section 4.1.)
- Antibodies that boost the activity of T cells (e.g., those that target checkpoint proteins or checkpoint protein ligands such as CTLA-4, PD-1, or PD-L1) are used to treat people with a wide variety of different solid tumors, and their use will no doubt expand further in the coming years. (These treatments are described in greater detail in Chapter 5.)
- Antibodies that deliver radioactive particles (called radiolabeled antibodies or radioimmunotherapies) or a toxin (immunotoxins) are used in a limited way to treat people with hematological cancers (mostly leukemias and lymphomas) but not solid tumors [24]. All white blood cells are extremely sensitive to radiation, and the cancer cells of leukemias and lymphomas retain this characteristic. This means that radiolabeled antibodies are ideal treatments for leukemias and lymphomas but cause too much immune suppression to be useful treatments for solid tumors. However, problems and complications with storage and delivery mean that, although these treatments are effective, they are only rarely used.

2.2.8 Antibody Biosimilars

Drugs such as aspirin or various forms of chemotherapy all have a relatively simple chemical structure. They generally contain around 20–100 atoms (mostly carbon, hydrogen, oxygen, and nitrogen). Because of their small size and relatively simple chemical structure, they can be manufactured by many different companies. All the company needs is an understanding of the chemical composition of the compound and the technology to manufacture

it. Thus, when a company's patent expires on one of these drugs, rival companies can quickly manufacture identical, generic versions.

However, antibodies are much, much bigger, and a lot more complicated. Each copy of an antibody contains around 1500 amino acids (each of which comprises 10–27 atoms – again carbon, hydrogen, oxygen, and nitrogen), which have been linked together to create four separate chains (2 larger, heavy chains and 2 shorter, light chains). Once the cell has made the four strings of amino acids that make up the antibody protein, it then has to fold them properly and pin them together with chemical bonds. Finally, the cell adds vital sugar molecules to the antibody's surface that help the antibody attract complement proteins and white blood cells.

Antibodies can only be manufactured by using living cells (no chemist could possibly make one from scratch). And, even if a company knows the precise amino acid makeup of an antibody such as rituximab, the cells they use to manufacture the antibody will attach a unique combination of sugar molecules to it [66]. Added to this are the complex processes needed to purify and manufacture the final product [17].

Because of the complexities involved, even if two companies set out to manufacture the exact same antibody, they would end up making antibodies with slightly different properties to each other. As a reflection of this diversity, copycat versions of antibodies are called "biosimilars" rather than generics [67].

Biosimilar versions of bevacizumab, rituximab, and trastuzumab have been approved for use in the United Kingdom, the European Union, and the United States. These approvals were based on trial results that proved that the biosimilars were no different from their originals in terms of their safety and effectiveness [68]. In many cases, the biosimilar trials involved more patients and were more rigorous than the trials conducted on the original treatment [69]. There's a vast amount of information on the biosimilar approval process on the EMA (European Medicines Agency) website [70].

2.3 SMALL MOLECULE CANCER TREATMENTS

The second major group of targeted cancer treatments are the small molecules. These are small chemical compounds (similar in size to many chemotherapies[9]) that block the activity of a protein target. The most common target of a small molecule cancer treatment is a kinase. Because kinases are such an important target, I will be telling you a lot more about them later in this chapter. But first, I'll talk about small molecule drugs in general.

2.3.1 Why Small Molecules Make Good Cancer Treatments

Probably the single most important property of small molecule drugs is their size. Small molecules and chemotherapies generally contain 20–100 atoms, whereas antibody-based therapies contain 5000–50,000 atoms (i.e., antibodies are roughly 200–500 times bigger).

I said earlier that the target of an antibody-based treatment must be something on the cell surface. But, because small molecules are physically so much smaller than antibodies, they can easily cross the cell membrane and enter the main body of the cell – the cytoplasm. It is therefore possible to use them to block internal (intracellular) proteins that are inaccessible to antibodies. This opens up thousands of opportunities in terms of being able to create treatments that block proteins that cancer cells are using to grow and multiply.

I've listed some other useful properties of small molecule therapies below:

- They can be used to disrupt the activity of powerful intracellular proteins (such as

kinases) that drive the proliferation and survival of cancer cells [71].

- Because of their relatively simple chemical structure, they are easy to manipulate, tweak, or redesign [72].
- If a new protein is discovered that drives the behavior of a type of cancer, it is quicker and cheaper to create a new small molecule drug than an antibody-based treatment [73].
- Using computer models and advances in biochemistry, it's now possible to visualize the structure of a protein, search its surface for useful nooks and crannies, and design a small molecule that will precisely block the protein's actions [74, 75].
- Small molecules are chemical compounds rather than proteins. This means that many of them can be taken in tablet form, making them much simpler, and less time-consuming, to administer. Patients can also take them in the comfort of their home rather than traveling to a hospital [76].
- They are often destroyed quickly in the body. This means that patients often have to take them as daily or twice-daily tablets, which is not necessarily a good thing. But it also means that if they are causing a worrying side effect then a quick solution is to simply lower the dose [76].
- Another benefit of their small size is that small molecules can travel around the body and penetrate organs, tissues, and tumors much more easily than antibodies. In addition, whereas antibodies and most chemotherapies are unable to cross the blood-brain barrier, small molecules are sometimes able to do so and can therefore attack brain metastases, including those from lung cancer and HER2-driven breast cancer [77, 78].
- These drugs are often less selective than antibody-based treatments and commonly block more than one protein. For example,

---

[9] Small molecules and chemotherapies generally contain 20–100 atoms, whereas antibody-based therapies contain 5000–50,000 atoms (i.e., antibodies are roughly 200–500 times bigger).

drugs that block VEGF receptors will almost always block some types of PDGF receptors and FGF receptors because of similarities between them.[10] The ability to block multiple kinases means that kinase inhibitors can be more potent treatments than monoclonal antibodies, which will only ever block one target. This same characteristic can also lead to unexpected additional uses for kinase inhibitors. For example, imatinib was created as a Bcr-Abl inhibitor for the treatment of chronic myeloid leukemia. However, imatinib was later discovered to block both PDGF receptors and KIT – both of which are involved in gastrointestinal stromal tumors (GISTs). Imatinib is now an important treatment for GISTs.

2.3.2 How Small Molecule Drugs Have Changed Over the Years

Greater Precision

One of the biggest advances in small molecule drug design has been the gradual development of drugs that are more precise in what they target. For example, the first small molecule drug to be approved as a treatment for cancer was imatinib [73]. Imatinib blocks a fusion protein called Bcr-Abl, which is found in the cancer cells of people with chronic myeloid leukemia. However, as I mentioned in the previous point, imatinib also blocks other proteins such as PDGF receptors and KIT. There are also many other examples of small molecule drugs that are relatively imprecise.

But, thanks to advances in computer technology and a better understanding of the 3-dimensional shape of proteins, scientists can create much more precise drugs. They can even create drugs that block one distinct, mutated version of a protein. For example, there are now multiple drugs, such as sotorasib and adagrasib that block the G12C[11] mutant version of the K-Ras protein. This mutant protein is found in the cancer cells of about 11%–16% of people with non-small cell lung cancer (NSCLC) [79].

Scientists are constantly creating new drugs that are more potent, and more precise, than their older counterparts [73, 75].

However, it's vitally important to remember that a treatment is only as good as its target. The effectiveness of a new small molecule cancer treatment largely comes down to:

- The precision of the drug. Whether it can block the desired target without affecting other proteins and processes
- The relative importance of the drug's target to cancer cells compared to healthy cells. This determines whether the drug can selectively kill cancer cells while leaving healthy cells unaffected

In Figure 2.15, I have tried to represent this in graphic form and given examples of drugs that fit into each of the four quadrants. However, please remember that this figure contains my personal opinions about these drugs – other people might disagree.

In addition, the usefulness of a targeted treatment is profoundly impacted by the degree of heterogeneity found within the person's tumor. If a person's tumor is homogenous (i.e., all their cancer cells are the same), then the target protein will be equally important to every cancer cell. But, if there's lots of variation from one cancer cell to the next, then there's likely to be cancer cells in the tumor that don't need the drug's target for their

---

[10] VEGF – vascular endothelial growth factor; FGF – fibroblast growth factor; PDGF – platelet-derived growth factor.
[11] "G12C" refers to the fact that the 12th codon of the *KRAS* gene has changed from the usual glycine to become a cysteine. A codon is a series of three base pairs in a gene that corresponds to one amino acid in the protein made from that gene. Watch this amazing animation to find out how proteins are made from our genes: https://www.youtube.com/watch?v=gG7uCskUOrA.

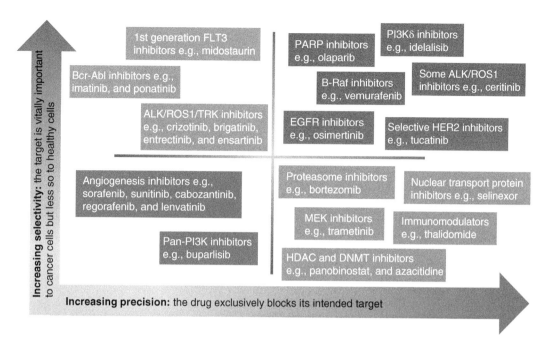

Figure 2.15 A small molecule drug's effectiveness depends both on the drug and its target. In the top-right quadrant are drugs that are both precise and selective. These treatments include the use of B-Raf inhibitors for people with *BRAF*-mutated melanoma skin cancer; PI3Kδ inhibitors for people with B cell-derived cancers; PARP inhibitors, when given to people whose tumors have a defect in a DNA repair mechanism; some ALK/ROS1 inhibitors given to people with *ALK*- or *ROS1*-mutated non-small cell lung cancer (NSCLC); and EGFR inhibitors for *EGFR*-mutated NSCLC. In each case, the drug is relatively precise, and the target is essential for cancer cell survival but much less important for healthy cells. In contrast, in the bottom-right quadrant are treatments that are precise in what they target, but that target is important both for healthy cells and for cancer cells (e.g., MEK) or has a variety of different functions (e.g., nuclear transport proteins). In the top-left quadrant are drugs whose target is essential for cancer cells, e.g., mutant FLT3, Bcr-Abl, or mutant versions of ALK, ROS1, or TRK proteins. However, the drugs are much less precise and block multiple proteins in addition to their intended target. In the bottom-left quadrant are treatments that block multiple proteins, and their target is less selective for cancer cells. *Source:* Adapted from Ref. [73].

survival. The more of these cells that exist, the less the treatment will help the patient.

Broadening the Range of Targets

I have already mentioned that kinases are the most common targets of small molecule cancer treatments. This is for two main reasons:

1. Kinases are powerful enzymes that control many different processes in our cells. Cancer cells often contain too much of a kinase (e.g., HER2), or they're making a faulty, overactive version of a kinase (e.g., mutant versions of EGFR in NSCLC).

In these situations, the cancer cells are dependent on the kinase – it tells them to keep multiplying and it keeps them alive.

2. Kinases are relatively easy to block with small molecules. All kinases have a groove in their surface where a molecule called ATP fits (more on this later). Drugs that mimic ATP block kinases.

Because of these features of kinases, they are the most common target of small molecule drugs. But, in recent years, scientists have made progress in creating drugs that block proteins other than kinases. For example, we now have drugs that block proteins such as PARP enzymes, Bcl-2, K-Ras, histone deacetylases (HDACs), Smoothened, IDH1, and IDH2.[12]

Drugs for Rarer Mutations

Perhaps unsurprisingly, when scientists (and companies) first set out to create small molecule cancer treatments, they focused on creating drugs for common cancers. Or, at the very least, they wanted to find a faulty, targetable protein found in the cancer cells of every patient with a particular type of cancer.

For example, the first small molecule drug to be licensed as a cancer treatment was a Bcr-Abl inhibitor. The Bcr-Abl protein is found in the cancer cells of virtually every patient with chronic myeloid leukemia (CML) [80].

Next came EGFR inhibitors for people with NSCLC. When scientists first created EGFR-targeted drugs, they thought they were creating drugs that would help anyone with NSCLC; it was only later they discovered these drugs only work for the portion of patients in whom the EGFR protein has been affected by a mutation [81].

More recently, we've seen drugs developed for rarer cancers, or for mutant versions of proteins only found in tiny proportions of cancer patients. Examples here include TRK inhibitors, which are effective against cancers with *NTRK* gene mutations. Roughly 1% of human cancers contain these mutations [82].

I'm now going to turn my attention to the targets and mechanisms of action of small molecule cancer drugs. I'll split them into two groups: small molecules that block kinases and small molecules with other targets.

2.3.3 Small Molecules that Block Kinases

I've mentioned kinases a few times in this chapter already, without explaining what they are. But we'll now turn to them properly.

Hopefully it will soon become clear why so many targeted cancer treatments are small chemical compounds that block kinases.

The first thing to know is that kinases are enzymes. Enzymes are catalysts that cause chemical reactions to take place in our body's cells. All our cells contain thousands of proteins that act as enzymes. The kinases are a group of more than 500 enzymes that all cause one particular chemical reaction to occur, namely phosphorylation [83].

To phosphorylate something is to add a phosphate chemical group to it (phosphate is the name for a phosphorous atom surrounded by oxygen atoms). Many of our cells' proteins are controlled by phosphorylation. Usually, adding a phosphate to a protein causes it to swing into action and start doing its job. Added phosphates can also create new bulges and dips in a protein's surface (kinases mostly attach phosphate to other proteins). These bulges and dips create interaction sites, allowing the altered protein to interact with other proteins or with DNA.

Kinases obtain phosphate from a molecule known as [84] adenosine triphosphate (ATP), which contains three phosphate groups (hence "tri"). ATP is the energy source in our cells. Our cells manufacture ATP from sugars, fats, and other high-energy molecules, which in turn come from the food we eat. High-energy chemical bonds hold together the phosphates in ATP; thus, ATP can be used to store and release a cell's energy.

So, kinases are enzymes that take a phosphate from ATP (which now becomes ADP – adenosine diphosphate) and transfer it to something else (see Figure 2.16). The most common thing that kinases attach phosphate to is another protein (often another kinase). Kinases are very selective about what they can attach phosphates to, and they tend to attach them to three particular amino acids in recipient

---

[12] PARP – poly(ADP-ribose)polymerase; Bcl-2 – B-cell lymphoma-2; HDAC – histone deacetylase; IDH – isocitrate dehydrogenase.

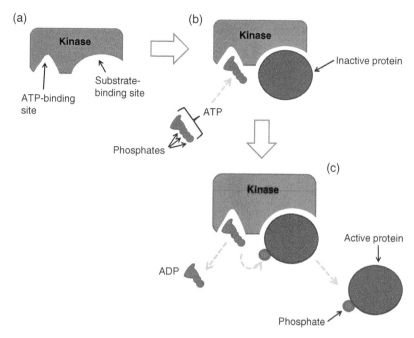

Figure 2.16 Kinases are catalysts that attach phosphates to other proteins and molecules in our cells.
(a) Kinases have docking sites for both ATP and one or more substrates (in this case, an inactive protein).
(b) Both ATP and the inactive protein dock with the kinase. **(c)** The kinase transfers one of the phosphates from ATP to a tyrosine, threonine, or serine amino acid in the protein. This activates the protein. What was ATP is now ADP. The active protein and ADP are released by the kinase.
Abbreviations: ADP – adenosine diphosphate; ATP – adenosine triphosphate.

proteins: tyrosine, threonine, or serine. For example, a kinase that attaches phosphates to tyrosine amino acids is referred to as a tyrosine kinase. Kinases that can attach phosphates to serine and threonine are serine/threonine kinases.[13]

The addition (phosphorylation) and removal (dephosphorylation) of phosphates is a common way through which our cells control the activity of many of their proteins – in fact, up to a third of the many thousands of different proteins in our cells are controlled through phosphorylation. By adding phosphates to

their targets, kinases exert a huge influence on how our cells behave [83, 85].

In many cancers, the cells' abnormal behavior is driven by overproduced or overactive kinases [3, 71, 86]. These include many kinases that would normally be under the control of growth factor receptors such as the EGFR (also known as HER1), HER2, or VEGF receptors.[14] In addition, growth factor receptors are themselves kinases (see Figure 2.17). You can read more about growth factor receptors and how they work in Chapter 3, Section 3.2. Because kinases play a central role in the

---

[13] This has ultimately become an unhelpful way of talking about kinases (at least outside of scientific circles). The problem comes from the fact that the first kinase inhibitors to be created were all drugs that blocked tyrosine kinases, giving rise to the label "tyrosine kinase inhibitor" or "TKI." However, ever since then, ANY drug that blocks a kinase, whether or not it's a tyrosine kinase, has also been referred to as a TKI. So, you find that inhibitors of serine/threonine kinases like B-Raf get called TKIs, even though they're no such thing.
[14] If you're not sure what a growth factor receptor is, turn to the introduction to Chapter 3 before you go any further.

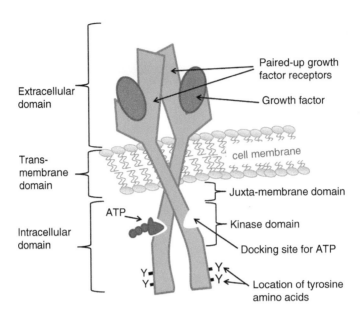

Figure 2.17 Growth factor receptors are kinases. Growth factor receptors are large proteins that sit in our cells' outer membrane. They have three main parts: an extracellular domain that sticks outside the cell, a transmembrane domain that spans the cell membrane, and an intracellular domain that protrudes into the cell cytoplasm. Growth factor receptors come together in pairs when a suitable growth factor is present. The intracellular domain of each receptor has two important features: a docking site for ATP and multiple tyrosine (Y) amino acids. When two receptors are paired up, and when ATP slots into their docking sites, the two receptors phosphorylate one another on tyrosine amino acids.
Abbreviation: ATP – adenosine triphosphate.

behavior of cancer cells, scientists have created many drugs that block them [75].

Lastly, it's important to know that kinases don't just phosphorylate proteins. In fact, a family of kinases that are overactive in a large proportion of breast, bowel, and lung cancers, and in some blood cancers, are kinases called phosphatidylinositol 3-kinases (PI3Ks). These kinases attach phosphate to a lipid – a fatty molecule – found in cell membranes. A variety of PI3K inhibitors have been developed by scientists, and some of them are licensed treatments (see Section 3.8.3).

2.3.4 Different Types of Kinase Inhibitors

Kinase inhibitors are classified according to how they block a kinase's activity, and whether or not the blockage is temporary or permanent. There are five main types of kinase inhibitors [73, 87, 88], summarized in Table 2.2.

Now, as far as you or I are concerned, it probably doesn't really matter to us exactly how any individual kinase inhibitor works. We might feel that we don't need to understand the intricacies of the shape of a kinase's ATP-binding site, or all the different shapes and contortions it can go through. But, there are a couple of things that it is helpful to know because they explain some of what patients experience when given these treatments.

Firstly, many kinase inhibitors in some way mimic the shape of ATP (see Figure 2.18a & b). But, because all kinases have an ATP-binding site, a drug that slots into the ATP-binding site of one kinase is likely to slot into the ATP-binding site of other kinases too. This means

Table 2.2   Comparison of different types of kinase inhibitors.

	Type of binding	Binding site on the kinase	Competes with ATP?	Examples
Type 1	Reversible	ATP-binding site of active kinases	Yes	Gefitinib, erlotinib, sunitinib, bosutinib, cabozantinib, ceritinib, crizotinib, pazopanib, ruxolitinib, and vandetanib
Types 1½ and 2	Reversible	ATP-binding site of inactive kinases	No	Imatinib, nilotinib, sorafenib, and axitinib
Types 3 and 4: Allosteric inhibitors	Reversible	Away from the ATP-binding site	No	Selumetinib, trametinib, and cobimetinib
Type 5: Covalent inhibitors	Irreversible	ATP-binding site	Yes	Afatinib, ibrutinib, dacomitinib, and neratinib

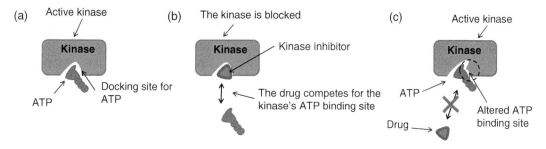

Figure 2.18 Many kinase inhibitors work by mimicking the shape of ATP in some way. (a) All kinases have a binding site for ATP. When the kinase is activated, the ATP-binding site becomes accessible, and ATP enters. The kinase is then able to phosphorylate its targets. **(b)** Kinases can be blocked by drugs that mimic the shape of ATP and that compete with ATP for the kinase's ATP-binding site. **(c)** In a cancer cell that is resistant to treatment with a kinase inhibitor, the gene for the target kinase has often sustained a mutation that has changed the binding site's shape. The mutation means that ATP can still enter its binding site, but the drug cannot; therefore, the kinase remains active, and the cancer cell survives. **Abbreviation:** ATP – adenosine triphosphate.

that many kinase inhibitors aren't very careful about what they block. The scientist might have planned to create a drug that only blocks one specific kinase. But, in fact, the drug blocks a whole series of kinases, and therefore giving it to patients has lots of unintended consequences. This can account for the sometimes strange side effects that kinase inhibitors cause.

Secondly, if a kinase inhibitor works by slotting a kinase's ATP-binding site, this makes it vulnerable to changes in the shape of the binding site. A common reason for drug resistance is when the gene for a target kinase

is mutated and the ATP-binding site has changed shape (Figure 2.18c). Often, these resistance-causing mutations affect gatekeeper amino acids that play a critical role in controlling access to small molecule drugs. For example, in the Bcr-Abl protein the 315th amino acid is the gatekeeper. It's normally a threonine (T), but if a point mutation causes it to change to an isoleucine (I), then imatinib and many other Bcr-Abl inhibitors can no longer access the ATP-binding site and block the protein [89].

I've included a bit of extra detail about the different types of kinase inhibitors below:

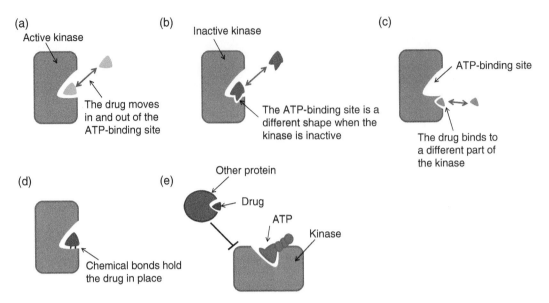

Figure 2.19 Different types of kinase inhibitors and the way they work. (a) Type 1 kinase inhibitors compete with ATP for the ATP-docking site of active kinases. **(b)** Type 1½ and type 2 kinase inhibitors can enter a kinase's ATP-binding site only when the kinase is inactive. **(c)** Allosteric inhibitors bind outside of the ATP-binding site. **(d)** Covalent inhibitors enter the kinase's ATP-binding site and form chemical bonds that hold the drug in place. **(e)** Indirect kinase inhibitors don't bind to the kinase directly; instead, they attach to a separate protein that only inhibits the kinase when the drug is present.
Abbreviation: ATP – adenosine triphosphate.

Type 1 Kinase Inhibitors

This is the most common type of kinase inhibitor. These drugs are small molecules that mimic ATP's shape and slot into the ATP-binding site of active kinases (Figure 2.19a). Thus, they compete with ATP for the binding site, blocking the kinase's activity. This blockage is only temporary – hence they are reversible (rather than irreversible) kinase inhibitors.

Type 1½ and Type 2 Kinase Inhibitors

These drugs are small molecules that bind to the ATP-binding site of kinases when the kinase is inactive (Figure 2.19b). These drugs can trap their target kinases in an inactive state. They don't compete with ATP. As with type 1 kinases, these are reversible inhibitors; that is, they get into the binding pocket and then drop out again – they don't stick.

Allosteric Inhibitors

These drugs bind to a site on the kinase that is separate from the ATP-binding site (Figure 2.19c); therefore the drug isn't competing with ATP. Many of these drugs are reversible inhibitors that enter a pocket in the target kinase that is involved in controlling the kinase's level of activity. The allosteric inhibitors include several MEK inhibitors.

Covalent Inhibitors

Some kinase inhibitors can chemically bond with the ATP-binding site, making them irreversible kinase inhibitors (also known as covalent inhibitors) (Figure 2.19d). They include pan-HER inhibitors,[15] such as dacomitinib and afatinib, and BTK (Bruton's tyrosine kinase) inhibitors such as ibrutinib.

[15]There are four *h*uman *e*pidermal growth factor *r*eceptors, and some drugs effectively block all four of them, making them pan-HER inhibitors.

Indirect Inhibitors

Some kinase inhibitors don't physically interact with the kinase they block. Instead, they work via another protein (Figure 2.19e). The most well-known examples are everolimus and temsirolimus, which are derivatives of a naturally occurring chemical called rapamycin (everolimus and temsirolimus are sometimes called "rapalogs"). Rapamycin and other rapalogs bind to a protein in our cells called FKBP12, which then interacts with and blocks some of the functions of a kinase called mTOR [73] (there is more about mTOR inhibitors in Section 3.8.6). So the drug doesn't have to directly come into contact with the target kinase in order to block it.

2.3.5 Common Targets and Uses of Kinase Inhibitors

Kinases are very popular with drug companies looking to create new cancer treatments. This is for two main reasons: (1) lots of cancers contain overactive kinases, and (2) drug companies have become very adept at creating drugs that block them (various kinases and examples of drugs that block them are summarized in Table 2.3). Because there are so many kinases being targeted for the treatment of cancer, I have grouped them below into various categories:

- Kinase inhibitors that block the kinase part of a growth factor receptor (such as EGFR, HER2, MET, FGFRs, and FLT3) [73, 94]. Growth factor receptors are used by our cells to communicate with one another. These cell surface receptors are also kinases; hence their other name – receptor tyrosine kinases. I'm going to say a lot more about them, and the drugs that block them, in the next chapter.
- Kinase inhibitors that block internal kinases that are controlled by growth factor receptors (e.g., B-Raf, MEK, PI3K, AKT, mTOR, and PI3K) [73, 94]. Again, I'll be saying a lot more about these drugs in the next chapter.

- Kinase inhibitors that block internal kinases controlled by other types of cell surface receptors [73]. These include JAK2 inhibitors, BTK inhibitors, and PI3K-delta (PI3Kδ) inhibitors. JAK2 and its colleagues, JAK1, JAK3, and TYK2, are controlled by various types of receptors found on the surface of white blood cells. BTK and PI3Kδ are activated by B cell receptors on B lymphocytes. JAK2, BTK, and PI3Kδ inhibitors are all used as treatments for hematological cancers (cancers caused by faulty white blood cells). JAK2 inhibitors are covered in Section 3.9; BTK and PI3Kδ inhibitors are described in Section 4.8.
- Kinase inhibitors that block fusion proteins [113]. Cancer cells sometimes make fusion proteins because of a chromosome translocation or gene rearrangement (for a refresher, look back at Section 1.2.2). Sometimes, one of the protein pieces in the fusion protein is a kinase, and the fusion protein is an overactive kinase. For example, in the cancer cells of NSCLC you sometimes find fusion proteins that contain the kinase portion of a growth factor receptor, such as ALK, ROS1, or RET. Another kinase fusion protein, Bcr-Abl, is found in the cells of CML. Again, I come back to these treatments in Chapter 3.
- Kinase inhibitors that target kinases involved in the cell cycle [73]. The cell cycle (the process our cells go through in order to multiply) involves an elaborate, tightly controlled series of events involving hundreds of proteins. Some of the proteins involved are kinases. For example, cyclin-dependent kinases (CDKs) are a family of proteins that control a cell's progress through the cell cycle. They in turn are controlled by another family of proteins called the cyclins. Two CDKs in particular, CDK4 and CDK6, are controlled by cyclin D, which is often overproduced by cancer

Table 2.3 Kinase inhibitors used as cancer treatments and their targets.

Target protein	Where is it found?	Treatment examples	Indications
Intact growth factor receptors (i.e., not one that's part of a fusion protein)			
EGFR (also called HER1 or ErbB1)	On cells of many cancers, including those of the bowel, ovaries, lungs, head and neck, esophagus, and brain; found on healthy cells of many tissues and organs [50, 51]. The kinase domain is sometimes mutated and overactive in lung cancer cells [90].	Gefitinib, erlotinib, afatinib[a], dacomitinib[a], osimertinib, mobocertinib, poziotinib, and lapatinib	Non-small cell lung cancer (NSCLC) containing various *EGFR* mutations
HER2 (also called EGFR2, ErBb2, or Neu)	A growth factor receptor often found in excessive amounts on breast cancer cells and stomach cancer cells; found in small amounts in other cancers [52]. Found in lower levels than EGFR on a variety of healthy cells and tissues [59, 60].	Lapatinib, neratinib[a], tucatinib, and poziotinib	HER2-positive breast cancer and stomach cancer
MET	Low levels found in most tissues. Thought to be important in various cancer types and cause resistance to various targeted treatments. Mutated and overactive in around 3% of people with NSCLC [91, 92].	Tivantinib, capmatinib, and tepotinib; also blocked by various multi-kinase inhibitors such as crizotinib and cabozantinib	NSCLC containing *MET* exon 14 mutations
FGFRs	FGFRs are found on endothelial cells that line blood vessels. In 10%–30% of bladder cancers and cholangiocarcinomas (and in smaller proportions of other cancers), mutated versions of FGFRs are found on the cell surface or as part of a fusion protein in the cell cytoplasm [93].	Erdafitinib, pemigatinib, and infigratinib	*FGFR*-mutated bladder cancer and bile duct cancer (cholangiocarcinoma)
KIT and PDGFR-alpha (PDGFRα)	KIT and PDGFRα are found on various cell types; 80%–90% of gastrointestinal stromal tumors (GISTs) produce mutated versions of KIT and/or PDGFRα [94, 95].	Imatinib[b], sunitinib[b], regorafenib[b], avapritinib, and ripretinib	GISTs that produce mutated versions of KIT and/or PDGFRα
FLT3	A growth factor receptor mutated in the cancer cells of around a third of people with acute myeloid leukemia (AML) and almost always overproduced by AML cells; also found on the surface of some immature white blood cells [96, 97].	Midostaurin, lestaurtinib, quizartinib, crenolanib, and gilteritinib	*FLT3*-mutated AML
Intracellular kinases normally controlled by growth factor receptors			
mTOR	Plays a central role in regulating many cell functions, such as cell growth, metabolism, survival, and immune responses. Overactive in many cancer types due to mutations affecting the PI3K/AKT/mTOR pathway, but rarely directly affected by mutations [98].	Temsirolimus and everolimus	Kidney cancer, hormone receptor-positive breast cancer, and pancreatic neuroendocrine tumors
B-Raf	Involved in the Ras/Raf/MEK/ERK signaling pathway and mutated in around 7% of all solid tumors, including 40%–50% of melanomas, 10% of bowel cancers, and around 2%–4% of NSCLC [99–101].	Vemurafenib, dabrafenib, and encorafenib	*BRAF*-mutated melanoma, bowel cancer, NSCLC, and thyroid cancer
MEK	Involved in the Ras/Raf/MEK/ERK signaling pathway and controlled by Raf proteins: A-Raf, B-Raf, and C-Raf. MEK gene mutations are rare [101].	Trametinib, selumetinib, cobimetinib, and binimetinib	*BRAF*-mutated melanoma, bowel cancer, NSCLC, and thyroid cancer

Phosphatidyl-inositol-3-kinase-alpha (PI3Kα)	The PI3K/AKT/mTOR pathway controls diverse cell functions, including cell metabolism, cell growth, and survival. It is the most commonly activated pathway in human cancer. PI3Kα is often overactive due to mutations affecting the *PIK3CA* gene [102].	Alpelisib	*PIK3CA*-mutated, hormone receptor-positive breast cancer
Intracellular kinases controlled by cell surface receptors found on white blood cells			
JAK2	A signaling protein found in cells throughout the body. Activated by various cytokine receptors on the surface of white blood cells. It activates a family of transcription factors known as STATs. JAK inhibitors have a wide range of applications, including rheumatoid arthritis and other immune-related diseases [103].	Ruxolitinib, momelotinib, pacritinib, and fedratinib	Myeloproliferative neoplasms such as myelofibrosis and polycythemia vera
Bruton's tyrosine kinase (BTK)	A signaling protein controlled by the B cell receptor (BCR), which is found on the surface of B lymphocytes [104].	Ibrutinib, acalabrutinib, zanubrutinib, tirabrutinib, pirtobrutinib, and orelabrutinib	Chronic lymphocytic leukemia and non-Hodgkin lymphoma
Phosphatidyl-inositol-3-kinase-delta (PI3Kδ)	Controlled by the BCR and implicated in various B cell leukemias and lymphomas [105].	Idelalisib, copanlisib, duvelisib, and umbralisib	Chronic lymphocytic leukemia and non-Hodgkin lymphoma
Fusion proteins that contain the kinase portion of a growth factor receptor			
ALK fusions	The normal protein is a growth factor receptor important during brain development. Fusion proteins containing the kinase portion of ALK plus a second protein such as EML4 or NPM1 have been found in some people with NSCLC, anaplastic large cell lymphoma (ALCL), and other cancer types. ALK is also overactive in some neuroblastomas and other cancers [106].	Crizotinib, alectinib, ceritinib, brigatinib, lorlatinib, and entrectinib	NSCLC or ALCL containing ALK fusion proteins (ALK positive)
ROS1 fusions	ROS1 is a growth factor receptor similar to ALK. ROS1 fusion proteins are found in 1%–2% of NSCLC [107].	Entrectinib, crizotinib, lorlatinib, and repotrectinib	NSCLC containing a ROS1 fusion protein
RET fusions	RET is a growth factor receptor with various functions in the developing embryo. RET fusion proteins have been found in NSCLC and thyroid cancer [108].	Pralsetinib and selpercatinib	Thyroid cancer or NSCLC containing ROS1 fusion proteins
TRK fusions	TRKA, TRKB, and TRKC are growth factor receptors predominantly found in the brain. TRK fusion proteins are caused by *NTRK* gene fusions. They are found in a high proportion of some rare cancers (e.g., secretory breast cancer and congenital mesoblastic nephroma) and in much smaller proportions of some common cancers, such as NSCLC, breast cancer, and bowel cancer [82].	Entrectinib and larotrectinib	Any solid tumor with an *NTRK* gene fusion

(Continued)

Table 2.3 (Continued)

Target protein	Where is it found?	Treatment examples	Indications
Other kinase fusion proteins			
Bcr-Abl	The natural Abelson (Abl) kinase controls various processes in nerve cells [109]. The Bcr-Abl fusion protein is found in all cases of CML and in a proportion of people with acute lymphoblastic leukemia (ALL) [80].	Imatinib, dasatinib, bosutinib, nilotinib, ponatinib, and asciminib	CML and Bcr-Abl-positive ALL
Kinases involved in the cell cycle			
CDK4 and CDK6	CDKs control progress through the cell cycle. CDK4 and CDK6 are the first to be activated as a cell enters the cell cycle. They are overactive in cancer cells because of the overproduction of cyclin D, loss of natural CDK inhibitors such as p16, or mutation of the CDK4 gene [110].	Palbociclib, ribociclib, and abemaciclib	Hormone receptor-positive breast cancer
Kinases involved in angiogenesis			
VEGFRs (PDGFRs and FGFRs)	These growth factor receptors are found on endothelial cells that line normal blood vessels and those found in tumors; they are also sometimes found on cancer cells, although the significance of this is unclear. Because the ATP-binding sites of VEGF, PDGF, and FGF receptors are similar to one another, many of the drugs listed have some ability to block all three sets of receptors. These drugs may also block various other kinases (e.g., MET, RET, ALK, KIT, and FLT3) [111]. They often give the best results when used as treatments for kidney cancer, in which *VHL* mutations (which lead to excessive angiogenesis) are common [112].	Sunitinib, sorafenib, pazopanib, axitinib, regorafenib, cabozantinib, vandetanib, cediranib, lenvatinib, vatalanib, and tivozanib	Various solid tumors, including bowel cancer, ovarian cancer, cervical cancer, and kidney cancer

[a] Afatinib, dacomitinib, and neratinib are pan-HER inhibitors that block all EGFR receptors.
[b] Imatinib, regorafenib, and sunitinib are all multi-kinase inhibitors that block various kinases and therefore also have other uses.

cells. I'll look at CDK inhibitors properly in Chapter 4.

- Kinase inhibitors that target angiogenesis [111]. Angiogenesis is when a blood vessel sprouts side branches that elongate to create new blood vessels. Kinases that control this process include various growth factor receptors, such as VEGF receptors, PDGF receptors, and FGF receptors. As with other growth factor receptors, the internal portion of these receptors is where their kinase activity resides. Drugs that block them are known as angiogenesis inhibitors. There's more detail about these treatments in Chapter 4.

For some of these kinase targets, the kinase being blocked is a mutated, overactive version of the kinase, i.e., one that doesn't normally exist in healthy cells. These mutated kinases are ideal as drug targets as there's likely to be a large therapeutic window; the dose at which the drug kills cancer cells is likely to be a lot lower than the dose that causes lots of side effects. This makes it possible to give patients a dose that they can tolerate, and that will also be very effective. I've listed a few examples below.

- Various mutated versions of EGFR found in NSCLC
- The V600E version of the B-Raf protein, found in melanoma skin cancer and in small proportions of other cancers (e.g., NSCLC and bowel cancer)
- The Bcr-Abl fusion protein found in the cancer cells of people with chronic myeloid leukemia, and other kinase fusion proteins found in the cells of some people with other cancers, such as NSCLC and thyroid cancer

Another useful situation is where the cancer cells are massively overproducing a kinase because the cells have accidentally made extra copies of the kinase's gene. This is the situation for some people with breast cancer, stomach cancer, or gastroesophageal junction cancer. In about 20% of people with these cancers, the gene for HER2 is amplified

(there are extra copies of it) and there is an excessive amount of HER2 on the cells' surface. Because there is so much less HER2 in the rest of the body, again there is a useful therapeutic window. HER2-targeted kinase inhibitors are helpful, especially when the disease has spread to the brain.

A less promising scenario is when a kinase is normal, but it's overactive because of the impact of a mutation affecting another protein. For example, if cancer cells contain a *KRAS* gene mutation, this has a knock-on effect on various kinases, such as B-Raf, PI3K, and MEK. We don't have drugs that block most K-Ras mutants, and targeting the downstream kinases hasn't been terribly effective in the trials conducted so far [114].

2.3.6 Limitations of Kinase Inhibitors and Reasons Why They Cause Side Effects

As with antibody-based treatments, kinase inhibitors have some important limitations. I've listed some of them below.

Reasons why they might not work at all or only work for a limited amount of time: [75, 115–117]

- Resistance to kinase inhibitors is commonly due to additional mutations in the gene for the target kinase. For example, the T790M mutation in the *EGFR* gene changes the shape of its ATP-binding site and causes resistance to some EGFR inhibitors [118]. Also, the C481S mutation in the *BTK* gene causes resistance to ibrutinib by removing the amino acid that ibrutinib binds to [119].
- Resistance might also be caused by mutations affecting a different pathway or protein that can substitute for the targeted protein. For example, mutations in *KRAS* cause resistance to EGFR inhibitors (Figure 3.10).
- Amplification of the gene (i.e., extra copies of the gene) for the target protein can lead to such high protein levels that the drug is overwhelmed – you simply cannot

give the patient a high enough dose of the drug for it to completely block its target.

- If the drug's target isn't essential for the survival of cancer cells, then the cells won't die. This might be intrinsic resistance, i.e., the cancer cells are configured in such a way that the target simply isn't that important to them. Or it could be acquired resistance, i.e., most cancer cells are killed by the treatment, but small pockets of cells contain mutations that cause resistance, and these cells multiply and cause the disease to return months or years later.

- There may be cancer cells in protected environments (e.g., brain or bone marrow) where the drug can't penetrate.

- Epigenetic changes and changes to the cancer cells' appearance and behavior can also cause resistance, although the precise reason isn't always obvious.

- If the drug isn't very targeted, and/or the target is on lots of healthy cells, then the dose needed to destroy cancer cells might be very similar to the dose that causes intolerable side effects. This means that you won't be able to give the patient a dose of treatment that would have the potential to cure them.

- There is a high degree of drug-to-drug and patient-to-patient variation in the concentration of these treatments in the blood, how long they remain there, how they get broken down, and what proportion is floating free (rather than being stuck to blood proteins). This can make it difficult to find the optimum dose for an individual patient.

Reasons why they cause side effects:

- Kinase inhibitors tend to be less precise compared to antibody treatments. For example, in laboratory experiments, sunitinib and pazopanib are each able to block the activity of at least 30 different kinases [120]. As mentioned earlier, the ability of kinase inhibitors to block more than one target can be an advantage. But this same ability also leads to a greater number of side effects.

- Like the antibody treatments, these drugs' targets will be present in healthy cells as well as cancer cells. Destruction of healthy cells and damage to tissues in which the drug's target is present will cause side effects.

Reasons why we don't have a kinase inhibitor suitable for every patient:

- Cell communication pathways involve lots of kinases (Figure 2.20). However, not every protein involved is a kinase. For example, cancer cells often contain overactive versions of Ras enzymes such as K-Ras. However, Ras enzymes are not kinases, and it has proven very difficult to create drugs that block them.

- If a patient's tumor is incredibly diverse, with lots of intratumoral heterogeneity and many pockets of cancer cells driven by different mutations, then finding a suitable kinase to block might be an impossible task.

- Although it might seem that there is an endless list of kinase inhibitors approved as treatments for cancer, the actual number of targets is pretty small. So, even if a person's cancer is driven by a powerful kinase, we might not have a drug that can block it.

- Many patients' cancers are driven by faults that have nothing to do with kinases. For example, the most common mutations in small cell lung cancer affect two tumor suppressor genes, *TP53* and *RB* [121, 122].

- The possibility of prescribing a patient a kinase inhibitor often rests on the results of a biopsy analysis. But sometimes it isn't safe to perform a biopsy. Other times, the biopsy sample obtained is too small for analysis, or it contains too few cancer cells. In these instances, you don't know whether a targetable kinase exists in the patient's cancer cells or not.

2.3.7 Small Molecules with Non-Kinase Targets

As you've gathered by now, most small molecule cancer drugs have been designed to block kinases. However, we do have some

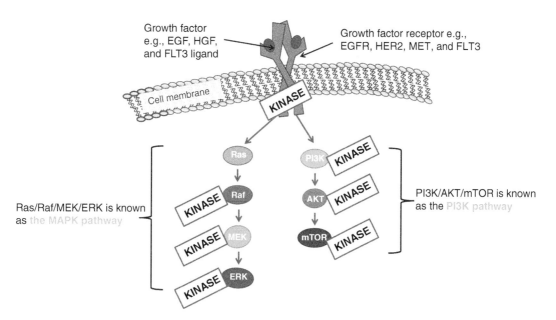

Figure 2.20 Cell communication pathways involve lots of kinases. Growth factor receptors on the cell surface have an internal kinase domain. Raf proteins (A-Raf, B-Raf, and C-Raf), MEK proteins (MEK1 and MEK2), and ERK proteins (ER1 and ERK2) are all kinases. As are the main components of the PI3K pathway: PI3K, AKT, and mTOR. The only proteins in this illustration that are not kinases are the Ras enzymes (K-Ras, N-Ras, and H-Ras).

Abbreviations: EGF – epidermal growth factor; EGFR – EGF receptor; ERK – extracellular-signal-regulated kinase; FLT3 – Fms-like tyrosine kinase; HER2 – human EGF receptor-2; HGF – hepatocyte growth factor; MAPK – mitogen-activated protein kinase; mTOR – mammalian target of rapamycin; PI3K – phosphatidylinositol 3-kinase.

drugs with non-kinase targets. As with the kinase inhibitors, some of these drugs are very precise, and some less so. Also, some of them have a target that is far more important for cancer cells than healthy cells. This means that when they work, it's obvious why this is the case, whereas for others, it can be difficult to unpick their effects and work out exactly why it is that they're helpful.

These drugs are summarized below and listed in Table 2.4:

• Drugs that block PARP enzymes [123]. Our cells use PARP enzymes to repair nicks – single-strand breaks – in their DNA. These nicks occur thousands of times a day in every cell in our body. If PARP enzymes are blocked with a PARP inhibitor, then some of these nicks become complete breaks (double-strand DNA breaks) that

need repairing quickly. Healthy cells quickly step in and repair these breaks. But in some cancers (notably ovarian cancer) the cancer cells have problems with double-strand break repair, making them vulnerable to PARP inhibitors. See Section 4.3 for more information on PARP inhibitors.

• Drugs that block Bcl-2 or other proteins that promote cell survival [124]. It seems an obvious thing to say that healthy cells don't want to die (see Section 4.7). However, at every moment, they're closely monitoring themselves for signs of irreparable damage or stress. And, if they find these things, they will trigger a self-destruct process called apoptosis. In contrast, cancer cells know that there's something wrong. They're aware that they contain DNA damage and toxic levels of faulty proteins, and

Table 2.4 Small molecules with non-kinase targets.

Target proteins	What is it? Where is it found? [40]	Treatment examples	Indications
PARP enzymes	They are important DNA repair enzymes found in cells throughout the body.	Olaparib, rucaparib, niraparib, talazoparib, and veliparib	Ovarian cancer, breast cancer, prostate cancer, and pancreatic cancer
Bcl-2	A powerful protein that can keep cells alive, even when damaged. Found in many tissues throughout the body.	Venetoclax	Some hematological cancers, e.g., chronic lymphocytic leukemia and acute myeloid leukemia (AML)
Epigenetic enzymes	A wide variety of enzymes found in all our cells; responsible for controlling gene activity by altering the way DNA is stored and manipulated.	HDAC inhibitors: vorinostat, belinostat, panobinostat, and romidepsin DNMT inhibitors: azacitidine and decitabine IDH1 and IDH2 inhibitors: ivosidenib and enasidenib	Some hematological cancers, e.g., cutaneous T cell lymphoma, AML, and myelodysplastic syndromes
Smoothened	Part of the Hedgehog pathway; found in many tissues and important in the developing embryo.	Vismodegib, sonidegib, glasdegib, saridegib, taladegib, and itraconazole	Basal cell carcinoma, and AML
Proteasomes	Found in all cells and tissues. Responsible for recycling proteins and releasing amino acids.	Bortezomib, carfilzomib, and ixazomib	Myeloma and mantle cell lymphoma
Cereblon	Found in most cells and tissues. Involved in tagging proteins ready for destruction by the proteasome.	Thalidomide, lenalidomide, and pomalidomide	Myeloma and various non-Hodgkin lymphomas
Exportin-1 (XPO-1)	Responsible for transporting hundreds of proteins and other complicated molecules out of the nucleus and into the cytoplasm.	Selinexor	Myeloma and diffuse large B cell lymphoma

they often live in a toxic, low oxygen environment. And yet, despite all of this, they stay alive. One of the "stay alive at all costs" proteins that cancer cells contain, and that protects them against apoptosis, is called Bcl-2. Perhaps not surprisingly, Bcl-2 inhibitors have proven to be helpful against some cancers, particularly those with extremely high levels of Bcl-2 inside them.

• Drugs that target enzymes involved in epigenetics [125], including inhibitors of histone deacetylase enzymes, IDH1 and IDH2 (isocitrate dehydrogenase 1/2), and DNA methyltransferases (DNMTs). (If you want to know about epigenetics, look at

Section 4.6). The epigenetic regulation of our genes involves over 700 different proteins. These proteins add and remove different chemical groups (e.g., methyl, acetyl, and phosphate) from DNA and from the histone proteins it is wrapped around. Scientists have found gene mutations affecting virtually every epigenetic protein in almost all types of cancer. But it's not clear what these mutations mean for cancer cells, or how they are affecting their behavior. There are some drugs that block epigenetic regulators that are licensed as cancer treatments, but it's often difficult to pinpoint their mechanism of action.

- Drugs that target the hedgehog pathway by blocking Smoothened [126, 127]. The hedgehog pathway involves proteins such as Sonic Hedgehog, Patched, and Smoothened (see Section 4.5). Scientists believe that these proteins, and this pathway, play an important role in normal embryo development in a wide range of organisms. The pathway is also overactive in basal cell carcinoma skin cancer (BCC), and two cancers that mostly affect children: medulloblastoma (a cancer that occurs in brain and spinal cord) and rhabdomyosarcoma (a cancer that usually occurs in muscles that are attached to bones). In addition, the Hedgehog pathway is active in AML, particularly in cancer cells resistant to chemotherapy [128]. Drugs that target the Smoothened protein block the Hedgehog pathway. At one point, scientists thought that Smoothened inhibitors would be helpful against a range of cancers, but they're mostly given to people with BCC or AML.

- Drugs that block proteasomes [129]. Each cell in our body contains up to 1 million proteasomes [130]. These cylindrical structures are made from layers of proteins stacked around a hollow core (see Section 4.10). Inside this core are many enzyme sites capable of chopping up proteins. In fact, every second of every day, our cells are using their ribosomes to manufacture proteins and using their proteasomes to destroy them. Many cancers rely on proteasomes to destroy tumor suppressor proteins or cell cycle proteins that might otherwise limit their ability to multiply. Myeloma cells in particular seem dependent on keeping their proteasomes working at full tilt to keep them alive. Not surprisingly then, proteasome inhibitors are staple myeloma treatments.

- Drugs that target cereblon and influence the immune system as well as affecting other processes (e.g., thalidomide, pomalidomide, and lenalidomide) [131]. If you know anything about thalidomide, you probably think of it as a morning sickness treatment that caused thousands of babies to be born with deformities in the 1950s. Since that time, thalidomide has become a useful treatment for some hematological cancers, such as myeloma, lymphomas, chronic lymphoblastic leukemia, and myelodysplastic syndromes. Thalidomide and its chemical cousins, lenalidomide and pomalidomide, all bind to a protein in our cells called cereblon. They have direct effects on cancer cells, as well as impacting the environment in which the cancer cells live. For example, they alter the actions of various types of white blood cells (hence being referred to as immunomodulators), and I cover them in Section 6.3.

- Drugs that affect the transport of proteins out of the nucleus [132]. Our cells have an inner nucleus that contains the cell's DNA. Surrounding the nucleus is the cytoplasm. Various transport proteins are responsible for escorting proteins and other complex molecules back and forth. One such protein, called XPO1, transports hundreds of different proteins out of the nucleus and into the cytoplasm. Overproduction of XPO1 is a common feature of many cancers, and various drugs that block XPO1 are in trials. One, selinexor, is an approved treatment for people with myeloma and is also in trials for other cancer types. I cover transport protein inhibitors in Section 4.9.

2.4 TREATMENT COMBINATIONS

So far in this chapter, I have described each treatment individually. However, people with cancer are often given combinations of treatments. In the past, they would most likely have been combinations of chemotherapy drugs. But these days, it might be a monoclonal antibody plus a kinase inhibitor, or another combination.

There are various reasons why a combination of treatments often works better than one on its own:

1. Cancer cell behavior is driven by a combination of different factors, such as the location, number, type, and combination of DNA mutations the cells contain; the influence of non-cancer cells close by; their access to a blood supply; whether they're attacked by the patient's immune system; and what other treatments the person might be taking to control other medical conditions. So, it makes sense to combine treatments that target cancer cells in different ways.

2. There is often diversity (heterogeneity) between populations of cancer cells in a tumor or blood cancer. Each population will vary in its sensitivity to different types of treatment. Therefore, it makes sense to combine treatments that work in different ways to kill as many cells as possible.

3. There may be cancer cells in protected locations in the body, such as the brain, bone marrow, or nerves. Each type of drug, particularly an antibody or a small molecule, varies in its ability to penetrate each environment. So, again, it makes sense to combine treatments that can reach cancer cells in different locations.

4. Every cancer drug causes side effects. These are often related to (1) the physical nature of the drug, (2) its target, and (3) its selectivity for that target. By combining drugs with different side effect profiles, you can increase the amount of treatment you can safely give to the patient, while keeping each side effect at a tolerable level.

5. Sometimes drugs enhance one another's effects, creating synergy. For example, a drug that helps white blood cells to mature and get in and out of blood vessels (a possible feature of angiogenesis inhibitors) might enhance the effects of a treatment that uses white blood cells to attack and destroy cancer cells (such as checkpoint inhibitors) [133, 134].

6. To prolong a treatment's effects. For example, B-Raf inhibitors are often effective against *BRAF*-mutated melanoma skin cancer (*BRAF* is the gene for making B-Raf protein). But giving a B-Raf inhibitor on its own only works for a few months. Combining together a B-Raf inhibitor with a MEK inhibitor results in longer-lasting disease control [100].

7. Sometimes there are predictable intrinsic resistance mechanisms that can be blocked or avoided using a treatment combination. For example, a proportion of bowel cancers contain *BRAF* mutations. But, unlike in melanoma skin cancer, B-Raf inhibitors don't affect *BRAF*-mutated bowel cancers because of a feedback loop involving the EGFR. So, instead, patients are given a combination of a B-Raf inhibitor plus an EGFR-targeted treatment.

8. Sometimes you don't know why it works. Drug combinations can be put together using scientific evidence to try and predict which drugs, in which combinations, will work best. But this often doesn't work. Also, drugs thought to work through one mechanism sometimes turn out later to work via a totally different mechanism [135]. In addition, many cancer treatments and cancer discoveries have come about through luck and serendipity [136]. So, sometimes it's worth giving a combination a try, even if there isn't a powerful scientific reason to do so.

2.5 FINAL THOUGHTS

Since the 1980s and 1990s, there has been a rapid increase in the number of cancer drugs that don't fit the traditional term, chemotherapy. Rather than working by killing any multiplying cell (how most chemotherapies work), these drugs have (mostly) been deliberately designed to target a specific protein or process. The targeted protein/process has been chosen because of its importance to cancer cells. The vast majority of these targeted treatments are either small chemical compounds, or they're based on the structure of antibodies made by our immune system to fight infections.

In this chapter, I've tried to describe these two groups of treatments and explain their advantages and drawbacks. Perhaps the biggest drawback (and one that's often downplayed or misunderstood) is that their targets are virtually always present in, or on, healthy cells as well as cancer cells. So, even if they precisely block or attach to their target, they will still cause side effects.

Another source of confusion is that fact that antibody-based treatments have an added dimension in that they can attract and activate white blood cells like macrophages and NK cells and generate immune responses. Antibodies that attach to checkpoint proteins or their ligands can also boost the number and activity of T cells. This means that antibody-based treatments can be referred to both as targeted treatments and as immunotherapies.

I hope it's also now clear to you that antibodies and small molecules are sometimes used to block the same targets, i.e., many of them block growth factor receptors (e.g., HER2, EGFR, MET, FGFRs, and VEGFRs) and the signaling pathways under the receptors' control (Figure 2.21). For this reason, they have an overlapping set of uses and side effects.

Two of the most important differences between monoclonal antibodies and small molecules are the following:

1. Their specificity for their target. Monoclonal antibody treatments, like the antibodies generated during our body's response to an infection, are incredibly precise. In contrast, for example, most small molecule kinase inhibitors work by entering ATP-binding sites on kinases, and many kinases have very similar ATP-binding sites. Hence, kinase inhibitors tend

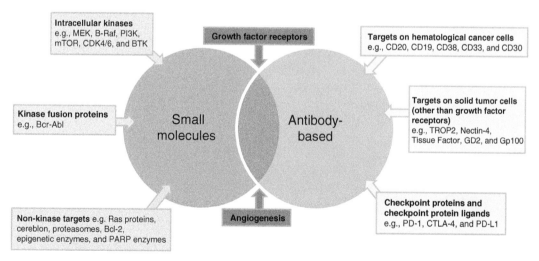

Figure 2.21 Targets of small molecule- and antibody-based cancer treatments. Small molecules easily cross the cell membrane, and therefore their targets are in the cell cytoplasm and nucleus. Antibodies are much larger, and the targets of antibody-based treatments are proteins on the cell surface. Growth factor receptors are cell surface receptors that span the cell membrane and have a cytoplasmic kinase domain. It is therefore possible to block growth factor receptors using both antibodies and small molecules. Angiogenesis, the growth of blood vessels, involves various growth factor receptors.
Abbreviations: BTK – Burton tyrosine kinase; PARP – poly(ADP-ribose)polymerase; PI3K – phosphoinositide 3-kinase.

to block many different kinases alongside the one they've been created to block. This adds to the toxicities caused by kinase inhibitors, but it can also boost their impact on tumors (in which many different kinases may be overactive for different reasons).

2. Their size. By their nature, antibodies (and even small segments of antibodies) are too big to diffuse across cell membranes. This means that the targets of antibodies are always cell surface proteins. In contrast, small molecules can block proteins in the cytoplasm and nucleus.

It's important to remember that we still only have a relatively small number of proteins and processes that we can target with treatments. Cancer cells are often driven by numerous mutations, and they exhibit many behaviors that it would theoretically be helpful to block. But even now, despite discovering and categorizing thousands of genes and proteins involved in driving cancer's behavior, we are still only able to successfully block a small handful of these potential targets.

Having said all of that, in this chapter I have mentioned well over a hundred drugs that target 50 or so different proteins found in or on cancer cells. In the following chapters, I will look at these treatments in greater detail.

REFERENCES

1 Drago JZ, Modi S, Chandarlapaty S (2021). Unlocking the potential of antibody–drug conjugates for cancer therapy. *Nat Rev Clin Oncol* **18**(6). doi: 10.1038/s41571-021-00470-8.

2 Lesterhuis WJ, Haanen JBAG, Punt CJA (2011). Cancer immunotherapy-revisited. *Nat Rev Drug Discovery* **10**(8). doi: 10.1038/nrd3500.

3 Cohen P (2002). Protein kinases – the major drug targets of the twenty-first century? *Nat Rev Drug Discovery* **1**(4). doi: 10.1038/nrd773.

4 Craig Jordan V (1997). Tamoxifen treatment for breast cancer: Concept to gold standard. *Oncology* **11**: 7.

5 Crawford ED (2004). Hormonal therapy in prostate cancer: Historical approaches. *Rev Urol* **6**(Suppl 7): S3.

6 DeVita VT, Chu E (2008). A history of cancer chemotherapy. *Cancer Res* **68**(21). doi: 10.1158/0008-5472.CAN-07-6611.

7 Thariat J *et al.* (2013). Past, present, and future of radiotherapy for the benefit of patients. *Nat Rev Clin Oncol* **10**(1). doi: 10.1038/nrclinonc.2012.203.

8 Zhang Y, Zhang Z (2020). The history and advances in cancer immunotherapy: Understanding the characteristics of tumor-infiltrating immune cells and their therapeutic implications. *Cell Mol Immunol* **17**: 807–821. doi: 10.1038/s41423-020-0488-6.

9 Liu JKH (2014). The history of monoclonal antibody development – progress, remaining challenges and future innovations. *Ann Med Surg* **3**(4) Elsevier Ltd: 113–116. doi: 10.1016/j.amsu.2014.09.001.

10 Vickers E (2018). *A Beginner's Guide to Targeted Cancer Treatments*, 1st ed. Wiley-Blackwell.

11 Sompayrac L (2019). Lecture 3 B Cells and Antibodies. In *How the Immune System Works*. 6th ed. Wiley-Blackwell. pp. 27–41.

12 Goydel RS, Rader C (2021). Antibody-based cancer therapy. *Oncogene* **40**(21). doi: 10.1038/s41388-021-01811-8.

13 Adams GP, Weiner LM (2005). Monoclonal antibody therapy of cancer. *Nat Biotechnol* **23**(9). doi: 10.1038/nbt1137.

14 Scott AM, Wolchok JD, Old LJ (2012). Antibody therapy of cancer. *Nat Rev Cancer* **12**(4): 278–287. doi: 10.1038/nrc3236.

15 Salles G *et al.* (2017). Rituximab in B-Cell hematologic malignancies: A review of 20 years of clinical experience. *Adv Ther* **34**(10). doi: 10.1007/s12325-017-0612-x.

16 Grillo-Lopez A *et al.* (2005). Rituximab the first monoclonal antibody approved for the treatment of lymphoma. *Curr Pharm Biotechnol* **1**(1). doi: 10.2174/1389201003379059.

17 Burke E Biomanufacturing: How biologics are made. *BiotechPrimer*. [Online] Available: https://weekly.biotechprimer.com/biomanufacturing-how-biologics-are-made/ [Accessed February 8, 2022].

18 Lu RM *et al.* (2020). Development of therapeutic antibodies for the treatment of diseases. *J Biomed Sci* **27**(1). doi: 10.1186/s12929-019-0592-z.

19 Zhou S *et al*. (2021). The landscape of bispecific T cell engager in cancer treatment. *Biomark. Res.* **9**(1). doi: 10.1186/s40364-021-00294-9.

20 Weiner GJ (2015). Building better monoclonal antibody-based therapeutics. *Nat Rev Cancer* **15**(6) Nature Publishing Group: 361–370. doi: 10.1038/nrc3930.

21 Gajria D, Chandarlapaty S (2011). HER2-amplified breast cancer: Mechanisms of trastuzumab resistance and novel targeted therapies. *Expert Rev Anticancer Ther* **11**(2). doi: 10.1586/era.10.226.

22 Zahavi D, Weiner L (2020). Monoclonal antibodies in cancer therapy. *Antibodies* **9**(3): 34. doi: 10.3390/antib9030034.

23 Scott AM, Allison JP, Wolchok JD (2012). Monoclonal antibodies in cancer therapy. *Cancer Immun* **12**: 34.

24 Larson SM *et al*. (2015). Radioimmunotherapy of human tumours. *Nat Rev Cancer* **15**(6). doi: 10.1038/nrc3925.

25 Smaglo BG, Aldeghaither D, Weiner LM (2014). The development of immunoconjugates for targeted cancer therapy. *Nat Rev Clin Oncol* **11**(11). doi: 10.1038/nrclinonc.2014.159.

26 Kreitman RJ, Pastan I (2011). Antibody fusion proteins: Anti-CD22 recombinant immunotoxin moxetumomab pasudotox. *Clin Cancer Res* **17**(20). doi: 10.1158/1078-0432.CCR-11-0487.

27 Tarantino P *et al*. (2023). Optimizing the safety of antibody–drug conjugates for patients with solid tumours. *Nat Rev Clin Oncol* **20**(8): 558–576. doi: 10.1038/s41571-023-00783-w.

28 Weiner L, Surana R, Wang S (2010). Antibodies and cancer therapy: Versatile platforms for cancer immunotherapy. *Nat Rev Immunol* **10**(5): 317.

29 van de Donk NWCJ, Usmani SZ (2018). CD38 antibodies in multiple myeloma: Mechanisms of action and modes of resistance. *Front Immunol* **9**(SEP). doi: 10.3389/fimmu.2018.02134.

30 Mandó P *et al*. (2021). Targeting ADCC: A different approach to HER2 breast cancer in the immunotherapy era. *Breast* **60**. doi: 10.1016/j.breast.2021.08.007.

31 Murata Y *et al*. (2020). Blockade of CD47 or SIRPα: A new cancer immunotherapy. *Expert Opin Ther Targets* **24**(10). doi: 10.1080/14728222.2020.1811855.

32 Tong B, Wang M (2018). CD47 is a novel potent immunotherapy target in human malignancies: Current studies and future promises. *Future Oncol* **14**(21). doi: 10.2217/fon-2018-0035.

33 Chao MP *et al*. (2020). Therapeutic targeting of the macrophage immune checkpoint CD47 in myeloid malignancies. *Future Oncol* **9**. doi: 10.3389/fonc.2019.01380.

34 Feins S *et al*. (2019). An introduction to chimeric antigen receptor (CAR) T-cell immunotherapy for human cancer. *Am J Hematol* **94**(S1). doi: 10.1002/ajh.25418.

35 Lee CM, Tannock IF (2010). The distribution of the therapeutic monoclonal antibodies cetuximab and trastuzumab within solid tumors. *BMC Cancer* **10**. doi: 10.1186/1471-2407-10-255.

36 Cai WQ *et al*. (2020). The latest battles between EGFR monoclonal antibodies and resistant tumor cells. *Front Oncol* **10**. doi: 10.3389/fonc.2020.01249.

37 Guan M *et al*. (2015). Adverse events of monoclonal antibodies used for cancer therapy. *Biomed Res Int* **2015**. doi: 10.1155/2015/428169.

38 Michot JM *et al*. (2016). Immune-related adverse events with immune checkpoint blockade: A comprehensive review. *Eur J Cancer* **54**. doi: 10.1016/j.ejca.2015.11.016.

39 Fu Z *et al*. (2022). Antibody drug conjugate: The 'biological missile' for targeted cancer therapy. *Signal Transduct Target Ther* **7**(1): 93. doi: 10.1038/s41392-022-00947-7.

40 Uhlén M *et al*. (2015). Tissue-based map of the human proteome. *Science (1979)* **347**(6220). doi: 10.1126/science.1260419.

41 Hammer O (2012). CD19 as an attractive target for antibody-based therapy. *mAbs* **4**(5). doi: 10.4161/mabs.21338.

42 Maloney DG (2012). Anti-CD20 antibody therapy for B-cell lymphomas. *N Engl J Med* **366**(21). doi: 10.1056/nejmct1114348.

43 Lanza F *et al*. (2020). CD22 expression in b-cell acute lymphoblastic leukemia: Biological significance and implications for inotuzumab therapy in adults. *Cancers* **12**(2). doi: 10.3390/cancers12020303.

44 Schirrmann T *et al*. (2014). CD30 as a therapeutic target for lymphoma. *BioDrugs* **28**(2). doi: 10.1007/s40259-013-0068-8.

45 Ehninger A *et al*. (2014). Distribution and levels of cell surface expression of CD33 and CD123 in acute myeloid leukemia. *Blood Cancer J* **4**(6). doi: 10.1038/bcj.2014.39.

46 Phipps C *et al.* (2015). Daratumumab and its potential in the treatment of multiple myeloma: Overview of the preclinical and clinical development. *Ther Adv Hematol* **6**(3). doi: 10.1177/2040620715572295.

47 Assi R *et al.* (2021). Polatuzumab vedotin: Current role and future applications in the treatment of patients with diffuse large B-cell lymphoma. *Clin Hematol Int* **3**(1). doi: 10.2991/chi.k.210305.001.

48 van de Donk NWCJ *et al.* (2016). Clinical efficacy and management of monoclonal antibodies targeting CD38 and SLAMF7 in multiple myeloma. *Blood* **127**(6). doi: 10.1182/blood-2015-10-646810.

49 Shah N *et al.* (2020). B-cell maturation antigen (BCMA) in multiple myeloma: Rationale for targeting and current therapeutic approaches. *Leukemia* **34**(4). doi: 10.1038/s41375-020-0734-z.

50 Bublil EM, Yarden Y (2007). The EGF receptor family: Spearheading a merger of signaling and therapeutics. *Curr Opin Cell Biol* **19**(2): 124.

51 Hynes NE, Lane HA (2005). ERBB receptors and cancer: The complexity of targeted inhibitors. *Nat Rev Cancer* **5**(5). doi: 10.1038/nrc1609.

52 Arguello D *et al.* (2014). HER2 distribution in diverse tumors: Analysis of 11,493 nonbreast, nongastric cancers. *J Clin Oncol* **32**(15_suppl). doi: 10.1200/jco.2014.32.15_suppl.e22200.

53 Press MF, Cordon-Cardo C, Slamon DJ (1990). Expression of the HER-2/neu proto-oncogene in normal human adult and fetal tissues. *Oncogene* **5**(7).

54 Natali PG *et al.* (1990). Expression of the p185 encoded by her2 oncogene in normal and transformed human tissues. *Int J Cancer* **45**(3). doi: 10.1002/ijc.2910450314.

55 Yang RK, Sondel PM (2010). Anti-GD2 strategy in the treatment of neuroblastoma. *Drugs Future* **35**(8). doi: 10.1358/dof.2010.035.08.1513490.

56 Martinez-Perez D *et al.* (2021). Gp-100 as a novel therapeutic target in uveal melanoma. *Cancers* **13**(23). doi: 10.3390/cancers13235968.

57 Recondo G *et al.* (2020). Targeting MET dysregulation in cancer. *Cancer Discov* **10**(7). doi: 10.1158/2159-8290.CD-19-1446.

58 Hisada Y, Mackman N (2019). Tissue factor and cancer: Regulation, tumor growth, and metastasis. *Semin Thromb Hemostasis* **45**(4). doi: 10.1055/s-0039-1687894.

59 Kasthuri RS, Taubman MB, Mackman N (2009). Role of tissue factor in cancer. *J Clin Oncol* **27**: 4834–4838. doi: 10.1200/JCO.2009.22.6324.

60 Trerotola M *et al.* (2013). Upregulation of Trop-2 quantitatively stimulates human cancer growth. *Oncogene* **32**: 222–233. doi: 10.1038/onc.2012.36.

61 Hicklin DJ, Ellis LM (2005). Role of the vascular endothelial growth factor pathway in tumor growth and angiogenesis. *J Clin Oncol* **23**(5). doi: 10.1200/JCO.2005.06.081.

62 Garcia J *et al.* (2020). Bevacizumab (Avastin®) in cancer treatment: A review of 15 years of clinical experience and future outlook. *Cancer Treat Rev* **86**. doi: 10.1016/j.ctrv.2020.102017.

63 Oyewole-Said D *et al.* (2020). Beyond T-Cells: functional characterization of CTLA-4 expression in immune and non-immune cell types. *Front Immunol* **11**. doi: 10.3389/fimmu.2020.608024.

64 Quezada SA, Peggs KS (2013). Exploiting CTLA-4, PD-1 and PD-L1 to reactivate the host immune response against cancer. *Br J Cancer* **108**(8). doi: 10.1038/bjc.2013.117.

65 Sun NY *et al.* (2019). Blockade of PD-L1 enhances cancer immunotherapy by regulating dendritic cell maturation and macrophage polarization. *Cancers (Basel)* **11**(9). doi: 10.3390/cancers11091400.

66 Zheng K, Bantog C, Bayer R (2011). The impact of glycosylation on monoclonal antibody conformation and stability. *MAbs* **3**(6). doi: 10.4161/mabs.3.6.17922.

67 Vulto AG, Jaquez OA (2017). The process defines the product: What really matters in biosimilar design and production? *Rheumatology (Oxford, England)* **56**(4). doi: 10.1093/rheumatology/kex278.

68 Konstantinidou S, Papaspiliou A, Kokkotou E (2020). Current and future roles of biosimilars in oncology practice (Review). *Oncol Lett* **19**(1). doi: 10.3892/ol.2019.11105.

69 Bloomfield D *et al.* (2022). Characteristics of clinical trials evaluating biosimilars in the treatment of cancer. *JAMA Oncol.* doi: 10.1001/jamaoncol.2021.7230.

70 Biosimilar medicines: Overview. *EMA website.* [Online] Available: https://www.ema.europa.eu/en/human-regulatory/overview/biosimilar-medicines-overview [Accessed November 10, 2023].

71 Zhang J, Yang PL, Gray NS (2009). Targeting cancer with small molecule kinase inhibitors. *Nat Rev Cancer* **9**(1): 28–39. doi: 10.1038/nrc2559.

72 Hoelder S, Clarke PA, Workman P (2012). Discovery of small molecule cancer drugs: Successes, challenges and opportunities. *Mol Oncol* **6**(2). doi: 10.1016/j.molonc.2012.02.004.

73 Zhong L *et al.* (2021). Small molecules in targeted cancer therapy: Advances, challenges, and future perspectives. *Signal Transduction Targeted Ther* **6**(1). doi: 10.1038/s41392-021-00572-w.

74 Sofi MY, Shafi A, Masoodi KZ (2022). Introduction to Computer-aided Drug Design. In *Bioinformatics for Everyone*. pp. 215–229. doi: 10.1016/B978-0-323-91128-3.00002-1.

75 Cohen P, Cross D, Jänne PA (2021). Kinase drug discovery 20 years after imatinib: Progress and future directions. *Nat Rev Drug Discov* **20**(7): 551–569. doi: 10.1038/s41573-021-00195-4.

76 Groenland SL *et al.* (2021). The right dose: From phase I to clinical practice. *Am Soc Clin Oncol Educ Book* **41**. doi: 10.1200/edbk_319567.

77 Fares J *et al.* (2020). Landscape of combination therapy trials in breast cancer brain metastasis. *Int J Cancer* **147**(7). doi: 10.1002/ijc.32937.

78 Goss G *et al.* (2018). CNS response to osimertinib in patients with T790M-positive advanced NSCLC: Pooled data from two phase II trials. *Ann Oncol* **29**(3). doi: 10.1093/annonc/mdx820.

79 Palma G *et al.* (2021). Selective KRAS G12C inhibitors in non-small cell lung cancer: Chemistry, concurrent pathway alterations, and clinical outcomes. *npj Precis Oncol* **5**(1). doi: 10.1038/s41698-021-00237-5.

80 Quintás-Cardama A, Cortes J (2009). Molecular biology of bcr-abl1-positive chronic myeloid leukemia. *Blood* **113**(8). doi: 10.1182/blood-2008-03-144790.

81 Armour AA, Watkins CL (2010). The challenge of targeting egfr: Experience with gefitinib in nonsmall cell lung cancer. *Eur Respir Rev* **19**(117). doi: 10.1183/09059180.00005110.

82 Cocco E, Scaltriti M, Drilon A (2018). NTRK fusion-positive cancers and TRK inhibitor therapy. *Nat Rev Clin Oncol* **15**(12). doi: 10.1038/s41571-018-0113-0.

83 Ardito F *et al.* (2017). The crucial role of protein phosphorylation in cell signalingand its use as targeted therapy (review). *Int J Mol Med* **40**(2). doi: 10.3892/ijmm.2017.3036.

84 The Editors (2024). Adenosine triphosphate. *The Encyclopaedia Britannica*. [Online] Available: https://www.britannica.com/science/adenosine-triphosphate [Accessed February 14, 2022].

85 Alberts B, Johnson A, Lewis J (2002). Protein Function. In *Molecular Biology of the Cell. 4th edition*. New York: Garland Science. [Online] Available: https://www.ncbi.nlm.nih.gov/books/NBK26911/#A503 [Accessed February 14, 2022].

86 Cicenas J *et al.* (2018). Kinases and cancer. *Cancers (Basel)* **10**(3): 63. doi: 10.3390/cancers10030063.

87 Bhullar KS *et al.* (2018). Kinase-targeted cancer therapies: Progress, challenges and future directions. *Mol Cancer* **17**(1). doi: 10.1186/s12943-018-0804-2.

88 Roskoski R (2016). Classification of small molecule protein kinase inhibitors based upon the structures of their drug-enzyme complexes. *Pharmacol Res* **103**. doi: 10.1016/j.phrs.2015.10.021.

89 Gibbons DL *et al.* (2012). The rise and fall of gatekeeper mutations? The BCR-ABL1 T315I paradigm. *Cancer* **118**(2). doi: 10.1002/cncr.26225.

90 Russo A *et al.* (2015). A decade of EGFR inhibition in EGFR-mutated non small cell lung cancer (NSCLC): Old successes and future perspectives. *Oncotarget* **6**(29). doi: 10.18632/oncotarget.4254.

91 Hong L *et al.* (2021). Current and future treatment options for MET exon 14 skipping alterations in non-small cell lung cancer. *Ther Adv Med Oncol* **13**. doi: 10.1177/1758835921992976.

92 Fu J *et al.* (2021). HGF/c-MET pathway in cancer: From molecular characterization to clinical evidence. *Oncogene* **40**(28). doi: 10.1038/s41388-021-01863-w.

93 Krook MA *et al.* (2021). Fibroblast growth factor receptors in cancer: Genetic alterations, diagnostics, therapeutic targets and mechanisms of resistance. *Br J Cancer* **124**(5). doi: 10.1038/s41416-020-01157-0.

94 Montor WR, Salas AROSE, de Melo FHM (2018). Receptor tyrosine kinases and downstream pathways as druggable targets for cancer treatment: The current arsenal of inhibitors. *Mol Cancer* **17**(1). doi: 10.1186/s12943-018-0792-2.

95 Wang MX *et al.* (2021). Current update on molecular cytogenetics, diagnosis and management of gastrointestinal stromal tumors. *World J Gastroenterol* **27**(41). doi: 10.3748/wjg. v27.i41.7125.

96 Small D (2006). FLT3 mutations: Biology and treatment. *Hematology Am Soc Hematol Educ Program*. doi: 10.1182/asheducation-2006. 1.178.

97 Smith CC (2019). The growing landscape of FLT3 inhibition in AML. *Hematology (United States)* **1**: 2019. doi: 10.1182/hematology. 2019000058.

98 Zou Z *et al.* (2020). MTOR signaling pathway and mTOR inhibitors in cancer: Progress and challenges. *Cell Biosci* **10**(1). doi: 10.1186/ s13578-020-00396-1.BioMed Central Ltd

99 Pisapia P *et al.* (2020). BRAF: A two-faced janus. *Cells* **9**(12). doi: 10.3390/cells9122549.

100 Zaman A, Wu W, Bivona TG (2019). Targeting oncogenic braf: Past, present, and future. *Cancers* **11**(8). doi: 10.3390/cancers11081197.

101 Degirmenci U, Wang M, Hu J (2020). Targeting aberrant RAS/RAF/MEK/ERK signaling for cancer therapy. *Cells* **9**(1). doi: 10.3390/cells 9010198.

102 Hoxhaj G, Manning BD (2020). The PI3K–AKT network at the interface of oncogenic signalling and cancer metabolism. *Nat Rev Cancer* **20**(2). doi: 10.1038/s41568-019-0216-7.

103 McLornan DP *et al.* (2021). Current and future status of JAK inhibitors. *The Lancet* **398**(10302). doi: 10.1016/S0140-6736(21)00438-4.

104 Wen T *et al.* (2021). Inhibitors targeting Bruton's tyrosine kinase in cancers: Drug development advances. *Leukemia* **35**(2). doi: 10.1038/s41375-020-01072-6.

105 Castel P *et al.* (2021). The present and future of PI3K inhibitors for cancer therapy. *Nat Cancer* **2**(6). doi: 10.1038/s43018-021-00218-4.

106 Holla VR *et al.* (2017). ALK: A tyrosine kinase target for cancer therapy. *Mol Case Stud* **3**(1). doi: 10.1101/mcs.a001115.

107 Sehgal K *et al.* (2020). Cases of ROS1-rearranged lung cancer: When to use crizotinib, entrectinib, lorlatinib, and beyond? *Precis Cancer Med* **3**(June). doi: 10.21037/pcm-2020-potb-02.

108 Thein KZ *et al.* (2021). Precision therapy for RET-altered cancers with RET inhibitors. *Trends Cancer* **7**(12). doi: 10.1016/j. trecan.2021.07.003.

109 Thompson CL, van Vactor D (2006). Abelson Family Protein Tyrosine Kinases and the Formation of Neuronal Connectivity. In *Abl Family Kinases in Development and Disease. Molecular Biology Intelligence Unit*. New York, NY:Springer.doi:10.1007/978-0-387-68744-5_9.

110 Du Q *et al.* (2020). The application and prospect of CDK4/6 inhibitors in malignant solid tumors. *J Hematol Oncol* **13**(1). doi: 10.1186/ s13045-020-00880-8.

111 Zirlik K, Duyster J (2018). Anti-angiogenics: Current situation and future perspectives. *Oncol Res Treat* **41**(4). doi: 10.1159/000488087.

112 Chung C (2020). From oxygen sensing to angiogenesis: Targeting the hypoxia signaling pathway in metastatic kidney cancer. *Am J Health Syst Pharm* **77**(24). doi: 10.1093/ajhp/ zxaa308.

113 Stransky N *et al.* (2014). The landscape of kinase fusions in cancer. *Nat Commun* **5**. doi: 10.1038/ncomms5846.

114 Jänne PA *et al.* (2017). Selumetinib plus docetaxel compared with docetaxel alone and progression-free survival in patients with KRAS-mutant advanced non-small cell lung cancer: The SELECT-1 randomized clinical trial. *J Am Med Assoc* **317**(18). doi: 10.1001/ jama.2017.3438.

115 Rubin BP, Duensing A (2006). Mechanisms of resistance to small molecule kinase inhibition in the treatment of solid tumors. *Lab Invest* **86**(10). doi: 10.1038/labinvest.3700466.

116 Xu XQ *et al.* (2021). Intrinsic and acquired resistance to CDK4/6 inhibitors and potential overcoming strategies. *Acta Pharmacol Sin* **42**(2). doi: 10.1038/s41401-020-0416-4.

117 Lovly CM, Shaw AT (2014). Molecular pathways: Resistance to kinase inhibitors and implications for therapeutic strategies. *Clin Cancer Res* **20**(9). doi: 10.1158/1078-0432.CCR-13-1610.

118 Yu HA *et al.* (2014). Poor response to erlotinib in patients with tumors containing baseline EGFR T790M mutations found by routine clinical molecular testing. *Ann Oncol* **25**(2). doi: 10.1093/annonc/mdt573.

119 Woyach JA *et al.* (2014). Resistance mechanisms for the Bruton's tyrosine kinase inhibitor

ibrutinib. *N Engl J Med* **370**(24). doi: 10.1056/nejmoa1400029.

120 Kitagawa D *et al*. (2013). Activity-based kinase profiling of approved tyrosine kinase inhibitors. *Genes to Cells* **18**(2). doi: 10.1111/gtc.12022.

121 Schulze AB *et al*. (2019). Future options of molecular-targeted therapy in small cell lung cancer. *Cancers* **11**(5). doi: 10.3390/cancers11050690.

122 Karachaliou N, Sosa AE, Rosell R (2016). Unraveling the genomic complexity of small cell lung cancer. *Transl Lung Cancer Res* **5**(4). doi: 10.21037/tlcr.2016.07.02.

123 Curtin N (2014). PARP inhibitors for anticancer therapy. *Biochem Soc Trans* **42**(1). doi: 10.1042/BST20130187.

124 Lee EF, Fairlie WD (2021). Discovery, development and application of drugs targeting BCL-2 pro-survival proteins in cancer. *Biochem Soc Trans* **49**(5). doi: 10.1042/BST20210749.

125 Bates SE (2020). Epigenetic therapies for cancer. *N Engl J Med* **383**(7). doi: 10.1056/nejmra1805035.

126 de Lartigue J (2020). Targeting the hedgehog pathway holds promises and pitfalls. *OncologyLive* **21**(2) [Online] Available: https://www.onclive.com/view/targeting-the-hedgehog-pathway-holds-promises-and-pitfalls [Accessed February 24, 2022].

127 Nguyen NM, Cho J (2022). Hedgehog pathway inhibitors as targeted cancer therapy and strategies to overcome drug resistance. *Int J Mol Sci* **23**(3): 1733. doi: 10.3390/ijms23031733.

128 Jamieson C *et al*. (2020). Hedgehog pathway inhibitors: A new therapeutic class for the treatment of acute myeloid leukemia. *Blood Cancer Discov* **1**(2). doi: 10.1158/2643-3230.bcd-20-0007.

129 Thibaudeau TA, Smith DM (2019). A practical review of proteasome pharmacology. *Pharmacol Rev* **71**(2). doi: 10.1124/pr.117.015370.

130 Milo R *et al*. (2010). BioNumbers–the database of key numbers in molecular and cell biology. *Nucleic Acids Res* **38**: D750–D753. doi: 10.1093/nar/gkp889.

131 Fuchs O (2017). Immunomodulatory drugs and their therapeutic effect in hematological malignancies through cereblon. *Hematol Med Oncol* **2**(3). doi: 10.15761/hmo.1000129.

132 Azizian NG *et al*. (2020). XPO1-dependent nuclear export as a target for cancer therapy. *J Hematol Oncol* **13**(1). doi: 10.1186/s13045-020-00903-4.

133 Hegde PS, Wallin JJ, Mancao C (2018). Predictive markers of anti-VEGF and emerging role of angiogenesis inhibitors as immunotherapeutics. *Semin Cancer Biol* **52**. doi: 10.1016/j.semcancer.2017.12.002.

134 Wallin JJ *et al*. (2016). Atezolizumab in combination with bevacizumab enhances antigen-specific T-cell migration in metastatic renal cell carcinoma. *Nat Commun* **7**. doi: 10.1038/ncomms12624.

135 Ledford H (2019). Many cancer drugs aim at the wrong molecular targets. *Nature*. doi: 10.1038/d41586-019-02701-6.

136 Hargrave-Thomas E, Yu B, Reynisson J (2012). The effect of serendipity in drug discovery and development. *Chem N Z* **76**(1).

137 Rogers J, Ajani J (2024). State of the art and upcoming trends in claudin-directed therapies in gastrointestinal malignancies. *Curr Op Oncol*. **36**(4): 308–312. doi: 10.1097/CCO.0000000000001041.

CHAPTER 3

Treatments that Target Cell Communication

IN BRIEF

Our cells communicate with each other constantly. One of the ways they do so is by releasing small proteins into their surroundings that attach to receptors on the surface of neighboring cells. These receptors then trigger internal chain reactions inside the cell: The receptor transmits a signal to one protein, which activates another, and then another. Finally, the signal reaches its conclusion and triggers a response. Maybe the cell grows, dies, or becomes dormant.

Communication pathways (sometimes called signaling pathways, or signal transduction cascades), and the receptors that control them, have virtually always gone awry in cancer cells. Drugs that block them have become important treatments for many cancer types.

In this chapter, I first provide a general introduction to how cells communicate. I'll then describe how various communication pathways operate, what goes wrong with them in cancer cells, and how these defects are targeted using treatments such as monoclonal antibodies and kinase inhibitors.

Many of the treatments described in this chapter block cell surface receptors called epidermal growth factor receptor (EGFR) and human epidermal growth factor receptor-2 (HER2). EGFR-targeted treatments are important treatments for people with lung cancer and bowel cancer. HER2-targeted treatments are predominantly given as a treatment for breast cancer. Increasingly though, they're finding a role as treatments for other cancers that overproduce HER2 or that make a faulty, overactive version of the HER2 protein.

I also describe the ways in which other growth factor receptors are defective in cancer. For example, fusion proteins that contain the kinase portion of a growth factor receptor such as RET, ALK, ROS1, or TRK are sometimes present in a person's cancer cells due to a chromosome defect. These fusion proteins are rare, but found in a range of cancer types.

I also describe in this chapter drugs that target three important signaling pathways triggered by cell surface receptors. These pathways are the mitogen-activated protein kinase (MAPK) pathway, the PI3K/AKT/mTOR pathway, and the JAK-STAT pathway. The MAPK pathway is perhaps the most well known. It involves proteins such as K-Ras, B-Raf, and MEK. B-Raf and MEK inhibitors are important treatments for many people with melanoma skin cancer, and for some people with bowel or lung cancer.

A Beginner's Guide to Targeted Cancer Treatments and Cancer Immunotherapy, Second Edition. Elaine Vickers.
© 2025 John Wiley & Sons Ltd. Published 2025 by John Wiley & Sons Ltd.

As yet, treatments that target the PI3K/AKT/mTOR pathway have had only moderate success as cancer treatments. mTOR inhibitors are sometimes given to people with breast or kidney cancer, and PI3K-delta (PI3Kδ) inhibitors are treatments for some B cell leukemias and lymphomas.

I've also included in this chapter the Bcr-Abl inhibitors. Bcr-Abl is a fusion protein created by a translocation that exists in the cancer cells of people with chronic myeloid leukemia and some acute lymphoblastic leukemias. I've included inhibitors of Bcr-Abl in this chapter because it is a kinase that activates various signaling pathways.

Finally, the JAK-STAT pathway is defective in many cancers and various autoimmune diseases. JAK2 inhibitors are approved as treatments for some myeloproliferative neoplasms, as well as for conditions such as rheumatoid arthritis.

An important limitation of treatments that target growth factor receptors and the signaling pathways under their control is their importance to healthy cells. Our cells all have these receptors on their surface, and the proteins they control are vitally important for the health of our organs and tissues. Hence, none of these treatments is without side effects.

However, receptors and internal signaling proteins have become important targets of cancer treatments.

3.1 INTRODUCTION

Our cells are constantly responding to signals and instructions from a variety of sources [1]. Depending on the messages they receive, cells alter their behavior or might even die. For example, cells use receptor proteins on their surface to detect levels of oxygen, proteins, amino acids, some hormones, and tiny proteins called growth factors. Our cells also have an array of receptors inside them that pick up other signals, such as fat-soluble hormones released by the brain, adrenal glands, and sex organs. Also, by forming physical connections with their neighbors, our cells can tell if there are too many, or too few, cells in their neighborhood. In addition, all our tissues and organs contain a network of complex proteins and sugars that our cells make connections with. This extracellular matrix (ECM) also provides cells with feedback about their surroundings.

If that wasn't enough, our cells also respond to signals sent out by white blood cells. Each type of white blood cell (and there are *lots* of different types) has a repertoire of signaling proteins called cytokines that it can release into its surroundings to coordinate immune responses and trigger healing [2, 3]. Finally, some of our cells have specialized receptors for light, sound, touch, or electrical signals (for a summary see Figure 3.1).

The largest group of receptors found on the surface of our cells are the G-protein-coupled receptors (GPCRs). In fact, there are over 1000 different GPCRs playing a vast array of different functions in our bodies [4, 5]. A much smaller group of receptors are the 58 different receptor tyrosine kinases (RTKs) [6–8]. These receptors usually respond to proteins called growth factors; thus another name for them is growth factor receptors.

Growth factors are tiny proteins that our cells use to communicate with their close neighbors. When a growth factor attaches to a growth factor receptor, this triggers a series of events inside a cell. This passing-on of a signal from a receptor on the cell surface to the

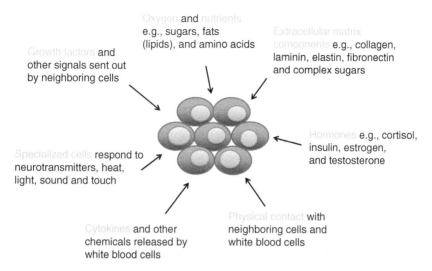

Oxygen and nutrients e.g., sugars, fats (lipids), and amino acids

Growth factors and other signals sent out by neighboring cells

Extracellular matrix components e.g., collagen, laminin, elastin, fibronectin and complex sugars

Hormones e.g., cortisol, insulin, estrogen, and testosterone

Specialized cells respond to neurotransmitters, heat, light, sound and touch

Cytokines and other chemicals released by white blood cells

Physical contact with neighboring cells and white blood cells

Figure 3.1 Our cells respond to a wide range of short-range and long-range signals. Short-range signals include growth factors, which travel short distances between cells. Our cells also respond to oxygen and nutrients, complex proteins and sugars in their immediate surroundings (called the extracellular matrix), and physical contact with neighboring cells. Long-range signals that cells respond to include hormones, which are produced and released by specialized glands throughout the body, such as the adrenal glands (that sit above each kidney), hypothalamus and pituitary gland in the brain, testes (in men), and ovaries (in women). Hormones travel throughout the body and affect distant cells. White blood cells that live in the bone marrow and lymphoid tissues, or that patrol the body and accumulate at the site of infections and injuries, send out a wide variety of signals in the form of proteins called cytokines. Finally, specialized cells, such as nerve cells (neurons), ear cells, eye cells, and other sensory cells, respond to signals such as neurotransmitters, sound, light, and touch.

nucleus is called a signaling pathway, cell communication pathway, or signal transduction cascade.

Many receptors and other proteins involved in signaling pathways are faulty in cancer cells. As a result, over the past 30 years, cell communication has become a major area of cancer research. Many of the small molecule- and antibody-based cancer treatments mentioned in this book work by blocking cell communication proteins.

Currently, most cancer drugs that target signaling pathways do this by:
1. Blocking growth factor receptors on the cell's surface (e.g., EGFR, HER2, HER3, or FLT3)
2. Blocking kinases inside the cell that are normally controlled by growth factor

receptors (e.g., B-Raf, MEK, mTOR, PI3K, and AKT)
3. Blocking faulty versions of growth factor receptors that are found in the cell cytoplasm (e.g., fusion proteins involving the kinase portion of RET, ALK1, ROS1, or TRK1, 2, or 3)

A handful of cancer drugs work by blocking proteins that are involved in other signaling pathways – ones that aren't controlled by growth factor receptors. These include drugs that target Hedgehog signaling, which I look at in Chapter 4.

There are yet other signaling pathways that scientists think are very important in some cancers, but that haven't as yet led to any licensed cancer treatments. One example is the WNT/β-catenin pathway, which is overactive in most bowel cancers [9].

Although human cells have a vast array of receptors on their surface, for the remainder of this chapter I will focus on growth factor receptors and three of the signaling pathways they control (the MAPK pathway, the PI3K/AKT/mTOR pathway, and the JAK-STAT pathway). My focus on growth factor receptor signaling is for two reasons: [7]

1. Many of the most common and most powerful genetic mutations that drive the behavior of cancer cells affect growth factor receptor signaling pathways.
2. A large proportion of licensed targeted treatments for cancer work by blocking these pathways.

Also included in this chapter are treatments that block the Bcr-Abl fusion protein, which is most often found in the cells of people with chronic myeloid leukemia (CML). The Bcr-Abl protein activates all three of the pathways covered in this chapter, which is why I've included it here.

3.2 GROWTH FACTOR-CONTROLLED SIGNALING PATHWAYS

Growth factor-controlled signaling involves a few main elements:

1. Growth factors released by cells into their surroundings.
2. Growth factor receptors that stick out from the cell surface and that pair up and attach phosphates to each other when a suitable growth factor is present.
3. Docking proteins that attach to phosphates on paired-up receptors.
4. Various kinases and other enzymes that are activated by docking proteins.
5. Many more kinases and other enzymes that gradually transmit the signal through the cell cytoplasm and potentially also into the cell nucleus (sometimes the signal reaches its conclusion in the cytoplasm).

6. Transcription factors and other proteins that alter gene activity or coordinate the cell's response to growth factors in other ways.

Finally, the cell responds. Maybe it simply stays alive, or perhaps it enters the cell cycle and multiplies. Or it might react by dying, or moving, or any number of other responses depending on the nature, duration, and strength of the signal it received.

Signaling pathways involve many kinases, which are the targets of a large number of kinase inhibitors. In addition, because growth factor receptors protrude from the cell surface, they are also the target of various antibody-based treatments, including antibody-drug conjugates (described in more detail in Chapter 4).

But, before I start working my way through all the cancer treatments that target cell signaling pathways, I'll first spend some time describing some of the proteins and pathways involved. I hope that this information will help you understand the treatments better and appreciate their uses and limitations.

3.2.1 Growth Factor Receptors: Some Basics

Growth factor receptors are large, complicated proteins. Thousands of them are embedded in the surface of our cells. Their other name, receptor tyrosine kinase (RTK), refers to the fact that the part of the receptor that protrudes inside the cell functions as a tyrosine kinase (Chapter 2, Figure 2.17). Different cells in our body have different types and numbers of RTKs on their surface [10].

The external (extracellular) portion of RTKs – the part that sticks out from the cell's surface – is shaped so that it provides an attachment site for one or more growth factors. Growth factors are typically small proteins produced and released by pretty much all our cells (e.g., EGF is 53 amino acids long; many other growth factors are a similar size [11]). Growth factors travel short distances between cells. When they attach to growth factor receptors on a cell's surface, the receptors pair up, and this triggers a chain reaction within the cell cytoplasm. Finally, the signal reaches the cell nucleus and transmits an instruction to the cell such as "stay alive," "it's time to multiply," or "it's time to mature and specialize" (Figure 3.2).

At any given time, most of the cells in our body are going about their daily business and have no need to multiply (Figure 3.3a). When this is the case, our cells use growth factors simply to provide a background hum of activity that keeps them alive [12]. However, cells sometimes become old or damaged and die. If this happens, nearby cells might change or increase the amount of growth factors they produce (Figure 3.3b). Cells close by that have the relevant receptors on their surface will then respond and create extra cells to fill the gap left by the dead cell [13].

For many years now, scientists have known that growth factor receptor signaling is seriously awry in cancer cells (Figure 3.3c), and we'll go into this in more detail later in this chapter.

3.2.2 Growth Factor Receptors Activate Signaling Pathways

Growth Factor Receptors Become Active When They Pair Up

As I outlined earlier, the first step in a signaling pathway is when growth factors attach to their receptors. When this happens, the receptors change shape and pair up with one another (a process known as dimerization) (Figure 3.4a & b). Once receptors have paired up, they phosphorylate each other – they take phosphates from ATP and attach them to their partner on tyrosine amino acids (Figure 3.4c). Phosphorylation of the two receptors changes their shape and creates docking sites for other proteins [13]. The exact number, and nature, of these docking sites varies from receptor to receptor, as does the precise way that the receptors pair up and phosphorylate one another [14].

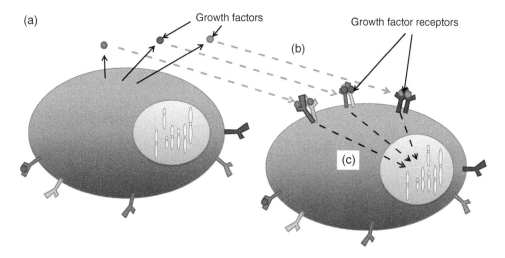

Figure 3.2 Growth factor receptors are activated by growth factors. **(a)** Cells produce and release growth factors into their surroundings. **(b)** Growth factors attach to growth factor receptors and cause them to pair up (shown with a dotted pink line). This pairing up activates the receptors' kinase domain, and they phosphorylate one another. **(c)** The paired-up receptors activate proteins that activate more proteins, and more proteins, and this transmits the signal through the cell's cytoplasm (shown with a dotted black line). Eventually, the signal reaches the nucleus.

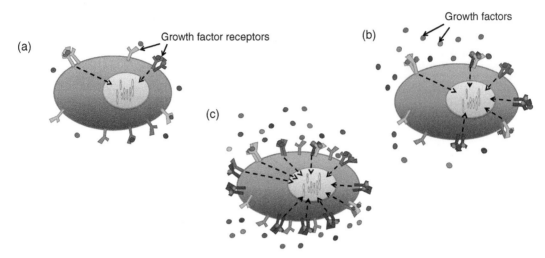

Figure 3.3 Growth factors can have a variety of different impacts on cells. (a) Healthy cells need growth factors to stay alive. **(b)** Changes to the amount and type of growth factors present give this healthy cell a signal to grow and multiply. **(c)** Mutations in cancer cells' DNA, and changes to the amount of growth factors and growth factor receptors on their surface, provide cancer cells with continuous signals to survive, cause them to multiply, increase their mobility, alter their metabolism, and trigger angiogenesis.

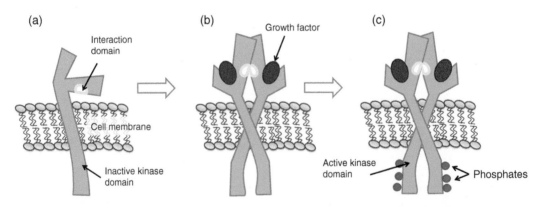

Figure 3.4 Growth factor receptors phosphorylate each other only when growth factors attach to them. **(a)** An un-paired growth factor receptor. The "interaction domain" through which it interacts with another receptor is hidden. **(b)** When suitable growth factors attach to the two receptors, they change shape, exposing their interaction domains. The two receptors then pair up (they dimerize). **(c)** The kinase domains of the paired receptors become active, and the two receptors phosphorylate each other.

Paired Receptors Trigger Signaling Pathways

Various proteins can dock with paired-up, phosphorylated receptors. Many of them are intermediaries that pass on the signal to other proteins. These other proteins are often themselves intermediaries that pass on the signal to others, and so the pathway continues. Finally, the signal is passed to proteins called transcription factors in the cell nucleus. These transcription factors then attach to genes and cause gene transcription and protein production.[1] So, when growth factors attach to receptors on a cell's surface, this ultimately causes the cell to alter what proteins it makes, which will impact the cell's behavior.

There are Many Signaling Pathways

Growth factor receptors control a wide variety of signaling pathways, involving hundreds of different proteins. Some of these proteins are kinases that amplify the signal as it passes through the cell. Some proteins act as scaffolds that hold other proteins in the right position for them to interact. Some of them are suppressor proteins that block a pathway. Others coordinate feedback loops, so that if one pathway becomes very active, others shut down. Some proteins work alone, others come together in pairs, and others form groupings containing many protein members.

All in all, this is such complicated stuff that it's virtually impossible to understand, never mind remembering it all. However, there are a few key pieces of information it's worth remembering. Among them are the identities of the main proteins involved in two powerful pathways triggered by growth factor receptors. These are the MAPK pathway and the PI3K/AKT/mTOR pathway (summarized in Figure 3.5[2] along with a few other proteins and pathways) [13–15]. These pathways control cell survival, proliferation, and cell movement, and they even influence the creation of blood vessels by angiogenesis. They are commonly overactive in cancer cells for a variety of different reasons, and they are the target of many cancer treatments.

3.2.3 A Few Extra Things to Know About Signaling Pathways

There are a few other properties of signaling pathways that I think it's useful to know: [10, 14, 15]

- Signaling pathways involve many different proteins, but they also involve small molecules such as phosphatidylinositol-3,4,5-triphosphate (PIP_3) – a little fatty molecule with some phosphates attached.
- There is generally more than one version of each protein in our cells. For example, there are three main Ras proteins (K-Ras, N-Ras, and H-Ras), three Raf proteins (A-Raf, B-Raf, and C-Raf), and seven MEK proteins (MEK1-7). Sometimes a single cell makes more than one version of a protein; sometimes the different versions are found in different cell types.
- Various pathways interact with and influence one another; this is known as cross-talk.
- Sometimes the activation of a pathway triggers a feedback loop that later shuts off the pathway or prevents it from becoming overactive.
- The activation of a signaling pathway can be all over in a matter of minutes, or it can last for many hours.
- The endpoint of a signaling pathway might be a change that occurs in the cell cytoplasm, such as rearrangement of scaffolding proteins, or it might be the activation of transcription factors in the nucleus that alter what proteins the cell makes.
- Most signaling pathways involve proteins that actively pass on the signal and proteins that block it; for example, PTEN blocks the

---

[1] If you are not sure how transcription factors cause the cell to produce proteins, I recommend looking at this page on the Khan Academy website: https://www.khanacademy.org/science/biology/gene-regulation/ene-regulation-in-eukaryotes/a/eukaryotic-transcription-factors.

[2] Although I provide many abbreviations in this figure, for the rest of the book I won't bother, as the names aren't useful. They sometimes reflect the proteins' history and how they were discovered, but the names don't describe what the proteins do. You might also notice that some proteins, such as AKT, B-Raf, and MEK, don't have a longer name, which again just adds to confusion.

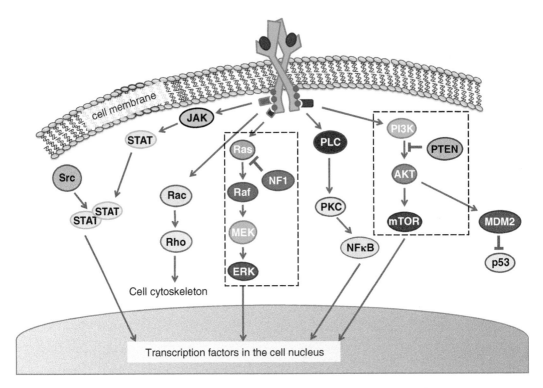

Figure 3.5 Some of the many proteins and pathways activated by growth factor receptors. When growth factor receptors pair up, they activate many different signaling proteins in the cell, which control processes such as proliferation, survival, growth, and the cell's ability to move. Some of the most important and well-known signaling pathways are those that involve Ras, Raf, MEK, and ERK (known as the MAPK pathway), and PI3K, AKT, and mTOR (highlighted). This latter pathway is kept under control by PTEN, which prevents the activation of AKT. Two other proteins also controlled by growth factor receptors are Rac and Rho, which control the cell's internal skeleton. NFκB is another powerful protein it's worth knowing about; it is a transcription factor that, once in the nucleus, prevents cell death. STAT proteins (there are numerous) are also transcription factors.

Abbreviations: ERK – extracellular-signal-regulated kinase; JAK – Janus kinase; mTOR – mechanistic target of rapamycin; NFκB – nuclear factor kappa-B; PI3K – phosphoinositide 3-kinase; PKC – protein kinase C; PLC – phospholipase C; PTEN – phosphatase and tensin homolog; STAT – signal transducer and activator of transcription.

PI3K/AKT/mTOR pathway and NF1 blocks the MAPK pathway.

- Which pathways are activated by a growth factor receptor depends on the type of cell it is, where the cell is, its access to oxygen, nutrients, and energy, which receptor was activated, how long the receptors remained paired up, which growth factor caused the receptors to pair up, and so on.
- Depending on which pathways become active, and for how long, the cell will choose its response.

- Most signaling pathways involve several kinases. Each kinase phosphorylates one or more other kinases, which then phosphorylate other kinases. Through this process, the signal received at the cell's surface is amplified as it passes through the cell.
- Pathways are generally switched off by removing the activated receptors from the cell surface or removing phosphates from activated kinases. Kinases are enzymes that add phosphates; phosphatases are enzymes that remove them.

- Some individual proteins are involved in more than one pathway, e.g., Ras proteins are involved in the MAPK pathway, but Ras also activates PI3K (and therefore also AKT and mTOR) [16].
- Some pathways are activated by various types of receptors and not just growth factor receptors, e.g., PI3K is also activated by lots of other receptors such as G-protein-coupled receptors and cytokine receptors [17].
- The pathways shown in Figure 3.5 are just a drop in the ocean. The pathways shown are vastly more complicated than the illustration, and there are many other pathways I haven't mentioned.

3.2.4 Signaling Pathways in Cancer Cells

Defects in the MAPK pathway and the PI3K/AKT/mTOR pathway have been found in pretty much every type of cancer ever studied. Sometimes, there's a mutation forcing the pathway into overdrive, such as *EGFR*, *HER2*, *KRAS*, *BRAF*, and *PIK3CA* mutations. Other times, mutations affect tumor suppressor genes like *PTEN* or *NF1*, and their protective, growth-limiting function is lost.

To put some numbers to this, scientists taking part in The Cancer Genome Atlas (TCGA) program[3] [18] have analyzed cancer samples from thousands of patients with different types of cancer. In one of their analyses (using 9125 samples from patients with 33 different types of cancer), they discovered that: [19]

- 46% of cancers contained a mutation affecting the gene for a growth factor receptor, and/or a gene involved in the MAPK pathway, including 94% of melanomas, 88% of genomically stable bowel cancers,[4] 78% of pancreatic cancers, and 74% of lung adenocarcinomas.
- Mutations affecting the PI3K/AKT/mTOR pathway were also very common. For example, they were found in 68% of lung squamous cell carcinomas, 80% of Epstein-Barr virus (EBV)-positive esophageal and stomach cancers, and over 85% of non-hypermutated uterine cancers.[5]
- The most commonly mutated genes involved in the MAPK pathway were *KRAS*, which was mutated in 9% of all samples (including 72% of pancreatic ductal adenocarcinomas and 69% of genomically stable bowel cancers), and *BRAF* in 7% of all samples (including 51% of melanomas and 62% of thyroid cancers).
- *EGFR* gene mutations were most common in glioblastoma (50%), human papillomavirus (HPV)-negative head and neck cancer (13%), lung adenocarcinoma (13%), and squamous cell cancers of the esophagus and stomach (14%).
- Mutations affecting the *HER2* gene (also called *ERBB2*) were found in 5% of all the cancers tested, being most common in breast cancer, chromosomal instability (CIN) stomach cancer,[6] and cervical cancer.
- In a separate, similar study, *PIK3CA* mutations (which cause the PI3K protein to be overactive), were found in 14% of all samples tested, and *PTEN* was mutated in 9% [22].

---

[3] I'm sure they'd love it if you noticed that their name comprises the one-letter abbreviations of the four DNA bases – adenine, thymine, guanine, and cytosine.
[4] Around 15% or so of bowel cancers contain mutations affecting a DNA repair process called **mismatch repair**; these cancers are also known as the **microsatellite-instability (MSI) bowel cancers,** and they are **genomically unstable.** The other 85% or so are **genomically stable** [20].
[5] Roughly 30% of uterine cancers are hypermutated – they either exhibit MSI or they have a mutation affecting DNA polymerase. The other ~70% are non-hypermutated [21].
[6] CIN refers to cancers that have lots of large-scale problems with their chromosomes, rather than the thousands of small-scale mutations that are typical of a microsatellite instability (MSI) cancer. Both CIN and MSI are forms of genome instability, but it's important to know the difference. MSI cancers tend to be very sensitive to immunotherapy, whereas CIN cancers are generally resistant.

- Some gene mutations coexist with each other, but others don't (they're said to be mutually exclusive). Scientists think that when mutations don't occur together in a tumor that's because either (1) once one of the genes is mutated, a mutation in the second gene doesn't confer any further advantage, or (2) if both mutations occurred together in a single cell, the cell would die. When two mutations do often occur together, it's presumed that they work together in some way. For example, you very rarely find a *KRAS* mutation and a *BRAF* mutation in the same person's bowel cancer. But you do often find mutations both in the *EGFR* gene and in the *PDGFRA* gene (the gene for another growth factor receptor) in glioblastoma.

As you can see by the footnotes I've included in the bulleted list earlier, scientists in TCGA program are drilling down into the types and subtypes of each cancer. That's because if you want to give each patient a treatment approach tailored toward the details of their disease, then the details really do matter. This should become even more apparent as I go through each mutation and its consequences. I'll then discuss the targeted treatments we have at our disposal.

I'll begin by looking at mutations affecting growth factor receptors. Then I'll look at those affecting the MAPK pathway, then those that affect the PI3K/AKT/mTOR pathway, and finally I'll look at the JAK-STAT pathway.

For each set of proteins, I'll describe how the normal protein works and the effect of any mutations found in cancer cells. I'll then discuss the treatments we have that target it.

3.3 GROWTH FACTOR RECEPTORS IN CANCER

As I've just mentioned, many cancers contain a mutation affecting the activity of a growth factor receptor, and many more have excessive amounts of one or more growth factor receptors on their surface. There are two receptors that dominate in terms of their importance across numerous cancer types: EGFR and HER2. However, numerous other growth factor receptors have been implicated in a wide variety of cancer types. I've listed some of the most important ones in Table 3.1.

3.3.1 Reasons for Overactive Growth Factor Receptors on Cancer Cells

One of the most common reasons that growth factor receptor signaling pathways are overactive in cancer cells is because of faults with the receptor (reviewed in [36–39] and summarized in Figure 3.6). For example:

Some cancer cells produce faulty, overactive versions of growth factor receptors (Figure 3.6a), for example:

- In the cancer cells of up to 40% of people with non-small cell lung cancer (NSCLC), the *EGFR* gene is mutated in such a way that the kinase portion of EGFR is overactive [40]. (To be more precise, the proportion is 10%–15% in a Caucasian population, but 30%–40% in people from countries such as China, Japan, and Korea.)
- In the cancer cells of over 50% of people with glioblastoma, a mutant version of EGFR is present that lacks part of the extracellular domain (the bit sticking out from the cell's surface). The mutated receptor (called EGFRvIII) is always in the right shape to pair up, even without a growth factor present [41].
- FGF receptor genes are mutated in around 50% of bladder cancers and in some cervical cancers, lung cancers, multiple myelomas, and prostate cancers [30].
- In around a third of people with acute myeloid leukemia (AML), their cancer cells are making an extra-long version of FLT3. Unlike normal FLT3, the mutated version of FLT3 is unable to regulate itself and is overactive. In a smaller proportion of

Table 3.1 Some growth factor receptors implicated in cancer.

Receptor	Ligand[a]/growth factor	Main cancers in which the receptor is implicated
EGFR: Epidermal growth factor receptor; ErbB1; HER1	EGF, transforming growth factor alpha (TGF-α), heparin-binding EGF-like growth factor (HB-EGF), amphiregulin, betacellulin, epigen, and epiregulin	Breast cancer, bowel cancer, non-small cell lung cancer (NSCLC), brain tumors, prostate cancer, ovarian cancer, stomach cancer, pancreatic cancer, head and neck squamous cell carcinomas (HNSCCs), anal cancer, esophageal cancer, and many more [23]
HER2: Human EGF receptor-2; ErbB2; Neu	No known ligand	Breast cancer, stomach cancer, esophageal cancer (also some lung, ovarian, uterine, bladder, and bowel cancers) [24]
HER3: Human EGF receptor-3; ErbB3	Neuregulin – NRG	Thought to be a common reason for drug resistance; frequently present alongside other EGF receptors on cancer cells, for example, those of breast, prostate, ovarian, bowel, and lung cancers [25]. Fusion proteins involving NRG are present in a small proportion of various cancer types [26].
HER4: Human EGF receptor-4; ErbB4	HB-EGF, betacellulin, epiregulin, and neuregulin	Melanoma, NSCLC, and medulloblastoma [27]
VEGFR1 and VEGFR2: vascular endothelial growth factor receptors 1 and 2	VEGF-A, VEGF-B, VEGF-C, VEGF-D, and placental growth factor (PlGF)	Any cancer with a blood supply – VEGFRs are on endothelial cells lining blood vessels [28]
PDGFRA and PDGFRB: platelet-derived growth factor receptor alpha and beta	PDGF-A, PDGF-B, PDGF-C, and PDGF-D	Glioblastoma, gastrointestinal stromal tumors (GISTs), and bone metastases from prostate cancer; also implicated in angiogenesis [29]
FGF-R1, 2, 3, 4, and 5: fibroblast growth factor receptors	FGFs (there are 22 different fibroblast growth factors)	Bladder cancer, squamous NSCLC, cervical cancer, multiple myeloma, prostate cancer, breast cancer, and stomach cancer; important in angiogenesis [30]
IGF1-R: insulin-like growth factor-1 receptor	Insulin-like growth factor 1 (IGF-1)	Bowel, prostate, breast, and lung cancer, and probably many others; associated with resistance to EGFR inhibitors [31]
MET[b]: hepatocyte growth factor receptor	Hepatocyte growth factor (HGF)	Kidney, lung, liver, and pancreatic cancer and bone metastases from prostate cancer; important in invasion and metastasis; associated with resistance of bowel cancer to EGFR inhibitors and VEGF-R inhibitors [32]
KIT[c]/CD117	Stem cell factor (SCF)	GIST, small cell lung cancer (SCLC), acute myeloid leukemia (AML), T cell lymphoma, testicular germ cell tumors, and melanoma skin cancer [33]
FLT3: FMS-like tyrosine kinase 3	FLT3 ligand	AML, acute lymphocytic leukemia, and chronic myeloid leukemia in blast crisis [34]
RET	Glial cell line-derived neurotrophic factor (GDNF) family ligands (GFLs), including neurturin (NRTN), artemin (ARTN), and persephin (PSPN)	Papillary thyroid cancer, medullary thyroid cancer, and NSCLC [35]

[a] A ligand is anything that attaches to a receptor; most receptors have one or more ligands.
[b] MET is sometimes called c-MET. Various other proteins implicated in cancer sometimes have "c-" in front of their name (e.g., c-KIT, c-SRC, c-Myc, and c-Raf). This was historically done in order to distinguish between the human, cellular (c-) version of a gene or protein compared to the viral version (v-) thought to be the cancer-causing version. However, our views of the relationship between viruses and cancer have now changed, and the c- prefix is gradually being dropped. Sadly, adding to the confusion is the fact that sometimes the c- refers to the version of the protein in situations where there are multiple versions. For example, there are three versions of Raf: A-Raf, B-Raf, and C-Raf; so, when you see c-Raf written down, the person might be referring to Raf proteins in general or just one of them.
[c] KIT is sometime called c-KIT. See note above about MET for the reason why. Confusingly, KIT is also sometimes called CD117. Every protein found on the surface of white blood cells is allocated a CD number when it is discovered; KIT's number is 117. CD stands for "cluster of differentiation"; it is a historical term coined by the first scientists who examined white blood cells decades ago.

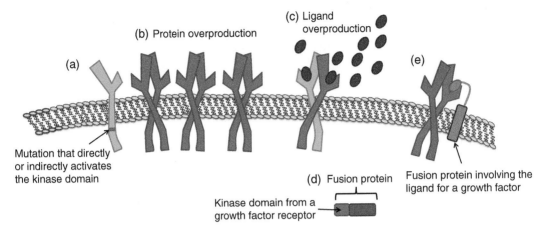

Figure 3.6 Growth factor receptors are overactive in cancer cells for a variety of reasons. (a) In some instances, the kinase domain of a receptor has been affected by a mutation, causing the receptor to be active in the absence of any ligand. **(b)** Cancer cells overproduce growth factor receptors due to gene amplification or increased gene transcription. **(c)** Cancer cells often overproduce growth factors, which activate receptors on their own surface and on the surface of cells nearby. **(d)** In some people, their cancer cells contain a chromosome translocation or other sort of gene rearrangement that has created a fusion gene. The gene contains the instructions to make the kinase portion of a growth factor receptor, plus part of another protein. The resulting fusion protein is an overactive kinase. **(e)** A fusion protein involving the ligand for a receptor and a membrane protein activates a growth factor receptor.

patients with AML, the kinase domain of FLT3 is mutated and overactive [34, 42].

- In rare cases, the whole kinase domain of a receptor has been duplicated, so that multiple kinase domains sit side-by-side [38].

Many cancers have excessive amounts of growth factor receptors on their surface (Figure 3.6b), including the following:

- Excess EGFR on the surface of the cancer cells in bowel cancer, lung cancer, esophageal cancer, thyroid cancer, and glioblastoma [38].
- Around 15%–20% of breast cancers and stomach cancers have extra copies (amplification) of the *HER2* gene. They therefore have more HER2 protein on their surface than normal. Overproduction of HER2 has also been found in various other solid tumors [43].

Many cancer cells and nearby non-cancer cells make and release large amounts of growth factors, which saturate growth factor receptors on the cancer cells' surface (Figure 3.6c) [38].

In some cancers, a translocation or other gene rearrangement is causing the cells to produce a fusion protein containing the kinase portion of a growth factor receptor (Figure 3.6d), for example:

- ALK fusion proteins are produced by around 5% of NSCLCs and more than 50% of anaplastic large cell lymphomas [44].
- RET fusion proteins are common in papillary thyroid cancer; they have been linked to exposure to radiation (they're more common in people living close to Chernobyl or Hiroshima[7]) [37].

---

[7] The Fukushima nuclear powerplant incident in Japan in 2011 caused much lower doses of radiation to leak, and this isn't thought to have led to increased cases of thyroid cancer – although there's been much anxiety in the population exposed [45].

Lastly, in 2014, scientists discovered a fusion protein called CD74-NRG1 in the cancer cells of some people with a rare form of NSCLC called mucinous adenocarcinoma [46]. This fusion protein contains a growth factor, NRG1, linked to a protein found in the cell membrane. NRG1 is a ligand for HER3, and the resulting fusion protein causes HER3 to pair up with HER2 and activate internal signaling pathways (Figure 3.6e).

3.4 DRUGS THAT TARGET EGFR

Licensed drugs mentioned in this section:		
Treatment class	**Drugs**	**Given to some people with:**
EGFR-targeted antibody therapies	Cetuximab, panitumumab, and necitumumab	• Bowel cancer • Squamous cell NSCLC
EGFR-targeted kinase inhibitors	Erlotinib, gefitinib, afatinib, dacomitinib, osimertinib, lazertinib, and mobocertinib	• NSCLC with activating *EGFR* mutations
Dual-targeted antibody against EGFR and MET	Amivantamab	• NSCLC with activating *EGFR* mutations

The EGFR was the first growth factor receptor discovered by scientists in the late 1970s [47], and it's still the one we know most about. This receptor is found on a wide range of cell types in many of our tissues and organs. It responds to the presence of at least seven different growth factors, the main one being epidermal growth factor (EGF) [48].

Like other growth factor receptors, when EGF attaches to EGFRs, the receptors change shape and pair up (you might want to look back at Figure 3.4). However, EGF receptors can also pair up with other members of the EGF receptor family. There are four family members: EGF receptor (also called EGFR, HER1, or ErbB1), HER2 (also called EGF receptor-2, Neu, or ErbB2), HER3 (EGF receptor-3; ErbB3), and HER4 (EGF receptor-4; ErbB4).

All four receptors can pair up with themselves or with any other member of the family (Figure 3.7) [49]. However, there are some important differences between them. For example, EGFR, HER3, and HER4 only pair up when a suitable growth factor is present. In contrast, HER2 doesn't need a growth factor to get into the correct shape for pairing – it's in the right shape all the time [27]. As a result, HER2 is constantly pairing up with

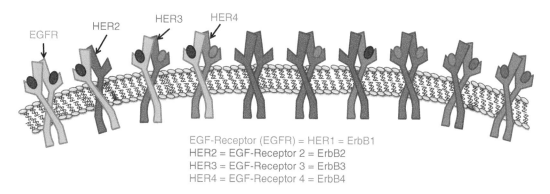

EGF-Receptor (EGFR) = HER1 = ErbB1
HER2 = EGF-Receptor 2 = ErbB2
HER3 = EGF-Receptor 3 = ErbB3
HER4 = EGF-Receptor 4 = ErbB4

Figure 3.7 All four EGF receptors can pair up to create homo- and heterodimers. A homodimer is when two identical receptors have paired up. A heterodimer contains two different receptors. HER2 is different from HER1, HER3, and HER4 in that it doesn't need a growth factor to be present to pair up.
Abbreviations: EGF – epidermal growth factor; HER – human epidermal growth factor receptor.

itself and with EGFR, HER3, or HER4. When it pairs up with other family members, it activates signaling pathways more strongly than pairings that don't contain HER2. HER2 is therefore the most active and most powerful member of the EGF receptor family [49].

The EGFR (HER1) is found on the surface of cancer cells in lots of different cancer types, and it is the target of many cancer treatments (see Table 3.2). However, just because there are lots of EGFRs on the surface of a person's cancer cells, that doesn't necessarily mean it would be helpful to target it. There are many cancer types in which you find excessive amounts of unmutated (or wild-type) EGFR on the cells' surface (such as ovarian cancer, triple-negative breast cancer, prostate cancer, liver cancer, and esophageal cancer). However, it's only in bowel cancer and head and neck cancer that targeting the unmutated receptor seems helpful [50].

Where it appears to be more helpful to target EGFRs is when the kinase portion of the receptor has been rendered overactive due to a mutation, as is the case in a proportion of people with NSCLC.

Drugs that target EGFRs can be split into two groups:

1. Monoclonal antibodies that attach to EGFRs from outside the cell and that are most used in the treatment of people with bowel cancer and head and neck cancer, for example, cetuximab, panitumumab, and necitumumab.
2. Kinase inhibitors that block EGFRs from inside the cell and that are mostly given to people whose cancer cells are making a mutated, overactive version of EGFR (most common in NSCLC), for example, gefitinib, erlotinib, afatinib, and osimertinib.

The goal of all these treatments is to block the receptor and prevent it from activating any internal signaling pathways. Hopefully, EGFR activity is vital to the person's cancer cells, both in terms of forcing them to multiply and in keeping them alive. If this is the case, then blocking the receptor will cause cancer cells to die.

3.4.1 Monoclonal Antibodies that Target EGFR

Physical Makeup and Differences Between Them

As you might have already noticed from the names: Cetuximab is a chimeric antibody, nimotuzumab is a humanized antibody, and panitumumab and necitumumab are fully human antibodies (see Figure 2.6). Because of this difference, panitumumab and necitumumab are theoretically less visible to the patient's immune system and less likely to cause infusion reactions [51]. See Figure 3.8 for a comparison between cetuximab and panitumumab.

Another difference between the antibodies is the type of antibody that they're made from. Our B cells can produce a variety of different classes of antibodies (called IgA, IgG, IgE, IgD, and IgM[8]), and within each class there are also numerous subclasses. All licensed antibody treatments are made from IgGs. Panitumumab is made from an IgG2 antibody, whereas cetuximab and necitumumab are made from IgG1 antibodies. Although this might seem like an excessive piece of detail, this subtle difference means that cetuximab and necitumumab are (at least in theory) better than panitumumab at attracting and activating white blood cells. Hence, cetuximab and necitumumab can create a cancer-fighting immune response [52].

---

[8] For a little bit more about what each class of antibody does, see https://microbiologyinfo.com/antibody-structure-classes-and-functions/.

Table 3.2 Treatments that target EGFR.

Treatment type and licensed examples	Who are they given to?	Why?
Antibody-based treatments		
Intact, "naked" antibodies[a]: cetuximab, panitumumab, necitumumab, and nimotuzumab	Cetuximab is a licensed treatment for bowel cancer and head and neck cancer; panitumumab is licensed for bowel cancer. Necitumumab is licensed for squamous cell NSCLCs that have high levels of EGFR.	In these cancers, EGFR is normal (wild-type), but there is too much of it. These antibodies prevent EGFRs from becoming active by blocking access to ligands; they also cause EGFRs to be internalized and destroyed. They have varying abilities to attract and activate white blood cells.
Bi-specific antibodies: amivantamab (targets both EGFR and MET)	People with NSCLC with *EGFR* exon 20 insertions.	NSCLCs with exon 20 insertions don't respond to first-, second-, or third-generation EGFR kinase inhibitors. Dual targeting of both EGFR and MET appears to block EGFR and MET activity; the antibody also recruits and activates white blood cells.
Antibody-drug conjugates:Several are in development, but none are licensed so far	In trials for people with triple-negative breast cancer, glioblastoma, pancreatic cancer, and other cancer types.	In these cancers, the cells have lots of EGFR on their surface and there is a massive need for effective new treatments. Naked antibodies haven't been successful in trials, but drug-conjugated antibodies might be more helpful.
Kinase inhibitors		
First-generation, reversible inhibitors: gefitinib and erlotinib. Second-generation, irreversible, pan-HER inhibitors: afatinib, dacomitinib, and neratinib	These are licensed treatments for • NSCLCs with sensitizing *EGFR* mutations. • HER2-positive breast cancer.	In about 10%–15% of NSCLCs, the EGF receptor is mutated and overactive; kinase inhibitors are far more likely to be effective when these mutations are present. Pan-HER inhibitors also block HER2, and neratinib is a treatment for HER2-positive breast cancer.
Third-generation, irreversible inhibitors: osimertinib and lazertinib	Licensed for NSCLCs containing sensitizing *EGFR* mutations, and those with the T790M mutant version of EGFR.	The T790M mutation causes resistance to first- and second-generation drugs; third-generation drugs have been designed to block EGFR even when the T790M mutation is present.
Kinase inhibitors active against EGFRs with exon 20 insertions: poziotinib, mobocertinib, and many more in development	People with NSCLC with *EGFR* exon 20 insertions.	Exon 20 insertions in the *EGFR* gene are rare, but they lead to versions of EGFR that are resistant to first-, second-, and third-generation EGFR inhibitors. Over 50 different exon 20 insertions have been found in the *EGFR* gene.

[a] A "naked" antibody is one where nothing has been added to or removed from the antibody's structure.

Who They Are Given To

Panitumumab and cetuximab are licensed as treatments for people with bowel cancer. Cetuximab is also licensed for some people with head and neck cancer. The cells of both these cancers tend to have lots of EGFRs on their surface.

However, these aren't the only cancers where the cancer cells have lots of EGFRs on their surface. Because of this, scientists have

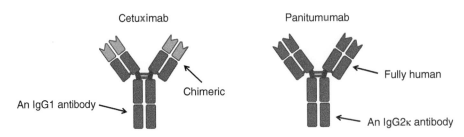

Figure 3.8 Comparison of panitumumab and cetuximab. Both treatments are monoclonal antibodies. However, cetuximab is chimeric – the back part of the antibody is a human IgG1 antibody, whereas the antigen-binding region is from a mouse antibody. Panitumumab is a fully human IgG2κ (IgG2-kappa) antibody.

conducted numerous clinical trials, involving thousands of people with cancer. In these trials, EGFR-targeted antibodies (and kinase inhibitors) have been given to people with many other cancer types (such as ovarian cancer, triple-negative breast cancer, pancreatic cancer, prostate cancer, primary liver cancer, esophageal cancer, and glioblastoma). But, aside from bowel cancer and head and neck cancer, EGFR-targeted antibodies haven't helped enough people to warrant being approved by regulators [50].

By the way, in case you're interested, necitumumab was licensed in Europe[9] as a treatment for people with squamous cell NSCLC in 2016, but it was withdrawn in 2021 [53]. Nimotuzumab is an approved treatment in an eclectic group of countries including India, Cuba, Argentina, and China (but not in the United States or Europe) [54].

How They Work

All EGFR-targeted antibodies attach to the external part of EGFR and prevent EGF or other EGFR ligands[10] attaching to the receptor. These antibodies also cause cells to destroy

their EGFRs [52]. Without any growth factors attached, the receptors can't pair up or become active. As I mentioned before, cetuximab can also attract and activate white blood cells (cetuximab's mechanisms of action are summarized in Figure 3.9). Despite their differences, cetuximab and panitumumab have given very similar results in clinical trials for people with bowel cancer [51].

Why They Can't Be Given to Everyone

Cetuximab and panitumumab don't work for everyone with bowel cancer (or head and neck cancer for that matter, but we have a lot more information about what happens in bowel cancer). An important discovery has been that in bowel cancer the cancer cells often contain mutations that make treatment with EGFR-targeted antibodies pointless. It seems that if intracellular proteins[11] such as K-Ras, N-Ras, or B-Raf are mutated and overactive (as is the case in roughly 50% of patients), then this leads to activation of the MAPK and PI3K/AKT/mTOR pathways and renders the receptor redundant. If you then block the receptor with an antibody, this

[9] Whenever I mention "Europe" in terms of where a treatment is licensed, I'm talking about decisions made by the European Medicines Authority (EMA), which approves treatments for use in countries in the European Union and the European Economic Area (Iceland, Liechtenstein, and Norway).

[10] As I've said before, ligands are molecules such as small proteins that attach to receptors. For example, EGF is a ligand that attaches to EGF receptors.

[11] That is, proteins that exist in the cytoplasm and/or nucleus of the cell.

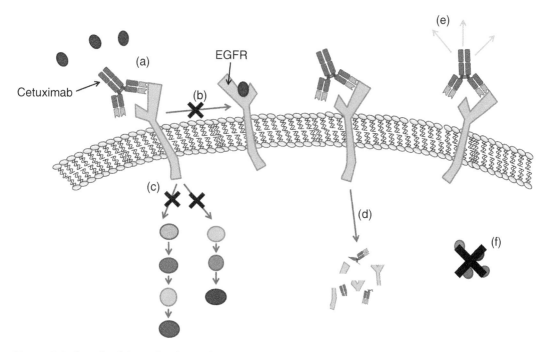

Figure 3.9 Cetuximab's mechanisms of action. **(a)** Cetuximab prevents ligands such as EGF from attaching to EGFRs. **(b)** It also physically prevents two EGFRs from pairing up, even if EGF has successfully attached. **(c)** Because EGFRs cannot pair up, internal signaling pathways don't become active. **(d)** The attachment of cetuximab causes EGFRs to be drawn inside the cell and destroyed. **(e)** Cetuximab attracts and activates white blood cells and complement proteins, which kill cancer cells. **(f)** Without the activation of EGFRs, the cell doesn't produce proteins that would protect it from death or trigger angiogenesis. **Abbreviation:** EGFR – epidermal growth factor receptor.

won't block the pathways or kill the cell, and the patient doesn't get any better [55, 56] (Figure 3.10).

Other, related reasons for resistance include overproduction of alternative growth factor receptors (such as MET, HER2, or PDGFRA), loss of PTEN (which naturally suppresses the PI3K/AKT/mTOR pathway), *MEK* mutations, alteration of the binding site for cetuximab on the EGFR, or the presence of a kinase fusion protein [55, 56].

Why They Sometimes Stop Working
Even when no *KRAS*, *NRAS*, or *BRAF* gene mutation is found when the patient's tumor is tested, cetuximab and panitumumab don't help everyone. Also, even if these treatments

do work initially, and the person's cancer shrinks or stops growing, this effect doesn't generally last forever [55–57].

Many scientists have examined cells from patients whose bowel cancer has stopped responding to cetuximab or panitumumab to understand what has happened. They've generally found that resistant cancers contain the same mutations as I've described before. Presumably, at the point that the person was diagnosed, cells with these mutations were in such a tiny minority that they weren't picked up by mutation testing. But, months or years later, the resistant cells have had the time and opportunity to multiply. Finally, there are enough cells to be picked up on a scan and the person is told that their cancer has come back.

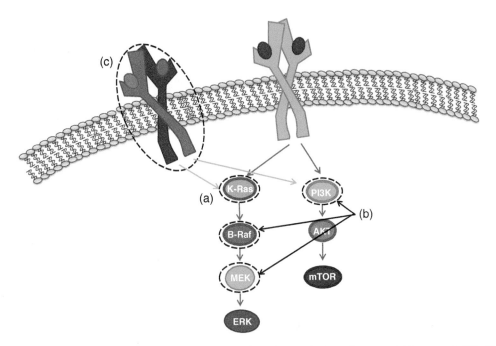

Figure 3.10 Reasons for resistance to EGFR-targeted antibodies in bowel cancer. (a) In around 40%–50% of bowel cancers, the cells contain a mutated, overactive version of K-Ras or, less commonly N-Ras. **(b)** Many mutations affecting B-Raf, PI3K, and MEK proteins also cause resistance. **(c)** Amplification of the genes for HER2, MET, or other growth factor receptors causes excessive amounts of these receptors on the cell surface, which cause resistance by activating Ras, PI3K, and other signaling pathways.
Abbreviations: See Figure 3.5

3.4.2 Kinase Inhibitors that Target EGFR

The first EGFR-targeted kinase inhibitors, gefitinib and erlotinib, entered clinical trials around the year 2000. Since that time, we've learned a huge amount about when, and when not, to prescribe these treatments. We've also seen the arrival of second-generation and third-generation drugs. Scientists have also created new inhibitors that target versions of EGFR that were previously un-blockable. All these treatments are almost exclusively used in the treatment of people with NSCLC. But they're only given to the 10%–15% of people whose cancer cells are producing a mutated, overactive version of the EGFR.

To understand that last sentence, it's worth knowing a bit about the *EGFR* gene and the EGFR protein made from it. I promise you that this isn't just random knowledge! Some of the language used to describe the various mutated versions of EGFR, and the problems faced when making EGFR inhibitors, only becomes clear when you understand how genes work.

The first bit of information I want you to know is that the *EGFR* gene contains 28 exons and 27 introns [58]. (Exons are regions of a gene whose information is used to make the final protein. Introns are regions of genes that initially get turned into mRNA, but whose information then gets cut out through a process called splicing.[12]) The kinase portion of

---

[12] There's a great explanation of this on the Khan Academy website: https://www.khanacademy.org/science/ap-biology/gene-expression-and-regulation/transcription-and-rna-processing/a/eukaryotic-pre-mrna-processing.

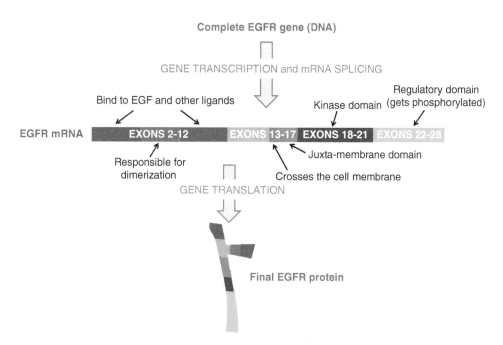

Figure 3.11 Structure of the *EGFR* gene and how it relates to EGFR protein. The complete *EGFR* gene contains 28 exons and 27 introns. Information in the gene's exons is used to make different parts of the EGFR protein. For example, exons 18-21 contain the information needed to construct the EGFR's kinase domain. The final protein is shown in its un-paired shape. When a ligand attaches to the receptor, it changes shape, exposing its dimerization domain. In its new shape, the receptor can pair up with a partner, which will be EGFR or another member of the HER family.
Abbreviation: EGFR – epidermal growth factor receptor.

the EGFR protein, the part that's inside the cell and is responsible for attaching phosphates to its partner receptor, is made from exons 18-21 in the *EGFR* gene (Figure 3.11).

Mutations in the *EGFR* gene that cause the EGFR protein to be overactive (and that drive the behavior of cancer cells with these mutations) affect this kinase domain. For example, the most common mutations affecting the kinase domain are deletions in exon 19 and the L858R substitution in exon 21 (instead of a leucine there is an arginine amino acid at position 858 in the EGFR protein). These cause the kinase domain to change shape in such a way that the EGFR is overactive and highly sensitive to EGFR inhibitors (these mutations are summarized in Figure 3.12).

First- and Second-Generation EGFR Inhibitors

EGFR is a cell surface protein accessible to antibodies like cetuximab and panitumumab. But it's also a kinase, and it can therefore be blocked with a kinase inhibitor.[13]

Several kinase inhibitors that block EGFR have been created. Erlotinib and gefitinib were two of the first. They are first-generation, reversible EGFR inhibitors that mimic ATP and block EGFR's kinase activity. Afatinib, dacomitinib, and neratinib, which are second-generation drugs, are slightly different. They are irreversible inhibitors that chemically bond with EGFR's ATP-binding site (see Section 2.3.4 and Figure 2.19d). In addition to blocking EGFR, they also block the kinase domains of

---

[13] For more about antibodies and kinase inhibitors, see Chapter 2.

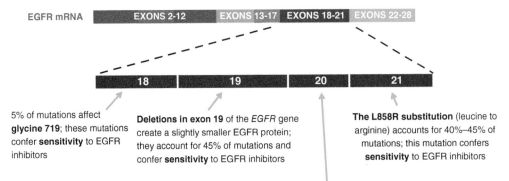

EGFR mRNA | EXONS 2-12 | EXONS 13-17 | EXONS 18-21 | EXONS 22-28 |

| 18 | 19 | 20 | 21 |

5% of mutations affect **glycine 719**; these mutations confer **sensitivity** to EGFR inhibitors

Deletions in exon 19 of the *EGFR* gene create a slightly smaller EGFR protein; they account for 45% of mutations and confer **sensitivity** to EGFR inhibitors

The L858R substitution (leucine to arginine) accounts for 40%–45% of mutations; this mutation confers **sensitivity** to EGFR inhibitors

Insertions in exon 20 and the **T790M mutation in exon 20** are found in **5%-10% of newly diagnosed** lung adenocarcinomas and confer **resistance** to first- and second-generation EGFR inhibitors (e.g., erlotinib, gefitinib, and afatinib); the **T790M mutation is also found in ~60% of tumors resistant** to first- and second-generation drugs and is **sensitive to third-generation drugs** (e.g., osimertinib)

Figure 3.12 **Location of mutations in the *EGFR* gene that cause overactivity of EGFRs and that determine sensitivity to EGFR-targeted kinase inhibitors.** *Source:* Khaddour et al. [59]/MDPI/Public Domain. **Abbreviation:** EGFR – epidermal growth factor receptor.

HER2 and HER4 (HER3 doesn't have kinase activity of its own, but it can pair up with and activate other family members [60]). Because they block multiple human EGF receptors, afatinib, dacomitinib, and neratinib are sometimes called pan-HER inhibitors [59].

All these treatments appear to work best when the cancer cells are producing a mutated, overactive version of EGFR. The cancer in which these kinase domain mutations are most common is NSCLC. The most common activating mutations are exon 19 deletions and the L858R mutation.

It seems that when the EGFR is mutated and overactive, lung cancer cells become more reliant on it for their survival than if they simply overproduce the normal, un-mutated version of the protein. Erlotinib and gefitinib (and later afatinib and dacomitinib) became standard treatments for people with *EGFR*-mutated NSCLC in the early 2000s. However, all four drugs have now largely been superseded by osimertinib (see below).

In 2017, neratinib became licensed in the United States as an adjuvant treatment for women with HER2-positive breast cancer [61].

Its effects against HER2-positive breast cancer are presumably because of its impact on HER2 rather than EGFR.

Third-Generation EGFR Kinase Inhibitors

When first- and second-generation EGFR kinase inhibitors were first created, they represented a huge step forward in the treatment of people with *EGFR*-mutated, advanced lung cancer. However, it soon became apparent that people weren't being cured by these treatments. Scientists figured out that resistance was often caused by cancer cells that had a further mutation in their *EGFR* gene [59]. This additional mutation, called the T790M mutation, changes the shape of EGFR's ATP-binding site. Drugs like gefitinib and erlotinib can no longer block the mutated protein. However, third-generation drugs such as osimertinib and lazertinib can block EGFRs with this mutation.

For a comparison of first-, second-, and third-generation EGFR inhibitors, see Table 3.3.

In addition to blocking EGFRs with the T790M mutation, third-generation EGFR

Table 3.3 Comparison of first-, second-, and third-generation EGFR kinase inhibitors.

	First generation	Second generation	Third generation
Type of inhibition	Reversible	Irreversible	Irreversible
Ability to block:			
Wild-type EGFR	Strong	Strong	Weak
Exon 19 deleted EGFR	Strong	Very strong	Very strong
L858R mutated EGFR	Strong	Very strong	Very strong
T790M mutated EGFR	nil	Moderate	Very strong
HER2	nil	Strong	nil
HER4	nil	Strong	nil
Examples of drugs	Gefitinib, erlotinib, and icotinib	Afatinib, dacomitinib, and pyrotinib	Osimertinib, olmutinib, lazertinib, EGF816, and ASP8273

Source: Ref. [59, 62, 63].

inhibitors have another strength – their relative inability to block wild-type EGFR. As a result, third-generation drugs like osimertinib cause less severe side effects than first- and second-generation drugs [64, 65]. Over the past few years, osimertinib has gradually been used more and more, and first- and second-generation drugs used less.

EGFRs with Exon 20 Insertions

In around 4%–12% of people with *EGFR*-mutated lung cancer, the mutation in the cancer cells' *EGFR* gene is an insertion of between 3 and 21 DNA base pairs in exon 20 (corresponding to between 1 and 7 extra amino acids in the EGFR protein) [66–68]. These mutations are also found in tiny proportions of people with bladder cancer, breast cancer, and central nervous system tumors [66]. Over 50 different exon 20 insertions have been discovered, and each mutation affects the EGFR protein in a different way [69, 70]. This creates its own problems. For example, each individual mutation is very rare, making it difficult to get a clear picture as to its impact in terms of sensitivity to different EGFR inhibitors.

In general, first-, second-, and third-generation EGFR inhibitors are ineffective against EGFRs with exon 20 insertions [69].

Thankfully, a few new drugs have been created that seem to be active against a range of different EGFRs with exon 20 insertions. These include amivantamab, poziotinib, and mobocertinib.

Amivantamab is the one that has so far been the most successful (see Figure 2.6 for its structure). It is a bi-specific antibody that attaches to both EGFR and MET. Scientists believe that in addition to blocking the activity of these receptors, the antibody also recruits and activates white blood cells [71]. Results from clinical trials have shown it can be an effective treatment for people with NSCLC with *EGFR* exon 20 insertion mutations [72].

Who They're Given To

EGFR kinase inhibitors are almost exclusively given to the 10%–15% or so of people with NSCLC whose cancer cells have mutated, overactive EGFRs on their surface. These mutations are usually found in people with adenocarcinoma NSCLC, who have little or no history of smoking. They're also much more common in people from East-Asian countries [73, 74].

Erlotinib, a first-generation EGFR kinase inhibitor, has also shown a degree of usefulness against pancreatic cancer, despite *EGFR* mutations being incredibly rare in this cancer [75]. It's important to say, though, that whereas EGFR inhibitors generally hold NSCLC at bay for 9–19 months, in pancreatic cancer they only add a week or two to survival times when added to standard chemotherapy [76]. The licensing of erlotinib for people with pancreatic cancer is therefore more of a reflection of how few effective treatment options we have for pancreatic cancer, rather than a belief that erlotinib will provide dramatic benefits [77].

Resistance to EGFR-Targeted Kinase Inhibitors

Almost all the detailed information we have about resistance mechanisms to EGFR kinase inhibitors comes from people with NSCLC, as they are the people most likely to be treated with one of these drugs. And, as I said earlier, a common reason why an NSCLC becomes resistant to a first- or second-generation EGFR kinase inhibitor is because of cancer cells that contain the T790M mutation in one of their *EGFR* genes [78].

Resistance mechanisms to third-generation drugs like osimertinib are more diverse (they are summarized in Figure 3.13). They include mutations or amplifications affecting the *EGFR* gene; mutations and/or amplification of other growth factor receptors such as MET or HER2; mutations affecting proteins involved in the MAPK or PI3K/AKT/mTOR pathways; the presence of kinase fusion proteins; activation of STAT or NFκB transcription factors; and

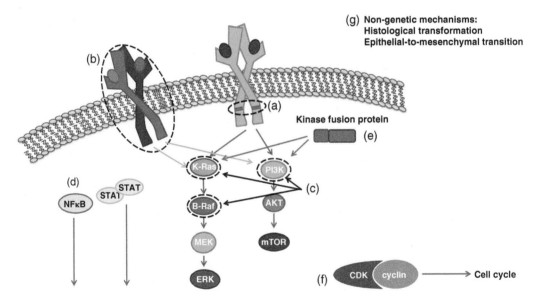

Figure 3.13 Reasons for resistance to osimertinib in EGFR-mutated NSCLC. (a) Mutations affecting the kinase domain of EGFR include C797S, L792X, and G796X. **(b)** Amplification or activating mutations affecting other growth factor receptors, such as HER2, FGFRs, or MET. **(c)** Many mutations affecting B-Raf, PI3K, and Ras proteins also cause resistance. **(d)** Mutations affecting STAT and NFκB transcription factors can promote cell survival and proliferation without activity of MAPK or PI3K signaling pathways.
(e) Sometimes the kinase portion of a growth factor receptor or other kinase is present as part of a fusion protein. **(f)** Mutations in the genes for cyclins or CDKs can force cells to multiply. **(g)** Some mechanisms of resistance have no known genetic cause, such as the epithelial-to-mesenchymal transition, or transformation to become a small cell lung cancer or squamous cell carcinoma.
Abbreviations: CDK – cyclin-dependent kinase. For other abbreviations see Figure 3.5.

mutations affecting cyclins and CDKs, which force cells into the cell cycle. Another reason for resistance is when NSCLC cells change shape and become much more like the cells that cause small cell lung cancer (SCLC) or squamous cell NSCLC [79].

Huge efforts are being made to overcome resistance to osimertinib using various targeted drugs and treatment combinations. Approaches include the following: [80–85]

- Combining osimertinib with a treatment that directly targets MET (e.g., tepotinib) in people with *EGFR*-mutated and *MET*-amplified NSCLC.
- A combination of amivantamab (the bispecific antibody targeting EGFR and MET) with another third-generation EGFR inhibitor, lazertinib, and chemotherapy.
- Osimertinib combined with chemotherapy. The reduced side effects of osimertinib versus first- and second-generation drugs make this a feasible combination.
- Combinations involving a checkpoint inhibitor. Over the course of various clinical trials, we've learned that people whose NSCLCs contain an *EGFR* mutation generally get very little benefit from checkpoint inhibitors. But, one combination, that of chemotherapy, atezolizumab, and bevacizumab (an angiogenesis inhibitor), did give positive results and is available to people with *EGFR* mutations.
- HER3-targeted treatments, such as the antibody-drug conjugate (ADC) patritumab deruxtecan, zenocutuzumab (a bispecific antibody targeting HER2 and HER3), patritumab, and seribantumab (naked antibodies that target HER3).
- Other ADCs being investigated include TROP2 treatments such as datopotamab deruxtecan.

Combinations are also being tested as a way of improving on osimertinib alone for newly diagnosed patients with sensitizing *EGFR* mutations. For example, in the MARIPOSA trial, the combination of lazertinib with amivantamab was directly compared to osimertinib in patients with newly diagnosed *EGFR*-mutated NSCLC. The percentage of people whose disease hadn't progressed after 2 years was 48% in patients given the combination versus 34% with osimertinib alone [86].

3.5 DRUGS THAT TARGET HER2

Licensed drugs mentioned in this section:		
Treatment class	**Drugs**	**Given to some people with:**
Naked antibody therapies	Trastuzumab, trastuzumab biosimilars, pertuzumab, and margetuximab	• HER2-positive breast cancer • HER2-positive stomach cancer or gastroesophageal junction cancer
Antibody-drug conjugates	Trastuzumab emtansine and trastuzumab deruxtecan	• HER2-positive breast cancer • HER2-low breast cancer • HER2-positive stomach cancer or gastroesophageal junction cancer • NSCLCs containing mutations in the *HER2* gene
HER2-targeted kinase inhibitors	Lapatinib, neratinib, and tucatinib	• HER2-positive breast cancer • HER2-positive bowel cancer

As with EGFR-targeted treatments, the drugs that target HER2 can be split into monoclonal antibodies and kinase inhibitors (see Table 3.4 for more detail):

1. Monoclonal antibodies that block HER2 from outside the cell
2. Drug-conjugated antibodies that block HER2 from outside the cell and that also deliver chemotherapy
3. Kinase inhibitors that block the kinase portion of HER2 from inside the cell

Table 3.4   Treatments that target HER2 [87–93].

Treatment type and examples	Who are they given to?	Why?
Antibody-based treatments		
Intact, "naked" antibodies: trastuzumab, pertuzumab, margetuximab, and trastuzumab biosimilars	These are licensed treatments for people with breast cancers and stomach cancers considered to be "HER2-postive."	These cancers depend on HER2 for growth and survival, and many clinical trials have proven trastuzumab and other HER2-targeted antibodies to be helpful treatments.
ADCs: trastuzumab emtansine and trastuzumab deruxtecan	Both treatments are licensed for people with *HER2*-amplified breast cancer. Trastuzumab deruxtecan is also licensed as a treatment for people with HER2-low breast cancer, HER2-positive stomach cancer, and people with *HER2*-mutated NSCLC.	ADCs deliver chemotherapy direct to cancer cells and combine the effects of the antibody with those of chemotherapy. The antibody's target must be present for the antibody to attach to.
Bi-specific antibodies: none licensed yet but several in trials, such as zenocutuzumab, which targets both HER2 and HER3	They may be useful for people with trastuzumab-resistant disease where resistance is driven by multiple different receptors.	There is a need for treatments that work in new ways for people who have already received existing HER2-targeted treatments. Bi-specific antibodies block the targeted receptors and provoke an immune response from macrophages and NK cells.
Kinase inhibitors		
Kinase inhibitors that selectively block HER2: tucatinib	People with HER2-positive breast cancer or bowel cancer.	Cancers in which the HER2 gene is amplified are thought to rely on HER2 for their survival.
Kinase inhibitors that block EGFR and HER2: lapatinib	People with HER2-positive breast cancer.	As mentioned earlier, the fact that lapatinib also blocks EGFR isn't thought to be part of its mechanism of action against breast cancer.
Drugs that block EGFR, HER2, and HER4 (irreversible, pan-HER inhibitors): neratinib, dacomitinib, and afatinib (poziotinib and pyrotinib)	Of these treatments, only neratinib is approved for HER2-positive breast cancer. Dacomitinib and afatinib are licensed for NSCLC with *EGFR* mutations.	As for lapatinib and tucatinib, the fact that these treatments block other HERs aside from HER2 isn't thought to add to their effectiveness.
Drugs with activity against *HER2* with exon 20 insertions: poziotinib and pyrotinib	These treatments are in trials for people with NSCLC, breast cancer, or other solid tumors, but only if their cancer cells contain exon 20 insertions in the *HER2* gene.	Exon 20 mutations in *HER2* are most common in people with NSCLC, although they still only account for 1%–2% of people. They're also found in ~1% of bladder cancers and breast cancers and even smaller percentages of other cancers. Exon 20 insertions render HER2 insensitive to most HER2-targeted kinase inhibitors

3.5.1 Monoclonal Antibodies that Target HER2

Five antibodies that target HER2 are licensed as cancer treatments: trastuzumab, pertuzumab, margetuximab, trastuzumab emtansine, and trastuzumab deruxtecan.

The first three of these antibodies are "naked" antibodies; that is, nothing has been added to, or removed from, the antibody's structure. The other two are ADCs that deliver chemotherapy to target cells.

Mechanisms of Action

Trastuzumab was the first HER2-targeted antibody to be licensed. It is thought to have several mechanisms of action, including the following [87, 88]:

- It prevents paired-up HER2s from activating signaling pathways, being most active against a pairing of HER2 with HER2 (HER2:HER2), and less active against HER2:HER3 or HER2:EGFR.
- It recruits white blood cells such as macrophages and natural killer cells, which then destroy HER2-positive cancer cells.
- It prevents the external part of HER2 from breaking off and being shed from the cell – if the HER2 protein is allowed to break, the part of HER2 that remains embedded in the cell membrane (called p95) is extremely active.
- It may have some ability to prevent HER2s from pairing up with one another or with other receptors.
- It causes destruction of HER2.

In contrast, pertuzumab's main mechanism of action is to prevent HER2 from pairing up with EGFR or HER3 [89]. The two antibodies therefore have slightly different, and complementary, mechanisms of action, and some clinical trials have shown that the two antibodies work well in combination [90].

Trastuzumab emtansine (T-DM1) and trastuzumab deruxtecan (T-Dx) are different again. They are ADCs made from trastuzumab linked to potent chemotherapies called emtansine (also called mertansine or DM1) or deruxtecan.

The mechanisms of action of trastuzumab and of other HER2-targeted antibodies are summarized in Figure 3.14 [43, 87, 89, 91–93]

Who They're Given To

Treatments that target HER2 are primarily given to people[14] with HER2-positive breast cancer, or HER2-positive stomach cancer – people whose cancer cells have very high levels of HER2 protein on their surface and/or contain extra copies (amplification) of the *HER2* gene (Figure. 3.15).

However, the precise meaning of "HER2-positive" depends on what tests were performed on the person's cancer and the type of cancer the person has. For example, if no genetic analysis was performed, the doctor simply won't know whether the *HER2* gene is amplified or not. In which case, "HER2-positive" will refer to the amount of HER2 protein on the cells' surface as determined by immunohistochemistry (IHC).

Trastuzumab was first licensed in Europe in 2000 for the treatment of people diagnosed with HER2-positive breast cancer. In 2010, its license was extended to include people with HER2-positive stomach cancer. Pertuzumab, T-DM1, T-Dx, and margetuximab are also licensed breast cancer treatments, as are some kinase inhibitors.

HER2-positive breast cancers are very aggressive and likely to spread and return following treatment. However, the association between HER2-positivity and poor prognosis has been reversed thanks to HER2-targeted treatments [94–96].

---

[14] Of course, the vast majority of breast cancers occur in people born with female sex organs (roughly 56,000 cases diagnosed per year in the United Kingdom), but around 400 or so develop in people born biologically male.

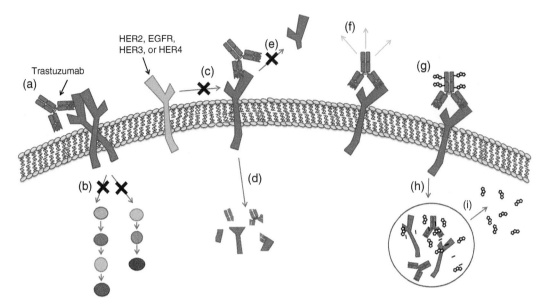

Figure 3.14 Mechanisms of action of HER2-targeted antibodies. (a) Trastuzumab attaches to HER2 near the cell membrane. **(b)** It prevents HER2 homodimers and heterodimers from activating signaling pathways. **(c)** Pertuzumab (and to some extent trastuzumab) prevents HER2 from pairing up with HER2, EGFR, or HER3 and thereby prevents the activation of signaling pathways (unpaired growth factor receptors cannot activate signaling pathways). **(d)** Trastuzumab triggers destruction of HER2 and **(e)** prevents breakage and shedding of HER2 from the cell surface. **(f)** Trastuzumab and pertuzumab can both activate white blood cells. Margetuximab has been designed to do this even better. **(g)** The ADCs, trastuzumab emtansine (T-DM1) and trastuzumab deruxtecan (T-Dx), do all the things that naked trastuzumab can do, but they also have chemotherapy linked to them. **(h)** Once inside the cell, T-DM1 and T-Dx break apart. **(i)** Chemotherapy leaks into the cell.
Abbreviations: ADC – antibody-drug conjugate; EGFR – epidermal growth factor receptor; HER2 – human epidermal growth factor receptor-2; HER3 – human epidermal growth factor receptor-3.

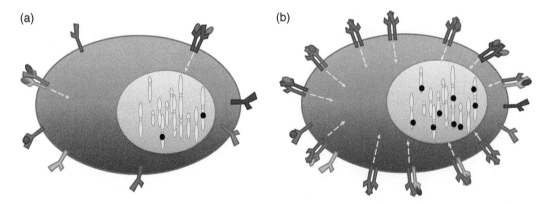

Figure 3.15 HER2-positive cancers have extra copies of the *HER2* gene and/or extra amounts of HER2 protein on their surface. (a) Normal cells have two copies of the *HER2* gene (on chromosome 17) and produce very little HER2 protein. Paired receptors on the cell surface provide just enough activation of signaling pathways to keep it alive. **(b)** *HER2* gene amplification leads to the overproduction of HER2 protein which pairs up with itself and other HER-family members (namely EGFR, HER3, and HER4). This causes increased activity of signaling pathways and drives cell proliferation and survival. Black dots denote the location of each copy of the *HER2* gene.
Abbreviations: EGFR– epidermal growth factor receptor; HER2 – human epidermal growth factor receptor-2; HER3 – human epidermal growth factor receptor-3; HER4 – human epidermal growth factor receptor-4.

Around 15%–20% of breast cancers and stomach cancers are HER2-positive [43]. But what "HER2-positive" means differs between the two cancer types. In stomach cancer, the amount of HER2 on the surface of cancer cells varies a lot from cell to cell. Also, when a person's cancer is tested for HER2, the results from immunohistochemistry (testing for HER2 protein) don't always match-up with the results obtained with in situ hybridization (testing for *HER2* gene amplification) [97]. Scientists think that this high degree of variation (referred to as heterogeneity) is why HER2-targeted treatments don't tend to work as well against stomach cancer compared to breast cancer.

Improvements in HER2-targeted Treatments

Trastuzumab deruxtecan (T-Dx) contains several improvements compared to trastuzumab emtansine (T-DM1). For example, T-Dx contains more copies of drug per antibody. In addition, the linker holding the drug (deruxtecan) to the antibody breaks more easily inside cancer cells. (For a more detailed look at the differences between the two treatments see Table 4.3 in Chapter 4.) As a result, T-Dx seems to be active even in situations where T-DM1 fails to make an impact [92, 93]. In 2022, regulators in America and Europe approved T-Dx as a treatment for HER2-low breast cancer based on the results of the DESTINY-Breast04 study [98, 99]. Around 50% or so of breast cancers are HER2-low (much greater than the proportion usually described as being HER2-positive).

HER2-low cancers are those that have some HER2 on their surface, but not enough to be considered HER2-positive, and they test negative for extra copies of the *HER2* gene. HER2-low cancers include around 50% of hormone receptor-positive breast cancers and around 30% of triple-negative breast cancers [98, 100].

The creation of drug conjugates like T-Dx also seems to be creating new opportunities for treating HER2-positive, and HER2-low,

cancers other than breast and stomach cancer. There are various cancers, such as NSCLC, salivary gland cancer, bowel cancer, biliary tract cancer, uterine cancer, ovarian cancer, and pancreatic cancer, where in a proportion of people there's at least some HER2 on the surface of their cancer cells, and/or HER2 is overactive [43, 101].

In the past, blocking HER2 with trastuzumab, lapatinib, or another HER2-targeted treatment didn't appear to bring a lot of benefit to these people. But, particularly because of the creation of T-Dx, the results from clinical trials with HER2-targeted treatments are looking better all the time [43]. In 2022, the FDA gave accelerated approval to trastuzumab deruxtecan for people with NSLC whose tumors contain a *HER2* mutation [102].

Why They Sometimes Don't Work

Although HER2-targeted antibodies have proven to be very helpful, particularly against HER2-positive breast cancer, they don't work for everyone. Also, for people with metastatic cancer, the benefit they bring is generally only temporary (although it can last for many months, if not years) [103].

Much of what we know about mechanisms of resistance to HER2-targeted antibodies comes from studying breast cancers that are resistant to trastuzumab. Various mechanisms of resistance have been found (summarized in Figure 3.16). They include the following: [88, 94, 103–106]

- Cancer cells in protected environments such as the brain survive treatment.
- Mutations that activate the PI3K/AKT/mTOR pathway make HER2 redundant; therefore, blocking HER2 has no impact.
- Changes to HER2. Sometimes a shortened version of HER2 called p95 is made by cancer cells, which lacks the binding site for trastuzumab. In other cancers, the kinase portion of HER2 has become overactive.
- The ability of trastuzumab to attract and activate white blood cells is important for maximum benefit – people whose tumors

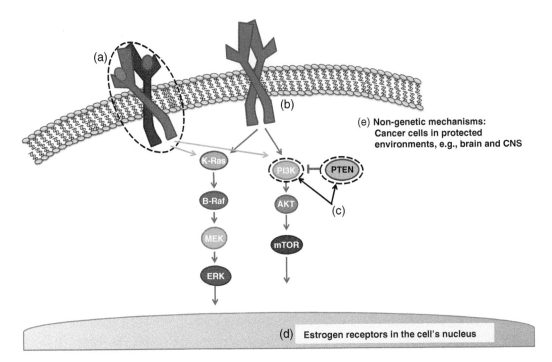

Figure 3.16 Some reasons for resistance to HER2-targeted antibodies in breast cancer cells.
(a) Some trastuzumab-resistant cells have mutations affecting the HER2 gene. They therefore manufacture overactive HER2, or they make a version of HER2 that lacks a binding site for trastuzumab. **(b)** Another cause of resistance is the presence of other growth factor receptors on the cell surface. **(c)** Mutations affecting the PI3K pathway, such as mutations in the *PIK3CA* gene that cause PI3K to be overactive, or loss of PTEN. **(d)** If there are lots of active estrogen receptors in the cell's nucleus, these can protect the cell from death. **(e)** Cancer cells in protected environments such as the brain are largely inaccessible to antibody treatments such as trastuzumab that struggle to cross the blood-brain barrier.
Abbreviations: See Figure 3.5. CNS – central nervous system.

contain low levels of infiltrating white blood cells, or high levels of immune-suppressing proteins, seem less likely to benefit from trastuzumab.
- If other growth factor receptors are present on the cancer cells' surface, such as EGFR, HER3, MET, IGF-1, and EphA2, these activate signaling pathways even when HER2 is blocked.
- Also, if EGFR or HER3 pairs up with HER2, this creates a pairing that can't be completely blocked by trastuzumab (these pairings can be prevented by pertuzumab or blocked by a kinase inhibitor such as lapatinib).

- If there are lots of estrogen receptors (ERs) in the cancer cells, these trigger the production of many growth factor receptors, and they activate various signaling pathways that can overcome the effects of trastuzumab.

Because of this knowledge, we have seen lots of clinical trials in which treatment combinations have been tried. For example, some trials have tested a combination of trastuzumab with pertuzumab or lapatinib. Other trials have combined trastuzumab with hormone therapies such as anastrozole or letrozole, or with mTOR, AKT, or PI3K inhibitors, or with immunotherapy.

3.5.2 Kinase Inhibitors that Target HER2

Like other growth factor receptors, the intracellular part of HER2 (the bit that extends inside the cell cytoplasm) is a kinase. When HER2 pairs up with another HER2 or with another HER family member, the receptors phosphorylate one another and activate various signaling pathways.

Because HER2 is a kinase, it has been possible to create kinase inhibitors that target it. However, it's the antibody-based treatments that have shown the greatest impact against HER2-positive breast cancer. As a result, antibodies that target HER2 are used much more widely than the kinase inhibitors.

Comparison of HER2-Targeted Kinase Inhibitors

In Europe, there are so far three kinase inhibitors licensed for people with HER2-positive breast cancer: lapatinib, neratinib, and tucatinib (see Table 3.5). Lapatinib, like many other kinase inhibitors, mimics ATP and reversibly blocks the ATP-binding site of its targets, EGFR and HER2. And, unlike antibodies targeted against HER2, it can block the broken, constantly active form of HER2 called p95 [109].

Neratinib, like afatinib and dacomitinib, is an irreversible, pan-HER inhibitor (it blocks all HER-family members, not just HER2 and EGFR). In September 2018, the European Medicines Agency (EMA) approved neratinib as an adjuvant treatment for people with early-stage, HER2-positive breast cancer, who have completed the standard year of treatment with trastuzumab following surgery.

Tucatinib is a more recent addition. It is a highly specific, reversible HER2 inhibitor [110]. So far, it is licensed for people with advanced HER2-positive breast cancer who have already received other HER2-targeted treatments. The FDA has also approved it for people with HER2-positive bowel cancer who have already received other treatments.

Activity Against Brain Metastases

Brain metastases occur in about 50% of patients with HER2-positive breast cancer. This is largely because antibody-based treatments destroy cancer cells elsewhere in the body, so patients now live long enough for brain metastases to develop.

One area in which kinase inhibitors have a theoretical advantage over antibody-based cancer treatments is their potential to cross the blood-brain barrier and either prevent or control brain metastases. Various trials have been conducted. These have showed that kinase inhibitors such as lapatinib, neratinib, and tucatinib can all benefit patients who either already have brain metastases or are at risk of developing them [108].

However, things are never that clear-cut, and there's clear evidence that some antibody-based treatments also have an effect on brain metastases. For example, in

Table 3.5 Comparison of HER2-targeted kinase inhibitors.

	Type of inhibition	Targets	Able to block HER2 with exon 20 insertions?
Lapatinib	reversible	EGFR, HER2	No
Neratinib, dacomitinib, and afatinib	irreversible	EGFR, HER2, and HER4[a]	No
Tucatinib	reversible	HER2	No
Poziotinib and pyrotinib	irreversible	EGFR, HER2, and HER4[a]	Yes

Source: Ref. [107, 108].
[a] HER3 doesn't have kinase activity so these drugs effectively block all HER family members.

the DESTINY-Breast03 trial, T-Dx (a drug-conjugated antibody), was clearly active against brain metastases [111].

Cancers with HER2 Exon 20 Insertions

Amplification of *HER2* is the most common type of mutation affecting the *HER2* gene in breast cancer and some other cancers. But in NSCLC, the most common type of mutation affecting the *HER2* gene is a mutation affecting the kinase portion of HER2. These mutations generally affect exon 20, and their impact is very similar to that of the exon 20 insertions found in the *EGFR* gene.

Trastuzumab deruxtecan (T-Dx) became the first licensed treatment for people with *HER2*-mutated NSCLC in 2022 thanks to the DESTINY-Lung02 trial [112]. In addition,

poziotinib and pyrotinib have given positive results in HER2-mutated NSCLC [113, 114]. These treatments might also be useful for the small proportions of people with other cancer types whose disease is also driven by a *HER2* exon 20 insertion. This includes some people with breast, bladder, and central nervous system cancer [66, 107, 115].

Resistance Mechanisms

Reasons for resistance to HER2-targeted kinase inhibitors are similar to those that cause resistance to antibody-based treatments. For example, mutations affecting the *HER2* gene, the presence of alternative growth factor receptors (such as HER3), and mutations affecting the PI3K/AKT/mTOR pathway all cause resistance to HER2-targeted kinase inhibitors [108].

3.6 DRUGS THAT BLOCK OTHER GROWTH FACTOR RECEPTORS

Licensed drugs mentioned in this section:		
Treatment class	**Drugs**	**Given to some people with:**
PDGFR and KIT inhibitors	Imatinib, sunitinib, avapritinib, ripretinib, and regorafenib	• Gastrointestinal stromal tumors
FGFR inhibitors	Erdafitinib, pemigatinib, futibatinib, and infigratinib	• Bladder cancer • Cholangiocarcinoma (bile duct cancer)
MET-targeted treatments	Capmatinib, tepotinib and telisotuzumab vedotin	• NSCLC
RET inhibitors	Pralsetinib and selpercatinib	• NSCLC • Thyroid cancer
ALK inhibitors	Crizotinib, alectinib, ceritinib, brigatinib, and lorlatinib	• NSCLC • Anaplastic large cell lymphoma
ROS1 inhibitors	Crizotinib and entrectinib	• NSCLC
TRK A/B/C inhibitors	Entrectinib and larotrectinib	• Any solid tumor with an *NTRK* gene fusion
FLT3 inhibitors	Midostaurin, gilteritinib, and quizartinib	• Acute myeloid leukemia

In addition to EGFR and HER2, many other growth factor receptors are sometimes found on the surface of cancer cells.

At this point, I'm going to look at licensed drugs that target two overlapping sets of growth factor receptors. These are the following:

• Receptors that are found intact on the surface of cancer cells. The receptor might be either present in high amounts due to gene amplification, and/or the receptor is affected by a mutation that increases its kinase activity.

Table 3.6 Treatments that target growth factor receptors other than EGFR or HER2.

Receptor	Type/s of mutation affecting this receptor	Examples of treatments
PDGF receptors (PDGFRs) [116]	• Mutations that increase the receptor's activity • Gene fusions containing the receptor's kinase domain	Imatinib, sunitinib, regorafenib, avapritinib, ripretinib, masitinib, and crenolanib
KIT [117]	• Mutations that increase the receptor's activity	Avapritinib, imatinib, ripretinib
FGF receptors (FGFRs) [118, 119]	• Gene amplification • Mutations that increase the receptor's activity • Gene fusions containing the receptor's kinase domain	Erdafitinib, pemigatinib, infigratinib, rogaratinib, futibatinib, bemarituzumab, and derazantinib
MET [120]	• Gene amplification • Mutations that increase the receptor's activity	Crizotinib, tivantinib, savolitinib, tepotinib, capmatinib, cabozantinib, foretinib, bozitinib, onartuzumab, ficlatuzumab, rilotumumab, telisotuzumab vedotin
RET [121]	• Gene fusions containing the receptor's kinase domain • Mutations that increase the receptor's activity	Selpercatinib and pralsetinib
ALK [122, 123]	• Gene fusions containing the receptor's kinase domain • Mutations that increase the receptor's activity (less common) • Gene amplification (less common)	Crizotinib, ceritinib, alectinib, lorlatinib, brigatinib, and ensartinib
ROS1 [124]	• Gene fusions containing the receptor's kinase domain	Crizotinib, ceritinib, lorlatinib, and entrectinib
TRKA/B/C [125]	• Gene fusions containing the receptors' kinase domains	Entrectinib, larotrectinib, selitrectinib, repotrectinib, and taletrectinib
HER3 [26, 126]	• Fusion protein involving a growth factor • Mutations that increase the receptor's activity • Gene amplification	Patritumab deruxtecan, seribantumab, lumretuzumab, elgemtumab, and zenocutuzumab
FLT3 [34, 42]	• Mutations that increase the receptor's activity	Midostaurin, gilteritinib, quizartinib, and crenolanib

• Receptors where the kinase portion of a receptor is part of an internal fusion protein.

For a summary of these receptors and the drugs that target them, see Table 3.6.

3.6.1 PDGFR and KIT Inhibitors

Inhibitors of PDGFRA (PDGF receptor-alpha) and KIT are licensed treatments for a rare type of cancer called gastrointestinal stromal tumor (GIST). Around 60% of GISTs start in the stomach, but they can arise anywhere in the digestive system [127].

Thanks to research in the late 1990s, we know that the vast majority of GISTs (around 90%) contain mutations either in the gene for KIT (75%–80%) or for PDGFRA (~10%) [128, 129]. Both PDGFRA and KIT are growth factor receptors and therefore have a kinase domain that protrudes inside the cell.

Mutations in the *KIT* gene generally affect the portion of the receptor that protrudes just inside the cell, close to the cell membrane (the juxtamembrane domain – see Figure 2.17). This domain normally exerts an inhibitory influence over the kinase domain, but mutations found in exon 11 of the *KIT* gene (such as those found in GIST) remove this influence [130].

Mutations in the *PDGFRA* gene often affect the second of the receptor's two kinase domains or, less commonly, its juxtamembrane domain [131].

PDGFRA and KIT are very closely related and have very similar ATP-binding sites. We have several drugs that can block both PDGFRA and KIT alongside their other targets (see Table 3.6).

Imatinib was approved as a treatment for people with advanced GIST in Europe in 2002. As a result, the median survival time for patients with metastatic GIST improved from about 20 months to 5 years (60 months) [132].

However, most patients with metastatic GIST do eventually relapse. The most common reason why imatinib stops working is that the gene for KIT has picked up another mutation. The extra mutation generally alters the shape of KIT's ATP-binding site [130]. Thankfully, various forms of KIT that are resistant to imatinib can still be blocked by sunitinib or regorafenib. Both these drugs are licensed treatments for imatinib-resistant GIST. Newer inhibitors, such as ripretinib and avapritinib, have come along in recent years [129].

In addition to being involved in GIST, KIT is also found on the surface of cancer cells in people with AML. Most *KIT* gene mutations in AML affect KIT's activation loop, which controls the protein's kinase activity, or the extracellular domain [133]. Various KIT inhibitors have been tested in patients with AML, including imatinib and dasatinib. However, the trials have been small, and the inhibitors tested don't only block KIT, so the results are difficult to interpret. It's still going to be a few more years before we know whether KIT inhibitors have a future as treatments for AML.

3.6.2 FGFR Inhibitors

Fibroblast growth factor receptors (FGFRs) are a family of four: FGFR1, FGFR2, FGFR3, and FGFR4. Mutations in the genes for these receptors have been found in people with a variety of different cancer types. Sometimes an *FGFR* gene is amplified or affected by a mutation that activates its kinase domain.

Other times, the kinase portion of an FGFR is present as part of an intracellular fusion protein [118].

For example, in a massive study of over 5000 people in China with a wide variety of tumor types, mutations affecting *FGFR* genes were most common in people with endometrial cancer (22%), followed by sarcoma (17%), breast cancer (13%), and gastric cancer (12%) [134]. Gene amplifications and activating mutations were more common than mutations that led to fusion proteins. In other studies, cancers of the bladder, lung, breast, and stomach were the most likely to contain *FGFR* gene mutations [118]. These conflicting results might reflect the size of the studies and the ethnic backgrounds of the people involved.

Amplification of genes for various fibroblast growth factors (there are 18 FGFs made by human cells) has also been discovered in many cancers, such as head and neck cancer, bladder cancer, and stomach cancer [96].

So far, FGFR inhibitors have given the most promising results against bladder cancer and cholangiocarcinoma. The first FGFR inhibitors were imprecise and blocked lots of other kinases. But newer inhibitors, like pemigatinib, erdafitinib, and rogaratinib, are much more precise and only block FGFRs [135].

Pemigatinib, futibatinib, and infigratinib are approved treatments for people with cholangiocarcinomas that contain mutations affecting the *FGFR2* gene. Erdafitinib is also available in the United States for people with bladder (urothelial) cancer containing mutations in either *FGFR2* or *FGFR3*.

Another way to block an FGFR is to use a monoclonal antibody such as vofatamab (which targets FGFR3) or bemarituzumab (which is selective for FGFR2b). Bemarituzumab is in trials for people with stomach or gastroesophageal junction cancers that overproduce FGFR2b [136].

3.6.3 MET Inhibitors

MET is the receptor for hepatocyte growth factor (HGF). Mutations affecting the *MET* gene have been found in various cancer types, but they are most common in people with NSCLC.

The most common types of mutations affecting *MET* are gene amplification (found in ~4% of people with newly diagnosed adenocarcinoma NSCLC) and exon 14 skipping mutations (also present in ~4%). You might remember that the exons of a gene are the bits that get stuck together to create a strand of mRNA, which is then used to make the final protein (the introns are the bits that get chopped out). If exon 14 doesn't make it into the mRNA (because it's been missed out or "skipped"), then the final MET protein is missing a bit, and it stays around in the cell too long. This is exacerbated by the fact the *MET* gene is often also amplified, and the cell makes excessive amounts of this shortened MET protein [137].

Where MET inhibitors are taking off is in the treatment of people with NSCLCs containing *MET* exon 14 skipping mutations. Kinase inhibitors such as tepotinib, capmatinib, and savolitinib have all given positive results in trials, and both tepotinib and capmatinib are licensed treatments. However, *MET* mutations often coexist with other mutations affecting genes such as *KRAS*, *EGFR*, *NF1*, *MDM2*, and *CDK4*. Mutations in these genes seem to cause resistance to MET inhibitors [137, 138]. Scientists have also created antibodies that target MET, including antibody-drug conjugates such as telisotuzumab vedotin, and amivantamab, a dual-targeted antibody that attaches to both MET and EGFR.

3.6.4 RET Inhibitors

RET is yet another growth factor receptor. It is mostly found on the surface of cells that help create an embryo's nerves, bones, cartilage, and other tissues in the very first few weeks of life [35]. RET fusion proteins are found in 10%–20% of papillary thyroid cancers (the most common type of thyroid cancer) and in ~2% of NSCLCs [121]. As with other kinase fusion proteins, RET fusion proteins always contain the kinase part of the RET protein. Over 20 different RET fusion proteins have been discovered [121].

As with other growth factor receptors, becoming part of a fusion protein is not the only way that RET can become dangerous. Point mutations in *RET* (particularly one known as the M918T mutation) are found in a rare form of thyroid cancer called medullary thyroid cancer. The M918T mutation changes the range of proteins that RET can phosphorylate [139].

Various drugs able to block RET are licensed treatments for medullary and/or papillary thyroid cancer, such as cabozantinib, vandetanib, lenvatinib, sorafenib, and sunitinib. However, as all these drugs also block VEGF receptors and other kinases (they are sometimes called multi-kinase inhibitors), it was initially impossible to know how much of their impact was due to inhibition of RET.

More recently, scientists have created much more selective RET inhibitors such as pralsetinib and selpercatinib [121]. The results of a clinical trial comparing selpercatinib to cabozantinib or vandetanib for people with *RET*-mutated medullary thyroid cancer suggest that the inhibition of RET is more important than any impact on angiogenesis. The response rate was almost 70% in people given selpercatinib versus 40% or so with either of the multi-kinase inhibitors [140].

Similarly impressive results have been reported in trials with RET inhibitors in people with NSCLC with RET fusion proteins [141].

Selpercatinib and pralsetinib are both licensed treatments for people with NSCLC or papillary thyroid cancer with a RET fusion protein, and for people with medullary thyroid cancer with the M918T mutation.

3.6.5 ALK and ROS1 Inhibitors

Again, ALK and ROS1 are growth factor receptors [116]. A diverse array of fusion proteins involving the kinase domains of these receptors have been discovered in human cancers. The kinase portions of ALK and ROS1 are very similar to one another, and various kinase inhibitors can block both proteins [124, 142].

The cancer in which ALK and ROS1 inhibitors are most used is NSCLC. However, they are only relevant to the small proportions of patients whose tumors contain an *ALK* (found in ~5% of patients) or *ROS1* (found in 1%–2% of patients) gene rearrangement. In NSCLC, the most common ALK fusion protein is ALK-EML4 (EML4 stands for a long name that doesn't bear including), but another 30 or so ALK fusion proteins have been discovered [44, 143].

Even before ALK fusion proteins were discovered in lung cancer cells, they had already been found in the cancer cells of a rare form of T cell non-Hodgkin lymphoma called anaplastic large cell lymphoma (ALCL). In ALCL, ALK fusions are found in about 50% of patients and NPM-ALK is the most common [44].

Aside from being found as part of fusion proteins in lung cancer and ALCL, ALK is important in some other cancers. For example, mutated, overactive versions of ALK have been found in 6%–8% of neuroblastomas (rare cancers that generally affect children). In addition, cancer cells of neuroblastomas and NSCLC occasionally contain extra copies of the *ALK* gene, forcing the cell to make more ALK protein than normal. *ALK* mutations have also been discovered in people with anaplastic thyroid cancer.

As with ALK, various ROS1 fusion proteins have been found in NSCLC. The most common is called CD74-ROS1 [124]. *ROS1* gene fusions are also found in glioblastoma and spitzoid neoplasms (a group of melanomas more common in childhood that are often benign); they are also occasionally found in other cancer types [144].

First-Generation ALK Inhibitors

The first ALK inhibitor was a drug called crizotinib; however, it was originally created to block MET, so it's not selective for ALK. Like many other kinase inhibitors, crizotinib works by competing with ATP for its targets' ATP-binding site. It's now known to have three main targets: MET, ALK, and ROS1. Crizotinib was first approved in Europe as a treatment for people with *ALK*-mutated NSCLC in 2012.

As with EGFR inhibitors, the benefits from crizotinib don't last forever – typically the cancer starts growing again after less than a year of treatment [145, 146]. One reason for treatment resistance is the presence of cancer cells with an additional mutation in the *ALK* fusion gene such as the C1156Y and L1196M mutations among others [147]. In other patients, the disease returns in their brain because crizotinib isn't very good at getting into brain tissue [148]. Other resistance mechanisms involve mutations that reactivate the MAPK or PI3K/AKT/mTOR pathways [147].

Second- and Third-Generation ALK Inhibitors

Second- and third-generation ALK inhibitors include alectinib, ceritinib, brigatinib, lorlatinib, and ensartinib. These drugs can block some of the mutated versions of the ALK fusion protein that cause resistance to crizotinib, and they're also better at penetrating the brain. In head-to-head trials, alectinib, lorlatinib, brigatinib, and ensartinib have all given better results than crizotinib in terms of response rates, duration of benefit, and control of brain metastases [149].

ROS1 Inhibitors

ROS1 gene rearrangements are found in about 1%–2% of NSCLCs and almost never coexist with *ALK* mutations or *EGFR* mutations. Crizotinib, ceritinib, lorlatinib, and entrectinib have all proven to be effective treatments for people with *ROS1*-mutated NSCLC [124].

Crizotinib is actually a more effective treatment for people with *ROS1*-mutated NSCLC than for people with *ALK*-mutated disease. In people with NSCLC with a *ROS1* fusion gene, crizotinib treatment is effective for a median of just over two years [150], compared to under a year for people with *ALK* fusion genes [145].

3.6.6 TRKA/B/C Inhibitors
Tropomyosin-related kinase-A (TRKA), TRKB, and TRKC are three growth factor receptors made from the *NTRK1*, *NTRK2*, and *NTRK3* genes. Fusion genes involving *NTRK1, 2,* or *3* are common in some rare cancers, and rare in some common cancers (see Table 3.7) [125, 151].

As with other receptors (such as RET, ALK, and ROS1), TRK fusion proteins contain the kinase part of the respective TRK protein. The fusion protein, like the natural receptor, activates various signaling pathways within the cell.

Entrectinib and larotrectinib were the first TRK inhibitors licensed as treatments for people whose cancer contains an *NTRK* gene fusion. (Entrectinib also blocks ROS1 and ALK and is given to people with *ROS1*-mutated lung cancer.) As with other kinase inhibitors, they don't work forever. Eventually, resistant cells multiply to the point where the cancer is deemed to have returned. Causes of resistance include additional mutations in the *NTRK* fusion gene and mutations that

affect other proteins involved in signaling pathways, such as *KRAS, MET, BRAF,* and *IGF1R* mutations [152].

Second-generation inhibitors, such as selitrectinib and repotrectinib, are more potent and can block TRK fusion proteins even when they have many of the additional mutations that render them resistant to entrectinib and larotrectinib [152].

3.6.7 HER3 Inhibitors
HER3 is overproduced by the cells of many cancers and is a reason for resistance to both EGFR- and HER2- targeted treatments and to hormone treatments [125]. Various HER3-targeted treatments are in clinical trials, and they work through a variety of mechanisms, such as preventing HER3 from pairing up with other HER family members; preventing its ligand, NRG, from binding to the receptor; or recruiting white blood cells. There are also HER3-targeted antibody-drug conjugates. (If you remember from earlier, the kinase domain of HER3 doesn't work, so a HER3-targeted kinase inhibitor wouldn't be helpful [126].)

In addition, in around 10%–30% of cases, the cells of a rare form of lung cancer (mucinous adenocarcinoma NSCLC) produce a fusion protein that involves part of NRG (the ligand for HER3) [46]. Similar fusion proteins are found very occasionally in other cancer types [26, 153]. The fusion protein involves a second protein that embeds itself in the cell membrane (Figure 3.6e). The final NRG fusion

Table 3.7 Cancers in which *NTRK* gene fusions are found.

Frequency of *NTRK* gene fusions		
Found in less than 5% of patients	**Found in 5%–25% of patients**	**Found in greater than 75% of patients**
Some brain tumors (including glioblastoma), lung cancer, bowel cancer, cholangiocarcinoma, GIST (with driver mutations), pancreatic cancer, melanoma, sarcoma, breast cancer, acute myeloid leukemia, and head and neck squamous cell carcinoma	Congenital mesoblastic nephroma, papillary thyroid cancer, pontine glioma, spitz tumors, and GIST (without driver mutations)	Mammary analog secretory carcinoma of the salivary gland, secretory breast carcinoma, and infantile fibrosarcoma

protein sits in the cell membrane, and the NRG portion attaches to HER3 and causes it to pair up with HER2. This activates HER2, which then activates internal signaling pathways. Both HER3-targeted treatments (such as zenocutuzumab) and pan-HER inhibitors (such as afatinib) are in trials for people with NRG fusion-positive cancers.

3.6.8 FLT3 Inhibitors

FLT3 is predominantly found on white blood cells such as immature myeloid white blood cells. It responds to the presence of a growth factor called FLT3 ligand. Mutant versions of FLT3, which activate signaling pathways even when no FLT3 ligand is present, are found in the cancer cells of about 30% of people with AML [154, 155]. The most common sort of mutation (found in around 25% of AML patients) is an internal tandem duplication (ITD) (Figure 3.17). ITDs occur when part of the *FLT3* gene is accidentally duplicated and then reinserted back into the gene. Point mutations, which affect just one amino acid in the kinase domain of FLT3, are found in a further 7%–10% of AML patients. In addition, wild-type (i.e., normal, unmutated FLT3) is overproduced in 70%–100% of AML patients.

The first FLT3 inhibitors tested in trials, such as sorafenib, sunitinib, lestaurtinib, and midostaurin, are imprecise and block a wide range of different kinases. Despite this, midostaurin became a licensed treatment in the United States and Europe for people with *FLT3*-mutated AML in 2017.

Newer drugs such as quizartinib, crenolanib, and gilteritinib are much more selective FLT3 inhibitors. One important detail about these drugs is the range of mutated versions of FLT3 they can block. Whereas gilteritinib and midostaurin can block versions of FLT3 with ITDs and kinase domain mutations, sorafenib and quizartinib can only block FLT3 with ITDs [155]. As with midostaurin, quizartinib and gilteritinib are both licensed treatments for people with FLT3-mutated AML.

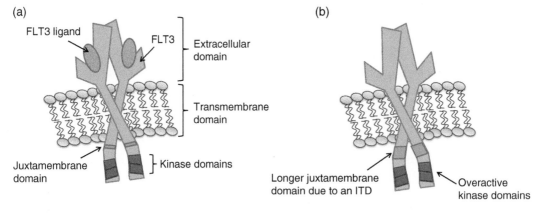

Figure 3.17 The structure of FLT3 showing the impact of internal tandem duplications. (a) The normal FLT3 protein is a growth factor receptor that responds to the presence of FLT3 ligand. FLT3 contains various different domains. The extracellular domain protrudes out of the cell and is where FLT3 ligand binds. The trans-membrane domain spans the cell membrane. The juxtamembrane domain is just inside the cell, close to the membrane, and the protein's two kinase domains are inside the cell and responsible for activating signaling pathways. **(b)** When the *FLT3* gene is affected by mutations known as internal tandem duplications (ITDs), the FLT3 protein contains a longer juxtamembrane domain. This change in the protein's shape causes its kinase domains to be constantly active.
Abbreviations: FLT3 – FMS-like tyrosine kinase; ITD – internal tandem duplication.

3.7 TARGETING THE MAPK SIGNALING PATHWAY

Licensed drugs mentioned in this section:		
Treatment class	Drugs	Given to some people with:
KRAS G12C inhibitors	Adagrasib and sotorasib	• NSCLC
B-Raf inhibitors	Vemurafenib, dabrafenib, encorafenib, tovorafenib	• Melanoma skin cancer • NSCLC • Bowel cancer • Other cancers with *BRAF* mutations (e.g., low-grade childhood glioma and anaplastic thyroid cancer)
MEK inhibitors	Cobimetinib, trametinib, and binimetinib	• As for B-Raf inhibitors • Histiocytic neoplasms

One of the most important signaling pathways controlled by growth factor receptors is the MAPK pathway (Figure 3.18). This involves growth factor receptors, docking proteins, and a series of enzymes in the cell cytoplasm (such as Ras, Raf, MEK, and ERK) [17, 156].

The mechanics of the MAPK pathway are illustrated in Figure 3.18. Some of the most important proteins in the pathway are the Ras proteins (N-Ras, H-Ras, or K-Ras). SOS activates Ras proteins by encouraging them to let go of the low-energy molecule, GDP, and swap it for high-energy GTP. With GTP bound to it, Ras gets into its active shape in which it can recruit and activate Raf proteins. Ras then turns GTP back into GDP.

Raf and MEK proteins are kinases that amplify the signal as it's transmitted through the cell. ERK, the final part of the pathway, is activated by MEK. When ERK is active, it phosphorylates some proteins in the cell cytoplasm (such as components of the cell's internal skeleton and various receptors), and it also moves into the cell's nucleus, where it activates transcription factors such as Elk-1 and Myc [157]. (In fact, ERK can phosphorylate over 200 different proteins.) It takes just a few minutes for the activation of a growth factor receptor on the surface of the cell to culminate in the activation of transcription factors in the nucleus [158].

3.7.1 Things to Remember

I've described the MAPK pathway as a linear series of events with one protein activating another and then another. In fact, the MAPK pathway has many branches and loops, and it interacts with other signaling pathways. For example, ERK can activate the JAK/STAT pathway, and the estrogen receptor can activate ERK.

It is also important to note that there are often several different versions of each protein. For example, there are three main Ras proteins in human cells (N-Ras, H-Ras, and K-Ras), three Raf proteins (A-Raf, B-Raf, and C-Raf), and seven MEKs (MEK 1-7). In addition, there are at least 14 MAPKs, split into three families: ERKs, JNKs, and p38 kinases [159].[15] Each cell type uses different versions of these proteins for different purposes and in response to different signals.

It's important to keep in mind how complicated and nuanced cell signaling is when we look at drugs that block various proteins involved. Although the drug might do its job properly and block the protein it is designed to, this can have unforeseen consequences. Some of these consequences can make the

---

[15] In general, ERK proteins coordinate a cell's response to mitogens – substances that cause cells to grow and multiply, whereas JNK and p38 proteins respond to stress signals, such as low oxygen or nutrient levels.

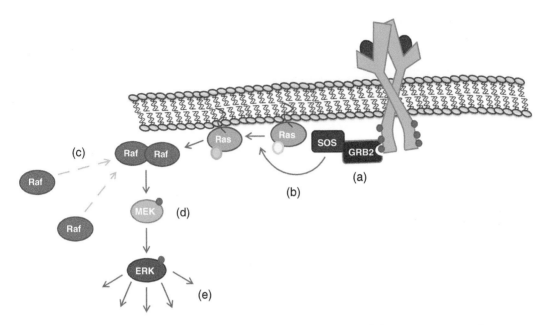

Figure 3.18 Fundamentals of the MAPK pathway. (a) Paired-up growth factor receptors attach phosphates to one another, creating attachment sites for various docking proteins such as GRB2, which then recruits SOS. **(b)** SOS activates Ras (K-Ras, N-Ras, or H-Ras) by causing it to let go of GDP (yellow circle) and take hold of GTP (green circle) instead. Ras is constantly in contact with the cell membrane. **(c)** Ras attracts Raf proteins to the cell membrane where they pair up and become active. **(d)** Raf proteins are kinases; they phosphorylate MEK, which in turn phosphorylates ERK. **(e)** ERK, another kinase, activates over a hundred different targets, some in the cell cytoplasm and some in the cell nucleus. **Abbreviations:** GDP – guanosine diphosphate; GTP – guanosine triphosphate; MAPK – mitogen-activated protein kinase; SOS – son of sevenless.

drug less effective, such as if it accidentally triggers a feedback loop that activates or blocks another pathway.

3.7.2 Defects in the MAPK Signaling Pathway in Cancer Cells

There are three main ways that the MAPK signaling pathway (i.e., Ras/Raf/MEK/ERK) becomes overactive in cancer cells [160]:

1. Because of the overactivity of growth factor receptors or other receptors on the cell surface [covered in the first half of this chapter].

2. Because a Ras protein is overactive. *RAS* genes (*KRAS*, *NRAS*, and *HRAS*) are mutated in around 20% of all human cancers, causing Ras proteins (K-Ras, N-Ras,

or H-Ras) to be overactive [161]. *KRAS* mutations are the most common. Ras proteins will also become overactive if a protein that would normally control them is missing. For example, neurofibromin (NF1) switches off Ras protein activity. NF1 protein is missing or unable to do its job in various cancer types [162].

3. Because B-Raf is faulty [163]. There are three different Raf proteins (A-Raf, B-Raf, and C-Raf), but it is usually B-Raf that is faulty in human cancers. The most common fault in the *BRAF* gene affects just one amino acid, the 600th in the B-Raf protein. In the normal B-Raf protein, this amino acid is a valine (V). But in the cancer-causing version of B-Raf, it's a glutamic acid (E). It is known as the V600E mutation. Less

commonly, V600 becomes a lysine (K), creating the V600K version of B-Raf.

Mutations in the genes for MEK and ERK proteins are much rarer in cancer cells [156].

3.7.3 Drugs that Block the MAPK Pathway

Out of the many proteins involved in the MAPK pathway, we only have licensed treatments that block a handful of them. They are the following:

- one particular mutant version of K-Ras (K-Ras G12C)
- the V600E and V600K mutant versions of B-Raf
- MEK1 and MEK2

The treatments are summarized in Table 3.8.

In summary:

Ras inhibitors. After many years of failures and dead ends, scientists are now making steady (if slow) progress in creating direct Ras inhibitors. The three *RAS* genes, *KRAS*, *NRAS*, and *HRAS* (and corresponding proteins), are often mutated in cancer cells and they are powerful drivers and controllers of cancer cell behavior. I can't underplay how amazing it would be to have a whole series of drugs that could together block all the different mutant versions of the three Ras proteins. But we're a long way from making that a reality.

Raf inhibitors. The V600E (and V600K) mutated forms of B-Raf are again powerful drivers of cancer cell behavior. Thankfully, we have selective drugs that block just the mutated protein, and, because the mutated protein is missing from healthy cells, they cause relatively mild side effects. However, there are other mutant forms of B-Raf that we're only just developing inhibitors for (such as tovorafenib, a pan-RAF inhibitor now licensed for some children with low-grade glioma).

MEK inhibitors. There are various forms of MEK, but only MEK1 and MEK2 are activated by Ras/Raf. The genes for MEK1 and MEK2 (called *MAP2K1* and *MAP2K2*) are only very rarely mutated in human cancers [19]. This means that MEK1 and MEK2 are their normal selves in cancer cells (although they're probably being constantly activated by Raf proteins). MEK proteins are also important to healthy cells. These mean that MEK inhibitors have limited usefulness as a stand-alone treatment – you're likely to kill lots of

Table 3.8   Summary of licensed drugs that block the MAPK pathway.

Drug target and examples	Used in what cancers?	Why?
K-Ras G12C inhibitors: sotorasib and adagrasib	Cancers in which the G12C K-Ras protein is present in a proportion of patients, such as NSCLC and bowel cancer.	The *KRAS* G12C mutation is present in about 14% of people with NSCLC and 3%–4% of people with metastatic bowel cancer; it is much rarer in other cancer types [164].
B-Raf inhibitors: vemurafenib, dabrafenib, encorafenib, tovorafenib	Almost exclusively given to people with the V600E or V600K mutated forms of B-Raf protein in their cancer cells. This mutated form of B-Raf is most common in melanoma skin cancer, thyroid cancer, bowel cancer, and NSCLC.	If V600E or V600K B-Raf is found in the person's cancer cells, these drugs are likely to be effective. However, these drugs don't work if these specific mutant forms of B-Raf are absent [163].
MEK inhibitors: trametinib, cobimetinib, selumetinib, and binimetinib	MEK inhibitors are mostly given in combination with B-Raf inhibitors to people with the V600E or V600K B-Raf protein in their cancer cells.	MEK inhibitors delay resistance to B-Raf inhibitors and overcome paradoxical activation of cells with *NRAS* and other mutations [165].

healthy cells, which creates side effects. Right now, their main use is in combination with B-Raf inhibitors.

ERK inhibitors. Scientists are working on ERK inhibitors, although it's still early days [166]. For many years, scientists didn't see any point in making ERK inhibitors because they didn't think they'd be any different in their effects from a MEK inhibitor. But they've since decided that an ERK inhibitor might be worth having because (1) cell signaling is so complicated that scientists' predictions have often been proved wrong, and (2) cancer cells that are resistant to both B-Raf and MEK inhibitors have often found a way to reactivate ERK [167].

There's more detail about Ras, Raf, and MEK inhibitors below.

3.7.4 K-Ras Inhibitors

When I wrote the first edition of this book, back in 2016–2018, there was very little I could say about Ras inhibitors except that we wished we had some! Thankfully since that time, scientists have made some exciting progress. However, although it's great to celebrate the first ever Ras inhibitors becoming licensed cancer treatments, there's still a long road ahead, as you'll see from the information below.

A Bit of Background on Ras Proteins

Ras proteins are immensely powerful. They are present in every cell in our body – similar proteins exist in everything from yeast to insects, birds, plants, and mollusks. Although Ras proteins are enzymes, they are not kinases – they don't phosphorylate anything. Instead, they activate Raf proteins through a complicated mechanism that includes recruiting them to the cell membrane and encouraging them to pair up [156].

I think of Ras proteins a bit like bumper cars in that they have a stalk, which constantly tethers them to the internal surface of the cell membrane. While attached by their stalk, they are free to buzz around, looking for activated receptors with docking proteins that they can attach to. If they become detached from the membrane, they can no longer do their job [168].

Because Ras proteins aren't kinases, they don't have a handy ATP-binding pocket that you can design a drug to fit into. Instead, they have a relatively smooth surface. They do, however, have a little pocket where GTP fits (see Figure 3.19), but they have such a high affinity for GTP that it's impossible to dislodge it with any drug [169].

So far, scientists have created drugs that block one specific mutated version of K-Ras, the G12C mutant. But there are many different mutated versions of all three Ras proteins found in cancer cells (some of the most common ones are listed in Table 3.9). Because of this diversity, we have a long way to go in having an effective treatment for everyone with a Ras-driven cancer [168].

Treatments that Target G12C K-Ras

The K-Ras protein is made from 188 amino acids [172]. The 12th amino acid is normally a glycine (G), but in the G12C mutant it has become a cysteine (C). This is handy, because scientists have worked out how to create drugs that chemically bond with cysteines. Adagrasib and sotorasib, two recently created K-Ras G12C inhibitors, do just this. The normal version of K-Ras (the wild-type version) doesn't have a cysteine controlling its activity, so it isn't blocked by these drugs. Instead, the drugs attach to the extra cysteine in K-Ras G12C and this traps mutant K-Ras in its inactive shape [169].

Adagrasib and sotorasib have both given positive results in clinical trials involving people with NSCLC whose cancer cells contain K-Ras G12C [173]. However, *KRAS* mutations are strongly associated with a history of smoking, and lung cancers in smokers tend to be genetically complicated

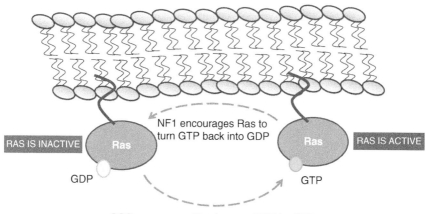

Figure 3.19 Ras proteins are active when bound to GTP. When growth factor receptors are activated, they recruit GRB2, which in turn activates proteins called guanosine exchange factors (GEFs). SOS is one of these GEFs. SOS assists Ras, enabling it to let go of GDP and grab hold of GTP. Ras then changes shape and becomes active. In its new, active shape, it can activate Raf and other proteins. Other proteins called GTPase-activating proteins (GAPs), such as NF1, activate Ras's own enzyme activity. Ras then turns guanosine triphosphate (GTP) into guanosine diphosphate (GDP) and switches itself off.

Table 3.9   Frequency and identity of *RAS* gene mutations in different cancer types.

Cancer type	Most frequently *RAS* gene in this cancer	Most frequently mutated amino acids in the corresponding Ras protein
Bowel cancer	*KRAS* – 41%	G12D: 45% G12V: 30%
Pancreatic ductal adenocarcinoma	*KRAS* – 86%	G12D: 45% G12V: 35% G12R: 17%
Melanoma skin cancer	*NRAS* – 29%	Q12R: 46% Q61K: 30% Q61L: 13%
Adenocarcinoma NSCLC	*KRAS* – 32%	**G12C: 46%** G12V: 23% G12D: 17%
Head and neck squamous cell carcinoma	*HRAS* – 5%	G12S: 29%
Urothelial bladder cancer[a]	*HRAS* – 4%	G13R[b] Q61R[b]

Source: Adapted from Ref. [168, 170, 171].
[a] Almost all bladder cancers are urothelial and begin in the urothelial cells that line the urethra, bladder, ureters, and other organs. A small number are squamous cell carcinomas, adenocarcinomas, or small cell carcinomas.
[b] The number of patients with these mutations is too small to have an accurate figure for their prevalence.

compared to lung cancers in never-smokers [174]. This genetic complexity goes hand in hand with a high degree of variation from one cancer cell to the next (intratumoral heterogeneity), and with rapid resistance to treatment [175]. In addition, some mutations, such as *EGFR* gene mutations, seem to be a very early event in the development of lung cancer, and the mutation is therefore present in every cancer cell. In contrast, *KRAS* mutations seem more likely to occur later in a cancer's development and are only present in a proportion of the person's cancer cells. Targeting a later, sub-clonal mutation isn't ideal, as only the proportion of cells with the mutation will be vulnerable to the targeted treatment [176].

Thus, even though sotorasib and adagrasib are potent and selective inhibitors of the K-Ras G12C protein, it's hard for them to keep lung cancer under control for long. You can see this in the results of a large clinical trial, the CodeBreak 200 trial, in which sotorasib was compared to docetaxel chemotherapy. The median overall survival time of people given sotorasib was 10.6 months, compared to 11.3 months in people who received docetaxel [177, 178].

The same G12C mutant version of K-Ras is found in the cancer cells of 3%–4% of people with bowel cancer [168, 179]. As with B-Raf inhibitors, K-Ras G12C inhibitors don't seem to work as a stand-alone treatment for bowel cancer. They appear to give better results when combined with an EGFR-targeted antibody such as panitumumab [180, 181].

Inhibitors of Other Mutant Ras Proteins
The mutation that creates K-Ras G12C is just one of the many mutant forms of K-Ras found in human cancer cells. K-Ras G12C is the only common mutant Ras protein with an extra cysteine (see Table 3.9 for other common mutations), which means that K-Ras G12C inhibitors can only block this one mutant version of K-Ras. Thankfully, drug companies are increasingly making progress in creating drugs that can block other mutant versions of Ras proteins, such as K-Ras G12D. They're also making progress with pan-K-Ras inhibitors, which block many mutant K-Ras proteins [182].

Another way to block Ras proteins is to create drugs that block SOS (which, if you

remember, activates Ras) and SHP2 (another protein needed for full Ras activity). There are also some encouraging signs that farnesyl transferase inhibitors (a group of failed Ras inhibitors from years gone by) might be able to block mutant H-Ras proteins [169, 183].

Lastly, in the absence of having any direct inhibitors for most Ras-driven cancers, doctors have investigated various ways of indirectly targeting overactive Ras proteins. For example, they've given people with *RAS*-mutated cancers MEK or ERK inhibitors (MEK and ERK are both lower down the MAPK pathway), CDK4/6 inhibitors (which target the cell cycle), and PI3K and mTOR inhibitors (these target the PI3K pathway, which is also activated by Ras). However, none of these approaches has yet given good enough results for it to become an approved treatment for people with *RAS*-mutated cancers [184].

3.7.5 B-Raf Inhibitors

A Bit of Background on Raf Proteins
Raf proteins (A-Raf, B-Raf, and C-Raf) are made from three RAF genes: *ARAF*, *BRAF*, and *RAF1* (*RAF1* codes for C-Raf; the others you can probably guess!). *BRAF* mutations are found in about 8% of all human cancers [163]. The two cancers in which *BRAF* mutations are most common are melanoma skin cancer (present in about 50%) and papillary thyroid cancer (again, present in about 50%). See Table 3.10 for the frequency of *BRAF* mutations in various cancer types. *ARAF* and *RAF1* mutations are rare.

The V600E mutant version of B-Raf protein (in which the valine [V] amino acid at position 600 has become a glutamic acid [E]) is the most common mutant form of B-Raf in human cancers. The V600K version (which has a lysine [K] instead) is similar [163].

Normal B-Raf proteins are only active when paired up. This only happens when they've been activated by Ras proteins. Instead, the

Table 3.10 Frequency of *BRAF* gene mutations in a range of cancer types.

Cancer	Frequency of *BRAF* mutations
Melanoma skin cancer	45%
Bowel cancer	12%
NSCLC	2%
Thyroid cancer	44%
Cancers of the central nervous system	8.5%
Cholangiocarcinoma (bile duct cancer)	4%
Hairy cell leukemia	Up to 100%
Multiple myeloma	5%
Prostate cancer	5%

Source: Adapted from Ref. [185–187].

V600E and V600K versions of B-Raf don't need to pair up to be active. They're active all the time (Figure 3.20) [163].

B-Raf Inhibitors: Drugs that Block V600E (and V600K)

These drugs include vemurafenib, dabrafenib, and encorafenib. All three can block the V600E and V600K mutant forms of B-Raf. However, they can't block normal Raf dimers (created when Ras persuades two Raf proteins to pair up – Figure 3.20). This is great news if you have a cancer driven by either the V600E or V600K forms of B-Raf, as the drug is likely to kill your cancer cells but leave healthy cells unharmed. But it means that these drugs won't help you if your cancer is driven by a different mechanism or by a different mutant form of B-Raf.

Vemurafenib, dabrafenib, and encorafenib have become important treatments for people with melanoma skin cancer driven by V600E/K mutant B-Raf. However, through a strange quirk, these drugs actually stabilize and increase the activity of healthy Raf dimers (this is called "the Raf-inhibitor paradox" – explained in Figure 3.21). This has two consequences. Firstly, these treatments have no impact on cancer cells that are not driven by V600E or V600K mutant B-Raf. Secondly, they sometimes cause additional skin cancers (and possibly also other new cancers) in people with lots of *RAS*-mutated cells. This is a common situation in people with a history of sun exposure. Their *RAS*-mutated skin cells, which were sitting quietly despite containing

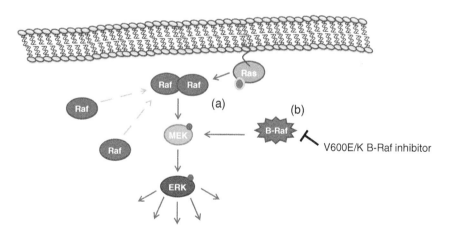

Figure 3.20 The V600E (and V600K) mutant versions of B-Raf are active as monomers. (a) Ras activates Raf proteins by attracting them to the cell membrane where they pair up and become active. A-Raf, B-Raf, and C-Raf proteins can all pair up with themselves or with one another. (b) The V600E and V600K versions of B-Raf found in some cancer cells are active as monomers (they don't need to pair up to be active). V600E/K inhibitors block unpaired B-Raf proteins, but they cannot block paired Raf proteins in healthy cells.

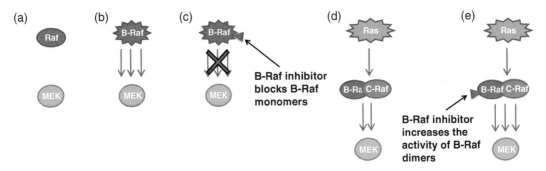

Figure 3.21 The Raf inhibitor paradox. (a) In healthy cells, most Raf proteins exist as un-paired monomers that cannot activate MEK. **(b)** In cancer cells containing the V600E or V600K B-Raf protein, the faulty B-Raf strongly activates MEK even as a monomer, which forces the cancer cell to grow, multiply, and survive. **(c)** V600E and V600K B-Raf monomers are blocked by a B-Raf inhibitor, causing cell death. **(d)** If a cell contains a *RAS* gene mutation, the overactive Ras protein creates lots of Raf dimers that activate MEK (Raf dimers could be made from any two Raf proteins). The cell is faulty, but not a cancer cell. **(e)** If a *RAS* mutant cell is exposed to a B-Raf inhibitor, the B-Raf inhibitor will activate Raf dimers even further. This causes *RAS*-mutant cells to become cancer cells and creates additional non-melanoma skin cancers.

lots of paired-up Raf proteins, become cancer cells when exposed to a B-Raf inhibitor [188].

Thankfully, by combining a B-Raf inhibitor with a MEK inhibitor, the problem of creating extra skin cancers is almost completely avoided. Dabrafenib, encorafenib, and vemurafenib are therefore usually given in combination with a MEK inhibitor such as trametinib, binimetinib, or cobimetinib.

Another advantage of giving a B-Raf inhibitor/MEK inhibitor combination to someone with *BRAF*-mutated melanoma is that the combination works for longer than a B-Raf inhibitor given alone [163].

Who They're Given To

People with BRAF-*Mutated Melanoma Skin Cancer*

B-Raf inhibitors (summarized in Table 3.11) are a treatment option for the 50% or so of people with melanoma skin cancer whose cancer contains the V600E (or V600K) version of B-Raf. They are usually given in combination with a MEK inhibitor due to the reasons given earlier.

Table 3.11   Summary of B-Raf inhibitors.

Type of inhibitor:	Examples:	Licensed for:
Drugs that block V600E and V600K mutated B-Raf protein	Vemurafenib, dabrafenib, and encorafenib	*BRAF*-mutated melanoma skin cancer, NSCLC, bowel cancer, and anaplastic thyroid cancer[a]
Pan-Raf inhibitors	Tovorafenib, exarafenib, BAL3833, LY3009120, lifirafenib, and belvarafenib	Tovorafenib was licenced by the FDA in April 2024 for children with low-grade gliomas whose cancer cells contain a *BRAF* mutation

Source: Adapted from Ref. [163, 189].
[a] Only 2% of thyroid cancers are "anaplastic thyroid cancer"; it is an extremely aggressive form of cancer, and in 45% of patients, the cancer cells contain the V600E mutation of the *BRAF* gene [190]. A B-Raf/MEK inhibitor combination was approved by the FDA for people with anaplastic thyroid cancer with the V600E *BRAF* mutation in America in 2018.

People with BRAF-*Mutated Bowel Cancer*
The V600E mutant version of B-Raf is found in the cancer cells of around 8%–10% of people with bowel cancer. However, unlike in people with *BRAF*-mutated melanoma skin cancer, a B-Raf inhibitor, or even a B-Raf inhibitor/MEK inhibitor combination, isn't effective against V600E B-Raf-driven bowel cancer. Scientists worked out the reason for this. They found that if you expose *BRAF*-mutated bowel cancer cells to a B-Raf inhibitor, they react by immediately upping the activity of their EGFRs. This activity then feeds down into c-Raf and activates ERK, which keeps the cells alive [191]. This doesn't happen in melanoma cells because they have different growth factor receptors on their surface such as KIT [192].

Through a mixture of laboratory science and clinical trials, a combination of a B-Raf inhibitor plus an EGFR inhibitor has been found to be an effective approach for people with V600E/K *BRAF*-mutated bowel cancer [193].

People with BRAF-*Mutated NSCLC*
BRAF mutations are found in the cancer cells of around 2%–4% of people with adenocarcinoma NSCLC. Around half of these mutations are the same V600E mutation found in the cancer cells of melanoma and bowel cancer. If this V600E mutation is present, a combination of B-Raf inhibitor and a MEK inhibitor is effective for around 70% of patients, with the effect lasting[16] for a median of around 10 months [194].

People with Other Cancers with the V600E BRAF *Mutation*
BRAF mutations are not unique to melanoma, bowel cancer, and NSCLC. There are some rare cancers in which *BRAF* mutations are very common, such as anaplastic thyroid cancer and hairy cell leukemia. There are also

some more common cancers that occasionally harbor a *BRAF* mutation, such as glioblastoma and ovarian cancer [195].

In some of these cancers, a B-Raf inhibitor has been tested as a monotherapy; in others, a combination of a B-Raf inhibitor with a MEK inhibitor has been tried. For example, a clinical trial involving 23 people with anaplastic thyroid cancer reported a response rate of 56% for a combination of a B-Raf inhibitor with a MEK inhibitor [196]. A second trial, involving people with various cancer types (all containing a *BRAF* mutation), reported results with a B-Raf inhibitor given alone. This included patients with *BRAF*-mutated ovarian cancer (response rate 50%), hairy cell leukemia (response rate 90%), ganglioglioma (response rate 67%), glioblastoma (response rate 33%), or cholangiocarcinoma (response rate 18%) [195].

Why B-Raf Inhibitors Stop Working
When patients with advanced, *BRAF*-mutated melanoma skin cancer are given a B-Raf inhibitor alone, the response rate is generally around 50%–60% [163]. If they're given a B-Raf inhibitor plus a MEK inhibitor, this climbs to 60%–80%. However, even with the combination, most people's cancer returns within a year or so [197].

Scientists have taken tumor samples from people who didn't benefit at all from a B-Raf inhibitor (those with primary resistance). They've also taken samples from people whose tumor initially responded (i.e., shrank) but is now growing again (secondary resistance).

Many of the mutations found in resistant cells either reactivate the MAPK pathway or they activate the PI3K/AKT/mTOR pathway [198] (see Figure 3.22).

---

[16] In terms of the person's cancer not beginning to grow or worsen again (called median progression-free survival).

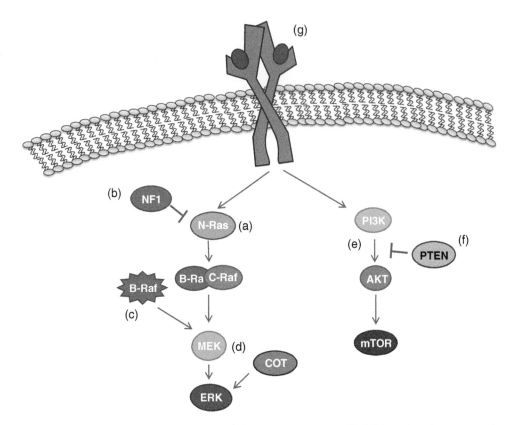

Figure 3.22 Some of the most common reasons for resistance to B-Raf inhibitors in *BRAF*-mutated melanoma skin cancer. (a) Mutations in *NRAS* or (b) loss of NF1 lead to overactive N-Ras protein, which activates unmutated Raf proteins. (c) The mutated *BRAF* gene is amplified, creating an amount of V600E B-Raf protein that overwhelms treatment. (d) Mutation or overexpression of MEK1, MEK2, or COT reactivates ERK. (e) Mutations affecting the PI3K protein (such *PIK3CA* mutations) or AKT, or (f) loss of PTEN, cause increased activation of mTOR, which can sustain cancer cell survival and proliferation in the absence of MAPK activity. (g) Increased levels of growth factor receptors on the cell surface, such as MET or PDGF receptors, activate both pathways.
Abbreviations: See Figure 3.5.

Overcoming Resistance to B-Raf and MEK Inhibitors

Strategies to avoid or overcome resistance to B-Raf/MEK inhibitor combinations include the following:

- Giving these treatments to patients immediately following surgery (if they are eligible for surgery). At this point in time, there's a much better chance of curing their disease compared to patients who have inoperable, metastatic disease [199].

- Developing pan-Raf inhibitors that can inhibit both B-Raf monomers and paired-up Raf proteins (although this raises the issue of increased toxicity due to the drug's impact on healthy cells) [198].

- Combining them with treatments that boost the immune system's response to cancer, such as checkpoint inhibitors or treatments that boost macrophages (I look at this approach in more detail in Section 5.7.5) [198].

3.7.6 A Bit Extra on MEK Inhibitors

How They Work

As with many of the other proteins in our cells, there are multiple different MEK proteins – seven in total. But just two of them, MEK1 and MEK2, are activated by the MAPK pathway controlled by growth factor receptors, Ras and Raf.

Unlike drugs that block growth factor receptors and Raf proteins, most MEK inhibitors are allosteric kinase inhibitors. That is, these drugs fit into a small pocket on MEK proteins that is adjacent to the ATP-binding site. When a MEK inhibitor is inside this pocket, MEK is locked into an inactive shape [200].

Who They're Given To

So far, MEK inhibitors have made their greatest impact in treating people with *BRAF*-mutated melanoma skin cancer. Numerous clinical trials have shown that, when used in combination with a B-Raf inhibitor, a MEK inhibitor can delay resistance and avoid secondary cancers caused by the B-Raf inhibitor [163]. They are also combined with B-Raf inhibitors in the treatment of people with V600E *BRAF*-mutated NSCLC for the same reason.

In addition to their importance as treatments for people with *BRAF*-mutated cancers, MEK inhibitors have also been investigated as stand-alone treatments for people with many different cancer types [165, 200]. However, MEK proteins are important for healthy cells, so blocking them is rapidly toxic to healthy tissues. Also, MEK mutations are rare, which generally means that a MEK inhibitor is being given in the hopes that it will overcome the effects of some other mutation, such as an *RAS* gene mutation.

Most trials in which a MEK inhibitor has been given to patients who have cancers with

RAS or other gene mutations have failed to show any improvement with the MEK inhibitor [165, 201].

However, there are two cancers in which a MEK inhibitor alone has made a difference. The first is in patients with low-grade serous ovarian cancer (SOC), which accounts for around 5% of ovarian cancers, and the second is a group of rare conditions called histiocytic neoplasms.

Low-grade SOCs commonly contain mutations affecting the MAPK pathway, such as *KRAS*, *NRAS*, or *BRAF* mutations. In a clinical trial of trametinib (a MEK inhibitor) versus standard care (which generally means chemotherapy), trametinib came out on top. However, it's important to say that in other, similar trials, MEK inhibitors (selumetinib and binimetinib) failed to improve survival times compared to chemotherapy [202].

Histiocytic neoplasms are a group of extremely rare conditions in which the body makes too many white blood cells such as macrophages or dendritic cells. The faulty cells often contain mutations affecting the MAPK pathway. In 2022, cobimetinib became an approved treatment option for people with histiocytic neoplasms based on a study that involved just 18 patients [203].

Lastly, there's also a theory that a MEK inhibitor could help T cells and other white blood cells gain access to tumors and enhance the effectiveness of immunotherapy with checkpoint inhibitors. However, although laboratory research backs this up, it hasn't yet been proven in clinical trials. For example, in one trial involving 170 people with bowel cancer, patients were given a combination of a checkpoint inhibitor plus cobimetinib (a MEK inhibitor) or the checkpoint inhibitor alone. There was no improvement with the addition of the MEK inhibitor.

3.8 TARGETING THE PI3K/AKT/ MTOR SIGNALING PATHWAY

Treatment class	Drugs	Given to some people with:
	Licensed drugs mentioned in this section:	
PI3Kα inhibitors	Alpelisib	• Hormone receptor-positive, *PIK3CA*-mutated breast cancer
PI3Kδ inhibitors	Idelalisib, copanlisib, and umbralisib	• Chronic lympho-cytic leukemia or B cell non-Hodgkin lym-phoma (there's more on these drugs in Section 4.7.6)
mTOR inhibitors	Everolimus and temsirolimus	• Hormone receptor-positive breast cancer • Neuroendocrine tumors • Kidney cancer (renal cell carcinoma) • Subependymal giant cell astrocytoma
AKT inhibitors	Capivasertib (not yet approved as of Nov '23)	Hormone receptor-positive breast cancer with a mutation in *PIK3CA, AKT1,* or *PTEN*

Box 3.1 The Greek Alphabet

Scientists are forever using letters from the Greek alphabet to distinguish between different versions of proteins. For example, in this chapter we meet PDGFRα; p38α, β and γ; p110α, β, γ, and δ; and PI3Kα, β, γ, and δ. So, it might be useful to know how to say them.

α – alpha
β – beta
γ – gamma
δ – delta

So far, I've just described the MAPK signaling pathway, but growth factor receptors also control other pathways. A second is the PI3K/AKT/mTOR pathway (see Figure 3.23 for an overview of this pathway and how it interlinks with the MAPK pathway). In fact, scientists believe that the PI3K/AKT/mTOR pathway is the most common pathway affected by mutations in human cancers [205, 206].

This is a complicated pathway with lots of components, so it might be helpful to break it apart as follows:

Step 1. *PI3K Becomes Active*

I first mentioned PI3K in Chapter 2 as an important kinase activated by growth factor receptors. However, whereas all the other kinases I've mentioned so far in this book phosphorylate other proteins, PI3K phospho-rylates a lipid molecule found in the cell membrane called phosphatidylinositol 4,5-bisphosphate (PIP_2). When a growth factor receptor is activated, it recruits PI3K (with additional help from Ras). Once it is con-nected to the receptor and close to the cell membrane, PI3K has easy access to supplies of PIP_2 and it can phosphorylate it to produce PIP_3.[17] PIP_3 then activates AKT [205, 206].

In addition to being activated by growth factor receptors (like EGFR and HER2), PI3K is also activated by various other types of receptors, such as G-protein-coupled recep-tors. It's also activated by the B cell receptor (BCR) found on the surface of B cells [17].

Step 2. *PI3K Activates AKT (counteracted By PTEN)*

As I've already said, PIP_3 activates AKT. To prevent overactivity of AKT, our cells nor-mally contain another protein called PTEN. This protein reverses the actions of PI3K by removing one of PIP_3's phosphates and turn-ing it back into PIP_2. PTEN is an immensely important protein and a powerful protector

---

[17] PIP_2 contains two phosphate groups, so when PI3K adds another phosphate it becomes phosphati-dylinositol 3,4,5-triphosphate (PIP_3).

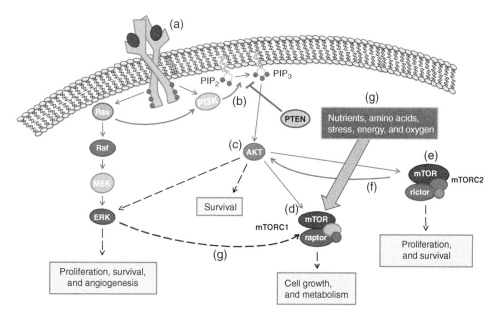

Figure 3.23 The basics of the PI3K/AKT/mTOR signaling pathway. (a) As with the MAPK pathway, the PI3K/AKT/mTOR pathway can be triggered by paired-up growth factor receptors that phosphorylate one another (phosphates are shown as red circles). **(b)** The paired receptors activate PI3K, which indirectly activates AKT by phosphorylating a lipid in the cell membrane called PIP$_2$ to create PIP$_3$. This phosphorylation is reversed by PTEN. **(c)** AKT has numerous impacts on the cell, including triggering cell proliferation, survival, and altered metabolism. AKT also activates mTOR, an important controller of cell growth, survival, motility, metabolism, and angiogenesis. **(d)** mTOR is active when it comes together with other proteins to form mTOR complex-1 (mTORC1) and **(e)** mTOR complex-2 (mTORC2). mTORC1 and mTORC2 have distinct, but overlapping, effects on the cell. **(f)** mTORC2 also causes further activation of AKT. **(g)** In addition, mTORC is influenced by the MAPK pathway and by proteins that respond to the cell's well-being and environment, such as changing levels of glucose, amino acids, energy, and oxygen. *Source:* Adapted from Ref. [204].
Abbreviations: ERK – extracellular-signal-regulated kinase; mTOR – mammalian target of rapamycin; PI3K – phosphatidylinositol 3-kinase; PIP2 – phosphatidylinositol 4,5-bisphosphate; PIP3 – phosphatidylinositol 3,4,5-triphosphate; PTEN – phosphatase and tensin homolog.

against cancer. In fact, loss of PTEN is a common feature of cancer cells.

AKT is yet another powerful kinase that controls numerous processes in our cells [207]. The net effect of AKT activation is to encourage the cell to multiply, protect it from cell death, and equip it with energy and proteins for growth. Some of AKT's actions are mediated by a kinase called mammalian target of rapamycin (mTOR).

Step 3. *AKT Activates mTOR*

Many people describe mTOR as a master switch or master regulator [208]. This is because, as well as responding to AKT – and therefore to growth factor receptors – mTOR is also influenced by lots of other receptors, and by the cell's energy, oxygen, amino acid, and nutrient supplies. On top of that, mTOR also responds to a variety of other signaling pathways, such as the Hippo, WNT, and Notch pathways. In fact, it seems that when a cell receives a signal to multiply via its growth factor receptors, it uses mTOR to make sure that it only complies if it's in good health and has the energy and other supplies necessary to do so. If that isn't the case, and there's an energy deficit, mTOR will trigger catabolism, in which the cell breaks down its large molecules (like proteins, lipids, and complex sugars) to release energy [205].

The many functions of mTOR in our body is a huge topic. Not only is mTOR important in terms of causing and driving the behavior of cancer cells, but it's also important in many other diseases such as arthritis, diabetes, and osteoporosis, as well as in the aging process [204, 209, 210].

In fact, it's hard to underestimate just how important mTOR is to our cells. To me, that means that mTOR comes with a health warning when it comes to creating mTOR inhibitors, or inhibitors of other components of the pathway. Given the importance of mTOR and its involvement in so many pivotal processes (such as cell growth, metabolism, and aging), it seems inevitable that when you block the PI3K/AKT/mTOR pathway, you're going to see lots of side effects.

Step 4: *mTOR Forms Complexes That Force the Cell to Grow and Multiply*

mTOR's activities are diverse and complicated. Importantly, it carries out its functions by forming groupings with numerous other proteins. In a grouping known as mTORC1 (mTOR complex 1), mTOR equips cells for rapid growth by increasing the production of lipids, mitochondria, DNA bases, and ribosomes, and by altering cell metabolism. In another grouping, known as mTORC2 (mTOR complex 2), mTOR can further activate AKT and control cell survival and proliferation [204].

There is considerable overlap, and some disagreement, over the precise function and control of mTORC1 and mTORC2. Also, do be aware that the information I've given here is a drastic simplification of the true situation.

3.8.1 Defects in the PI3K/AKT/mTOR Pathway in Cancer Cells

There are various reasons why the PI3K/AKT/mTOR pathway is overactive in cancer cells: [22, 204, 206, 211, 212]

1. Overactivity of growth factor receptors and other receptors on the cell surface. Many different growth factor receptors (e.g., EGFR, HER2, MET, and FLT3) are either overproduced or overactive in cancer cells. They all activate PI3K.
2. Overactivity of the MAPK signaling pathways. Overactive Ras proteins trigger both PI3K and AKT activity.
3. Overactivity of PI3Kα. PIK3CA mutations are common in many solid tumors (see Table 3.12 for some examples). PIK3CA is the gene for the catalytic subunit of PI3Kα, and PIK3CA mutations cause PI3Kα to become overactive (see Section 3.8.3).
4. Loss of PTEN protein. PTEN is the second most mutated gene in human cancer [214] (the most commonly mutated is TP53, the gene for p53). There are many reasons why PTEN is missing from cancer cells,

Table 3.12 Frequency of *PIK3CA* and *PTEN* gene mutations in various tumor types.

	PIK3CA mutated	PTEN lost or mutated
Overall	13%	36%
Endometrial cancer	37%	**82%**
Breast cancer	31%	39%
Cervical cancer	29%	34%
Bladder cancer	22%	35%
Bowel (colorectal) cancer	17%	**51%**
Head and neck squamous cell carcinoma	14%	36%
Ovarian cancer	8%	24%
Prostate cancer	7%	**66%**
Non-small cell lung cancer	5%	33%
Esophageal and gastroesophageal junction cancer	5%	37%
Kidney (renal cell) cancer	5%	47%
Liver (hepatocellular) cancer	4%	**59%**
Melanoma	2%	29%

Source: Adapted from Ref. [213].

including deletion, suppression, or mutation of the *PTEN* gene or instability of the PTEN protein. Whatever the reason, without the counterbalance of PTEN, the PI3K pathway is overactive.

5. Overactivity of AKT. Mutations in the three *AKT* genes (*AKT1*, *AKT2*, and *AKT3*) are less common than *PIK3CA* and *PTEN* mutations. However, amplification of *AKT* genes and other mutations have been found in various cancer types, including breast cancers, head and neck squamous cell carcinomas, endometrial cancer, NSCLC, and renal cancers [215].

6. Absence of mTOR suppressor proteins. Proteins such as the TSC1/TSC2 complex, STK11 (also called LKB1), and neurofibromin 1/2 (NF1/2) suppress the PI3K pathway. As with PTEN, the absence of these proteins causes overactivity of the pathway. For example, STK11 is missing from the cells of about 5%–15% of adenocarcinoma NSCLCs [216].

7. Mutations directly affecting the *MTOR* gene. Mutations that directly affect the *MTOR* gene and that cause mTOR protein to be overactive are less common than the mutations listed earlier. However, various mutated versions of mTOR have been discovered in human cancers.

3.8.2 Drugs that Block the PI3K/ AKT/mTOR Pathway

Scientists have developed drugs that can block all three of the main proteins in the PI3K/AKT/mTOR pathway. These include drugs that are highly specific and block just one form of PI3K, as well as some that block both PI3K and mTOR together (summarized in Tables 3.11 and 3.13). So far, two mTOR inhibitors, everolimus and temsirolimus, and various PI3Kδ inhibitors, e.g., idelalisib and copanlisib, have become licensed treatments. Many more are in trials.

At one point, scientists were optimistic that drugs targeting the pathway would be effective treatments for huge numbers of people affected by cancer. However, this hasn't (yet) become a reality and may never happen. The biggest obstacles are the following: [211, 212]

1. The enormous number of ways in which the PI3K/AKT/mTOR pathway can be activated and the way the cell compensates for the inhibition of one protein by upregulating others. This means that it's incredibly difficult to completely shut down the pathway, even with a combination of treatments.

2. Cross talk between the PI3K/AKT/mTOR pathway and the MAPK pathway means that if you block one, the other simply takes over.

3. Cancer cells often contain mutations that cause resistance to treatments that target components of the PI3K/AKT/mTOR pathway. For example, *MYC* and *HRAS* mutations both cause resistance.

4. The PI3K/AKT/mTOR pathway plays a central role in many vital physiological functions. Not surprisingly, blocking the pathway causes lots of side effects, including hyperglycemia (high blood sugar levels), bone marrow suppression, liver damage, and many other problems. The central issue is that the more effective you are in shutting down the pathway, the more severe the toxicities become.

5. As with all targeted treatments, intratumoral heterogeneity is an enormous obstacle. If there is diversity among a person's cancer cells (as there virtually always is), then it's likely that cancer cells exist that have mutations or other adaptations that render them resistant to treatment.

Because of the problems with side effects and lack of therapeutic window (the dose that works vs. the dose that causes intolerable side effects), the goal of entirely shutting down the PI3K pathway is being revised. The current direction of travel is to create more precise drugs (e.g., to create drugs that perhaps block

Table 3.13   A selection of PI3K, AKT, and mTOR inhibitors that have made it into clinical trials.

Drug target and examples	Used in what cancers?	Why?
Selective PI3Kα inhibitors: alpelisib, taselisib, inavolisib, and serabelisib	In trials for breast cancer and many other cancer types. Alpelisib is an approved treatment for *PIK3CA*-mutated breast cancer.	PI3Kα is commonly overactive in breast cancer and other solid tumors due to mutations in the *PIK3CA* gene.
PI3Kδ inhibitors: idelalisib, duvelisib, umbralisib, and copanlisib[a]	B cell chronic lymphocytic leukemia, and some B cell non-Hodgkin lymphomas.	PI3Kδ is found in white blood cells. It is overactive in many B cell leukemias, lymphomas, and other hematological cancers due to overactivity of B cell receptors.
PI3Kγ inhibitors: eganelisib	In early trials for various solid tumors.	May enhance the effectiveness of some immunotherapies by making the tumor environment less immune suppressing [217].
Dual mTOR/PI3K inhibitors: bimiralisib, dactolisib, gedatolisib, and GDC-0084	Being explored in a variety of cancers.	Dual targeting of mTOR and PI3K together may overcome some resistance mechanisms to drugs that only target mTOR. However, toxicity is a big obstacle.
AKT inhibitors: ipatasertib, capivasertib, afuresertib, and uprosertib	Being explored in a variety of cancers.	Many cancers have overactive PI3K/AKT/mTOR pathway. Most clinical trials of AKT inhibitor are in people with breast cancer or prostate cancer.
mTOR inhibitors: rapamycin, everolimus, temsirolimus, sapanisertib (TAK-228), vistausertib (AZD2014), CC-223, BI860585, DS-3078a, ME-344, GDC-0349, OSI-027, and P529	Everolimus is an approved treatment for kidney cancer, breast cancer, and neuroendocrine tumors (NETs). Temsirolimus is approved for people with kidney cancer. Other mTOR inhibitors are in trials for many other cancer types.	*VHL* gene mutations are common in kidney cancer; this mutation, together with overactive mTOR, drives angiogenesis and the growth of these cancers. In breast cancer, there is interplay between estrogen receptor signaling and the PI3K/AKT/mTOR pathway. PNETs[b] often contain mutations affecting mTOR activity.

Source: Adapted from Ref. [218].
[a] copanlisib is a pan-PI3K inhibitor.
[b] PNETs – pancreatic neuroendocrine tumors – these are a group of slow growing pancreatic cancers in which the cancer cells may produce hormones such as insulin or glucagon.

only one form of PI3K) or to give them only to very select groups of patients (e.g., people whose tumors contain a *PIK3CA* mutation). Or, of course, you can combine both strategies, e.g., giving a PI3Kα inhibitor only to patients whose tumors have *PIK3CA* mutations [219, 220].

Having said that though, there are still plenty of trials in which mTOR, PI3K, and AKT inhibitors are being investigated as treatments for people with a diverse range of cancers.

I'll now run through some of the treatments that have made it into clinical trials.

3.8.3 PI3K Inhibitors

Two important features of PI3K proteins are that there's a whole bunch of them and that they are actually made from two separate protein parts. The two parts are known as the regulatory subunit and the catalytic subunit (the catalytic subunit is the bit that phosphorylates PIP$_2$). Just to add more confusion, there are four different versions of the catalytic

Catalytic subunit   Regulatory subunit

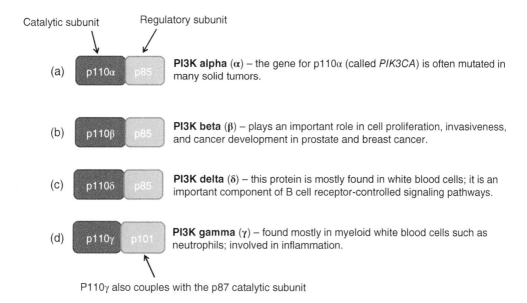

(a) **PI3K alpha** (α) – the gene for p110α (called *PIK3CA*) is often mutated in many solid tumors.

(b) **PI3K beta** (β) – plays an important role in cell proliferation, invasiveness, and cancer development in prostate and breast cancer.

(c) **PI3K delta** (δ) – this protein is mostly found in white blood cells; it is an important component of B cell receptor-controlled signaling pathways.

(d) **PI3K gamma** (γ) – found mostly in myeloid white blood cells such as neutrophils; involved in inflammation.

P110γ also couples with the p87 catalytic subunit

Figure 3.24 PI3K comes in various forms. There are numerous versions of the two subunits that come together to create each PI3K enzyme. Each subunit is encoded by a different gene. **(a)** The most commonly mutated gene for a PI3K subunit in cancer cells is *PIK3CA*, which is the gene for the p110-alpha subunit of PI3K-α. A wide variety of mutations in *PIK3CA* have been found in numerous solid tumors. **(b)** PI3K-β has overlapping roles with PI3K-α and seems to be particularly important to cancer cells that have lost PTEN, which includes the majority of prostate cancers. **(c)** PI3K-δ is predominantly found in white blood cells; it is often overactive in cancers that develop from faulty B cells. **(d)** PI3K-γ is activated by G protein-coupled receptors rather than by growth factor receptors.
Abbreviations: PI3K – phosphatidylinositol 3-kinase; PTEN – phosphatase and tensin homolog.

subunit (called p110α, β, δ, and γ), and eight regulatory subunits. These subunits can pair up in various different combinations[18] to create different versions of PI3K (see Figure 3.24) [212, 221].

An enormous number of PI3K inhibitors have been created and tested in clinical trials. Virtually all PI3K inhibitors are ATP mimics that competitively bind PI3K's ATP-binding site [222]. Some of these drugs block all four versions of PI3K illustrated in Figure 3.24 – these are called pan-PI3K inhibitors. Others

are more selective and block just one or two PI3Ks (see Table 3.14) [219].

Pan-PI3K inhibitors
Pan-PI3K inhibitors block the α, β, γ, and δ forms of PI3K. Some of these drugs, such as buparlisib (BKM120), have been the subject of numerous clinical trials. However, side effects have been a pretty insurmountable problem. Thus far, only copanlisib has become a licensed treatment. It blocks all four versions of PI3K but is most potent against PI3Kα

---

[18] If you really want to know, five of the regulatory subunits (p85α, p85β, p55α, p55γ, and p50α) will pair with p110α, β, and δ. The other three regulatory subunits (p101, p84, and p87PIKAP) will only pair with p110γ.

Table 3.14 Summary of selected PI3K inhibitors.

PI3K inhibitor	Relative ability to block each form of PI3K[a]				Comments
	α	β	δ	γ	
Pan-PI3K inhibitors					
Buparlisib	✓		✓	✓	Beset by problems with toxicities and lack of effectiveness. Buparlisib is still in trials.
Pictilisib	✓	(✓)	✓	(✓)	
PI3Kδ inhibitors					
Copanlisib	✓	(✓)	✓	(✓)	Given to people with some B cell-derived cancers (such as chronic lymphocytic leukemia) due to their ability to block B cell receptor-controlled signaling pathways.
Idelalisib			✓		
Umbralisib			✓		
Duvelisib			✓	(✓)	
Parsaclisib			✓		
PI3Kα inhibitors					
Taselisib	✓		✓	✓	Alpelisib is an approved treatment for people with *PIK3CA*-mutated, hormone receptor-positive breast cancer
Alpelisib	✓				
Inavolisib	✓				
PI3Kγ inhibitors					
Eganelisib			✓		

Source: Adapted from Ref. [219, 223, 224].
[a] Each drug's relative ability to inhibit each form of PI3K is depicted with a tick for strong inhibition; a lesser level of inhibition is shown by a tick in brackets.
Abbreviations: PI3K – phosphatidylinositol 3-kinase.

and PI3Kδ. Its efficacy against B cell cancers is presumably because of its ability to block PI3Kδ (see below).

PI3Kα Inhibitors

PIK3CA gene mutations are found in the cancer cells of people with a wide range of solid tumors (see Table 3.10) including around 30% of breast cancers [213]. The three most common mutations in the *PIK3CA* gene are E545K, E542K, and H1047R (see Figure 3.25) [225–227].

The initial focus of clinical trials with PI3Kα inhibitors has been in the treatment of people with hormone receptor (HR)-positive breast cancer. However, although *PIK3CA* mutations are most common in HR-positive breast cancer (present in 42%), they're also present in 16% of triple-negative breast cancers and 31% of HER2-positive/HR-negative breast cancers [227].

Alpelisib was the first PI3Kα to become an approved treatment option for people with HR-positive breast cancer. It can block all the various mutated versions of PI3Kα found in breast cancer cells. In addition, in some people, their cancer cells contain a version of the *PIK3CA* gene containing two or more different mutations. This seems to do two things: (1) It makes the PI3K protein even more active, and (2) it renders the person's tumor extra-sensitive to a PI3Kα inhibitor [226].

Most clinical trials of PI3Kα inhibitors have been for people with *PIK3CA*-mutated HR-positive breast cancer. However, alpelisib and other PI3Kα inhibitors are also in trials for people with *PIK3CA*-mutated triple-negative breast cancer, bowel cancer, ovarian cancer, endometrial cancer, head and neck cancer, and others. There's also evidence that PI3K inhibitors can inhibit homologous recombination (an important DNA repair process) and synergize with PARP inhibitors [219].

PI3Kδ Inhibitors

PI3Kδ is mostly found in B lymphocytes (I'll refer to them from now on as B cells). Its activity is controlled by BCRs and by other cell surface receptors and signaling pathways [228]. When idelalisib, the first PI3Kδ inhibitor, was first approved in 2014, scientists and doctors were optimistic about its effectiveness as a treatment for chronic

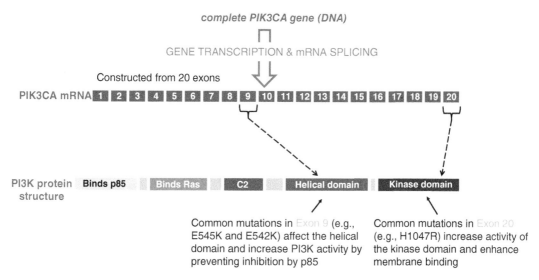

Figure 3.25 The location of mutations in the *PIK3CA* gene found in various solid tumors [22, 225].

lymphocytic leukemia and follicular lymphoma (a type of B cell non-Hodgkin lymphoma). However, toxicity problems and the risk of severe infections with idelalisib and other PI3Kδ inhibitors have led to various treatments being withdrawn from use [228].

BCR-controlled signaling pathways can also be blocked by another group of treatments called Bruton's tyrosine kinase (BTK) inhibitors. These treatments are much more widely used than PI3Kδ inhibitors, and I cover them in Section 4.8, when I look at BCR-controlled signaling pathway inhibitors in more detail.

3.8.4 Dual PI3K and mTOR Inhibitors

The ATP-binding sites on PI3K and mTOR are very similar to one another, making it possible to create chemical compounds that block both proteins. Early research suggested that these drugs would be more potent, and more difficult for cancer cells to be resistant to, than inhibitors of either PI3K or mTOR. A long list of dual inhibitors have made it into clinical trials. However, their development has generally been halted due to a lack of effectiveness and problems with side effects [219, 229].

3.8.5 AKT Inhibitors

AKT inhibitors have been in development as cancer treatments for roughly 20 years (the earliest published papers date from around 2002 [230]). However, despite decades of research and numerous clinical trials, the first approval only came at the end of 2023 when capivasertib was approved for advanced, HR-positive breast cancer.

AKT (also known as protein kinase B – PKB) comes in three main forms: AKT1, AKT2, and AKT3. AKT proteins have a diverse range of functions in human cells, just one of which is to activate mTOR. One of their main functions is to promote cell survival. They do this by inactivating proteins known to trigger cell death, such as Bad, and activating proteins that promote survival, such as MDM2. AKT proteins also block various proteins that would otherwise prevent the cell from multiplying [231].

AKT gene mutations are rare in human cancers, but AKT proteins are often overactive due to mutations affecting various cell surface receptors, *PIK3CA* mutations, or loss of functional PTEN protein (due to *PTEN* gene mutation or suppression) [215].

AKT inhibitors have been put through their paces in numerous clinical trials. But there's still no clear picture as to who they work best for. For example, in the clinical trial (called CAPItello-291) that led to the approval of capivasertib for HR-positive breast cancer, the results were similar between patients whose cancer did or didn't contain a mutation affecting the PI3K/AKT/mTOR pathway [232]. Despite this, the approvals only relate to patients whose cancers contain a *PIK3CA, AKT1,* or *PTEN* mutation [233].

AKT inhibitors have also been investigated in numerous other studies. For example:

- The IPATential150 study involved over 1000 patients with advanced, hormone therapy-resistant prostate cancer, who received hormone therapy (abiraterone) with or without an AKT inhibitor (ipatasertib). The study found that patients given ipatasertib lived longer without their disease progressing than if they were given abiraterone alone. This was particularly true if their cancer was missing the PTEN protein [234].
- Capivasertib and ipatasertib have both given promising results as a treatment for people whose cancer cells contain the E17K mutated form of AKT1, which is most common in breast cancer [231, 235]
- In addition to the CAPItello-291 trial, numerous other clinical trials are exploring AKT inhibitors as treatments for HR-positive and triple-negative breast cancer [235].

3.8.6 mTOR Inhibitors

The first mTOR inhibitors used as cancer treatments were derivatives of a naturally occurring chemical compound called rapamycin (also known as sirolimus). This chemical is produced by a bacterium discovered on Easter Island over 40 years ago [236].

Rapamycin can suppress our immune system and is used to prevent the body from rejecting transplanted organs. Scientists investigating rapamycin's properties also discovered that it can kill cancer cells. Two drugs created from rapamycin, temsirolimus, and everolimus (collectively known as rapalogs)

are used as treatments for people with kidney cancer, pancreatic neuroendocrine cancer (PNET), and mantle cell lymphoma (a form of B cell non-Hodgkin lymphoma). These drugs are also used as breast cancer treatments in combination with hormone therapies.

Rapamycin, temsirolimus, and everolimus are thus three closely related drugs that have been created from a natural compound. Unlike many drugs that block kinases, they do not mimic the shape of ATP, nor do they directly inhibit mTOR's kinase activity. Instead, these drugs attach to a protein called FKBP12. The drug–FKBP12 combination then blocks mTORC1 (but not mTORC2) [237].

The inability of rapamycin, everolimus, and temsirolimus to block mTORC2 gave rise to the question of whether drugs that blocked mTOR directly would be more effective as they'd block both mTOR complexes.

We now do have ATP-competitive drugs that block mTOR's catalytic activity and thereby block the actions of both mTORC1 and mTORC2. In addition, there are various ATP-competitive drugs that block both mTOR and PI3K. However, none of these drugs has yet proven its worth in clinical trials, mostly because of problems with toxicities [238].

3.9 TARGETING THE JAK-STAT PATHWAY

Licensed drugs mentioned in this section:		
Treatment class	Drugs	Given to some people with:
JAK2 inhibitors	Ruxolitinib, pacritinib, momelotinib, and fedratinib	Myeloproliferative neoplasms: myelofibrosis and polycythemia vera

The final signaling pathway I want to mention is the JAK-STAT pathway. As with other pathways, activation of the JAK-STAT pathway usually begins with the activation of a receptor on a cell's surface. Typically, the receptor is a cytokine receptor, which is responding to a cytokine [239]. Cytokines are small signaling molecules that our white blood cells use to give one another instructions. They include interferons, interleukins, chemokines, and tumor necrosis factor (TNF) [240].

When a cytokine attaches to a cytokine receptor, the receptors pair up. As JAK proteins are constantly attached to the receptors, this means that the JAK proteins come together inside the cell as well (Figure 3.26a-c).

JAK proteins are kinases, and when they're brought together, two JAK proteins will phosphorylate one another. Once this has happened, the phosphorylated JAK proteins then phosphorylate STATs. STATs are transcription factors that spend most of the time sitting in the cell cytoplasm. But when JAK phosphorylates them, they pair up and move into the nucleus. In the nucleus, they attach to genes in the cell's DNA and trigger the production of various proteins (Figure 3.26d) [239].

In addition, when JAK becomes active, it can activate both the MAPK pathway and the PI3K pathway. Consequently, all three pathways (JAK-STAT, MAPK, and PI3K/AKT/mTOR) add to each other's activity [102, 105].

As in other pathways, there are various versions of the proteins involved. There are four members of the JAK family: JAK1, JAK2, JAK3, and TYK2. There are also seven members of the STAT family, STATs 1, 2, 3, 4, 5a, 5b, and 6. JAK2 is particularly important in the response of white blood cells to some growth factors and interleukins.

3.9.1 Defects in the JAK-STAT Pathway in Cancer Cells

There are four main reasons why the JAK-STAT pathway can be overactive in cancer cells:

1. Overactive growth factor receptors, cytokine receptors, and other receptors on the cell surface. For example, mutated, overactive cytokine receptors have been

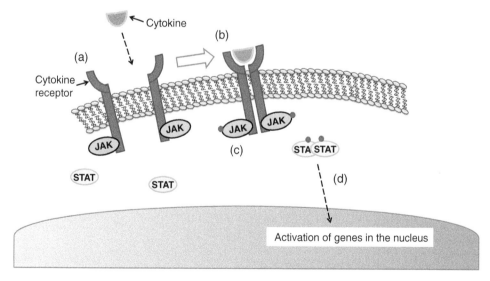

Figure 3.26 The basics of the JAK-STAT signaling pathway. (a) In the absence of a suitable cytokine, cytokine receptors remain separate and JAK proteins are kept apart. (b) Two or more cytokine receptors come together due to the presence of a cytokine. (c) JAK proteins are brought together. They phosphorylate each other, and then they phosphorylate STAT transcription factors in the cytoplasm. (d) Phosphorylated STATs pair up and move into the nucleus. In the nucleus, STATs control the production of a variety of proteins that between them encourage the cell to multiply and control other cell functions.
Abbreviations: JAK – Janus kinase, STAT – signal transducer and activator of transcription.

found on the surface of cancer cells in some myeloproliferative neoplasms (MPNs) and acute leukemias [241]. MPNs are a group of often slow-growing cancers affecting white blood cells.

2. *Mutations affecting JAK genes.* *JAK2* mutations are very common in MPNs such as polycythemia vera, essential thrombocythemia, and primary myelofibrosis [242]. Additionally, the *JAK2* gene is amplified in a high proportion of Hodgkin lymphomas [243]. JAK2 fusion proteins and other *JAK2* gene mutations are found occasionally in acute leukemia and lymphoma cells, and in some solid tumors [244]. Mutations in *JAK1, JAK3,* and *TYK2* are mostly found in the cells of T cell acute lymphoblastic leukemias and lymphomas [241]. *JAK1* mutations are also found in some solid tumors, such as primary liver cancer and bowel cancer [245]. JAK fusion proteins have found in some leukemias [246].

3. *Absence of proteins that would normally block the pathway,* such as SOCS1, SOCS2, and SOCS3, in a variety of solid tumors [244, 247].

4. *Mutations in STAT genes.* *STAT* gene mutations are relatively rare, but mutations in *STAT3* and *STAT5* have been found in some solid tumors as well as in rheumatoid arthritis [246]. *STAT6* mutations have been found in primary mediastinal large B cell lymphoma, a rare type of non-Hodgkin lymphoma [245].

In addition to being important in cancer (particularly in hematological cancers), the JAK-STAT pathway has also been implicated in various inflammatory conditions and autoimmune diseases [245].

3.9.2 JAK2 Inhibitors

JAK inhibitors are the only JAK-STAT pathway inhibitors to have been approved as cancer treatments (for myelofibrosis and polycythemia vera). In addition to being approved for cancer, some JAK inhibitors are also licensed as treatments for rheumatoid arthritis and other autoimmune conditions (Table 3.15) [245, 246].

The first JAK inhibitor to be licensed as a treatment was ruxolitinib, which blocks JAK1 and JAK2 [245]. As with many of the other JAK inhibitors created so far, ruxolitinib is a reversible inhibitor that competes for the enzyme's ATP-binding site. However, the most common mutation in JAK2 found in MPN cells is the V617F mutation, which does not affect the ATP-binding site [246]. Hence, ruxolitinib does not selectively block the mutated form of the protein. Because of its relative lack of specificity, ruxolitinib suppresses the normal creation of white blood cells in the bone marrow.

Table 3.15 Approved JAK inhibitors. Treatments licensed for people with cancer are highlighted in orange.

Disease	Drug
Myelofibrosis	Ruxolitinib, pacritinib, momelotinib, **and** fedratinib
Polycythemia vera	Ruxolitinib
Rheumatoid arthritis	Tofacitinib, baricitinib, upadacitinib, filgotinib, and peficitinib
Psoriatic arthritis	Tofacitinib and upadacitinib
Juvenile arthritis	Tofacitinib
Ankylosing spondyloarthritis	Tofacitinib and upadacitinib
Ulcerative colitis	Tofacitinib and filgotinib
Atopic dermatitis	Baricitinib, upadacitinib, abrocitinib, delgocitinib (topical), and ruxolitinib (topical)
Alopecia areata	Baricitinib
Graft versus host disease	Ruxolitinib
COVID-19	Baricitinib
Vitiligo	Ruxolitinib (topical)
Plaque psoriasis	Deucravacitinib

Source: Adapted from Ref. [245, 246].

Three other JAK2 inhibitors are approved as treatments for myelofibrosis: Fedratinib, which blocks JAK2 and FLT3, pacritinib, which blocks JAK2 and IRAK1 (interleukin-1 receptor-associated kinase 1), and momelotinib, which blocks JAK1, JAK2, and activin A receptor, type I (ACVR1) [248].

JAK inhibitors have not been licensed as treatments for any solid tumors. This is despite the JAK-STAT pathway being active in many cancer types. The issue might be that in solid tumors the reason why the JAK/STAT pathway is overactive is generally because of the overactivity of STAT transcription factors rather than defects directly affecting JAK proteins [249].

3.10 BCR-ABL INHIBITORS

Licensed drugs mentioned in this section:		
Treatment class	Drugs	Given to some people with:
Bcr-Abl inhibitors	Imatinib, dasatinib, nilotinib, bosutinib, ponatinib, and asciminib	• Chronic myeloid leukemia • Acute lymphoblastic leukemia • Gastrointestinal stromal tumors (GIST)[a]

[a] Imatinib is a treatment for GIST because in addition to inhibiting Bcr-Abl it also blocks PDGFRA and KIT, which are often overactive in GIST cells – see Section 3.6.1.

I mentioned Bcr-Abl and the inhibitors that block it several times in Chapter 2. The Bcr-Abl fusion protein exists in the cancer cells of virtually everyone with CML. The *BCR-ABL* fusion gene that causes cells to make Bcr-Abl is created by a translocation involving chromosomes 9 and 22. This translocation also creates an extra-short version of chromosome 22 known as the Philadelphia chromosome [250, 251].

Over the past 25 years, thousands of people with CML have been treated with Bcr-Abl

inhibitors. In fact, because of Bcr-Abl inhibitors, the life expectancy of people with CML is now approaching that of the general population [252, 253].

Bcr-Abl inhibitors are also given to people with acute lymphoblastic leukemia (ALL) if a Bcr-Abl protein is present in the person's cancer cells (called Philadelphia chromosome-positive ALL, or simply Ph+ ALL) [254]. In addition, they're sometimes given to people with "BCR/ABL1-like" ALL – these are forms of the disease that have similarities to Ph+ ALL, but where the Bcr-Abl protein isn't present [255].

3.10.1 The Bcr-Abl Protein

It might not seem obvious that I should include Bcr-Abl inhibitors in this chapter. However, Bcr-Abl is a kinase that activates numerous signaling pathways, including those involving Ras proteins, PI3K proteins, and JAK proteins [256, 257]. As with many other kinase inhibitors, most Bcr-Abl inhibitors fit into the ATP-binding site of the Abl part of the protein.

In case you were wondering, the break cluster region (*BCR*) gene on chromosome 22 involved in *BCR-ABL* translocation has nothing to do with the B cell receptor that I mention elsewhere in this book.

3.10.2 Imatinib: The First Bcr-Abl Inhibitor

Imatinib was the first small molecule kinase inhibitor ever given to patients as a cancer treatment. It is a "Type 2" kinase inhibitor (see Section 2.3.4 and Figure 2.19b). This means that it can only block Bcr-Abl when its ATP-binding site is empty, and the kinase is in its inactive shape [258].

When given to people with CML, the benefits of imatinib often last for many years, particularly for people whose cancer is in the "chronic phase" (i.e., very slow growing) when their treatment starts. However, some patients' cancers do eventually become resistant. This typically happens because of cancer cells with additional mutations in their *BCR-ABL* fusion gene [256, 258–261].

Scientists have now identified more than 50 different mutations affecting the kinase section of Bcr-Abl in the cancer cells of people whose disease has become resistant to imatinib. Many of these mutations trap the kinase in its active shape. Imatinib, which can only bind to the inactive enzyme, can therefore no longer do its job.

3.10.3 Second- and Third-Generation Bcr-Abl Inhibitors

Second-generation Bcr-Abl inhibitors such as nilotinib and dasatinib were designed to block many of the mutant versions of Bcr-Abl that imatinib can't block.

Nilotinib, like imatinib, can only bind to inactive Bcr-Abl, but it is 20 to 30 times better than imatinib at doing this. Dasatinib is about 325 times more potent than imatinib, and it can block Bcr-Abl when it's in a variety of different shapes [256, 261]. Other Bcr-Abl inhibitors developed in recent years include bosutinib, which inhibits both the Abl and SRC kinases [262].

One drawback of nilotinib, dasatinib, and bosutinib is that none of these drugs can block an important drug-resistant form of Bcr-Abl

known as the T315I mutant (the 315th amino acid in the Bcr-Abl protein has changed from being a threonine (T) to become an isoleucine (I)). The only licensed ATP-competitive drug able to block the T315I mutant is a third-generation Bcr-Abl inhibitor called ponatinib [263] (Table 3.16).

3.10.4 Allosteric Inhibitors of Bcr-Abl

Normal Abl protein (i.e., when it's not part of a Bcr-Abl fusion protein) can inhibit its own activity. It does this by sticking part of itself (a bit called the myristoyl group) into a little internal pocket called the myristoyl-binding pocket [265]. In contrast, the Bcr-Abl protein doesn't have the myristoyl group, so it can't stop itself from being active.

A new set of Bcr-Abl inhibitors created in recent years are the allosteric inhibitors that mimic the myristoyl group and slot into the myristoyl-binding pocket (Figure 3.27). This forces the Bcr-Abl protein into an inactive shape [265].

Because they don't interact with the ATP-binding site, myristoyl inhibitors aren't affected by mutations that distort the ATP-binding site (including the T315I mutation that renders Bcr-Abl insensitive to so many of our other Bcr-Abl inhibitors). The first licensed allosteric Bcr-Abl inhibitor is asciminib. So far, scientists have identified two possible reasons

Table 3.16   A comparison of ATP-competitive Bcr-Abl inhibitors.

	Imatinib	Dasatinib	Nilotinib	Bosutinib	Ponatinib
Binds the inactive or active form of Bcr-Abl?	inactive	active	inactive	both	inactive
Half-life (hours)	18	3–5	17	22.5	24
Mutations in Bcr-Abl that cause resistance	>100 different mutations, e.g., T315I, E255K, Y253H, F359V, G250E, and L387M	V299L, T315I, T315A, F317L, and F317I	Y253H, E255K, T315I, F359C, and F359V	T315I, E255K, and V299L	Y253H + T315I, and E255V+T315I

Source: Adapted from Ref. [258–261, 264].

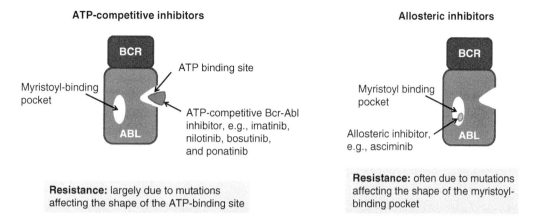

Figure 3.27 The mechanisms of action of ATP-competitive vs. allosteric Bcr-Abl inhibitors.
Abbreviation: ATP – adenosine triphosphate.

for asciminib resistance: a change in shape of the myristoyl-binding pocket, or the drug's expulsion from the cell by a protein called the ABCG2 protein pump [266].

As I've said before, the reasons why a cancer cell might be resistant to an ATP-competitive drug like ponatinib, or to an allosteric inhibitor like asciminib, are different. This might mean that giving a patient a combination that includes both drugs would be more effective than giving either treatment alone [264].

3.11 FINAL THOUGHTS

In this chapter, I have described some of the growth factor receptors found on the surface of cancer cells and the pathways under their control. These receptors and signaling pathways are faulty and overactive in cancer cells for a wide variety of reasons, and drugs that block them have become important cancer treatments.

However, as you're probably aware, results from clinical trials with signaling pathway inhibitors don't always give positive results. And, even when someone does benefit from one of these treatments, perhaps even for several years, their cancer almost always returns later, particularly if they have advanced, meta-

static cancer. There appear to be many reasons why a cancer might be intrinsically resistant to treatment with a signaling pathway inhibitor or can become resistant over time.

Reasons for this resistance include the following [115–117]:

1. The cancer was never dependent on the protein being blocked by the inhibitor. For example, just because EGFR is on the surface of a person's cancer cells, this doesn't necessarily mean that the cancer cells are reliant on EGFR for their survival.

2. A tumor is made of multiple populations of cancer cells that contain different combinations of mutations. It appears to be inevitable that among all those millions of cells, there will be some that contain mutations or other adaptations that enable them to survive a treatment that blocks a single protein or pathway. Given time to grow, these resistant cells cause the cancer to recur.

3. Most kinase inhibitors work by mimicking the shape of ATP and slotting into a kinase's ATP-binding site. Perhaps not surprisingly, these drugs become ineffective if their target's ATP-binding site changes shape.

4. Because signaling pathways are so important to our cells, there's lots of redundancy

built into them. This means that various cell surface receptors and signaling pathways can stand in for one another. And this in turn increases the likelihood that cancer cells will survive treatment with a drug that blocks just one receptor or pathway.

5. Signaling pathways are used by all healthy cells. Hence, sometimes a signaling pathway inhibitor causes almost as much damage to healthy cells as cancer cells, and it causes so much toxicity that it can't be given in a dose that would eradicate a cancer.

6. Non-cancer cells within the cancer environment participate in cell signaling. They sometimes protect cancer cells from the effects of an inhibitor.

7. Some cancer cells have access to protective mechanisms through which they become dormant and stop multiplying (called senescence), or through which they become more resilient (such as going through the epithelial-to-mesenchymal transition – see Chapter 1, Section 1.6.3). Cells that trigger these mechanisms can often survive treatment.

8. Tumors often contain regions with a poor blood supply due to leaky, tangled, and malformed blood vessels. Hence, a drug may simply not be able to get where it's needed.

9. Cancer cells sometimes have proteins in their cell membrane that can actively pump a drug out of the cell.

Of course, many of these resistance mechanisms also apply to other treatments included in this book, such as Bcr-Abl inhibitors, PARP inhibitors, and the other approaches covered in Chapter 4. Perhaps the only treatments for which many of these mechanisms don't apply are immunotherapies: treatments that work by activating or creating immune responses against cancer cells.

Another thing to keep in mind is just how complicated signaling pathways are. Back in Figure 3.5, when I illustrated some of the many proteins and pathways controlled by growth factor receptors, I included various proteins that I haven't mentioned elsewhere in the chapter. These include Rac, Rho, Src, phospholipase C (PLC), and NFκB. However, they are important proteins and often implicated in drug resistance. For example, Src overactivity is a known drug resistance mechanism to HER2-targeted treatments [267].

Thankfully, despite the daunting complexity of signaling pathways, we have seen a huge number of signaling pathway inhibitors become licensed cancer treatments. Efforts continue to make these treatments even more effective, using strategies such as:

• Combining signaling pathway inhibitors with one another to shut off feedback loops and to block signaling pathways at multiple points.

• Combining treatments that block different pathways (although toxicity is always a problem when you do this).

• Combining signaling pathway inhibitors with immunotherapy – this approach has several potential advantages: increasing the effectiveness of treatment; overcoming some resistance mechanisms; and minimizing side effects (because the two different sets of treatments cause very different toxicities and can therefore potentially be safely combined).

• Creating kinase inhibitors that are designed to specific mutant forms of kinases – such as osimertinib and mobocertinib, which block various mutant forms of EGFR.

• Using biomarker tests to predict which treatment is most likely to work for each patient.

• Using biopsy samples or extracting circulating tumor DNA (ctDNA) from the blood, to check for gene mutations likely to cause resistance. It may then be possible to change the person's treatment accordingly.

With all these potential strategies, hopefully signaling pathway inhibitors will become even more effective for an even greater number of people.

REFERENCES

1 Scitable. Cell signaling. *Nature Education*. [Online] Available: https://www.nature.com/scitable/topicpage/cell-signaling-14047077/ [Accessed March 1, 2022].

2 Testar J Cytokines: Introduction. *British Society for Immunology*. [Online] Available: https://www.immunology.org/public-information/bitesized-immunology/receptors-and-molecules/cytokines-introduction [Accessed March 1, 2022].

3 Manoylov M. What are cytokines? *LiveScience*. [Online] Available: https://www.livescience.com/what-are-cytokines.html [Accessed March 1, 2022].

4 Dorsam RT, Gutkind JS (2007). G-protein-coupled receptors and cancer. *Nat. Rev. Cancer* **7**(2). doi: 10.1038/nrc2069.

5 Scitable. GPCR. *Nature Education*. [Online] Available: https://www.nature.com/scitable/topicpage/gpcr-14047471/ [Accessed March 4, 2022].

6 Wintheiser GA, Silberstein P (2019). Physiology, tyrosine kinase receptors. [Online] Available: https://www.ncbi.nlm.nih.gov/books/NBK538532/ [Accessed March 1, 2022].

7 Blume-Jensen P, Hunter T (2001). Oncogenic kinase signalling. *Nature* **411**(6835). doi: 10.1038/35077225.

8 Robinson DR, Wu YM, Lin SF (2000). The protein tyrosine kinase family of the human genome. *Oncogene* **19**(49). doi: 10.1038/sj.onc.1203957.

9 Zhan T, Rindtorff N, Boutros M (2017). Wnt signaling in cancer. *Oncogene* **36**(11). doi: 10.1038/onc.2016.304.

10 Alberts B, Johnson A, Lewis J (2002). Signaling through Enzyme-Linked Cell-Surface Receptors. In *Molecular Biology of the Cell*. 4th ed. New York: Garland Science [Online] Available: https://www.ncbi.nlm.nih.gov/books/NBK26822/ [Accessed March 4, 2022].

11 Safran M *et al*. (2021). The GeneCards Suite. In *Practical Guide to Life Science Databases*. Singapore: Springer Singapore. pp. 27–56 doi: 10.1007/978-981-16-5812-9_2.

12 Henson ES, Gibson SB (2006). Surviving cell death through epidermal growth factor (EGF) signal transduction pathways: Implications for cancer therapy. *Cell. Signal.* **18**(12). doi: 10.1016/j.cellsig.2006.05.015.

13 Chen J *et al*. (2016). Expression and function of the epidermal growth factor receptor in physiology and disease. *Physiol. Rev.* **96**(3). doi: 10.1152/physrev.00030.2015.

14 Lemmon MA, Schlessinger J (2010). Cell signaling by receptor tyrosine kinases. *Cell* **141**(7). doi: 10.1016/j.cell.2010.06.011.

15 Wee P, Wang Z (2017). Epidermal growth factor receptor cell proliferation signaling pathways. *Cancers* **9**(5). doi: 10.3390/cancers9050052.

16 Castellano E, Downward J (2011). Ras interaction with PI3K: More than just another effector pathway. *Genes Cancer* **2**(3). doi: 10.1177/1947601911408079.

17 He Y *et al*. (2021). Targeting PI3K/Akt signal transduction for cancer therapy. *Signal Transduction Targeted Ther.* **6**(1): 425. doi: 10.1038/s41392-021-00828-5.

18 The cancer genome atlas program. *National Cancer Institute*. [Online] Available: https://www.cancer.gov/about-nci/organization/ccg/research/structural-genomics/tcga [Accessed March 7, 2022].

19 Sanchez-Vega F *et al*. (2018). Oncogenic signaling pathways in the cancer genome atlas. *Cell* **173**(2). doi: 10.1016/j.cell.2018.03.035.

20 Kawakami H, Zaanan A, Sinicrope F (2015). MSI testing and its role in the management of colorectal cancer. *Curr. Treat. Options in Oncol.* **16**(7).

21 Talhouk A, McAlpine JN (2016). New classification of endometrial cancers: The development and potential applications of genomic-based classification in research and clinical care. *Gynecol. Oncol. Res. Pract.* **3**(1). doi: 10.1186/s40661-016-0035-4.

22 Zhang Y *et al*. (2017). A pan-cancer proteogenomic atlas of PI3K/AKT/mTOR pathway alterations. *Cancer Cell* **31**(6). doi: 10.1016/j.ccell.2017.04.013.

23 Salomon DS *et al*. (1995). Epidermal growth factor-related peptides and their receptors in human malignancies. *Crit. Rev. Oncol. Hematol.* **19**(3). doi: 10.1016/1040-8428(94)00144-I.

24 Yan M *et al*. (2014). HER2 aberrations in cancer: Implications for therapy. *Cancer Treat. Rev.* **40**(6). doi: 10.1016/j.ctrv.2014.02.008.

25 Ma J *et al.* (2014). Targeting of erbB3 receptor to overcome resistance in cancer treatment. *Mol. Cancer* **13**(1). doi: 10.1186/1476-4598-13-105.

26 Benayed R, Liu S (2021). Neuregulin-1 (NRG1): An emerging tumor-agnostic target. *Clinical Care Options, Oncology*. [Online] Available: https://www.clinicaloptions.com/oncology/programs/2021/nrg1-fusions/text-module/nrg1-text-module/page-1 [Accessed March 24, 2022].

27 Arteaga CL, Engelman JA (2014). ERBB receptors: From oncogene discovery to basic science to mechanism-based cancer therapeutics. *Cancer Cell* **25**(3). doi: 10.1016/j.ccr.2014.02.025.

28 Sharma PS, Sharma R, Tyagi T (2012). VEGF/VEGFR pathway inhibitors as anti-angiogenic agents: Present and future. *Curr. Cancer Drug Targets* **11**(5). doi: 10.2174/156800911795655985.

29 Heldin CH (2013). Targeting the PDGF signaling pathway in tumor treatment. *Cell Commun. Signaling* **11**(1). doi: 10.1186/1478-811X-11-97.

30 Wesche J, Haglund K, Haugsten EM (2011). Fibroblast growth factors and their receptors in cancer. *Biochem. J.* **437**(2). doi: 10.1042/BJ20101603.

31 Pollak M (2008). Insulin and insulin-like growth factor signalling in neoplasia. *Nat. Rev. Cancer* **8**(12). doi: 10.1038/nrc2536.

32 Smyth EC, Sclafani F, Cunningham D (2014). Emerging molecular targets in oncology: Clinical potential of MEeT/hepatocyte growth-factor inhibitors. *Onco. Targets Ther.* **7**. doi: 10.2147/OTT.S44941.

33 Lennartsson J, Rönnstrand L (2012). Stem cell factor receptor/c-Kit: From basic Science to clinical implications. *Physiol. Rev.* **92**(4). doi: 10.1152/physrev.00046.2011.

34 Small D (2006). FLT3 mutations: Biology and treatment. *Hematol./Educ. Program Am. Soc. Hematol. Am. Soc. Hematol. Educ. Program.* doi: 10.1182/asheducation-2006.1.178.

35 Mulligan LM (2014). RET revisited: Expanding the oncogenic portfolio. *Nat. Rev. Cancer* **14**(3). doi: 10.1038/nrc3680.

36 Tebbutt N, Pedersen MW, Johns TG (2013). Targeting the ERBB family in cancer: Couples therapy. *Nat. Rev. Cancer* **13**(9). doi: 10.1038/nrc3559.

37 Yarden Y, Pines G (2012). The ERBB network: At last, cancer therapy meets systems biology. *Nat. Rev. Cancer* **12**(8). doi: 10.1038/nrc3309.

38 Du Z, Lovly CM (2018). Mechanisms of receptor tyrosine kinase activation in cancer. *Mol. Cancer* **17**(1). doi: 10.1186/s12943-018-0782-4.

39 Regad T (2015). Targeting RTK signaling pathways in cancer. *Cancers* **7**(3). doi: 10.3390/cancers7030860.

40 Zhang YL *et al.* (2016). The prevalence of EGFR mutation in patients with non-small cell lung cancer: A systematic review and meta-analysis. *Oncotarget* **7**(48). doi: 10.18632/oncotarget.12587.

41 Mishra R, Hanker AB, Garrett JT (2017). Genomic alterations of ERBB receptors in cancer: Clinical implications. *Oncotarget* **8**(69). doi: 10.18632/oncotarget.22825.

42 Kennedy VE, Smith CC (2020). FLT3 mutations in acute myeloid leukemia: Key concepts and emerging controversies. *Front. Oncol.* **10**. doi: 10.3389/fonc.2020.612880.

43 Oh DY, Bang YJ (2020). HER2-targeted therapies – a role beyond breast cancer. *Nat. Rev. Clin. Oncol.* **17**(1). doi: 10.1038/s41571-019-0268-3.

44 Hallberg B, Palmer RH (2016). The role of the ALK receptor in cancer biology. *Ann. Oncol.* **27**: iii4–iii15. doi: 10.1093/annonc/mdw301.

45 Yamashita S *et al.* (2018). Lessons from fukushima: Latest findings of thyroid cancer after the fukushima nuclear power plant accident. *Thyroid* **28**(1): 11–22. doi: 10.1089/thy.2017.0283.

46 Fernandez-Cuesta L *et al.* (2014). CD74-NRG1 fusions in lung adenocarcinoma. *Cancer Discov.* **4**(4). doi: 10.1158/2159-8290.CD-13-0633.

47 Gschwind A, Fischer OM, Ullrich A (2004). The discovery of receptor tyrosine kinases: Targets for cancer therapy. *Nat. Rev. Cancer* **4**(5). doi: 10.1038/nrc1360.

48 Chong CR, Jänne PA (2013). The quest to overcome resistance to EGFR-targeted therapies in cancer. *Nat. Med.* **19**(11). doi: 10.1038/nm.3388.

49 Rubin I, Yarden Y (2001). The basic biology of HER2. *Ann. Oncol.* **12**(SUPPL. 1). doi: 10.1093/annonc/12.suppl_1.S3.

50 Thomas R, Weihua Z (2019). Rethink of EGFR in cancer with its kinase independent function on board. *Front. Oncol.* **9**. doi: 10.3389/fonc.2019.00800.

51 Price TJ *et al*. (2014). Panitumumab versus cetuximab in patients with chemotherapy-refractory wild-type KRAS exon 2 metastatic colorectal cancer (ASPECCT): A randomised, multicentre, open-label, non-inferiority phase 3 study. *Lancet Oncol*. **15**(6). doi: 10.1016/S1470-2045(14)70118-4.

52 Cai WQ *et al*. (2020). The latest battles between EGFR monoclonal antibodies and resistant tumor cells. *Front. Oncol*. **10**. doi: 10.3389/fonc.2020.01249.

53 European Medicines Agency (2021). Portrazza: Expiry of the marketing authorisation in the European Union. [Online] Available: https://www.ema.europa.eu/en/documents/public-statement/public-statement-portrazza-expiry-marketing-authorisation-european-union_en.pdf [Accessed March 8, 2022].

54 Ramakrishnan MS *et al*. (2009). Nimotuzumab, a promising therapeutic monoclonal for treatment of tumors of epithelial origin. *MAbs* **1**(1): 41–48. doi: 10.4161/mabs.1.1.7509.

55 Bray SM *et al*. (2019). Genomic characterization of intrinsic and acquired resistance to cetuximab in colorectal cancer patients. *Sci. Rep*. **9**(1). doi: 10.1038/s41598-019-51981-5.

56 Parseghian CM *et al*. (2019). Mechanisms of innate and acquired resistance to anti-EGFR therapy: A review of current knowledge with a focus on rechallenge therapies. *Clin. Cancer Res*. **25**(23). doi: 10.1158/1078-0432.CCR-19-0823.

57 Bronte G *et al*. (2015). New findings on primary and acquired resistance to anti-EGFR therapy in metastatic colorectal cancer: Do all roads lead to RAS? *Oncotarget* **6**(28). doi: 10.18632/oncotarget.4959.

58 Hatil A *et al*. (2019). EGFR (epidermal growth factor receptor). *Atlas of Genetics and Cytogenetics in Oncology and Haematology*. [Online] Available: https://atlasgeneticsoncology.org/gene/147/egfr-(epidermal-growth-factor-receptor)/ [Accessed March 8, 2022].

59 Khaddour K *et al*. (2021). Targeting the epidermal growth factor receptor in egfr-mutated lung cancer: Current and emerging therapies. *Cancers* **13**(13). doi: 10.3390/cancers13133164.

60 Jura N *et al*. (2009). Structural analysis of the catalytically inactive kinase domain of the human EGF receptor 3. *Proc. Natl. Acad. Sci*. **106**(51): 21608–21613. doi: 10.1073/pnas.0912101106.

61 NCI Staff (2017). Neratinib approved by FDA for HER2-positive breast cancer. *National Cancer Institute*. [Online] Available: https://www.cancer.gov/news-events/cancer-currents-blog/2017/neratinib-breast-cancer-fda [Accessed November 3, 2023].

62 Ke EE, Wu YL (2016). EGFR as a pharmacological target in EGFR-mutant non-small-cell lung cancer: Where do we stand now? *Trends Pharmacol. Sci*. **37**(11). doi: 10.1016/j.tips.2016.09.003.

63 Costa DB (2016). Kinase inhibitor-responsive genotypes in EGFR mutated lung adenocarcinomas: Moving past common point mutations or indels into uncommon kinase domain duplications and rearrangements. *Transl. Lung Cancer Res*. **5**(3). doi: 10.21037/tlcr.2016.06.04.

64 Soria J-C *et al*. (2018). Osimertinib in untreated EGFR -mutated advanced non–small-cell lung cancer. *N. Engl. J. Med*. **378**(2). doi: 10.1056/nejmoa1713137.

65 Zhao Y *et al*. (2019). Efficacy and safety of first line treatments for patients with advanced epidermal growth factor receptor mutated, non-small cell lung cancer: Systematic review and network meta-analysis. *BMJ* **367**. doi: 10.1136/bmj.l5460.

66 Friedlaender A *et al*. (2022). EGFR and HER2 exon 20 insertions in solid tumours: From biology to treatment. *Nat. Rev. Clin. Oncol*. **19**(1). doi: 10.1038/s41571-021-00558-1.

67 Vyse S, Huang PH (2019). Targeting EGFR exon 20 insertion mutations in non-small cell lung cancer. *Signal Transduction Targeted Ther*. **4**(1). doi: 10.1038/s41392-019-0038-9.

68 Gonzalvez F *et al*. (2021). Mobocertinib (Tak-788): A targeted inhibitor of egfr exon 20 insertion mutants in non–small cell lung cancer. *Cancer Discov*. **11**(7). doi: 10.1158/2159-8290.CD-20-1683.

69 Robichaux JP *et al*. (2021). Structure-based classification predicts drug response in EGFR-mutant NSCLC. *Nature* **597**(7878). doi: 10.1038/s41586-021-03898-1.

70 Zhang SS, Zhu VW (2021). Spotlight on mobocertinib (TAK-788) in NSCLC with EGFR exon

20 insertion mutations. *Lung Cancer: Targets Ther.* **12**. doi: 10.2147/LCTT.S307321.

71 Cho BC *et al.* (2023). Amivantamab, an epidermal growth factor receptor (EGFR) and mesenchymal-epithelial transition factor (MET) bispecific antibody, designed to enable multiple mechanisms of action and broad clinical applications. *Clin. Lung Cancer* **24**(2): 89–97. doi: 10.1016/j.cllc.2022.11.004.

72 Zhou C *et al.* (2023). Amivantamab plus chemotherapy in NSCLC with *EGFR* Exon 20 insertions. *N. Engl. J. Med.* doi: 10.1056/NEJMoa2306441.

73 Midha A, Dearden S, McCormack R (2015). EGFR mutation incidence in non-Small-cell lung cancer of adenocarcinoma histology: A systematic review and global map by ethnicity (mutMapII). *Am. J. Cancer Res.* **5**(9): 2892.

74 D'Angelo SP *et al.* Incidence of EGFR Exon 19 deletions and 1858R in tumor specimens from men and cigarette smokers with lung adenocarcinomas. *J. Clin. Oncol.* **29**(15): 2011. doi: 10.1200/JCO.2010.32.6181.

75 Kelley RK, Ko AH (2008). Erlotinib in the treatment of advanced pancreatic cancer. *Biol.: Targets Ther.* **2**(1). doi: 10.2147/btt.s1832.

76 Moore MJ *et al.* (2007). Erlotinib plus gemcitabine compared with gemcitabine alone in patients with advanced pancreatic cancer: A phase III trial of the national cancer institute of canada clinical trials group. *J. Clin. Oncol.* **25**(15): 1960–1966. doi: 10.1200/JCO.2006.07.9525.

77 Ko AH (2007). Erlotinib in pancreatic cancer: A major breakthrough? *Oncology* **21**(14): 1706.

78 Passaro A *et al.* (2021). Overcoming therapy resistance in EGFR-mutant lung cancer. *Nat. Can.* **2**(4). doi: 10.1038/s43018-021-00195-8.

79 Leonetti A *et al.* (2019). Resistance mechanisms to osimertinib in EGFR-mutated non-small cell lung cancer. *Br. J. Cancer* **121**(9): 725–737. doi: 10.1038/s41416-019-0573-8.

80 Passaro A *et al.* (2023). Amivantamab plus chemotherapy with and without lazertinib in EGFR-mutant advanced NSCLC after disease progression on osimertinib: Primary results from the phase 3 MARIPOSA-2 study. *Ann. Oncol.* doi: 10.1016/j.annonc.2023.10.117.

81 Cho BC *et al.* (2023). Amivantamab plus lazertinib in osimertinib-relapsed EGFR-mutant advanced non-small cell lung cancer: A phase 1

trial. *Nat. Med.* **29**(10): 2577–2585. doi: 10.1038/s41591-023-02554-7.

82 Goodman A (2023) FLAURA2 trial: Osimertinib plus chemotherapy improves outcomes in advanced EGFR-positive NSCLC. *The ASCO Post.* [Online] Available: https://ascopost.com/issues/october-10-2023/flaura2-trial-osimertinib-plus-chemotherapy-improves-outcomes-in-advanced-egfr-positive-nsclc/ [Accessed November 3, 2023].

83 Reck M *et al.* (2019). Atezolizumab plus bevacizumab and chemotherapy in non-small-cell lung cancer (IMpower150): Key subgroup analyses of patients with EGFR mutations or baseline liver metastases in a randomised, open-label phase 3 trial. *Lancet Respir. Med.* **7**(5). doi: 10.1016/S2213-2600(19)30084-0.

84 Girard N (2022). New strategies and novel combinations in EGFR TKI-resistant non-small cell lung cancer. *Curr. Treat. Options in Oncol.* **23**(11): 1626–1644. doi: 10.1007/s11864-022-01022-7.

85 Gomatou G, Syrigos N, Kotteas E (2023). Osimertinib resistance: Molecular mechanisms and emerging treatment options. *Cancers (Basel)* **15**(3): 841. doi: 10.3390/cancers15030841.

86 Cho BC *et al.* (2023). LBA14 amivantamab plus lazertinib vs osimertinib as first-line treatment in patients with EGFR-mutated, advanced non-small cell lung cancer (NSCLC): Primary results from MARIPOSA, a phase III, global, randomized, controlled trial. *Ann. Oncol.* **34**: S1306. doi: 10.1016/j.annonc.2023.10.062.

87 Hudis CA (2007). Trastuzumab – mechanism of action and use in clinical practice. *N. Engl. J. Med.* **357**(1). doi: 10.1056/nejmra043186.

88 Kreutzfeldt J *et al.* (2020). The trastuzumab era: Current and upcoming targeted HER2+ breast cancer therapies. *Am. J. Cancer Res.* **10**(4): 1045.

89 Harbeck N *et al.* (2013). HER2 dimerization inhibitor pertuzumab – mode of action and clinical data in breast cancer. *Breast Care* **8**(1). doi: 10.1159/000346837.

90 Richard S *et al.* (2016). Pertuzumab and trastuzumab: The rationale way to synergy. *An. Acad. Bras. Cienc.* **88**. doi: 10.1590/0001-3765201620150178.

91 Verma S *et al.* (2012). Trastuzumab emtansine for HER2-positive advanced breast cancer.

N. Engl. J. Med. **367**(19). doi: 10.1056/nejmoa 1209124.

92 Indini A, Rijavec E, Grossi F (2021). Trastuzumab deruxtecan: Changing the destiny of her2 expressing solid tumors. *Int. J. Mol. Sci.* **22**(9). doi: 10.3390/ijms22094774.

93 Díaz-Rodríguez E *et al.* (2021). Novel ADCs and strategies to overcome resistance to anti-HER2 ADCs. *Cancers (Basel)* **14**(1): 154. doi: 10.3390/cancers14010154.

94 Luque-Cabal M *et al.* (2016). Mechanisms behind the resistance to trastuzumab in HER2-amplified breast cancer and strategies to overcome It. *Clin. Med. Insights Oncol.* **10**. doi: 10.4137/CMO.S34537.

95 Slamon DJ *et al.* (1987). Human breast cancer: Correlation of relapse and survival with amplification of the HER-2/neu oncogene. *Science 1979* **235**(4785). doi: 10.1126/science. 3798106.

96 Gómez HL *et al.* (2010). Prognostic effect of hormone receptor status in early HER2 positive breast cancer patients. *Hematol. Oncol. Stem Cell Ther.* **3**(3). doi: 10.5144/1658-3876. 2010.109.

97 Grillo F *et al.* (2016). HER2 heterogeneity in gastric/gastroesophageal cancers: From benchside to practice. *World J. Gastroenterol.* **22**(26): 5879. doi: 10.3748/wjg.v22.i26.5879.

98 Modi S *et al.* (2022). Trastuzumab deruxtecan in previously treated HER2-low advanced breast cancer. *N. Engl. J. Med.* **387**(1): 9–20. doi: 10.1056/NEJMoa2203690.

99 FDA (2022). FDA approves fam-trastuzumab deruxtecan-nxki for HER2-low breast cancer. [Online] Available: https://www.fda.gov/drugs/resources-information-approved-drugs/fda-approves-fam-trastuzumab-deruxtecan-nxki-her2-low-breast-cancer [Accessed October 17, 2023].

100 Gampenrieder SP *et al.* (2021). Landscape of HER2-low metastatic breast cancer (MBC): Results from the Austrian AGMT_MBC-Registry. *Breast Cancer Res.* **23**(1): 112. doi: 10.1186/s13058-021-01492-x.

101 Uzunparmak B *et al.* (2023). HER2-low expression in patients with advanced or metastatic solid tumors. *Ann. Oncol.* doi: 10.1016/j. annonc.2023.08.005.

102 Jaber N Enhertu marks first targeted therapy for HER2-mutant lung cancer. *National Cancer Institute.* [Online] Available: https://www. cancer.gov/news-events/cancer-currents-blog/2022/fda-lung-cancer-enhertu-her2#:~:text=On%20August%2011%2C%20 the%20Food,this%20kind%20of%20HER2%20 mutation [Accessed August 18, 2023].

103 Gu G, Dustin D, Fuqua SA (2016). Targeted therapy for breast cancer and molecular mechanisms of resistance to treatment. *Curr. Opin. Pharmacol.* **31**. doi: 10.1016/j.coph.2016.11.005.

104 Pieńkowski T, Zielinski CC (2009). Trastuzumab treatment in patients with breast cancer and metastatic CNS disease. *Ann. Oncol.* **21**(5). doi: 10.1093/annonc/mdp353.

105 Shmueli E, Wigler N, Inbar M (2004). Central nervous system progression among patients with metastatic breast cancer responding to trastuzumab treatment. *Eur. J. Cancer* **40**(3). doi: 10.1016/j.ejca.2003.09.018.

106 Rimawi MF, de Angelis C, Schiff R (2015). Resistance to anti-HER2 therapies in breast cancer. *Am. Soc. Clin. Oncol. Educ. Book* **35**. doi: 10.14694/edbook_am.2015.35.e157.

107 Son J *et al.* (2022). A novel HER2-selective kinase inhibitor is effective in HER2 mutant and amplified non-small cell lung cancer. *Cancer Res.,* p. canres.2693.2021. doi: 10.1158/0008-5472.CAN-21-2693.

108 Schlam I, Swain SM (2021). HER2-positive breast cancer and tyrosine kinase inhibitors: The time is now. *npj Breast Cancer* **7**(1). doi: 10.1038/s41523-021-00265-1.

109 Segovia-Mendoza M *et al.* (2015). Efficacy and mechanism of action of the tyrosine kinase inhibitors gefitinib, lapatinib and neratinib in the treatment of her2-positive breast cancer: Preclinical and clinical evidence. *Am. J. Cancer Res.* **5**(9).

110 Simmons C *et al.* (2022). Current and future landscape of targeted therapy in HER2-positive advanced breast cancer: Redrawing the lines. *Ther. Adv. Med. Oncol.* **14**: 175883592110666. doi: 10.1177/17588359211066677.

111 Jacobson A (2022). Trastuzumab deruxtecan improves progression-free survival and intracranial response in patients with HER2-positive metastatic breast cancer and brain metastases.

Oncologist **27**(Supplement_1): S3–S4. doi: 10.1093/oncolo/oyac009.

112 Goto K *et al*. (2023). Trastuzumab deruxtecan in patients with *HER2*-mutant metastatic non–small-cell lung cancer: Primary results from the randomized, phase II DESTINY-Lung02 trial. *J. Clin. Oncol.* **41**(31): 4852–4863. doi: 10.1200/JCO.23.01361.

113 Song Z *et al*. (2022). Efficacy and safety of pyrotinib in advanced lung adenocarcinoma with HER2 mutations: A multicenter, single-arm, phase II trial. *BMC Med.* **20**(1): 42. doi: 10.1186/s12916-022-02245-z.

114 Le X *et al*. (2022). Poziotinib in non–small-cell lung cancer harboring *HER2* exon 20 insertion mutations after prior therapies: ZENITH20-2 trial. *J. Clin. Oncol.* **40**(7): 710–718. doi: 10.1200/JCO.21.01323.

115 Wu HX, Zhuo KQ, Wang K (2021). Efficacy of targeted therapy in patients with HER2-positive non-small cell lung cancer: A systematic review and meta-analysis. *Br. J. Clin. Pharmacol.* doi: 10.1111/bcp.15155.

116 Guérit E *et al*. (2021). PDGF receptor mutations in human diseases. *Cell. Mol. Life Sci.* **78**(8). doi: 10.1007/s00018-020-03753-y.

117 Doma V *et al*. (2020). KIT mutation incidence and pattern of melanoma in central europe. *Pathol. Oncol. Res.* **26**(1). doi: 10.1007/s12253-019-00788-w.

118 Helsten T, Schwaederle M, Kurzrock R (2015). Fibroblast growth factor receptor signaling in hereditary and neoplastic disease: Biologic and clinical implications. *Cancer Metastasis Rev.* **34**(3). doi: 10.1007/s10555-015-9579-8.

119 Lengyel CG *et al*. (2022). FGFR pathway inhibition in gastric cancer: The golden era of an old target? *Life* **12**(1): 81. doi: 10.3390/life12010081.

120 Wang Q *et al*. (2019). MET inhibitors for targeted therapy of EGFR TKI-resistant lung cancer. *J. Hematol. Oncol.* **12**(1). doi: 10.1186/s13045-019-0759-9.

121 Thein KZ *et al*. (2021). Precision therapy for RET-altered cancers with RET inhibitors. *Trends Cancer* **7**(12). doi: 10.1016/j.trecan.2021.07.003.

122 Lin JJ, Riely GJ, Shaw AT (2017). Targeting ALK: Precision medicine takes on drug resistance. *Cancer Discov.* **7**(2). doi: 10.1158/2159-8290.CD-16-1123.

123 Takita J (2017). The role of anaplastic lymphoma kinase in pediatric cancers. *Cancer Sci.* **108**(10). doi: 10.1111/cas.13333.

124 Azelby CM, Sakamoto MR, Bowles DW (2021). ROS1 targeted therapies: Current status. *Curr. Oncol. Rep.* **23**(8). doi: 10.1007/S11912-021-01078-Y.

125 Cocco E, Scaltriti M, Drilon A (2018). NTRK fusion-positive cancers and TRK inhibitor therapy. *Nat. Rev. Clin. Oncol.* **15**(12). doi: 10.1038/s41571-018-0113-0.

126 Mishra R *et al*. (2018). HER3 signaling and targeted therapy in cancer. *Oncol. Rev.* **12**(1). doi: 10.4081/oncol.2018.355.

127 Cancer Research UK (2021). Gastrointestinal stromal tumour (GIST). *Cancer Research UK.* [Online] Available: https://www.cancerresearchuk.org/about-cancer/soft-tissue-sarcoma/types/gastrointestinal-stromal-tumour [Accessed March 22, 2022].

128 Bauer S, Joensuu H (2015). Emerging agents for the treatment of advanced, imatinib-resistant gastrointestinal stromal tumors: Current status and future directions. *Drugs* **75**(12). doi: 10.1007/s40265-015-0440-8.

129 Kelly CM, Gutierrez Sainz L, Chi P (2021). The management of metastatic GIST: Current standard and investigational therapeutics. *J. Hematol. Oncol.* **14**(1). doi: 10.1186/s13045-020-01026-6.

130 Italiano A KIT in gastrointestinal stromal tumor (GIST): ESMO biomarker factsheet. *ESMO Oncology Pro.* [Online] Available: https://oncologypro.esmo.org/education-library/factsheets-on-biomarkers/kit-in-gastrointestinal-stromal-tumours-gist [Accessed March 22, 2022].

131 Italiano A (2018). PDGFRA in gastrointestinal stromal tumor (GIST): ESMO biomarker factsheet. *ESMO Oncology Pro.* [Online] Available: https://oncologypro.esmo.org/education-library/factsheets-on-biomarkers/pdgfra-in-gastrointestinal-stromal-tumours-gist [Accessed March 22, 2022].

132 Call J *et al*. (2012). Survival of gastrointestinal stromal tumor patients in the imatinib era: Life

raft group observational registry. *BMC Cancer* **12**. doi: 10.1186/1471-2407-12-90.

133 Katagiri S *et al*. (2022). Mutated KIT tyrosine kinase as a novel molecular target in acute myeloid leukemia. *Int. J. Mol. Sci.* **23**(9): 4694. doi: 10.3390/ijms23094694.

134 Gu W *et al*. (2021). Comprehensive identification of FGFR1-4 alterations in 5 557 Chinese patients with solid tumors by next-generation sequencing. *Am. J. Cancer Res.* **11**(8): 3893.

135 Lee AJX, Waterhouse JV, Linch M. Changing paradigms in the treatment of advanced urothelial carcinoma: A 2020 update. *EMJ Oncol.* **2020**. doi: 10.33590/emj/20-00044.

136 Wainberg ZA *et al*. (2022). Bemarituzumab in patients with FGFR2b-selected gastric or gastro-oesophageal junction adenocarcinoma (FIGHT): A randomised, double-blind, placebo-controlled, phase 2 study. *Lancet Oncol.* **23**(11): 1430–1440. doi: 10.1016/S1470-2045(22)00603-9.

137 Garcia-Robledo JE *et al*. (2022). KRAS and MET in non-small-cell lung cancer: Two of the new kids on the 'drivers' block. *Ther. Adv. Respir. Dis.* **16**: 175346662110660. doi: 10.1177/17534666211066064.

138 Awad MM *et al*. (2020). Characterization of 1,387 NSCLCs with MET exon 14 (METex14) skipping alterations (SA) and potential acquired resistance (AR) mechanisms. *J. Clin. Oncol.* **38**(15_suppl): 9511–9511. doi: 10.1200/JCO.2020.38.15_suppl.9511.

139 Prescott JD, Zeiger MA (2015). The RET oncogene in papillary thyroid carcinoma. *Cancer* **121**(13). doi: 10.1002/cncr.29044.

140 Hadoux J *et al*. (2023). Phase 3 trial of selpercatinib in advanced *RET* -mutant medullary thyroid cancer. *N. Engl. J. Med.* doi: 10.1056/NEJMoa2309719.

141 Mudad R (2023). Selective RET inhibitors for RET fusion-positive non-small cell lung cancer. *Cancer Therapy Advisor*. [Online] Available: https://www.cancertherapyadvisor.com/clinicianpov/ret-inhibitors-selpercatinib-pralsetinib-non-small-cell-lung-cancer/ [Accessed November 2, 2023].

142 Ye M *et al*. (2016). ALK and ROS1 as targeted therapy paradigms and clinical implications to overcome crizotinib resistance. *Oncotarget* **7**(11). doi: 10.18632/oncotarget.6935.

143 Soda M *et al*. (2007). Identification of the transforming EML4-ALK fusion gene in non-small-cell lung cancer. *Nature* **448**(7153). doi: 10.1038/nature05945.

144 Yan D *et al*. (2022). Analysis of *ROS1* fusions in nonlung solid tumors. *J. Clin. Oncol.* **40, no. 16_suppl**: e15124–e15124. doi: 10.1200/JCO.2022.40.16_suppl.e15124.

145 Solomon BJ *et al*. (2014). First-line crizotinib versus chemotherapy in ALK -positive lung cancer. *N. Engl. J. Med.* **371**(23). doi: 10.1056/nejmoa1408440.

146 Dagogo-Jack I, Shaw AT, Riely GJ (2017). Optimizing treatment for patients with anaplastic lymphoma kinase-positive lung cancer. *Clin. Pharmacol. Ther.* **101**(5). doi: 10.1002/cpt.653.

147 Wu J, Savooji J, Liu D (2016). Second- and third-generation ALK inhibitors for non-small cell lung cancer. *J. Hematol. Oncol.* **9**(1). doi: 10.1186/s13045-016-0251-8.

148 Camidge DR, Doebele RC (2012). Treating ALK-positive lung cancer-early successes and future challenges. *Nat. Rev. Clin. Oncol.* **9**(5). doi: 10.1038/nrclinonc.2012.43.

149 Fukui T *et al*. (2022). Review of therapeutic strategies for anaplastic lymphoma kinase-rearranged non-small cell lung cancer. *Cancers (Basel)* **14**(5): 1184. doi: 10.3390/cancers14051184.

150 Shaw AT *et al*. (2019). Crizotinib in ROS1-rearranged advanced non-small-cell lung cancer (NSCLC): Updated results, including overall survival, from PROFILE 1001. *Ann. Oncol.* **30**(7): 1121–1126. doi: 10.1093/annonc/mdz131.

151 Kheder ES, Hong DS (2018). Emerging targeted therapy for tumors with NTRK fusion proteins. *Clin. Cancer Res.* **24**(23). doi: 10.1158/1078-0432.CCR-18-1156.

152 Drilon A (2019). TRK inhibitors in TRK fusion-positive cancers. *Ann. Oncol.* **30**. doi: 10.1093/annonc/mdz282.

153 Laskin J *et al*. (2020). NRG1 fusion-driven tumors: Biology, detection, and the therapeutic role of afatinib and other ErbB-targeting

agents. *Ann. Oncol.* **31**(12). doi: 10.1016/j.annonc. 2020.08.2335.

154 Perrone S *et al.* (2023). How acute myeloid leukemia (AML) escapes from FMS-related tyrosine kinase 3 (FLT3) inhibitors? Still an overrated complication? *Cancer Drug Resistance* **6**(2): 223–238. doi: 10.20517/cdr.2022.130.

155 Fedorov K, Maiti A, Konopleva M (2023). Targeting FLT3 mutation in acute myeloid leukemia: Current strategies and future directions. *Cancers (Basel)* **15**(8): 2312. doi: 10.3390/cancers15082312.

156 Degirmenci U, Wang M, Hu J (2020). Targeting aberrant RAS/RAF/MEK/ERK signaling for cancer therapy. *Cells* **9**(1). doi: 10.3390/cells9010198.

157 Roskoski R (2012). ERK1/2 MAP kinases: Structure, function, and regulation. *Pharmacol. Res.* **66**(2). doi: 10.1016/j.phrs.2012.04.005.

158 Bahrami S, Drabløs F (2016). Gene regulation in the immediate-early response process. *Adv. Biol. Regul.* **62**. doi: 10.1016/j.jbior.2016.05.001.

159 Yang SH, Sharrocks AD, Whitmarsh AJ (2013). MAP kinase signalling cascades and transcriptional regulation. *Gene* **513**(1). doi: 10.1016/j.gene.2012.10.033.

160 Santarpia L, Lippman SM, El-Naggar AK (2012). Targeting the MAPK–RAS–RAF signaling pathway in cancer therapy. *Expert Opin. Ther. Targets* **16**(1): 103–119. doi: 10.1517/14728222.2011.645805.

161 Prior IA, Hood FE, Hartley JL (2020). The frequency of ras mutations in cancer. *Cancer Res.* **80**(14). doi: 10.1158/0008-5472.CAN-19-3682.

162 Philpott C *et al.* (2017). The NF1 somatic mutational landscape in sporadic human cancers. *Hum. Genet.* **11**(1). doi: 10.1186/s40246-017-0109-3.

163 Halle BR, Johnson DB (2021). Defining and targeting BRAF mutations in solid tumors. *Curr. Treat. Options in Oncol.* **22**(4). doi: 10.1007/s11864-021-00827-2.

164 Désage A-L *et al.* (2022). Targeting KRAS mutant in non-small cell lung cancer: Novel insights into therapeutic strategies. *Front. Oncol.* **12**. doi: 10.3389/fonc.2022.796832.

165 Cheng Y, Tian H (2017). Current development status of MEK inhibitors. *Molecules* **22**(10). doi: 10.3390/molecules22101551.

166 Chin HM, Lai DK, Falchook GS (2019). Extracellular signal-regulated kinase (Erk) inhibitors in oncology clinical trials. *J. Immunother. Precis. Oncol.* **2**(1). doi: 10.4103/JIPO.JIPO_17_18.

167 Samatar AA, Poulikakos PI (2014). Targeting RAS-ERK signalling in cancer: Promises and challenges. *Nat. Rev. Drug Discov.* **13**(12). doi: 10.1038/nrd4281.

168 Moore AR *et al.* (2020). RAS-targeted therapies: Is the undruggable drugged? *Nat. Rev. Drug Discov.* **19**(8). doi: 10.1038/s41573-020-0068-6.

169 Cox AD *et al.* (2014). Drugging the undruggable RAS: Mission possible? *Nat. Rev. Drug Discov.* **13**(11). doi: 10.1038/nrd4389.

170 Moore AR, Malek S (2021). The promise and peril of KRAS G12C inhibitors. *Cancer Cell* **39**(8): 1059–1061. doi: 10.1016/j.ccell.2021.07.011.

171 Coleman N *et al.* (2023). *HRAS* mutations define a distinct subgroup in head and neck squamous cell carcinoma. *JCO Precis. Oncol.* **7**. doi: 10.1200/PO.22.00211.

172 Pantsar T (2020). The current understanding of KRAS protein structure and dynamics. *Comput. Struct. Biotechnol. J.* **18**. doi: 10.1016/j.csbj.2019.12.004.

173 O'Sullivan É *et al.* (2023). Treatment strategies for KRAS-mutated non-small-cell lung cancer. *Cancers (Basel)* **15**(6): 1635. doi: 10.3390/cancers15061635. PMID: 36980522; PMCID: PMC10046549.

174 Swanton C, Govindan R (2016). Clinical implications of genomic discoveries in lung cancer. *N. Engl. J. Med.* **374**(19). doi: 10.1056/nejmra1504688.

175 Jamal-Hanjani M *et al.* (2015). Translational implications of tumor heterogeneity. *Clin. Cancer Res.* **21**(6). doi: 10.1158/1078-0432.CCR-14-1429.

176 Jamal-Hanjani M *et al.* (2017). Tracking the evolution of non–small-cell lung cancer. *N. Engl. J. Med.* **376**(22): 2109–2121. doi: 10.1056/NEJMoa1616288.

177 Gyawali B The codebreak trial: We broke the code in more ways than one. *Medscape.* [Online] Available: https://www.medscape.com/viewarticle/991083 [Accessed May 3, 2023].

178 de Langen AJ *et al.* (2023). Sotorasib versus docetaxel for previously treated non-small-cell lung cancer with KRASG12C mutation: A randomised, open-label, phase 3 trial. *Lancet* **401**(10378): 733–746. doi: 10.1016/S0140-6736(23)00221-0.

179 Salem M *et al.* (2021). Characterization of KRAS mutation variants and prevalence of KRAS-G12C in gastrointestinal malignancies. *Ann. Oncol.* **32**. doi: 10.1016/j.annonc.2021.05.007.

180 Personeni N *et al.* (2021). Tackling refractory metastatic colorectal cancer: Future perspectives. *Cancers* **13**(18). doi: 10.3390/cancers13184506.

181 Fakih MG *et al.* (2023). Sotorasib plus panitumumab in refractory colorectal cancer with mutated *KRAS* G12C. *N. Engl. J. Med.* doi: 10.1056/NEJMoa2308795.

182 Kim D *et al.* (2023). Pan-KRAS inhibitor disables oncogenic signalling and tumour growth. *Nature* **619**(7968): 160–166. doi: 10.1038/s41586-023-06123-3.

183 Lee HW *et al.* (2020). A phase II trial of tipifarnib for patients with previously treated, metastatic urothelial carcinoma harboring *HRAS* mutations. *Clin. Cancer Res.* **26**(19): 5113–5119. doi: 10.1158/1078-0432.CCR-20-1246.

184 Chen K *et al.* (2021). Emerging strategies to target RAS signaling in human cancer therapy. *J. Hematol. Oncol.* **14**(1). doi: 10.1186/s13045-021-01127-w.

185 Rustad EH *et al.* (2015). BRAF V600E mutation in early-stage multiple myeloma: Good response to broad acting drugs and no relation to prognosis. *Blood Cancer J.* **5**(3). doi: 10.1038/bcj.2015.24.

186 Ahmadzadeh A *et al.* (2014). BRAF mutation in hairy cell leukemia. *Oncol. Rev.* **8**(2). doi: 10.4081/oncol.2014.253.

187 Tate JG *et al.* (2019). COSMIC: The catalogue of somatic mutations in cancer. *Nucleic Acids Res.* **47**(D1). doi: 10.1093/nar/gky1015.

188 Holderfield M, Nagel TE, Stuart DD (2014). Mechanism and consequences of RAF kinase activation by small-molecule inhibitors. *Br. J. Cancer* **111**(4). doi: 10.1038/bjc.2014.139.

189 Degirmenci U *et al.* (2021). Drug resistance in targeted cancer therapies with RAF inhibitors.

190 Ferrari SM *et al.* (2020). Novel treatments for anaplastic thyroid carcinoma. *Gland Surg.* **9**. doi: 10.21037/gs.2019.10.18.

191 Corcoran RB *et al.* (2012). EGFR-mediated reactivation of MAPK signaling contributes to insensitivity of *BRAF* -mutant colorectal cancers to RAF inhibition with vemurafenib. *Cancer Discov.* **2**(3): 227–235. doi: 10.1158/2159-8290.CD-11-0341.

192 Pham DDM, Guhan S, Tsao H (2020). KIT and melanoma: Biological insights and clinical implications. *Yonsei Med. J.* **61**(7): 562. doi: 10.3349/ymj.2020.61.7.562.

193 Kopetz S *et al.* (2019). Encorafenib, binimetinib, and cetuximab in *BRAF* V600E–mutated colorectal cancer. *N. Engl. J. Med.* **381**(17): 1632–1643. doi: 10.1056/NEJMoa1908075.

194 Planchard D *et al.* (2022). Phase 2 study of dabrafenib plus trametinib in patients with BRAF V600E-mutant metastatic NSCLC: Updated 5-year survival rates and genomic analysis. *J. Thorac. Oncol.* **17**(1): 103–115. doi: 10.1016/j.jtho.2021.08.011.

195 Blay JY *et al.* (2023). Long term activity of vemurafenib in cancers with BRAF mutations: The ACSE basket study for advanced cancers other than BRAFV600-mutated melanoma. *ESMO Open* **8**(6): 102038. doi: 10.1016/j.esmoop.2023.102038.

196 Subbiah V *et al.* (2022). Dabrafenib plus trametinib in patients with BRAF V600E-mutant anaplastic thyroid cancer: Updated analysis from the phase II ROAR basket study. *Ann. Oncol.* **33**(4): 406–415. doi: 10.1016/j.annonc.2021.12.014.

197 Grimaldi AM *et al.* (2017). Combined BRAF and MEK inhibition with vemurafenib and cobimetinib for patients with advanced melanoma. *Eur. Oncol. Haematol.* **13**(1). doi: 10.17925/eoh.2017.13.01.1a.

198 Kakadia S *et al.* (2018). Mechanisms of resistance to BRAF and MEK inhibitors and clinical update of us food and drug administration-approved targeted therapy in advanced melanoma. *Onco. Targets Ther.* **11**. doi: 10.2147/OTT.S182721.

199 Trojaniello C, Luke JJ, Ascierto PA (2021). Therapeutic advancements across clinical

Cancer Drug Resistance **4**(3). doi: 10.20517/cdr.2021.36.

stages in melanoma, with a focus on targeted immunotherapy. *Front. Oncol.* **11**. doi: 10.3389/fonc.2021.670726.

200 Zhao Y, Adjei AA (2014). The clinical development of MEK inhibitors. *Nat. Rev. Clin. Oncol.* **11**(7). doi: 10.1038/nrclinonc.2014.83.

201 Jänne PA *et al.* (2017). Selumetinib plus docetaxel compared with docetaxel alone and progression-free survival in patients with *KRAS* -mutant advanced non–small cell lung cancer. *JAMA* **317**(18): 1844. doi: 10.1001/jama.2017.3438.

202 Gershenson DM *et al.* (2022). Trametinib versus standard of care in patients with recurrent low-grade serous ovarian cancer (GOG 281/LOGS): An international, randomised, open-label, multicentre, phase 2/3 trial. *Lancet* **399** (10324): 541–553. doi: 10.1016/S0140-6736(21)02175-9.

203 Diamond EL *et al.* (2019). Efficacy of MEK inhibition in patients with histiocytic neoplasms. *Nature* **567**(7749): 521–524. doi: 10.1038/s41586-019-1012-y.

204 Saxton RA, Sabatini DM (2017). mTOR signaling in growth, metabolism, and disease. *Cell* **168**(6). doi: 10.1016/j.cell.2017.02.004.

205 Zou Z *et al.* (2020). MTOR signaling pathway and mTOR inhibitors in cancer: Progress and challenges. *Cell Biosci.* **10**(1). doi: 10.1186/s13578-020-00396-1.

206 Fruman DA, Rommel C (2014). PI3K and cancer: Lessons, challenges and opportunities. *Nat. Rev. Drug Discov.* **13**(2). doi: 10.1038/nrd4204.

207 Hemmings BA, Restuccia DF (2012). PI3K-PKB/Akt pathway. *Cold Spring Harb. Perspect. Biol.* **4**(9). doi: 10.1101/cshperspect.a011189.

208 Hosking R (2012). mTOR: The master regulator. *Cell* **149**(5). doi: 10.1016/j.cell.2012.05.011.

209 Mossmann D, Park S, Hall MN (2018). mTOR signalling and cellular metabolism are mutual determinants in cancer. *Nat. Rev. Cancer* **18**(12). doi: 10.1038/s41568-018-0074-8.

210 Zoncu R, Efeyan A, Sabatini DM (2011). MTOR: From growth signal integration to cancer, diabetes and ageing. *Nat. Rev. Mol. Cell Biol.* **12**(1). doi: 10.1038/nrm3025.

211 Fruman DA *et al.* (2017). The PI3K pathway in human disease. *Cell* **170**(4). doi: 10.1016/j.cell.2017.07.029.

212 Yang J *et al.* (2019). Targeting PI3K in cancer: Mechanisms and advances in clinical trials. *Mol. Cancer* **18**(1). doi: 10.1186/s12943-019-0954-x.

213 Millis SZ *et al.* (2016). Landscape of phosphatidylinositol-3-kinase pathway alterations across 19 784 diverse solid tumors. *JAMA Oncol.* **2**(12). doi: 10.1001/jamaoncol.2016.0891.

214 Yin Y, Shen WH (2008). PTEN: A new guardian of the genome. *Oncogene* **27**(41). doi: 10.1038/onc.2008.241.

215 Mundi PS *et al.* (2016). AKT in cancer: New molecular insights and advances in drug development. *Br. J. Clin. Pharmacol.* doi: 10.1111/bcp.13021.

216 Gill RK *et al.* (2011). Frequent homozygous deletion of the LKB1/STK11 gene in non-small cell lung cancer. *Oncogene* **30**(35). doi: 10.1038/onc.2011.98.

217 Dwyer CJ *et al.* (2020). Ex vivo blockade of PI3K gamma or delta signaling enhances the antitumor potency of adoptively transferred CD8+ T cells. *Eur. J. Immunol.* **50**(9): 1386–1399. doi: 10.1002/EJI.201948455.

218 Zhong L *et al.* (2021). Small molecules in targeted cancer therapy: Advances, challenges, and future perspectives. *Signal Transduction Targeted Ther.* **6**(1). doi: 10.1038/s41392-021-00572-w.

219 Vanhaesebroeck B *et al.* (2021). PI3K inhibitors are finally coming of age. *Nat. Rev. Drug Discov.* **20**(10). doi: 10.1038/s41573-021-00209-1.

220 Chang DY, Ma WL, Lu YS (2021). Role of alpelisib in the treatment of pik3ca-mutated breast cancer: Patient selection and clinical perspectives. *Ther. Clin. Risk Manag.* **17**. doi: 10.2147/TCRM.S251668.

221 Thorpe LM, Yuzugullu H, Zhao JJ (2015). PI3K in cancer: Divergent roles of isoforms, modes of activation and therapeutic targeting. *Nat. Rev. Cancer* **15**(1). doi: 10.1038/nrc3860.

222 Yap TA *et al.* (2015). Drugging PI3K in cancer: Refining targets and therapeutic strategies. *Curr. Opin. Pharmacol.* **23**. doi: 10.1016/j.coph.2015.05.016.

223 Castel P *et al.* (2021). The present and future of PI3K inhibitors for cancer therapy. *Nat. Can.* **2**(6). doi: 10.1038/s43018-021-00218-4.

224 Glaviano A *et al.* (2023). PI3K/AKT/mTOR signaling transduction pathway and targeted

therapies in cancer. *Mol. Cancer* **22**(1): 138. doi: 10.1186/s12943-023-01827-6.

225 Keraite I *et al.* (2020). PIK3CA mutation enrichment and quantitation from blood and tissue. *Sci. Rep.* **10**(1). doi: 10.1038/s41598-020-74086-w.

226 Fusco N *et al.* (2021). PIK3CA mutations as a molecular target for hormone receptor-positive, HER2-negative metastatic breast cancer. *Front. Oncol.* **11**. doi: 10.3389/fonc.2021.644737.

227 Martínez-Saéz O *et al.* (2020). Frequency and spectrum of PIK3CA somatic mutations in breast cancer. *Breast Cancer Res.* **22**(1). doi: 10.1186/s13058-020-01284-9.

228 Bou Zeid N, Yazbeck V (2023). PI3k inhibitors in NHL and CLL: An unfulfilled promise. *Blood Lymphat Cancer* **13**: 1–12. doi: 10.2147/BLCTT.S309171.

229 Tarantelli C *et al.* (2020). Is there a role for dual PI3K/mTOR inhibitors for patients affected with lymphoma? *Int. J. Mol. Sci.* **21**(3): 1060. doi: 10.3390/ijms21031060.

230 Nitulescu GM *et al.* (2016). Akt inhibitors in cancer treatment: The long journey from drug discovery to clinical use (review). *Int. J. Oncol.* **48**(3). doi: 10.3892/ijo.2015.3306.

231 Coleman N *et al.* (2021). Clinical development of AKT inhibitors and associated predictive biomarkers to guide patient treatment in cancer medicine. *Curr. Pharmacogenomics Pers. Med.* **14**. doi: 10.2147/PGPM.S305068.

232 Turner NC *et al.* (2023). Capivasertib in hormone receptor–positive advanced breast cancer. *N. Engl. J. Med.* **388**(22): 2058–2070. doi: 10.1056/NEJMoa2214131.

233 AstraZeneca (2023). Truqap (capivasertib) plus Faslodex approved in the US for patients with advanced HR-positive breast cancer. *AstraZeneca*. [Online] Available: https://www.astrazeneca.com/media-centre/press-releases/2023/truqap-approved-in-us-for-hr-plus-breast-cancer.html [Accessed December 12, 2023].

234 Sweeney C *et al.* (2021). Ipatasertib plus abiraterone and prednisolone in metastatic castration-resistant prostate cancer (IPATential150): A multicentre, randomised, double-blind, phase 3 trial. *Lancet* **398**(10295). doi: 10.1016/S0140-6736(21)00580-8.

235 Martorana F *et al.* (2021). AKT inhibitors: New weapons in the fight against breast cancer?

Front. Pharmacol. **12**. doi: 10.3389/fphar.2021.662232.

236 Garber K (2001). Rapamycin's resurrection: A new way to target the cancer cell cycle. *J. Natl. Cancer Inst.* **93**(20). doi: 10.1093/jnci/93.20.1517.

237 Yuan R *et al.* (2009). Targeting tumorigenesis: Development and use of mTOR inhibitors in cancer therapy. *J. Hematol. Oncol.* **2**. doi: 10.1186/1756-8722-2-45.

238 Teng QX *et al.* (2019). Revisiting mTOR inhibitors as anticancer agents. *Drug Discov. Today* **24**(10). doi: 10.1016/j.drudis.2019.05.030.

239 Rawlings JS, Rosler KM, Harrison DA (2004). The JAK/STAT signaling pathway. *J. Cell Sci.* **117**(8): 1281–1283. doi: 10.1242/jcs.00963.

240 Zhang J-M, An J (2007). Cytokines, inflammation, and pain. *Int. Anesthesiol. Clin.* **45**(2): 27–37. doi: 10.1097/AIA.0b013e318034194e.

241 Vainchenker W, Constantinescu SN (2013). JAK/STAT signaling in hematological malignancies. *Oncogene* **32**(21): 2601–2613. doi: 10.1038/onc.2012.347.

242 Tefferi A (2016). Myeloproliferative neoplasms: A decade of discoveries and treatment advances. *Am. J. Hematol.* **91**(1): 50–58. doi: 10.1002/ajh.24221.

243 Green MR *et al.* (2010). Integrative analysis reveals selective 9p24.1 amplification, increased PD-1 ligand expression, and further induction via JAK2 in nodular sclerosing Hodgkin lymphoma and primary mediastinal large B-cell lymphoma. *Blood* **116**(17): 3268–3277. doi: 10.1182/blood-2010-05-282780.

244 Thomas SJ *et al.* (2015). The role of JAK/STAT signalling in the pathogenesis, prognosis and treatment of solid tumours. *Br. J. Cancer* **113**(3): 365–371. doi: 10.1038/bjc.2015.233.

245 Hu X *et al.* (2021). The JAK/STAT signaling pathway: From bench to clinic. *Signal Transduction Targeted Ther.* **6**(1): 402. doi: 10.1038/s41392-021-00791-1.

246 Philips RL *et al.* (2022). The JAK-STAT pathway at 30: Much learned, much more to do. *Cell* **185**(21): 3857–3876. doi: 10.1016/j.cell.2022.09.023.

247 Buchert M, Burns CJ, Ernst M (2016). Targeting JAK kinase in solid tumors: Emerging opportunities and challenges. *Oncogene* **35**(8): 939–951. doi: 10.1038/onc.2015.150.

248 Mascarenhas J (2022). Pacritinib for the treatment of patients with myelofibrosis and thrombocytopenia. *Expert Rev. Hematol.* **15**(8): 671–684. doi: 10.1080/17474086.2022.2112565.

249 Qureshy Z, Johnson DE, Grandis JR (2020). Targeting the JAK/STAT pathway in solid tumors. *J. Cancer Metastasis Treat.* **6**.

250 Quintás-Cardama A, Cortes J (2009). Molecular biology of bcr-abl1-positive chronic myeloid leukemia. *Blood* **113**(8). doi: 10.1182/blood-2008-03-144790.

251 Quintás-Cardama A, Cortes JE (2006). Chronic myeloid leukemia: Diagnosis and treatment. *Mayo Clin. Proc.* doi: 10.4065/81.7.973.

252 Bower H *et al.* (2016). Life expectancy of patients with chronic myeloid leukemia approaches the life expectancy of the general population. *J. Clin. Oncol.* **34**(24): 2851–2857. doi: 10.1200/JCO.2015.66.2866.

253 Gambacorti-Passerini C *et al.* (2011). Multicenter independent assessment of outcomes in chronic myeloid leukemia patients treated with imatinib. *JNCI J. Natl. Cancer Inst.* **103**(7): 553–561. doi: 10.1093/jnci/djr060.

254 Abou Dalle I *et al.* (2019). Treatment of philadelphia chromosome-positive acute lymphoblastic leukemia. *Curr. Treat. Options in Oncol.* **20**(1): 4. doi: 10.1007/s11864-019-0603-z.

255 Chiaretti S, Messina M, Foà R (2019). BCR/ABL1 – like acute lymphoblastic leukemia: How to diagnose and treat? *Cancer* **125**(2): 194–204. doi: 10.1002/cncr.31848.

256 Braun TP, Eide CA, Druker BJ (2020). Response and resistance to BCR-ABL1-targeted therapies. *Cancer Cell* **37**(4): 530–542. doi: 10.1016/j.ccell.2020.03.006.

257 Amarante-Mendes GP *et al.* (2022). BCR-ABL1 tyrosine kinase complex signaling transduction: Challenges to overcome resistance in chronic myeloid leukemia. *Pharmaceutics* **14**(1): 215. doi: 10.3390/pharmaceutics14010215.

258 Soverini S *et al.* (2011). BCR-ABL kinase domain mutation analysis in chronic myeloid leukemia patients treated with tyrosine kinase inhibitors: Recommendations from an expert panel on behalf of European LeukemiaNet. *Blood* **118**(5): 1208–1215. doi: 10.1182/blood-2010-12-326405.

259 Soverini S *et al.* (2014). Drug resistance and BCR-ABL kinase domain mutations in Philadelphia chromosome–positive acute lymphoblastic leukemia from the imatinib to the second-generation tyrosine kinase inhibitor era: The main changes are in the type of mutations, but not in the frequency of mutation involvement. *Cancer* **120**(7): 1002–1009. doi: 10.1002/cncr.28522.

260 Kuroda J (2013). Principles and current topics concerning management of tyrosine kinase inhibitor therapy for chronic myelogenous leukemia. *Transl. Med.* **01**(S2). doi: 10.4172/2161-1025.S2-001.

261 Pophali PA, Patnaik MM (2016). The role of new tyrosine kinase inhibitors in chronic myeloid leukemia. *Cancer J.* **22**(1): 40–50. doi: 10.1097/PPO.0000000000000165.

262 Khoury J, Rassi E (2013). Bosutinib: A SRC/ABL tyrosine kinase inhibitor for treatment of chronic myeloid leukemia. *Pharmacogenomics Pers. Med.*: 57. doi: 10.2147/PGPM.S32145.

263 Cortes JE *et al.* (2012). Ponatinib in refractory philadelphia chromosome–positive leukemias. *N. Engl. J. Med.* **367**(22): 2075–2088. doi: 10.1056/NEJMoa1205127.

264 Poudel G *et al.* (2022). Mechanisms of resistance and implications for treatment strategies in chronic myeloid leukaemia. *Cancers (Basel)* **14**(14): 3300. doi: 10.3390/cancers14143300.

265 Réa D, Hughes TP (2022). Development of asciminib, a novel allosteric inhibitor of BCR-ABL1. *Crit. Rev. Oncol. Hematol.* **171**: 103580. doi: 10.1016/j.critrevonc.2022.103580.

266 Qiang W *et al.* (2017). Mechanisms of resistance to the BCR-ABL1 allosteric inhibitor asciminib. *Leukemia* **31**(12): 2844–2847. doi: 10.1038/leu.2017.264.

267 Peiró G *et al.* (2014). Src, a potential target for overcoming trastuzumab resistance in HER2-positive breast carcinoma. *Br. J. Cancer* **111**(4). doi: 10.1038/bjc.2014.327.

CHAPTER 4

More Targets and Treatments

In Chapter 3, all the drugs I mentioned fitted neatly together under one heading as they all targeted the same process, namely cell communication. In this chapter, however, I cover a range of treatments that target diverse cell processes and proteins.

First, I'm going to walk you through a group of treatments that target angiogenesis – the process through which new blood vessels are formed. Numerous angiogenesis inhibitors have been put through trials, both monoclonal antibodies and kinase inhibitors. Often, the results of these trials weren't as positive as people had hoped. However, the benefits of angiogenesis inhibitors for people with kidney cancer are very clear. There are also lots of ideas as to how these treatments might be improved or used in combinations to boost the effects of other treatments.

Antibody-drug conjugates (ADCs) are the next set of treatments I look at. I pondered long and hard over where in this book to include this group of treatments. They are defined not by what they target, but by their physical makeup: the combination of an antibody, a linker, and a drug. Thus, they don't fit easily into a chapter where every other treatment is defined by what it targets. However, I wanted to include them near the beginning of this chapter, partly because they don't easily fit anywhere (so why not here?), and partly because they are (in the Spring of 2024 as I write this) what the cancer research community is buzzing about. It might be that we have reached peak optimism regarding ADCs, or maybe we're only at the beginning of this journey. Only time will tell.

Next, we'll look at PARP inhibitors. PARP is neither on the cell surface, nor is it a kinase. So, for the first time in this book, we'll be looking at a group of treatments that aren't antibodies or kinase inhibitors. Instead, they're small molecules that block proteins called PARP enzymes. PARP inhibitors are particularly effective against ovarian cancers that contain defects in *BRCA* genes (or some other genes) and that cannot perform a DNA repair process called homologous recombination. We've learned that these treatments are also useful against other cancers that occur in people with mutated *BRCA* genes, and they're being explored as treatments for a range of other cancer types.

After PARP, I'll look at CDK inhibitors and other treatments that block proteins involved in the cell cycle. I've included plenty of diagrams that unpack the cell cycle and illustrate how these drugs are designed to work.

A Beginner's Guide to Targeted Cancer Treatments and Cancer Immunotherapy, Second Edition. Elaine Vickers.
© 2025 John Wiley & Sons Ltd. Published 2025 by John Wiley & Sons Ltd.

Then we turn to the Hedgehog pathway. This pathway is vital for embryonic and adult stem cells. Two cancers, basal cell carcinoma skin cancer and medulloblastoma, commonly contain gene defects that activate this pathway.

Lastly, I'll turn to a variety of targets and treatments that will be most familiar to anyone involved in the care of people with hematological cancers. However, these treatments – nuclear transport inhibitors, epigenetic modifiers, proteasome inhibitors, and treatments that target cell survival proteins – could have wider applications in the coming years.

4.1 ANGIOGENESIS INHIBITORS

Licensed drugs mentioned in this section:		
Treatment class	**Drugs**	**Given to some people with:**
Antibody therapies	Bevacizumab and ramucirumab	• Kidney cancer, bowel cancer, NSCLC, ovarian cancer, cervical cancer, breast cancer, glioblastoma, liver cancer, and stomach cancer
Other antibody-based treatments	Aflibercept	• Bowel cancer
Kinase inhibitors	Axitinib, cabozantinib, fruquitinib, lenvatinib, nintedanib, pazopanib, regorafenib, sorafenib, sunitinib, tivozanib, vandetanib, everolimus, and temsirolimus	• Kidney cancer, liver cancer, thyroid cancer, endometrial cancer, NSCLC, soft tissue sarcoma, GIST, and PNET
Other small molecules	Belzutifan	• Cancers linked to von Hippel-Lindau (VHL) disease, including central nervous system hemangioblastoma, PNETs, and kidney cancer

Abbreviations: GIST – gastrointestinal stromal tumors; NSCLC – non-small cell lung cancer; PNETs – pancreatic neuroendocrine tumors.

I began explaining angiogenesis in Chapter 1, Section 1.6.3, where I described it as the formation of new blood vessels. When this process is triggered within a tumor, it can help the tumor to grow and spread. In fact, all solid tumors require a blood supply, and they usually achieve this by triggering angiogenesis (see Chapter 1, Figure 1.19 for an illustration of how angiogenesis often takes place) [1, 2].

Back in the early 1970s, scientists started discussing the possibility of starving a tumor by attacking its blood supply [3]. Since that time, many companies have created drugs designed to do just that (see Table 4.1 for a summary of licensed angiogenesis inhibitors). These drugs predominantly work by targeting a growth factor called vascular endothelial growth factor (VEGF) or one or more of its receptors (VEGFRs).[1] Some of these treatments

---

[1] There are actually five versions of VEGF in the human body (VEGF-A, VEGF-B, VEGF-C, VEGF-D, and placental growth factor – PlGF) and three VEGF receptors (VEGF-R1, VEGF-R2, and VEGF-R3).

Table 4.1 Angiogenesis inhibitors licensed for use against cancer in the United States, the United Kingdom, or Europe.

Drug name	Mechanism of action [4]	Cancer types it is licensed for [5–7]
Antibody-based treatments		
Aflibercept	A modified antibody (part-antibody, part-VEGF receptor) that attaches to three forms of VEGF (VEGF-A, VEGF-B, and placental growth factor). It keeps VEGF away from VEGF receptors.	Bowel cancer
Bevacizumab	A monoclonal antibody that attaches to VEGF-A and keeps it away from VEGF receptors	Kidney cancer, bowel cancer, NSCLC, ovarian cancer, cervical cancer, breast cancer, glioblastoma, and liver cancer
Ramucirumab	A monoclonal antibody that attaches to, and blocks, VEGF receptor-2	Stomach cancer[a], bowel cancer, liver cancer, and NSCLC
Small molecule kinase inhibitors		
Axitinib	Blocks multiple targets, including VEGF receptors, PDGF receptors, and KIT	Kidney cancer
Cabozantinib	Blocks multiple targets, including VEGF receptors, MET, RET, KIT, FLT-3, TIE-2, TRKB, and AXL	Kidney cancer, liver cancer, and thyroid cancer[b]
Fruquitinib	Blocks VEGF receptors	Bowel cancer
Lenvatinib	Blocks multiple targets, including VEGF receptors, PDGF receptors, FGF receptors, and RET	Kidney cancer, endometrial cancer, thyroid cancer[b], and liver cancer
Nintedanib	Blocks multiple targets, including VEGF receptors, PDGF receptors, FGF receptors, Src, Lck, Lyn, and FLT-3	NSCLC
Pazopanib	Blocks multiple targets, including VEGF receptors and PDGF receptors; it also has some ability to block FGF receptors	Kidney cancer and soft tissue sarcoma
Regorafenib	Blocks multiple targets, including VEGF receptors and other kinases such as RET, KIT, PDGF receptors, and Raf	Bowel cancer, liver cancer, and GIST[c]
Sorafenib	Blocks multiple targets, including Raf-1, B-Raf, VEGF receptor-2, VEGF receptor-3, PDGF receptors, RET, FLT3, and KIT	Kidney cancer, liver cancer, and thyroid cancer[b]
Sunitinib	Blocks multiple targets, including VEGF receptors, PDGF receptors, KIT, and FLT3	Kidney cancer, PNET[d], and GIST[c]
Tivozanib	Blocks VEGF receptors	Kidney cancer
Vandetanib	Blocks multiple targets, including VEGF receptors, EGF receptors, and RET	Thyroid cancer[b]
Other angiogenesis inhibitors		
Everolimus	An indirect inhibitor of mTOR; it binds to FKBP12, which then partially blocks mTOR activity (see Chapter 3, Section 3.8.4 for further details)	Breast cancer, kidney cancer, neuroendocrine tumors, and subependymal giant cell astrocytoma
Temsirolimus	As for everolimus	Kidney cancer and mantle cell lymphoma
Belzutifan	Blocks HIF-2-alpha (HIF2α), a subunit of hypoxia-inducible factor-2 (HIF-2)	Kidney cancer and other cancers that arise in people with VHL disease

[a] Including cancer that is at the junction between the stomach and the esophagus – called gastroesophageal junction cancer.
[b] A common theme is that drugs used in thyroid cancer are those that can block RET, a growth factor receptor that is often overproduced, and sometimes mutated, in thyroid cancer cells.
[c] Gastrointestinal stromal tumors (GISTs) often contain mutations in KIT (also called CD117) or platelet-derived growth factor receptor-alpha (PDGFRα) – therefore kinase inhibitors that block KIT and PDGFRα are effective against GISTs, irrespective of their impact on angiogenesis.
[d] PNET – pancreatic neuroendocrine tumor.
As I said in Chapter 3, whenever I mention "Europe" in terms of where a treatment is licensed, I'm talking about decisions made by the EMA (European Medicines Agency), which approves treatments for use in countries in the European Union and the European Economic Area (Iceland, Liechtenstein and Norway).

are licensed for a number of different cancers, including kidney cancer, bowel cancer, non-small cell lung cancer (NSCLC), pancreatic neuroendocrine tumors (PNETs),[2] ovarian cancer,[3] cervical cancer, and liver cancer.

When angiogenesis inhibitors were first suggested as a way to treat cancer, scientists and doctors were extremely hopeful that they would benefit virtually anyone with a solid tumor. However, as with many treatments, the benefits of angiogenesis inhibitors are generally much more modest than initially predicted [1, 2]. Although some patients benefit a lot, most patients benefit very little, if at all. Also, the amount of angiogenesis and the characteristics of tumor blood vessels vary greatly from cancer to cancer, from patient to patient, between primary tumors and their metastases, and even from one part of a tumor to another. This means that angiogenesis inhibitors can have varying degrees of impact that are difficult to predict.

One cancer in which angiogenesis inhibitors have made a big difference is kidney cancer. The survival time of a person with metastatic kidney cancer doubled from a median of one year to two years after the introduction of angiogenesis inhibitors [8]. It has since improved even further thanks to the combined use of angiogenesis inhibitors plus checkpoint inhibitor immunotherapy [9].

4.1.1 How Tumors Trigger Angiogenesis

As a cluster of cancer cells grows and multiplies, the cells soon start running short of oxygen. They automatically respond to low oxygen levels (known as hypoxia) in the same way that a healthy cell would; that is, they start to produce a range of growth factors such as VEGF, fibroblast growth factor (FGF), platelet-derived growth factor (PDGF), and angiopoietins [10]. When these growth factors attach to receptors on the surface of nearby endothelial cells, the endothelial cells (which line our blood vessels) respond. As with other growth factor receptors, attachment of VEGF, FGF, or PDGF to their receptors triggers the activity of the MAPK cascade (Ras/Raf/MEK/ERK, described in Section 3.7), and the PI3K/AKT/mTOR pathway (described in Section 3.8). This encourages the cells to survive, but also causes endothelial cells to reorganize themselves, become more mobile, and multiply. In consequence, the blood vessels sprout side branches and grow.

The most important and powerful trigger of tumor angiogenesis is VEGF-A, which predominantly attaches to the VEGF receptor-2 (VEGFR2) [2, 10]. However, other forms of VEGF (such as VEGF-C, VEGF-D, and PlGF) are also released by cancer cells. Many other growth factors and signaling molecules, such as PDGF and FGF, angiopoietins, neuropilins, semaphorins, and ephrins are also involved.

More angiogenesis occurs in some cancers than others. For example, some tumors gain a blood supply by co-opting existing blood vessels or by moving and ordering cancer cells so that they form channels through which blood cells can move [1]. Tumors that are less reliant on angiogenesis are less affected by angiogenesis inhibitors.

---

[2] These are very different from the more common and much more aggressive pancreatic ductal adenocarcinomas; PNETs develop from exocrine cells that produce digestive enzymes and fluids.
[3] As it turns out, most "ovarian cancers" do not actually start in the ovaries, so we now tend to describe them collectively as "ovarian epithelial, fallopian tube, or primary peritoneal cancer."

4.1.2 Tumor Blood Vessels Are Weird

The endothelial cells that line healthy blood vessels are highly organized, well connected to one another, and well supported by pericytes.[4] Healthy blood vessels are also evenly distributed through the tissue to ensure that every cell gets a blood supply. In contrast, the endothelial cells that line a tumor's blood vessels are altered by their cancer neighbors: They are chaotic, irregular in shape, and strangely arranged. In consequence, a tumor's blood vessels are leaky, lumpy, and unstable. As a result, the blood flow is irregular [10]. They also double-back on themselves, creating areas where there are lots of blood vessels and areas where there are none. The weirdness of tumor blood vessels has a number of consequences [11]:

- Areas of a tumor that completely lack blood vessels become chronically hypoxic (short of oxygen). In the hypoxic areas, some cancer cells die, but others adapt by becoming dormant, or by becoming more aggressive and invasive.
- The blood vessels' leakiness allows cancer cells to squeeze into them and travel elsewhere in the body, eventually causing metastasis.
- The chaotic and irregular blood flow through a tumor can make it difficult for chemotherapy or other drugs to penetrate.

Overall, the number and density of blood vessels in a tumor seem to correlate with the aggressiveness of the cancer. In general, people whose tumors have a high density of blood vessels tend to fare worse than (and not live as long as) people whose tumors have fewer blood vessels [2].

4.1.3 Why Block VEGF?

VEGF is by far the most powerful trigger of angiogenesis, and it also sustains and supports tumor blood vessels (see Figure 4.1 for a brief overview and Figure 4.2 for an illustration). In summary, VEGF can: [2, 12–14]

Why block VEGF?

How important is it?	VEGF is the most important molecule responsible for **angiogenesis**
How does it work?	Various versions of VEGF activate **VEGF receptors** found on the surface of endothelial cells that line blood vessels
What does it do?	It triggers existing blood vessels to grow new side branches that then elongate to create new blood vessels (angiogenesis); activation of VEGF receptors also keeps existing blood vessels alive
When do tumors need it?	It is needed by tumors throughout their growth and development
Where does it come from?	VEGF is secreted by cancer cells and other cells in the tumor microenvironment, especially white blood cells
What are the benefits of blocking it?	Blocking VEGF or blocking VEGF receptors could destroy existing blood vessels, inhibit metastasis, and increase sensitivity to chemotherapy

Figure 4.1 **A summary of some of the functions of VEGF and its importance as a treatment target**. **Abbreviation:** VEGF – vascular endothelial growth factor.

---

[4] Pericytes wrap themselves around endothelial cells and provide physical support, as well as producing a range of growth factors and other molecules.

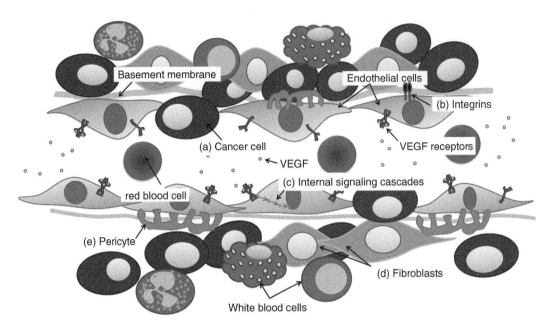

Figure 4.2 Longitudinal illustration of a tumor blood vessel. Healthy blood vessels are lined by endothelial cells, which should create an orderly, continuous layer. In a tumor blood vessel, the endothelial cells are less orderly, and there are gaps between them. **(a)** In places, cancer cells take the place of endothelial cells. **(b)** Integrins on the surface of endothelial cells connect with the basement membrane and with proteins in the extracellular matrix. **(c)** Binding of VEGF to its receptors activates the Ras/Raf/MEK/ERK pathway, PI3K/AKT/mTOR pathway, and other pathways. **(d)** The tumor microenvironment contains numerous cell types, including fibroblasts and white blood cells. **(e)** Pericytes provide support to endothelial cells and participate in angiogenesis.

Abbreviations: ERK – extracellular signal-regulated kinase; mTOR – mechanistic target of rapamycin; PI3K – phosphoinositide 3-kinase; VEGF – vascular endothelial growth factor.

- Cause endothelial cells to multiply.
- Help endothelial cells survive adverse conditions such as low oxygen or the presence of chemotherapy or radiotherapy.
- Help endothelial cells move into new positions.
- Increase the permeability of blood vessels.
- Attract cells from the bone marrow that cause continual angiogenesis in growing tumors.
- Cause tumor blood vessels to dilate.
- Prevent white blood cells (specifically dendritic cells) from maturing properly; therefore, VEGF can protect cancer cells from destruction by the immune system.

However, sometimes the changes in blood vessel diameter and permeability caused by VEGF seem to disrupt the flow of blood. So, increased VEGF levels don't necessarily help the cancer cells get more blood [15].

4.1.4 Why Angiogenesis Inhibitors Sometimes Work

As I said earlier, most angiogenesis inhibitors target VEGF in some way. There are various reasons why blocking VEGF can be helpful:[15]

- It can stop the growth of new blood vessels, hopefully starving cancer cells of oxygen and nutrients and halting further growth and spread.

- It can cause endothelial cells to die and potentially destroy existing tumor blood vessels.
- It can cause blood vessels to constrict (become narrower) and reduce the flow of blood.
- Some of the strangeness and leakiness of tumor blood vessels is driven by the excessive production of VEGF. So, blocking VEGF can sometimes return the endothelial cells to a more normal arrangement, helping blood flow through the tumor more easily. This in turn can improve the transport and distribution of chemotherapy (or other drugs) and make it more effective. It can also make radiotherapy more effective because it works better when there's more oxygen around.
- Tumor cells sometimes have VEGF receptors on their surface; in which case, VEGF blockers might affect them directly.
- Suppression of VEGF might help the patient's immune system attack and destroy cancer cells by allowing their white blood cells to mature properly.
- Treatment with chemotherapy or radiotherapy destroys many cancer cells and causes damage to millions of others. It also causes other stresses, such as a drop in oxygen and poorer nutrient supplies. Cells typically adapt to damage and stress by releasing VEGF. So, treating a patient with a VEGF blocker alongside their other treatment might prevent the cancer from adapting to its altered environment and improve the treatment's effectiveness.

Blocking angiogenesis may have different effects on different parts of the tumor. The net result may be very helpful and bring the patient many months, or occasionally even years, of additional life. But for other patients, the net result is no improvement at all (see Section 4.1.7 for more about drug resistance mechanisms).

4.1.5 Drugs that Target VEGF or VEGF Receptors

I will group these drugs into three categories: (1) drugs that prevent VEGF from attaching to its receptors, (2) drugs that directly block the activity of VEGF receptors, and (3) drugs that work through other mechanisms.

However, I will focus my attention largely on groups 1 and 2, as only two treatments in group 3 are licensed treatments: everolimus and temsirolimus (we met these drugs previously as mTOR inhibitors in Chapter 3, Section 3.8.6).

Drugs that Prevent VEGF from Attaching to its Receptors

There are two licensed drugs that fall into this category: bevacizumab and aflibercept (ziv-aflibercept). These drugs both attach to VEGF and keep it away from its receptors (see Figure 4.3).

Bevacizumab, as you would expect from its name, is a humanized monoclonal antibody. It attaches to VEGF-A and can't bind to the other forms of VEGF (VEGF-B, VEGF-C, VEGF-D, or PlGF). Bevacizumab works by keeping VEGF-A away from VEGF receptor-2 (VEGFR2) – the predominant VEGF receptor on tumor endothelial cells [16]. Because bevacizumab was the first angiogenesis inhibitor created (it first entered trials in 1997), it has been investigated in more trials than any other. It is also licensed for use against more types of cancer than any other angiogenesis inhibitor (see Table 4.1).

Aflibercept is a bioengineered protein – one that would never normally exist in nature. It is made from the back end of an antibody that has been fused to part of the external, VEGF-binding section of VEGFR1 and a similar section of VEGFR2 (see Figures 4.3 and 4.4). It is made by stitching together the necessary parts of the genes for the three proteins. When the final amalgamated gene is inserted into living cells, they are forced to make the desired aflibercept protein, which is harvested and purified. Because it contains part of VEGFR1 and VEGFR2, aflibercept can attach to VEGF-A, VEGF-B, and PlGF [17].

Mouse experiments to compare the effectiveness of bevacizumab and aflibercept appeared to show that aflibercept is the more powerful treatment [18], presumably because of its ability to block PlGF and other VEGF forms as well as blocking VEGF-A. However, in clinical trials, it seems that these drugs are probably roughly equivalent to one another[5] [19].

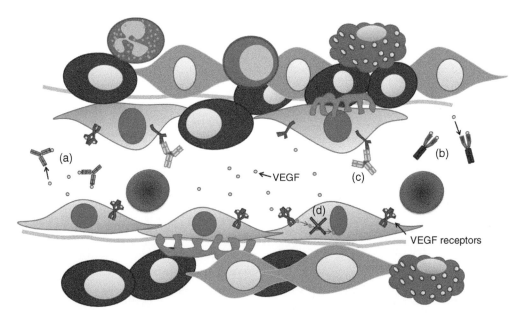

Figure 4.3 Mechanism of action of various angiogenesis inhibitors. (a) Bevacizumab, a humanized monoclonal antibody, attaches to VEGF-A and keeps it away from VEGF receptors. **(b)** Aflibercept, a bioengineered protein, attaches to VEGF-A, VEGF-B, and PlGF, keeping them away from VEGF receptors. **(c)** Ramucirumab is a fully human antibody that directly attaches to VEGF receptor 2. **(d)** Various kinase inhibitors block the kinase portion of VEGF receptors and those of other growth factor receptors.
Abbreviations: PlGF – placental growth factor; VEGF – vascular endothelial growth factor.

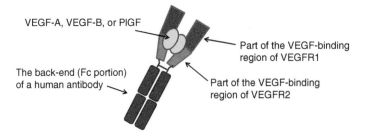

Figure 4.4 Structure of aflibercept (ziv-aflibercept). Aflibercept is made from parts taken from three separate proteins: VEGFR1, VEGFR2, and an antibody.
Abbreviations: PlGF – placental growth factor; VEGF – vascular endothelial growth factor; VEGFR – VEGF receptor.

---

[5] It's impossible to get a definitive answer as the drugs haven't been tested against one another in a clinical trial, so the only way of comparing them is by using statistics to compare different trials, which is tricky to do.

Monoclonal Antibodies that Directly Attach to VEGF Receptors

The only licensed monoclonal antibody that directly attaches to VEGF receptors is ramucirumab. Ramucirumab is a fully human monoclonal antibody that attaches to VEGFR2 and prevents any form of VEGF from attaching to it[6] [20]. It is a licensed treatment for some people with bowel cancer, primary liver cancer, NSCLC, stomach adenocarcinoma, or adeno-carcinoma of the gastroesophageal junction.

Small Molecule Kinase Inhibitors that Block VEGF Receptors

Many drug companies have created kinase inhibitors that enter cells and block the intra-cellular, kinase domain of VEGF receptors. There are numerous such drugs licensed for use in the United States and elsewhere (see Table 4.1 for summary information on these drugs).

Back in Chapter 2, I told you a bit about various different types of kinase inhibitors. Kinase inhibitors that block VEGF receptors tend to be highly promiscuous drugs; that is, they block numerous kinases and not just VEGF receptors [21] (see Figure 2.20 for an illustration of the basic mechanism of action of kinase inhibitors).

The ability of these drugs to block multiple kinases[7] can be helpful as it means you can block other receptors involved in angiogenesis with a single drug (such as PDGF receptors and FGF receptors). However, it also means that they are likely to block kinases that are essential to healthy cells, causing side effects [22, 23].

Seven of the licensed kinase inhibitors are approved for the treatment of people with kidney cancer – I'll explain why in Section 4.1.7.

In addition, four of them – vandetanib, cabozantinib, sorafenib, and lenvatinib – are licensed for the treatment of people with thyroid cancer. Their usefulness as thyroid cancer treatments probably owes as much, if not more, to their ability to block RET [24, 25] (RET stands for "rearranged during trans-fection"). RET is a growth factor receptor, and *RET* gene mutations are common in thyroid cancer cells [26].

4.1.6 Everolimus and Temsirolimus

As you can see in Table 4.1, everolimus and temsirolimus are also sometimes classed as angiogenesis inhibitors. I've mentioned these drugs before (in Chapter 3, Section 3.8.6). They work by blocking some of the actions of mTOR, which is part of the signaling pathway involving PI3K, AKT, mTOR, and PTEN. mTOR is involved both in controlling the growth and survival of cells and in controlling angiogenesis.

mTOR inhibitors seem able to (1) block the growth of cancer cells, (2) prevent cancer cells from releasing VEGF, and (3) block the growth of endothelial cells [27]. In kidney cancers and PNETs, mTOR inhibitors can improve patients' survival times by many months [28]. Everolimus is also licensed as a treatment for women with hormone receptor-positive breast cancer.

4.1.7 Kidney Cancer – A Special Case

Many angiogenesis inhibitors are licensed as treatments for people with kidney cancer. There is a very specific reason why angiogenesis inhibitors work well in kidney cancer: Up to 75% of clear cell renal cell carcinomas (the most common type of kidney cancer) contain a mutation affecting a protein called VHL [29].

---

[6] VEGF-A, VEGF-C, and VEGF-D can all attach to VEGFR2, but VEGF-B and PlGF cannot.
[7] These drugs are often referred to as "multi-kinase inhibitors."

In healthy cells with sufficient oxygen, VHL causes the destruction of two proteins called hypoxia-inducible factor (HIF)-1α and HIF-2α, which would otherwise trigger angiogenesis [30]. Because of mutations affecting the *VHL* gene, kidney cancer cells generally lack VHL protein. Without VHL, there's nothing to destroy the two HIF proteins, and hence they trigger the release of VEGF and cause angiogenesis (see Figure 4.5) [31]. As a result, kidney cancers have lots of blood vessels [32] and are the most sensitive of any cancer to angiogenesis inhibitors [2]. Hence, in kidney cancer, we are using angiogenesis inhibitors as a true, targeted treatment – we are specifically targeting the consequences of a mutation.

4.1.8 HIF-2alpha Inhibitor – Belzutifan

A newer type of angiogenesis inhibitor is belzutifan, which inhibits HIF-2α and prevents it from pairing with HIF-2β/ARNT. Belzutifan was approved in 2021 as a treatment for people with kidney cancer who have a genetic disease called VHL disease. People with this condition have a high chance of developing kidney cancer (and also other cancers) due to an inherited defect in the *VHL* gene [33]. Belzutifan is also approved as a treatment for people with kidney cancer not linked to inherited mutations in *VHL*, and it is being investigated as a treatment for other cancers [34, 35].

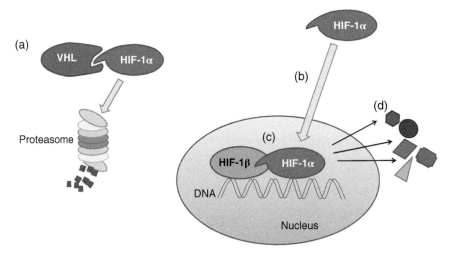

Figure 4.5 Mutations in VHL trigger angiogenesis. (a) In healthy cells, and in normal oxygen conditions, VHL interacts with HIF-1α and HIF-2α (for simplicity, only HIF-1α is shown). This interaction leads to the destruction of HIF-1α - by the cell's proteasomes. **(b)** In clear cell renal cell carcinoma cells, VHL is generally faulty or completely missing. Thus, HIF proteins aren't destroyed. Levels of HIF proteins therefore increase, and they move into the nucleus where they join with a partner protein called HIF-1β. **(c)** Together, HIF proteins and HIF-1β (which is also called ARNT) form a transcription factor called HIF-1, which attaches to the control regions (promoters) of a variety of genes, causing their transcription. **(d)** As a result, the cell produces more than 60 different proteins, including VEGF (which drives angiogenesis), EPO (which tells the bone marrow to produce more red blood cells), GLUT1 (which transports glucose into the cell), ADM (which protects the cell from apoptosis), and TGF-α (which activates EGF receptors).
Abbreviations: ADM – adrenomedullin; ARNT – aryl hydrocarbon receptor nuclear translocator; EPO – erythropoietin; GLUT1 – glucose transporter-1; HIF – hypoxia-inducible factor; TGF – transforming growth factor; VEGF – vascular endothelial growth factor; VHL – von Hippel-Lindau.

4.1.9 Why Angiogenesis Inhibitors Don't Always Work

Angiogenesis inhibitors have substantially improved the survival times of people with kidney cancer, and they have benefited thousands of people with other types of cancer. However, angiogenesis inhibitors haven't been as effective as was initially hoped [2, 13]. Sometimes, it looks as though the treatment is working, and the cancer stops growing, only to start growing again a few weeks or months later. In other cases, the tumor seems completely unaffected.

One of the main problems with blocking angiogenesis as a strategy to treat cancer is that we currently have no way of knowing who it's going to work for. In a single tumor, there may be areas where there is a good blood supply and areas where there is a very poor supply. There might also be areas where an inefficient blood supply is hindering the tumor's growth, and other areas where the same low oxygen levels are helping the tumor spread and helping it avoid destruction by the patient's immune system.

The impact of an angiogenesis inhibitor could therefore go either way: It might starve the tumor and slow its growth; it might normalize some blood vessels and increase blood flow; it might help the delivery of chemotherapy; it might help the cancer spread; it might increase or decrease the cancer's aggressiveness; and it might help or hinder the patient's immune system to destroy cancer cells. As a result, doctors cannot tell what the overall impact of the angiogenesis inhibitor is going to be when they prescribe it for their patients [36].

Sometimes treatment with an angiogenesis inhibitor can be beneficial to a patient, and it stops their tumor from growing. However, even then, it is only a matter of time before the effect wears off (do remember, though, that sometimes the beneficial effects can last for many months, especially for people with kidney cancer).

Scientists have discovered various ways through which tumors resist treatment with an angiogenesis inhibitor. I've summarized a few of these mechanisms in Figure 4.6 and in the list below, but this is by no means exhaustive: [2, 13, 37]

1. The tumor finds other ways to gain a blood supply, for example, by co-opting or growing along existing blood vessels (Figure 4.6a).
2. Pericytes multiply and surround the endothelial cells, increasing their stability and reducing their requirement for VEGF (Figure 4.6b).
3. Immature endothelial cells are recruited to the tumor (Figure 4.6c)
4. Angiogenesis inhibition causes oxygen levels to drop to levels that are toxic to most cells. However, any cells in the tumor that contain DNA mutations or other changes that allow them to survive low oxygen levels will survive (Figure 4.6d).
5. Influenced by their environment, some cancer cells take on the appearance and other properties of endothelial cells and take their place (Figure 4.6e).
6. The tumor cells produce alternative growth factors (such as FGF, PDGF, ephrins, and angiopoietins) that trigger and sustain angiogenesis via numerous signaling pathways even when VEGF or VEGF receptors have been blocked (Figure 4.6f).
7. Cancer cells release chemicals that attract cells from the bone marrow – these cells produce growth factors and cytokines that support existing blood vessels and help new blood vessels form (Figure 4.6g).

4.1.10 The Search for Biomarkers

Hundreds of scientists have attempted to discover a predictive biomarker for angiogenesis inhibitors (I am using the words "predictive biomarker" to mean something

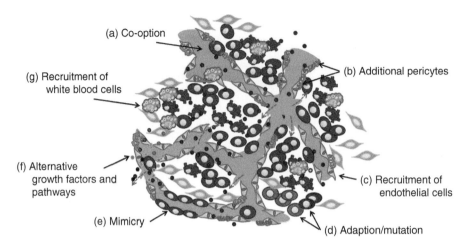

Figure 4.6 Various reasons for resistance to angiogenesis inhibitors. **(a)** Some cancers co-opt existing blood vessels rather than using angiogenesis. **(b)** Additional pericytes stabilize blood vessels. **(c)** Recruitment of immature endothelial cells to line growing blood vessels. **(d)** Additional mutations and adaptations of cancer cells allow them to survive in hypoxic conditions. **(e)** Some cancer cells acquire the physical properties of endothelial cells and take their place. **(f)** Various alternative growth factors are supplied by numerous cell types; endothelial cells use alternative signaling pathways to sustain their growth and survival. **(g)** Recruited white blood cells of various types support angiogenesis in the absence of VEGF signaling. **Abbreviation:** VEGF – vascular endothelial growth factor.

that scientists can measure before or soon after giving a patient treatment, which can be used to predict whether the treatment is going to be effective). So far, the search has been unsuccessful. However, many possible biomarkers are still being investigated.

Potential biomarkers that scientists have studied include the following: [2]

1. Using sophisticated scanners to monitor changes to the way blood flows through a patient's tumor to get a rapid idea of whether treatment is working.
2. Measuring changes in a patient's blood pressure.
3. Measuring the levels of various proteins in the patient's bloodstream, such as various forms of VEGF, or measuring the number of tumor cells or endothelial cells that end up in the person's blood.
4. Looking for inherited variations in genes that correlate with successful angiogenesis inhibitor treatment.

5. Looking inside tumors – at the levels of various proteins, at the presence or absence of white blood cells, at the number of blood vessels, and whether they are healthy.

If this search for biomarkers is successful, it would mean that only patients who benefit from angiogenesis inhibitors would receive them, allowing other patients to avoid the side effects of unnecessary treatment.

4.1.11 Combining Angiogenesis Inhibitors with Immunotherapy

In addition to affecting blood flow in a tumor, VEGF also affects the relationship between cancer cells and the immune system [9, 38]. For example, VEGF prevents dendritic cells from maturing and specializing, leading to immature dendritic cells becoming trapped in the tumor microenvironment. There's also a suggestion that VEGF can cause T cells to become exhausted and inactive and to become stuck inside abnormal tumor blood vessels.

It's therefore logical to think that an angiogenesis inhibitor would enhance the effects of an immunotherapy such as an immune checkpoint inhibitor and bring greater benefits to patients than either used alone.

However, achieving synergy is an immense challenge. In fact, an analysis of trials involving

checkpoint inhibitor combinations found little or no evidence of synergy in any trial [39]. The analysis included combinations involving two checkpoint inhibitors, checkpoint inhibitors combined with angiogenesis inhibitors, and checkpoint inhibitors combined with chemotherapy.

In Chapter 5, I explore various immune checkpoint inhibitor combinations in greater detail.

4.2 ANTIBODY CONJUGATES

Licensed drugs mentioned in this section:		
Treatment class	**Drugs**	**Given to some people with:**
ADC targeting HER2	Trastuzumab emtansine and trastuzumab deruxtecan	• HER2-positive breast cancer • HER2-low breast cancer • HER2-positive stomach cancer or gastroesophageal junction cancer • NSCLC containing mutations in the HER2 gene
ADC targeting TROP2	Sacituzumab govitecan	• Triple-negative breast cancer • HER2-negative breast cancer • Bladder cancer
ADC targeting nectin-4	Enfortumab vedotin	• Bladder cancer
ADC targeting folate receptor-alpha	Mirvetuximab soravtansine	• Ovarian cancer
ADC targeting tissue factor	Tisotumab vedotin	• Cervical cancer
ADC targeting CD33	Gemtuzumab ozogamicin	• Acute myeloid leukemia
ADC targeting CD22	Inotuzumab ozogamicin	• Acute lymphoblastic leukemia
ADC targeting CD30	Brentuximab vedotin	• Hodgkin lymphoma • Anaplastic large cell lymphoma • Cutaneous anaplastic large cell lymphoma • Peripheral T cell lymphoma • Cutaneous T cell lymphoma
ADC targeting CD19	Loncastuximab tesirine	• Some B cell NHLs
ADC targeting CD79B	Polatuzumab vedotin	• Some B cell NHLs
ADC targeting BCMA	Belantamab mafodotin	• Myeloma
Other types of conjugate		
Radiolabeled ligand	177Lu-labeled PSMA-617	• Prostate cancer
Radiolabeled antibody	90Y-Ibritumomab tiuxetan	• B cell follicular NHL
Immunotoxin	Tagraxofusp	• Blastic plasmacytoid dendritic cell neoplasm
Radiolabeled peptide	Lu-177-Dotatate	• Neuroendocrine tumors in the pancreas or other parts of the digestive tract

Abbreviations: ADC – antibody-drug conjugate; HER2 – human EGF receptor-2; NHL – non-Hodgkin lymphoma; NSCLC – non-small cell lung cancer.

I introduced the antibody-drug conjugates (ADCs) in Section 2.2.4, including Figures 2.11a and 2.12. In these treatments, the antibody is used as a delivery device to transport chemotherapy directly to the person's cancer cells.

Before I go into more detail, there are a few things about ADCs to bear in mind: [40, 41]

• In addition to delivering chemotherapy, the antibody might also trigger an immune response involving macrophages, natural killer (NK) cells, and complement proteins.

• Depending on the antibody's target, the ADC might kill some cancer cells without needing to release chemotherapy (for example, all antibodies that target HER2 are potentially lethal to HER2-positive cancer cells).

• Unless the antibody's target is exclusively present on the person's cancer cells, it will cause some destruction of healthy cells.

• Only a tiny fraction of the ADC's drug ever makes it into the person's cancer cells. The patient is therefore likely to experience toxicities caused by the chemotherapy payload.

I describe other forms of antibody conjugate in Section 4.2.8.

4.2.1 The Structure of ADCs

There are three main parts to an ADC: the antibody, the drug, and the linker (Table 4.2).

Drug selection is an area where there's been a shift in focus in recent years. Newer ADCs often include a topoisomerase inhibitor such as Dxd (the ADC's name ends in deruxtecan) or SN-38 (the ADC's name ends in govitecan). Topoisomerase inhibitors are less potent than the maytansinoids or calicheamicin and they are therefore designed to cause milder side effects. Initially, their lack of potency was considered a problem, but this has been overcome by increasing the number of copies of the chemotherapy attached to each antibody [42].

4.2.2 How ADCs Are Being Improved

Over recent years, scientists have gradually improved the properties of the ADCs they create (summarized in Figure 4.7).

Table 4.2 The key elements of ADCs and their properties.

Element	Description
Antibody	• Often a humanized or fully human antibody to reduce immunogenicity and limit infusion reactions. • Targeted against a cell surface protein found on the person's cancer cells. • Scientists hope to **find the perfect level of affinity** of the antibody for its target: too low and the antibody doesn't attach to cancer cells; too high and the antibody attaches to cancer cells near blood vessels and never penetrates deeper into the tumor.
Linker	• **Cleavable linkers** (pH-sensitive, protease-cleavable, or glutathione concentration-sensitive) break (cleave) inside cancer cells. • **Non-cleavable linkers** requiring proteasomal degradation in order to release the chemotherapy (i.e., the drug is only released when the ADC has been completely broken up inside the cell).
Drug	• Needs to be highly potent due to the relatively low concentration reached inside target cells. Common choices are topoisomerase inhibitors (Dxd and SN-38), microtubule inhibitors (maytansinoids or auristatins), and DNA-damaging agents (mainly calicheamicins). • The drug chosen is generally too potent (and therefore too toxic) to be given to patients unless it forms part of an ADC. • It's important to **find a balance between toxicity and potency**: too potent and it causes side effects for the patient; not potent enough and it fails to kill cancer cells.

Source: [41, 42].

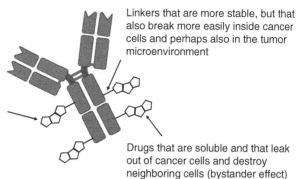

Linkers that are more stable, but that also break more easily inside cancer cells and perhaps also in the tumor microenvironment

Better control and consistency over the number of copies of the drug per antibody, and where on the antibody they are attached

Drugs that are soluble and that leak out of cancer cells and destroy neighboring cells (bystander effect)

Figure 4.7 Scientists are improving ADCs by making a number of changes. *Source:* [41, 43–46].

Table 4.3   Properties of trastuzumab emtansine compared to trastuzumab deruxtecan.

Trastuzumab emtansine	Trastuzumab deruxtecan
Attaches to HER2, killing cancer cells directly and recruiting and activating white blood cells; also delivers chemotherapy	Attaches to HER2, killing cancer cells directly and recruiting and activating white blood cells; also delivers chemotherapy
The linker is non-cleavable, meaning the cell must destroy the ADC for the drug to be released	The linker is easily cleavable by enzymes (cathepsins) found in high levels inside cancer cells
The chemotherapy it delivers is emtansine (DM1), which attacks the cell's microtubules, causing cell death	The chemotherapy it delivers is deruxtecan (Dxd), a topoisomerase inhibitor that causes DNA damage and cell death
Three or four copies of the drug are attached to each copy of the antibody	On average, eight copies of the drug are attached to each copy of the antibody
Emtansine has a relatively long half-life	Deruxtecan has a relatively short half-life to reduce toxicity to non-cancer cells
Emtansine is non-permeable; once released inside a cancer cell, it is trapped there	Deruxtecan is soluble – it leaks out of cancer cells and kills neighboring cells
Very high levels of HER2 must be present on the cancer cells' surface for the treatment to be helpful	Appears to be effective even against cancers with relatively low levels of HER2 on the surface of cancer cells

Source: Adapted from [47, 48].

4.2.3 An Example: Trastuzumab Deruxtecan

A comparison that illustrates this progress is that between trastuzumab emtansine and the newer ADC, trastuzumab deruxtecan (Table 4.3) [49, 50]. As you can tell from the names, both ADCs are modified versions of trastuzumab, a HER2-targeted antibody first approved as a treatment for HER2-positive breast cancer in 1998.

Trastuzumab deruxtecan has various improved properties that appear to be responsible for outperforming trastuzumab emtansine in trials such as the DESTINY-Breast03 study [47, 51].

4.2.4 Common Targets of ADCs and Treatment Examples

The target of an ADC doesn't need to be something that the cell is relying on for its survival (however, it's probably helpful if it is). The plan is that the drug carried by the antibody will take care of killing any cell it is delivered to. However, targets do need to be present on the surface of the person's cancer cells and hopefully absent, or only present at low levels, on healthy cells [41].

As the number of ADCs approved as cancer treatments increases, so does the number of targets. I've listed some of the most common ones in Table 4.4.

Judging by the enormous number of ADCs in clinical trials, no doubt this list of drugs and targets will get longer in the coming years.

Table 4.4 Current and emerging targets of antibody-drug conjugates. Antibodies highlighted in orange are approved treatments for one or more types of cancer as of March 2024.

Target	Treatment examples	Comments
Solid tumors		
HER2	**Trastuzumab emtansine, trastuzumab deruxtecan**, trastuzumab duocarmazine, and disitamab vedotin	• ADCs are established treatments for HER2-positive breast cancer and stomach/gastroesophageal junction cancer • Trastuzumab deruxtecan is also licensed for patients with "HER2-low" breast cancer, where in the past there would have been insufficient data to support the use of a HER2-targeted treatment • They may also be useful for individual patients with some other cancer types, where their cancer cells are found to be HER2-postive or HER2-low (e.g., endometrial or cervical cancer)
TROP2	**Sacituzumab govitecan** and datopotamab deruxtecan	• Sacituzumab govitecan is approved for triple-negative breast cancer, HER2-negative breast cancer, and bladder cancer • High levels of TROP2 are found in many epithelial cancers, including breast cancer, bladder cancer, NSCLC, small cell lung cancer, and gynecological and gastrointestinal cancers
Nectin-4	**Enfortumab vedotin**	• Enfortumab vedotin is approved for bladder cancer • High levels of nectin-4 are also found in some breast, lung, ovarian, and stomach cancers
Folate receptor-alpha (FRα)	**Mirvetuximab soravtansine**, luveltamab tazevibulin, and farletuzumab ecteribulin	• Mirvetuximab soravtansine is approved for ovarian cancer • FRα is also found in mesothelioma, NSCLC, and triple-negative breast cancer
Tissue factor (TF)	**Tisotumab vedotin**	• Tisotumab vedotin is approved for cervical cancer • Tissue factor is found in many cancer types, including gastrointestinal cancers, urogenital cancers, glioma, melanoma, and lung cancer
Claudin 18.2	CMG-901, CPO102, SHR-A1904, RC118, LM-302, and SOT102	• Claudin 18.2 is found in stomach, gastroesophageal junction, esophageal, and pancreatic cancers
Delta-like ligand-3 (DLL3)	Rovalpituzumab tesirine	• DLL3 is found in small cell lung cancer
LIV1	Ladiratuzumab vedotin	• LIV1 is found in breast cancer and a range of other solid tumors, including stomach, gastroesophageal junction, esophageal, and small cell lung cancer, and NSCLC
Carcinoembryonic antigen-related cell adhesion molecule 5 (CEACAM5)	Labetuzumab govitecan and tusamitamab ravtansine	• CEACAM5 is found in several cancers, including bowel, lung, and stomach cancers

Table 4.4 (Continued)

EGFR	Losatuxizumab vedotin and depatuxizumab mafodotin	• Overexpressed in a wide variety of cancer types, including lung, head and neck, breast, kidney, gastric, colon, pancreatic, ovary, prostate, and bladder cancers
HER3	Patritumab deruxtecan	• HER3 is overproduced by a wide variety of cancers
Mesothelin	Anetumab ravtansine	• Mesothelin is found in mesothelioma, ovarian cancer, NSCLC, pancreatic cancer, breast cancer, gastric cancer, and cholangiocarcinoma
MET	Telisotuzumab vedotin	• MET is implicated in many cancer types, including NSCLC
B7-H4	SGN-B7H4V and AZD8205	• B7-H4 is overexpressed by a variety of solid tumors, including breast, ovarian, and endometrial cancers
CD44v6	Bivatuzumab mertansine	• Overexpressed by numerous cancer types, including head and neck, ovarian, colorectal, and thyroid cancers

Hematological cancers

CD33	**Gemtuzumab ozogamicin**	• CD33 is found on various types of myeloid white blood cells • Gemtuzumab ozogamicin is an approved treatment for acute myeloid leukemia
CD22	**Inotuzumab ozogamicin,** pinatuzumab vedotin, and moxetumomab pasudotox	• CD22 is found on the surface of immature B cells • Inotuzumab ozogamicin is an approved treatment for acute lymphoblastic leukemia
CD30	**Brentuximab vedotin**	• CD30 is found on the cancer cells of Hodgkin lymphoma and some other rare lymphoma types • Brentuximab vedotin is a licensed treatment for Hodgkin lymphoma and various T cell non-Hodgkin lymphomas (NHLs)
CD19	**Loncastuximab tesirine** and coltuximab ravtansine	• CD19 is found on the surface of most B cells • Loncastuximab tesirine is an approved treatment for some B cell NHLs
CD79B	**Polatuzumab vedotin**	• CD79B is found on the surface of B cells in conjunction with the B cell receptor • Polatuzumab vedotin is approved for some B cell NHLs
B cell maturation antigen (BCMA)	**Belantamab mafodotin**	• High levels of BCMA found on antibody-secreting plasma cells • Belantamab mafodotin is an approved treatment for myeloma

Source: Adapted from [41, 48, 52–57].
Abbreviations: ADC – antibody-drug conjugate; NHL – non-Hodgkin lymphoma; NSCLC – non-small cell lung cancer.

4.2.5 Who Are They Given to?

We're still at the beginning of the era of ADCs as cancer treatments. This means that researchers and drug companies are still figuring out who to give these treatments to, and whether to select recipients based on the presence of the target protein on their cancer cells.

Whether biomarker selection is used will depend on the following:

• How reliable the targets' presence is on the surface of cancer cells of the type of cancer being treated. If it's only present in a small proportion of patients, then it's likely a biomarker test is needed to find them.

- How potent the ADC is, and how much of the target needs to be present for it to kill cancer cells.
- What the results of trials look like, and how accurately the presence of the target protein predicts the level of patient benefit – if there's a tight correlation and a lack of benefit when the target isn't present, this suggests that implementing a biomarker test would be useful.

A couple of examples for you to illustrate my point:

- Enfortumab vedotin, which targets nectin-4, is approved for some people with advanced bladder cancer without any patient selection based on nectin-4 levels. However, the degree of benefit patients derive from enfortumab vedotin does appear to correlate with the amount of nectin-4 on their cancer cells. Loss of nectin-4 also appears to be a reason for treatment resistance [58].
- Mirvetuximab soravtansine, which targets the folate receptor-alpha (FRα), is an approved treatment for advanced, "FRα positive," ovarian cancer. The level of FRα that needed to be on a person's cancer cells for it to be designated "FRα positive" changed over time as the clinical trials progressed [59]. The approval (by the FDA) was based on the results from a clinical trial called SORAYA [60]. In this trial, "FRα positive" cancers were those with FRα on at least 75% of the person's cancer cells, with a staining intensity of PS2+ (deemed a moderate/strong level of FRα) as determined by immunohistochemistry[8] [61].

4.2.6 Reasons for Resistance to ADCs

Resistance to an ADC can be for many reasons: [62]

- Loss of the target from the cancer cells' surface. This could be due to a mutation in the gene for the target protein or reduced production of the protein.
- The ADC is no longer able to bind its target. Possibly due to a change in the target protein's shape, or something that masks the target and prevents the ADC from binding.
- Not enough ADC getting inside cancer cells. Due to the ADC no longer being drawn inside cancer cells, or quickly being returned to the surface.
- Not enough drug being released. Perhaps the drug is being expelled from cancer cells as quickly as it's released.
- The drug no longer kills cancer cells. The cancer cells are protected from death by an increased amount of survival proteins, enhanced DNA repair, or other changes to the drug's target.

4.2.7 Side Effects of ADCs

I don't often comment on side effects. However, ADCs are often lauded in the medical press for their improved ability to target cancer cells, and terms such as "magic bullet" get mentioned. So, it may come as a surprise that many ADCs have failed to prove effective in trials, and the development of numerous ADCs has been halted due to excessive and dangerous side effects [40, 63].

If you remember, scientists estimate that only 0.1% (one in every thousand copies) of an

---

[8] Immunohistochemistry is when a pathologist takes a wafer-thin slice of tumor tissue and uses an antibody to hunt for the presence of a particular protein. The antibody is modified so that it creates a colored stain wherever it sticks. The intensity of the staining therefore reflects the amount of the target protein that is present. The staining intensity typically has four categories: negative (0), weak (1), moderate (2), and strong (3). PS2+ means that the staining intensity is at least 2.

ADC ever reaches a person's cancer cells. Most of it is gradually broken down in the circulation and in other organs and tissues. This means that the bulk of the toxicities of ADCs are driven by the release of drug into the body. Thus, regardless of an ADC's target, its side effects will be very similar to those caused by other ADCs that incorporate the same form of chemotherapy. For example, polatuzumab vedotin, enfortumab vedotin, and tisotumab vedotin, all cause similar side effects [63].

It's also worth noting that, in general, ADCs with non-cleavable linkers cause milder side effects than those with cleavable linkers, because less of the drug is released in the blood. However, ADCs with cleavable linkers are generally more effective and produce better results [63]. In addition, highly stable linkers have been linked to toxicities affecting the eyes, such as conjunctivitis, dry eye, and corneal inflammation. Eye toxicities are also more likely with ADCs that incorporate monomethyl auristatin F (such as tisotumab vedotin), or the maytansinoid DM4 (such as mirvetuximab soravtansine) [64].

That's not to say that ADCs can't cause on-target, but off-cancer toxicity. For example, any treatment that targets HER2 is likely to cause cardiac toxicity because of HER2 on cardiac cells. Another example is enfortumab vedotin, which targets nectin-4. It is liable to change a person's sense of taste (called dysgeusia) and cause skin problems because of the presence of nectin-4 in salivary glands and on skin cells [40, 63].

If you'd like to know more about the side effects of ADCs, I would suggest looking up the Tarantino [40] and Nguyen [63] references I have referred to several times in this section.

4.2.8 Other Types of Conjugate

An ADC is not the only way of delivering a drug to cancer cells. In addition, drugs are not the only thing that antibodies can potentially deliver. Hence, there are additional strategies to deliver toxic entities directly to cancer cells, such as:

1. Radioactively-labeled antibodies
2. Radioactively-labeled ligands for cell surface proteins
3. Drug-conjugated small molecules
4. Drug-conjugated peptides
5. Immunotoxins

Radioactively-labeled Ligands, Peptides, and Antibodies

Radiotherapy is beyond the scope of this book. However, there are a variety of different ways of introducing radiotherapy into the body as a systemic treatment. The goal is to introduce it in a form that preferentially affects cancer cells [65].

In general, these radioactively-labeled (radiolabeled) treatments are most relevant to people with cancers that are already known to be sensitive to radiation and that are relatively easy for both drugs and antibodies to penetrate. These include hematological cancers, prostate cancer, and some neuroendocrine tumors.

The radioactive isotope that forms part of the treatment is generally either a beta particle emitter (such as Lutetium-177, Yttrium-90, or Samarium-153) or an alpha particle emitter (such as Actinium-225, Radium-223, and Thorium-227).

Alpha- and beta-emitters have contrasting properties. For example, alpha particles travel shorter distances but release more energy. Thus, alpha emitters do more damage, and they can deliver effective doses of radiation inside small tumors. Beta emitters travel further (and might therefore damage sensitive structures away from tumors), but release less energy [66, 67].

The targeting element is generally supplied by an antibody, or by some sort of small molecule, such as a ligand for a receptor, or a short peptide known to bind to a specific target.

For example, a prostate cancer treatment called Lu177-PSMA-617 (also referred to as

^{177}Lu-labeled PSMA-617 and as Lutetium-177 vipivotide tetraxetan) includes PSMA-617, a small molecule known to bind to prostate-specific membrane antigen (PSMA). PSMA-617 is linked to the beta-emitting radioactive isotope, Lutetium-177. The intention is that Lu177-PSMA-617 attaches to cancer cells inside prostate tumors and any metastases and delivers a cell-killing dose of radiation [67].

Radioactively labeled antibodies (also called radioimmunoconjugates or radioimmunotherapies) have a long history as cancer treatments (see Figure 2.11b). The first one, ^{90}Y-Ibritumomab tiuxetan, became a licensed treatment in 2002. However, issues around side effects, staff and patient safety, containment, staff training, and other practicalities have limited their use [66, 68, 69].

Drug-conjugated Small Molecules and Peptides

As with ADCs, these include a targeting component, this time in the form of a peptide (a short piece of protein, made from amino acids) or a small molecule. This is chemically linked to a form of chemotherapy [70–73].

As with ADCs, the key to an effective treatment is the design of the cleavable linker between the peptide (or small molecule) and the drug. This linker would ideally only break when the whole structure is inside a cancer cell. One advantage that something like a peptide-drug conjugate (PDC) has over an ADC is its size. PDCs are much smaller. They can therefore penetrate deeper into tumors to deliver their payload.

Immunotoxins

These treatments again combine a targeting component with a toxic payload (Figure 2.11c). This time the targeting component is fused to a toxic protein. The toxic protein is often something produced naturally by a bacterium, such as the diphtheria toxin.

One immunotoxin that became a licensed treatment for hairy cell leukemia (a rare leukemia), although it has now been withdrawn

due to low uptake, was moxetumomab pasudotox. This treatment comprises the tip of an antibody targeted against CD22, fused to a fragment of Pseudomonas exotoxin [74].

Another immunotoxin that made it through to approval, but was later discontinued, is denileukin diftitox, a treatment for rare T cell lymphomas. This fusion protein combines a portion of interleukin-2 with a fragment of the diphtheria toxin. In a twist of fortune, a purified and reformulated version of denileukin diftitox was resubmitted to the FDA for approval at the end of 2022 [75].

An immunotoxin that is still in use is tagraxofusp. This treatment consists of interleukin-3 (IL-3) fused to a shortened version of the diphtheria toxin. It is given to people with a rare hematological cancer called blastic plasmacytoid dendritic cell neoplasm. The cells of this cancer have high levels of IL-3 receptors on their surface [76].

Sadly, there's a long list of immunotoxins that entered patient trials but that failed to become licensed treatments. Some of the main problems are (1) side effects caused by the release of toxins outside of cancer cells, (2) destruction of the treatment by the patient's immune system, and (3) poor penetration of the treatment into tumors [77].

4.3 PARP INHIBITORS

Licensed drugs mentioned in this section:		
Treatment class	**Drugs**	**Given to some people with:**
PARP inhibitors	Niraparib, olaparib, rucaparib, and talazoparib	• Ovarian cancer • Breast cancer • Prostate cancer • Pancreatic cancer

Poly ADP ribose polymerase (PARP) inhibitors were originally expected to benefit one particular group of people: People who have inherited a mutation in one of their *BRCA* (breast cancer associated) genes and who have subsequently developed breast or ovarian cancer. Since their creation, we've discovered that they benefit a much broader range of women[9] with ovarian cancer. These drugs have also been explored for people with other cancers.

I'll firstly explain why PARP inhibitors were proposed as treatments for breast or ovarian cancers in people with inherited *BRCA* mutations. Then I'll talk more widely about ovarian cancer and other cancers.

To explain PARP inhibitors, I need to work through a few different concepts:
- What is PARP?
- How do PARP inhibitors work?
- What are *BRCA* genes and BRCA proteins?

- Why are people with inherited *BRCA* mutations so likely to develop cancer?
- Why might PARP inhibitors be effective against cancers in people with inherited *BRCA* gene mutations?
- What about PARP inhibitors for patients with ovarian cancer who don't have an inherited *BRCA* mutation?
- Why might PARP be effective against pancreatic cancer and prostate cancer?

4.3.1 What is PARP?

PARP proteins play a vital role in the repair of single-strand breaks in our cells' DNA [78, 79] (see Figure 4.8). These little nicks to our DNA happen every day of our lives in each one of the billions of cells in our body. As I mentioned

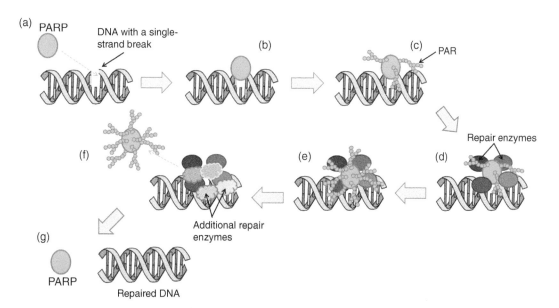

Figure 4.8 Function of PARP enzymes. (a) PARP detects a single-strand break in a chromosome and **(b)** attaches to the damaged DNA. **(c)** PARP uses NAD+ to create long strings of a polymer called PAR, which it attaches to itself to become active. **(d)** Active PARP recruits other proteins to the damaged DNA; these proteins start the repair process. **(e)** More PAR is added to PARP, and its affinity for DNA reduces. **(f)** PARP leaves the repair site, allowing additional repair proteins to gain access and complete the repair process. **(g)** The DNA repair process is complete, and PAR is removed from PARP's surface. **Abbreviations:** NAD – nicotinamide adenine dinucleotide; PAR – poly(ADP-ribose); PARP – poly (ADP ribose) polymerase.

---

[9] Or anyone born with ovaries.

in Chapter 1, DNA damage is often caused by oxygen free radicals: high-energy oxygen atoms that are created by our cells as they produce energy. The creation of oxygen free radicals is unavoidable, and they are often responsible for these little nicks in our DNA [80].

Happily, thanks to PARP and other proteins, our cells are well equipped to repair single-strand DNA breaks.

4.3.2 How do PARP Inhibitors Work?

PARP proteins (there are at least 18 family members) are not kinases; therefore, you can't use a kinase inhibitor to block them. Instead, PARP inhibitors are small chemical compounds that do two things to varying degrees (see Figure 4.9): [81, 82]

1. They compete with a chemical called NAD+[10] for a binding site on the PARP protein. PARP needs NAD+ to create poly ADP ribose (PAR) and recruit other repair proteins. Without access to NAD+, PARP is blocked, and the damaged DNA isn't repaired.
2. Once PARP has attached to damaged DNA, PARP inhibitors prevent it from letting go.

Scientists refer to this as "PARP trapping," and it's highly toxic to cells. PARP is effectively stuck to the DNA double helix. If the cell tries to multiply with PARP still in place, it can't do so, and it causes a complete break in the cell's DNA.

Many scientists think PARP inhibitors cause cells to accumulate double-strand breaks in their DNA (when a chromosome snaps in two). However, not all scientists agree on this. What they can agree on, though, is that PARP inhibitors cause problems that healthy cells can overcome, but that cause cells with defects in their *BRCA* genes to die [81].

4.3.3 What Are *BRCA* Genes and BRCA Proteins?

BRCA proteins (BRCA1 and BRCA2) are just two of a whole series of different proteins involved in a process called homologous recombination (HR). HR is a very accurate and efficient process that our cells use for repairing double-strand DNA breaks [84]. Both BRCA1 and BRCA2 are essential for HR, but they perform very different roles in the process. If a cell is missing either of its BRCA proteins, it's unable to perform HR.

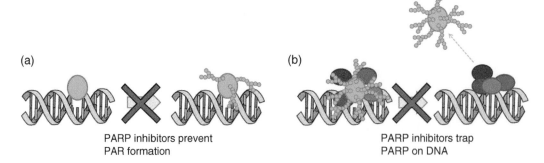

(a) PARP inhibitors prevent PAR formation

(b) PARP inhibitors trap PARP on DNA

Figure 4.9 Mechanisms of action of PARP inhibitors. (a) PARP inhibitors prevent PAR formation and (b) cause PARP enzymes to become trapped on DNA.
Abbreviation: PARP – poly(ADP-ribose)polymerase.

---

[10] Nicotinamide adenine dinucleotide (NAD+) is a complicated chemical found in our cells. It is necessary for the function of lots of different enzymes, including PARP [83].

Maybe not surprisingly, the two genes our cells use to make BRCA1 and BRCA2 proteins are called *BRCA1* and *BRCA2*.

The two *BRCA* genes were discovered by scientists in the mid-1990s when they were trying to work out why breast and ovarian cancers sometimes run in families. We have two copies of every gene – one from each biological parent. The scientists discovered that if you inherit a fault in one of your copies of either *BRCA1* or *BRCA2*, then your risk of developing breast cancer and/or ovarian cancer[11] is much higher than for other people: [85]

- Around 70% of biological females with a faulty *BRCA1* or *BRCA2* gene will develop breast cancer by the age of 80.
- Almost 45% of biological females with a faulty *BRCA1* gene, and around 20% with a faulty *BRCA2* gene, will develop ovarian cancer by the age of 80.

People who inherit a *BRCA1* or *BRCA2* mutation[12] are also more at risk of pancreatic cancer, stomach cancer, laryngeal cancer, and prostate cancer [87].

4.3.4 Why Are People with Inherited *BRCA* Mutations so Likely to Develop Cancer?

If someone has inherited a fault in one of their *BRCA* genes, then the fault is present in every cell in their body. But, because we have two copies of every gene, a fault in one copy isn't necessarily disastrous. In fact, even if our cells only have one functioning copy of *BRCA1* or *BRCA2*, then we develop normally. A high-profile example is the actor and director Angelina Jolie. She has said very publicly that she inherited a faulty copy of *BRCA1* and

lost her mother, grandmother, and aunt to cancer [88–90].

Despite being healthy at birth, people born with a *BRCA1* or *BRCA2* gene mutation have a much higher risk of cancer than most people. The problem is that our cells' DNA is getting damaged every day of our lives, and this damage affects the entire genome. In someone with an inherited *BRCA1* or *BRCA2* mutation, there is always a chance that a cell will pick up a second mutation, this time affecting its healthy copy of the affected *BRCA* gene. If this happens in a breast or ovary (or fallopian tube) cell, the results can be devastating (see Figure 4.10). Cells that were getting on quite happily have now lost their one healthy copy of *BRCA1* or *BRCA2*. The BRCA1 and BRCA2 proteins, being so different from one another physically, cannot stand in for each other. Therefore, if either of its BRCA proteins is completely missing, the cell can't perform HR. When this is the case, the cell is forced to rely on other methods to repair double-strand DNA breaks, and these other methods aren't as accurate.

The main fallback method that cells have for repairing double-strand DNA breaks is called non-homologous end joining (NHEJ). In NHEJ, the cell essentially takes two ends of DNA and jams them together [91]. A cell that is reliant on NHEJ is liable to make lots of mistakes, and it accumulates DNA mutations quickly. In fact, cells that lack one of their BRCA proteins and have to rely on NHEJ are genomically unstable (see Chapter 1 for more about this). They end up with lots of huge mistakes in their chromosomes and are liable to become cancer

---

[11] I have mentioned before that "ovarian cancers" often develop from faulty cells in the fallopian tubes, so I'm using the term "ovarian cancer" to mean a cancer that starts in the ovaries or fallopian tubes. See this Medscape article for more information: http://www.medscape.com/viewarticle/843469 (accessed July 28, 2022).

[12] It's incredibly rare for someone to inherit a mutation in **both** *BRCA1* and *BRCA2*, but it does occasionally happen [86].

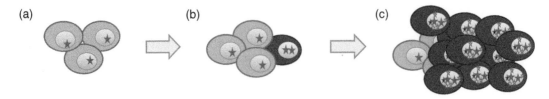

Figure 4.10 The path from *BRCA* gene mutations to cancer. (a) If a person is born with a fault in one of their *BRCA* genes (one red star), then every cell in their body will contain the fault. But the second, healthy copy of the gene in each cell is enough to keep them healthy (orange cells). **(b)** If the second copy of the affected *BRCA* gene gets damaged (two red stars) in a breast or ovary/fallopian tube cell, this cell will be completely unable to perform homologous recombination (dark red cell). Instead, the cell will have to rely on an error-prone method (called non-homologous end joining – NHEJ) to repair double-strand breaks to its DNA. **(c)** Because it's relying on NHEJ, the cell gradually picks up more and more DNA damage – it is genomically unstable. It accumulates damage to many important genes and becomes a cancer cell; it multiplies rapidly, and a tumor develops.
Abbreviations: BRCA – BRCA, DNA repair associated; NHEJ – non-homologous end joining.

Table 4.5 Characteristics of *BRCA*-mutated cancers in mutation carriers.

Cancer	Characteristics
Breast cancers in people with inherited *BRCA1* mutations	The majority (69%) of breast cancers diagnosed in people who are biologically female, and who have an inherited mutation in *BRCA1*, are "triple negative"; however, triple-negative breast cancer is very rare in people who are biologically male. Triple-negative breast cancers do not contain estrogen or progesterone receptors, nor do they have HER2 on their surface. They are likely to be aggressive and difficult to treat.
Breast cancers in people with inherited *BRCA2* mutations	The characteristics of these cancers vary a lot from person to person, but in both biological females and males they generally do contain estrogen and progesterone receptors. Only around 16% are triple negative.
Ovarian cancers in people with inherited *BRCA1* or *BRCA2* mutations	These tend to be high-grade (i.e., very aggressive) serous ovarian cancers[a]. The cancer sometimes starts in the ovaries, but it could have started in the fallopian tubes. These cancers tend to be very sensitive to chemotherapy, at least to begin with. But they are also genomically unstable and quickly become resistant to treatment.

Source: Adapted from [93, 94].
[a] The most common type of ovarian cancer.

cells [92]. In Table 4.5, I've summarized a couple of other characteristics of the cancers that develop in people with inherited faults in *BRCA* genes.

One aspect of *BRCA* mutations and cancer that puzzles scientists is why mutations in *BRCA* genes particularly cause breast and ovarian cancers rather than any other type. Despite lots of scientists having investigated this, there's still no agreement as to why this is the case, except a general acceptance of a probable link between *BRCA* genes, sex hormones (such as estrogen), and DNA damage [95].

4.3.5 PARP Inhibitors for People with Inherited *BRCA* Gene Mutations and Breast or Ovarian Cancer

So far, I've said that both BRCA and PARP proteins are involved in DNA repair. PARP enzymes are important for the repair of single-strand DNA breaks. BRCA proteins are involved in HR, an error-free method of repairing double-strand breaks. But you might be asking yourself: What does this have to do with PARP inhibitors?

Well, it seems that when a healthy cell is exposed to a PARP inhibitor (such as olaparib, rucaparib, niraparib, or talazoparib) it survives. But, if the cell is completely missing one of its BRCA proteins, then exposure to a PARP inhibitor is enough to kill it. In someone with an inherited *BRCA* gene mutation, it's only their cancer cells that are completely missing one of their BRCA proteins, and so it should be only these cells that die (see Figure 4.11).

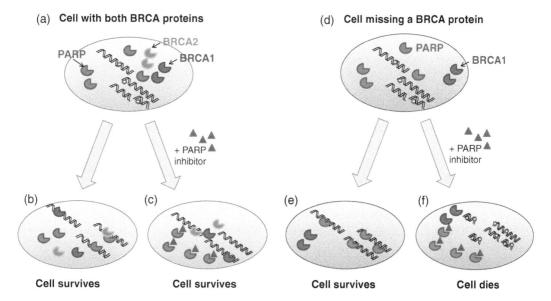

Figure 4.11 **PARP inhibitors kill cells that are missing one of their BRCA proteins.** **(a)** The blue oval represents the nucleus of a healthy cell, in which you find PARP and both BRCA proteins (and all the other proteins necessary for DNA repair). This cell's DNA is constantly getting damaged (represented by yellow spiky circles and broken black DNA strands). **(b)** Single-strand breaks are repaired by a PARP-dependent process; double-strand breaks are repaired using HR, which depends on BRCA proteins. **(c)** Exposing the cell to a PARP inhibitor (red triangles) prevents it from repairing single-strand breaks, which ultimately become double-strand breaks. However, double-strand breaks are repaired using HR, and the cell survives. **(d)** The burgundy oval represents the nucleus of a cancer cell in a person who has inherited a *BRCA* gene mutation (in this case affecting *BRCA2*). This cell contains PARP, but it is completely missing the BRCA2 protein. With only BRCA1 left, the cell cannot perform HR. This has led the cell to become genomically unstable, which has ultimately caused it to become a cancer cell. **(e)** When the cancer cell sustains damage to its DNA, it repairs the damage using PARP (to repair single-strand breaks) or non-homologous end joining (NHEJ) to repair double-strand breaks, and this is sufficient to keep the cell alive. **(f)** If the person is treated with a PARP inhibitor, this prevents all their cells from using PARP to repair single-strand breaks. These breaks ultimately become double-strand breaks, which the person's cancer cells can only repair using an error-prone method such as NHEJ. The cell quickly accumulates critical levels of DNA damage, and the cell dies. The other cells in their body, which still retain a healthy copy of the affected *BRCA* gene, can perform sufficient HR to stay alive (not shown).
Abbreviations: BRCA1/BRCA2 – BRCA1/BRCA2, DNA repair associated; HR – homologous recombination; NHEJ – non-homologous end joining; PARP – poly(ADP-ribose)polymerase.

Scientists often refer to the use of PARP inhibitors in people with cancers linked to faulty *BRCA* genes as an example of "synthetic lethality." They're referring to the fact that a combination (a synthesis) of the cancer cells' inability to perform HR plus exposure to a PARP inhibitor causes them to die.

Inherited pathogenic (i.e., disease-causing) mutations in either *BRCA1* or *BRCA2* are found in around:[93]

- 2%–5% of people with breast cancer (up to 20% in patients with triple-negative breast cancer)
- 10%–15% of people with ovarian cancer

These are the proportions of people with known pathogenic variants in a *BRCA* gene. What does get rather confusing is the sheer number of variations in *BRCA* genes that have been discovered. Over 3000 different variations on *BRCA1* and *BRCA2* have been found in the human population, and we don't know the significance of all of them [96]. For some of them, it's very clear-cut and the inherited variant clearly puts the person at a high risk of cancer. But for other variants it's much less easy to tell whether they're dangerous mutations or harmless variations. These variants are usually referred to as variants of uncertain significance (VUS).

4.3.6 PARP Inhibitors for Ovarian Cancers in People Who Haven't Inherited a *BRCA* Gene Mutation

I've hopefully established why PARP inhibitors are effective against breast and ovarian cancers in which the cells are missing one of their BRCA proteins and therefore can't perform HR. This is the reason why some of the first PARP inhibitor trials only included patients with inherited *BRCA* gene mutations. However, the important thing here is not that the cancer cells lack a BRCA protein, but that they can't perform HR. In fact, although roughly 10%–15% of ovarian cancers occur in people with inherited *BRCA* gene mutations, in around 50% of ovarian cancers, the cancer cells can't perform HR (Figure 4.12) [97, 98].

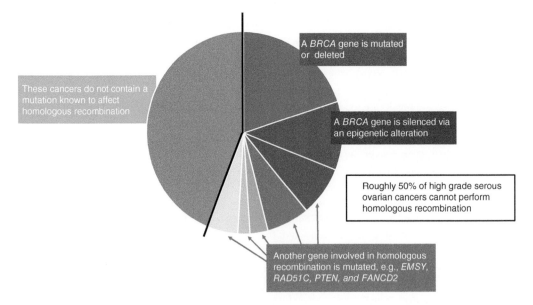

Figure 4.12 Roughly half of high-grade serous ovarian cancers can't perform homologous recombination. This is due to a defect in a *BRCA* gene or suppression of a *BRCA* gene, or due to a mutation in another gene involved in the process.
Abbreviation: BRCA – BRCA, DNA repair associated.

This is either due to inherited (germline) mutations affecting genes involved in HR, or due to mutations that have occurred during the person's lifetime (somatic mutations).

Several large trials have included both people with HR-deficient (HRD) and HR-proficient ovarian cancers. The results from these trials clearly show that it's the patients with HRD cancers who benefit the most from PARP inhibitors (see Figure 4.13 for an example of one of these trials) [99–101].

There's also a link between sensitivity to platinum-based chemotherapy and PARP inhibitors. These chemotherapies (such as cisplatin and carboplatin) work by causing DNA breaks. Cells unable to perform HR have difficulty repairing this damage. So, HR deficiency is a cause of sensitivity to both platinum-based chemotherapy and to PARP inhibitors [102]. Because of this, if a patient's cancer is sensitive to platinum-based chemotherapy, this suggests it will also be sensitive to a PARP inhibitor.

4.3.7 PARP Inhibitors as Treatments for Other Cancers

So far, I've talked about giving PARP inhibitors to people with breast or ovarian cancer who have an inherited *BRCA* gene defect, and to a wider group of people whose ovarian cancers are HR-deficient.

But they also have wider application: [103–107]

- They have been approved as a treatment for people with pancreatic cancer who have an inherited *BRCA* mutation (this accounts for about 4%–7% of people diagnosed with pancreatic cancer [108]).

- They have also been approved as a treatment for prostate cancer if there is a germline (an inherited mutation) or somatic (a non-inherited mutation found just in the cancer cells) mutation in a *BRCA* gene or in another gene involved in homologous recombination. These mutations are found in roughly 20% of cases of metastatic prostate cancer [109].

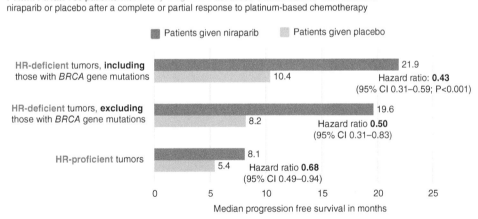

Figure 4.13 People with HR-deficient cancers benefit more from PARP inhibitors than people with HR-proficient cancers. Data from the PRIMA trial demonstrate that this is the case whether the HR defect is due to a *BRCA* gene mutation or another defect in the HR process. Patients with HR-proficient cancers still gained some benefit with the PARP inhibitor (niraparib) but the benefit wasn't as great as for patients with HR-deficient cancers, as shown by the longer progression free survival time.

Abbreviations: BRCA – BRCA, DNA repair associated; CI – confidence interval; HR – homologous recombination; PARP – poly(ADP-ribose)polymerase.

Table 4.6　Summary of licensed PARP inhibitors as of March 2024 (listed in alphabetical order; information taken from the FDA, EMA, and MHRA).

Drug	Licensed for:
Niraparib	• Ovarian cancer in people who have responded to platinum-based chemotherapy
Olaparib	• Ovarian cancer in people with a germline or somatic *BRCA* gene mutation, and for people whose ovarian cancer is sensitive to platinum-based chemotherapy • Breast cancer and pancreatic cancer in people with a germline *BRCA* mutation • Prostate cancer in people with a germline or somatic mutation in a *BRCA* gene or other HR gene • Pancreatic cancer in people with a germline *BRCA* gene mutation
Rucaparib	• Ovarian cancer in people who have responded to platinum-based chemotherapy • Prostate cancer in people with a germline or somatic mutation in an HR gene
Talazoparib	• Breast cancer in people with a germline *BRCA* mutation • Prostate cancer if the cancer has a mutation in an HR gene

Abbreviations: BRCA – breast cancer associated; EMA – European Medicines Agency; FDA – US Food & Drug Administration; HR – homologous recombination; MHRA – The Medicines and Healthcare products Regulatory Agency; NSCLC – non-small cell lung cancer.

• They might also be helpful for people with other cancers that contain a *BRCA* mutation or that are HR-deficient for another reason, such as cancers containing mutations in *ATM, ATR, PALB2,* or the *FANC* gene family (all these genes are involved in HR) [107]

• They are also in trials for cancers that are sensitive to platinum-based chemotherapy, or in combination with an immune check-point inhibitor.

Four PARP inhibitors have so far been licensed as cancer treatments either in the United States or Europe/the United Kingdom (listed in Table 4.6).

4.3.8 Biomarkers of Response to PARP Inhibitors

As I've outlined earlier, there are various situations that can cause a person to develop a cancer that is (probably) sensitive to treatment with a PARP inhibitor:

• When the person has inherited a mutation in a *BRCA* gene (a germline mutation).

• When mutations that have occurred during the person's lifetime (somatic mutations) have caused them to develop a cancer in which a BRCA protein is missing.

• When germline or somatic mutations (other than *BRCA* gene mutations) have led to a cancer in which the cancer cells are HR-deficient.

But that leaves the question of how best to test for these various scenarios and therefore predict who is going to benefit from a PARP inhibitor and who won't.

There are several potential methods: [103]

1. Test for germline BRCA mutations using healthy cells from a blood or saliva sample.

2. Test for somatic BRCA mutations using cancer cells from a biopsy or other tumor sample.

3. Test for various mutations in a range of genes involved in HR such as A*TM, ATR, PALB2,* and *FANC* genes.

4. Measure the cancer cells' ability to perform HR.

5. Look for patterns of DNA damage indicative of a defect in HR.

6. Look at the cancer's sensitivity to platinum-based chemotherapy.

7. Test for mutations that cause resistance to PARP inhibitors.

The most common methods used to select people to receive PARP inhibitor treatment are to test for various germline or somatic mutations, to look for patterns of DNA damage, or to use platinum sensitivity.

4.3.9 Resistance Mechanisms to PARP Inhibitors

For some people given a PARP inhibitor as an add-on treatment after surgery for ovarian cancer, the PARP inhibitor successfully prevents their cancer from coming back [110]. However, as with virtually all cancer treatments, some people's cancers are inherently resistant to PARP inhibitors (intrinsic resistance), and other peoples' cancers respond to treatment initially and then start growing again (acquired resistance).

Reasons for resistance to PARP inhibitors can be split into two groups: mechanisms of resistance that involve the restoration of the cells' ability to perform HR and mechanisms that don't involve the restoration of HR [111].

Examples of Mechanisms that Involve Restoration of HR

- Sometimes an additional mutation can restore the cell's ability to produce a protein (such as a BRCA protein) that it had initially lost the ability to make.
- Sometimes a more subtle, epigenetic change to an HR gene can restore the production of the missing protein.

Examples of Mechanisms that Don't Involve Restoration of HR

- In some people, their cancer cells reduce their dependence on whatever HR protein is missing or not working by switching to alternative repair mechanisms.
- The cells might have upped their production of PARP proteins or might be making mutated PARP proteins that can't be blocked by PARP inhibitors.
- Sometimes cancer cells expel a drug just as quickly as it enters, and they avoid the drug's effects.

4.3.10 Overcoming Resistance to PARP Inhibitors

The most common strategies to overcome resistance to PARP inhibitors appear to be to give them in some sort of combination, for example: [103]

- Combining a PARP inhibitor with chemotherapy or radiotherapy.
- Combining a PARP inhibitor with a targeted therapy such as a WEE1 inhibitor (Section 4.4.6), PI3K inhibitor (Section 3.8.3), or an angiogenesis inhibitor (Section 4.1).
- Combining a PARP inhibitor with an immune checkpoint inhibitor.
- Combining a PARP inhibitor with a hormone therapy (for people with prostate cancer).

However, so far none of these combination strategies has become an approved treatment option.

4.4 CDK INHIBITORS AND OTHER CELL CYCLE-TARGETED TREATMENTS

Licensed drugs mentioned in this section:		
Treatment class	**Drugs**	**Given to some people with:**
CDK4/6 inhibitors	Palbociclib, ribociclib, and abemaciclib	• Breast cancer
	Trilaciclib	• Small cell lung cancer

We now turn our attention to a group of treatments that target the cell cycle: the step-by-step series of events our cells go through when they multiply (see Figure 4.14 for an overview of the process) [112].

Many of you might have learned about the cell cycle in biology classes or during an undergraduate degree. Or you might have learned about it when being taught how various forms of chemotherapy exert their effects.

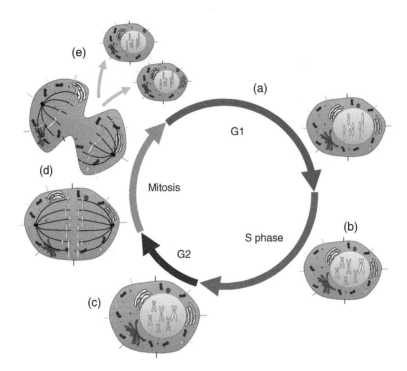

Figure 4.14 The cell cycle in a human cell. (a) The first stage in the cell cycle is G1, during which the cell grows bigger and duplicates many of its proteins and other contents, such as the Golgi body, endoplasmic reticulum, and mitochondria. **(b)** In S phase, the cell replicates all 46 of its chromosomes so that it now has a duplicate set, which exist in the cell as sister chromatids. **(c)** In G2 phase, the cell checks its new chromosomes for mistakes and prepares for mitosis. **(d)** In mitosis, the sister chromatids line up on a newly made protein structure called the spindle. The spindle fibers then retract, and the chromatids are pulled apart. **(e)** The cell finally splits into two to create two identical cells, each with a full set of chromosomes.

However, although many chemotherapies work by targeting one or more aspects of the cell cycle, they kill any cell that is multiplying, and they are therefore relatively nonspecific (see Figure 4.15 for the points in the cell cycle they commonly target).

To create more precise drugs that target the cell cycle, scientists have investigated exactly what parts of the cell cycle have gone wrong in cancer cells. They have focused much of their attention on a group of enzymes called cyclin-dependent kinases (CDKs). CDKs are a group of kinases that control a cell's transition from one phase of the cell cycle to the next (see Figure 4.16). The focus of scientists on CDKs is for a couple of reasons: (1) Several CDKs are overactive in many different cancer types, and (2) being kinases, they have a binding site for ATP that can be blocked with a kinase inhibitor [115, 116].

4.4.1 CDKs that Control the Cell Cycle

As you can see in Figure 4.16, CDKs are controlled by a second group of proteins called the cyclins. Different cyclins are made by cells as they enter each stage of the cycle. In turn, the cyclins activate various CDKs and the cell cycle continues [112].

When a cyclin attaches to a CDK, this causes the CDK to become active. CDKs, like all kinases, can attach phosphate chemical groups (phosphorus atoms surrounded by oxygen atoms) to a target. In the case of CDKs, their

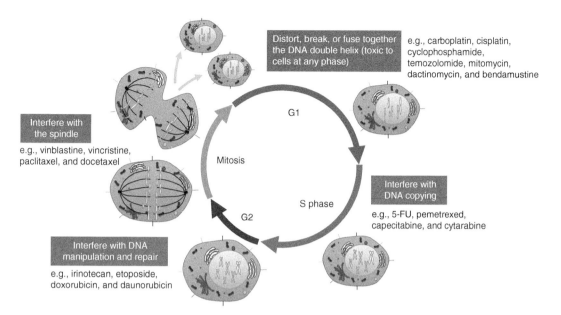

Figure 4.15 Chemotherapies often kill cells that are at certain stages of the cell cycle. *Source:* Adapted from [113, 114].
Abbreviation: 5-FU – 5-fluorouracil.

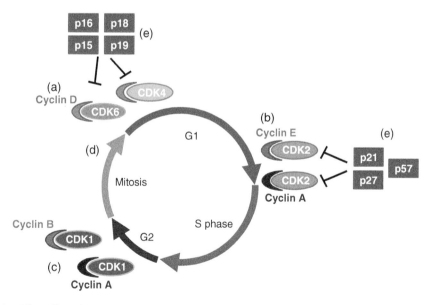

Figure 4.16 The cell cycle is controlled by CDKs, cyclins, and CDK inhibitors. (a) When a cell receives a signal to enter the cell cycle, it responds by producing cyclin D (shown as an orange crescent). Cyclin D activates two CDKs: CDK4 and CDK6, which cause the cell to enter the G1 phase of the cell cycle.
(b) The cell then produces two more cyclins, cyclin E and cyclin A, which activate CDK2. Activated CDK2 tells the cell to enter S phase and duplicate its chromosomes. **(c)** When all the cell's chromosomes have been copied and checked for mistakes, CDK1 becomes active due to the actions of cyclin A and cyclin B, and the cell enters mitosis. **(d)** Finally, once cyclin B has been destroyed, the cell can split in two. **(e)** If something goes wrong with the cell cycle, the cell will halt its progress through the cycle using a series of proteins that function as CDK inhibitors, such as p16, p15, p18, p19, p21, and p27.
Abbreviation: CDK – cyclin-dependent kinase.

most important target is a tumor suppressor protein called retinoblastoma protein (RB).

When RB doesn't have any phosphates attached to it, it clings to a group of transcription factors called the E2F proteins, and this blocks the cell from entering the cell cycle. But when RB is phosphorylated by CDKs, it lets go of E2F proteins (Figure 4.17). When E2F proteins are free of RB, they trigger the production of numerous proteins that force the cell into the cell cycle. As the cell moves through the cell cycle, more CDKs attach more phosphates to RB, making sure that the E2F proteins are free to drive the cell cycle through each of its stages [116].

The cell cycle is a vital process that enables us to grow, to replace dead cells, to heal wounds, and to replace cells that brush off from the surface of our skin and the lining of our gut. It is also vital that our white blood cells multiply when fighting off infections. However, it's also vital that our cells only enter the cell cycle under strict conditions, so that they don't become cancer cells. Also, if

something goes wrong during the cell cycle, it's essential that our cells can stop the process and put right whatever is awry. As a result, the cell cycle is very tightly regulated: CDKs are subject to numerous controls, and there are many additional checks and balances.

CDK inhibitors exert control over CDKs. CDK inhibitors are a set of proteins produced by our cells when they need to halt, or prevent, the cell cycle. They include proteins such as p16, p15, p18, p19, p21, and p27 (these proteins also get called $p16^{INK4a}$, $p15^{INK4b}$, $p18^{INK4c}$, $p19^{INK4d}$, $p21^{CIP1}$, and $p27^{KIP1}$) (see Figure 4.16e). Scientists have also discovered how to make small molecule drugs that block CDKs, and these also are referred to as CDK inhibitors.

4.4.2 Other CDKs

In all, our cells produce around 20 different CDK proteins [115]. Many of these proteins control the cell cycle, such as CDK4, CDK6, CDK1, and CDK2. However, some of them have completely different functions.[13] For example, CDK8, CDK7, CDK9, and CDK11

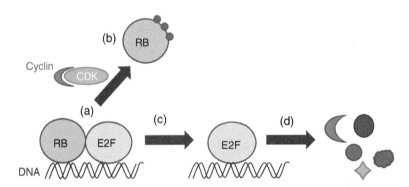

Figure 4.17 CDKs phosphorylate RB. (a) In a cell that isn't multiplying, RB and E2F sit together on the cell's DNA. **(b)** When the cell receives a signal to enter the cell cycle, the cell's CDKs become active due to the presence of cyclin proteins. Active CDKs phosphorylate RB. **(c)** Once phosphorylated, RB can no longer hold onto E2F and it lets go. **(d)** Free E2F proteins (which are transcription factors) then trigger the transcription of numerous genes, causing the cell to make proteins that force it through the cell cycle. **Abbreviations:** CDK – cyclin-dependent kinase; RB – retinoblastoma protein.

---

[13] Scientists believe that gene duplication is one of the driving forces of evolution and the creation of new species. There are many examples of where our genome (and that of other species) contains many different versions of a gene. These versions have evolved separately to take on different functions over time [117].

are part of the general transcription machinery that our cells use to read the information in our genes and make mRNA (which is then used to make proteins). CDK5 has numerous functions, including an important role in nerve cells (neurons) [115].

There are a couple of consequences to this complexity:

1. It can make it difficult to create CDK inhibitors that truly only affect the cell cycle.
2. If you block too many CDKs, you will affect many different cell functions. This can lead to unexpected, severe toxicities.

4.4.3 Why Cell Cycle CDKs Are Overactive in Cancer Cells

Various CDKs that control the cell cycle (most importantly, CDK4 and CDK6) are overactive in cancer cells for a variety of reasons: [116, 118–122]

1. Overactivity of signaling pathways controlled by growth factors. Both the MAPK pathway and the PI3K/AKT/mTOR pathway can force cells to produce cyclin D and cause the cell to enter the cell cycle (Figure 4.18a). As we learned in Chapter 3, these pathways are overactive in most cancers.

2. Amplification[14] of cyclin D genes (usually *CCND1*) is common in many cancers, causing the cells to produce high levels of cyclin D (usually cyclin D1) protein (Figure 4.18b). (There are three different versions of cyclin D, called cyclin D1, D2, and D3.) Cancers in which this has been found include head and neck cancer, breast cancer, NSCLC, esophageal cancer, malignant melanoma, endometrial cancer, pancreatic cancer, and glioblastoma.

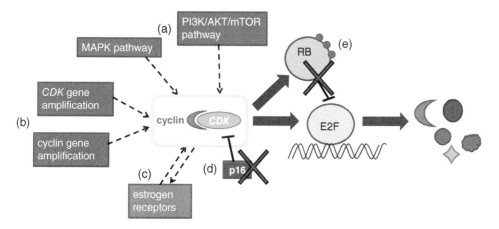

Figure 4.18 Reasons why CDKs are overactive and E2F proteins are uncontrolled in cancer cells.
(a) Signaling pathways such as the MAPK and PI3K/AKT/mTOR pathways are overactive in the majority of cancers, leading to increased production of cyclin D. **(b)** Many cancers contain extra copies of the genes for cyclins or CDKs, leading to increased production of these proteins. **(c)** The majority of breast cancers contain estrogen receptors, which force the cell to produce high levels of cyclin D1. In turn, cyclin D1 boosts the actions of estrogen receptors. **(d)** Many cancers lack important CDK inhibitors such as p16. **(e)** In some cancers, RB is missing, meaning that there is nothing to block E2F activity.
Abbreviations: CDK – cyclin-dependent kinase; MAPK – mitogen-activated protein kinase; mTOR – mammalian target of rapamycin; PI3K – phosphatidylinositol 3-kinase; RB – retinoblastoma protein.

---

[14] Amplification is when a cell has accidentally made extra copies of a gene.

3. Overproduction of CDK4, CDK6, cyclin E1, or cyclin E2 (Figure 4.18b). The genes for these proteins are amplified in many cancers, leading to high levels of the corresponding protein. Cancers in which this has been found include sarcomas, malignant melanoma, and esophageal, head and neck, uterine, ovarian, liver, breast, and bladder cancers.

4. Overproduction of cyclin D1 caused by the activity of estrogen receptors. Most breast cancers contain estrogen receptors. The estrogen receptor is an estrogen-sensitive transcription factor that triggers the transcription of many genes, including the cyclin D1 gene (*CCND1*). In return, cyclin D1 boosts the activity of estrogen receptors, reinforcing the link between the two proteins (Figure 4.18c).

5. Loss of p16 due to its gene (called *CDKN2A*) being either deleted or mutated. Loss of p16 leads to uncontrolled CDK4 and CDK6 activity (Figure 4.18d). Cancers in which this has been found include those of the pancreas, bladder, breast, prostate, stomach, head and neck, and in glioblastoma and melanoma.

6. A chromosome translocation is forcing the cells to produce high levels of cyclin D1. A translocation[15] between chromosomes 11 and 14 is found in the vast majority of mantle cell lymphomas (a type of non-Hodgkin lymphoma (NHL)). The translocation forces the cell to produce high levels of cyclin D1. The same translocation, and other translocations that force overproduction of cyclin D1, is often found in myeloma.

In addition, many cancers lack RB, which means that E2F proteins are overactive irrespective of what the cell's CDKs are doing (Figure 4.18e). Cancers in which this has been found include lung, ovarian, prostate, uterine, and bladder cancer.

Cyclin D controls the activity of CDK4 and CDK6 (usually abbreviated to CDK4/6). So, although cyclin D is unappealing as a drug target (there's no easy pocket to slot a drug into), it can be targeted indirectly by targeting CDK4/6 with a kinase inhibitor that blocks both proteins. (However, in cells that lack RB, a CDK4/6 inhibitor will have no effect.)

4.4.4 CDK4/6 Inhibitors as Cancer Treatments

When scientists set out to create CDK inhibitors, the first set of drugs they created were relatively unselective and blocked many CDKs (referred to as pan-CDK inhibitors). These drugs have limited usefulness because of the severe side effects they cause [116, 123].

Instead, the recent focus has been on CDK4/6 inhibitors, particularly as treatments for hormone receptor (HR)-positive breast cancers, which contain high levels of estrogen receptors [120–122]. Estrogen receptors force breast cancer cells to grow, multiply, and survive, partly by triggering cyclin D1 production.

Three CDK4/6 inhibitors, ribociclib, palbociclib, and abemaciclib, are licensed treatments for people with HR-positive breast cancer. Abemaciclib is the least specific of the three drugs and also blocks other kinases [121]. All three drugs are given in combination with hormone therapy to get the most out of both types of drugs (see Figure 4.19).

Although CDK4/6 inhibitors are primarily given as treatments for HR-positive breast cancer, they've also been investigated in trials involving people with an enormous range of different cancers. Most of these trials have given disappointing results, and only a handful of large trials in cancers other than HR-positive breast cancer are ongoing.

The one exception to this focus on breast cancer is the FDA approval in 2021 for trilaciclib. This CDK4/6 inhibitor was approved as

---

[15] The precise translocation is t(11;14)(q13;q32).

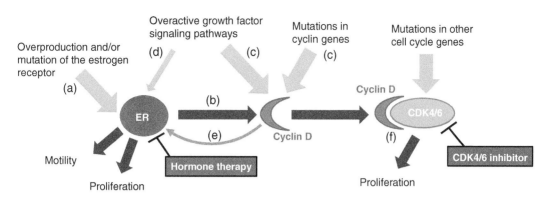

Figure 4.19 Combined hormone therapy + CDK4/6 inhibitor therapy for the treatment of HR-positive breast cancer. **(a)** Overproduction and overactivity of estrogen receptors (ERs) is a defining feature of HR-positive breast cancer. **(b)** ERs are transcription factors that activate >100 target genes, including the gene for cyclin D1 (*CCND1*) [124]. **(c)** Cyclin D production is also increased due to mutations in cyclin genes (such as *CCND1*) and the activity of growth factor-controlled signaling pathways. **(d)** Growth-factor controlled signaling pathways also enhance the activity of ERs. **(e)** Cyclin D also enhances the activity of ERs. **(f)** Cyclin D activates CDK4 and CDK6 causing entry into the cell cycle and cell proliferation. **Abbreviations:** ER – estrogen receptor; CDK – cyclin-dependent kinase; HR – hormone receptor. *Source:* Adapted from [125, 126].

a way of lessening the immune-suppressing effects of chemotherapy in patients with small cell lung cancer [127]. The idea is that the CDK4/6 inhibitor will halt white blood cells during the cell cycle and protect them from chemotherapy's toxic effects. However, there are concerns the drug might protect cancer cells from the effects of chemotherapy too and that there might be better ways of protecting white blood cells [128]. In fact, a large clinical trial involving people with bowel cancer was halted early. The researchers found that although trilaciclib protected patients' white blood cells, people receiving a placebo (rather than trilaciclib) did better in terms of tumor shrinkage and survival times [129].

4.4.5 Resistance to CDK4/6 Inhibitors

There are various reasons why an HR-positive breast cancer might keep growing despite treatment with a CDK4/6 inhibitor or becomes resistant after an initial response [121, 122, 130]. Many of these mechanisms involve

proteins involved in the cell cycle (summarized in Figure 4.20).

Other reasons for resistance include mutations and overactivity of proteins involved in growth factor-controlled signaling pathways, and the activation of Aurora kinase, an enzyme important for mitosis [121, 131].

The most common idea being explored to overcome resistance to CDK4/6 inhibitors is to use them in some sort of combination. They are being investigated combined with treatments such as chemotherapy, WEE1 inhibitors (see below for more on these treatments), signaling pathway inhibitors (e.g., MEK, mTOR, AKT, or PI3K inhibitors), or with immunotherapy [130, 132].

4.4.6 Treatments that Target Other Cell Cycle Proteins

Many proteins involved in the cell cycle are overproduced, overactive, or dysfunctional in cancer cells. However, only a few of them can be exploited as potential treatment targets [123, 133]. As ever, the most promising

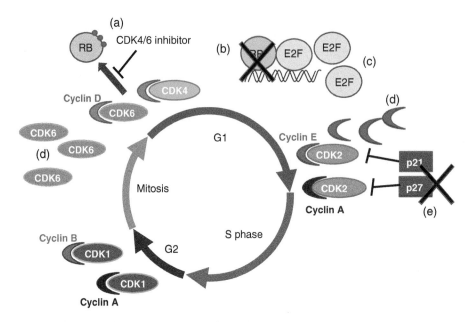

Figure 4.20 Mechanisms of resistance to CDK4/6 inhibitors. **(a)** CDK4/6 inhibitors work by blocking CDK4 and CDK6 and preventing them from phosphorylating RB. **(b)** However, if RB isn't present, perhaps because both of the cell's copies of the *RB* gene are deleted or suppressed, then a CDK4/6 inhibitor will have no impact on the cell. **(c)** Similarly, overproduction of E2F overwhelms the available RB. **(d)** Another cause of resistance is if the cell overproduces cyclin E or CDK6, or **(e)** if it lacks the CDK inhibitors, p21 or p27. **Abbreviations:** CDK – cyclin-dependent kinase; RB – retinoblastoma protein.

targets are kinase enzymes, as these are generally the most straightforward to block with a suitable small molecule.

Kinases involved in the cell cycle include all the CDKs, checkpoint kinase 1 (CHK1), CHK2, WEE1, polo-like kinase-1 (PLK1), and Aurora kinases.

CHK1 and WEE1 are involved in cell cycle checkpoints [134]. These are points in the cell cycle when the cell stops, checks itself, and makes sure that it only continues through the cycle if everything has gone well so far. CHK1 and WEE1 inhibitors allow faulty cells to continue through the cycle despite having accumulated lots of DNA damage. Eventually (so the theory goes) the cell accumulates so much damage that it dies.

PLK1 and the Aurora kinases play essential roles in mitosis and in the mobility of cells and cancer metastasis [135]. They are often overproduced by cancer cells.

All these kinases have been explored as potential treatment targets, and numerous small molecule inhibitors have been investigated in clinical trials (see Table 4.7). However, reading through research articles on these drugs makes for underwhelming reading, with lack of effectiveness and side effects being common problems. Also, a quick check on the clinical trials database, ClinicalTrials.gov (which lists thousands of trials going on around the world), reveals relatively few active trials, and none of these treatments has yet been approved for use.

Another potential cell cycle target (but not a kinase) is *Ataxia telangiectasia* and *Rad3*-related (ATR). This protein is activated by DNA damage and halts the cell cycle at the G2/M transition. The first ATR inhibitor was created in 2011. As with CHK1 and WEE1 inhibitors, the idea behind ATR inhibitors is that they will force unstable cancer cells with

Table 4.7 Cell cycle targets other than CDKs.

Target	Function	Examples of treatments
WEE1	Halts the cell cycle at the G2/M checkpoint (the boundary between the G2 phase and mitosis) in response to DNA damage. Present in high amounts in many cancers. Directly controls the activity of CDK1 and CDK2.	Adavosertib (AZD1775) and PD0166285
CHK1	Activated by ATR in response to DNA damage. Coordinates with WEE1 to prevent damaged cells from multiplying.	LY2606368
PLK1	Important for mitosis. It is necessary for various things that happen, such as creating the spindle (see Figure 4.14), separating duplicated chromosomes and cytokinesis – when the cell finally cleaves in two to create two new cells.	Rigosertib and volasertib
Aurora kinases	Important for entry into mitosis and progression through it (in a similar way to PLK1).	Alisertib, ENMD-2076, danusertib, and AMG-900
ATR	Required for cells to halt the cell cycle in response to DNA damage.	Berzosertib, ceralasertib, gartisertib, tuvusertib, elimusertib, and camonsertib

Source: Adapted from [133, 134, 136–139].

damaged DNA to multiply and then die due to excessive DNA damage [136].

In addition to the targets listed in Table 4.7, many more cell cycle proteins are being investigated by scientists as possible drug targets [123].

4.5 HEDGEHOG PATHWAY INHIBITORS

Licensed drugs mentioned in this section:		
Treatment class	Drugs	Given to some people with:
Smoothened inhibitors	Glasdegib, sonidegib, and vismodegib	• Acute myeloid leukemia • Basal cell carcinoma (a non-melanoma skin cancer)

In Chapter 3, I mentioned lots of drugs that block growth factor receptors and cell

signaling pathways such as the MAPK pathway and the PI3K/AKT/mTOR pathway. However, many other proteins and pathways influence how cells behave and influence whether they survive.

One such pathway is the Hedgehog pathway (so named because fruit fly larvae in which the Hedgehog pathway is faulty are balled up and extra bristly [140]). This pathway is highly active in mammalian embryos. It helps ensure that we have two arms, two legs, two eyes, and so on. It also helps our cells move and makes sure they all end up in the right place [140]. In addition to being vital for developing embryos, the pathway is also active in *adult* stem cells[16] in the skin, hair follicles, brain, bone marrow, prostate, bladder, and other locations [141]. Lastly, the Hedgehog pathway is activated when we get injured – it activates repair pathways and helps tissues regenerate [140].

Faults in various proteins involved in the Hedgehog pathway have been found in the

---

[16] Adult stem cells are rare cells found in many of our organs and tissues. When they multiply, they create specialized cells of different types. They replace dead cells and help our tissues regenerate after sustaining damage.

cancer cells of basal cell carcinoma skin cancer, and medulloblastoma. The pathway is also overactive in other cancer cell types [142].

4.5.1 Components of the Hedgehog Pathway

The Hedgehog pathway involves two receptors, Patched and Smoothened, and a ligand called Hedgehog. As ever, there are multiple versions of each protein. For example, there are three Hedgehog proteins in our bodies: Sonic Hedgehog, Indian Hedgehog, and Desert Hedgehog.

The Patched receptor's default behavior is to block the activity of the Smoothened receptor. However, if a Hedgehog (Hh) protein is present, Patched is blocked, and it can't inhibit Smoothened any longer. As a result, Smoothened is now free to act, and it in turn activates GLI transcription factors (see Figure 4.21 for an overview). Genes controlled by GLI transcription factors include many oncogenes, such as the genes for cyclin D1, Myc, and Bcl-2 [142–144].

4.5.2 Hedgehog Pathway Inhibitors

Almost all Hedgehog pathway inhibitors work by blocking Smoothened. The first Hedgehog pathway inhibitor discovered by scientists was a molecule called cyclopamine. This chemical is found in a poisonous plant common in the United States called the California false hellebore[17] (*Veratrum californicum*). In the 1950s, scientists in Idaho discovered that sheep that ate this plant often gave birth to lambs with only one eye (hence its name – cyclopamine) [145].

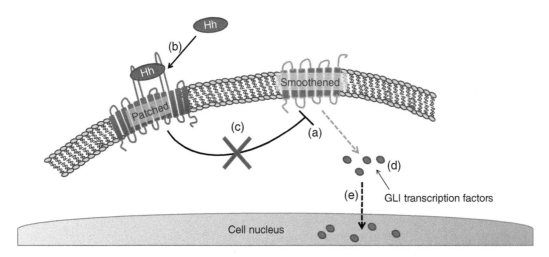

Figure 4.21 The basics of the hedgehog signaling pathway. (a) In the absence of Hh proteins, the Patched receptor blocks the hedgehog pathway by suppressing Smoothened (another receptor).
(b) Hh proteins attach to Patched. (c) With Hh attached to it, Patched no longer blocks Smoothened, and Smoothened becomes active. (d) Increased Smoothened activity indirectly leads to the activation of GLI transcription factors. (e) These transcription factors enter the cell's nucleus, attach to numerous genes, and switch on the production of various proteins, including cyclin D1, Myc, and Bcl-2, which encourage the cell to survive and multiply.
Abbreviations: GLI – glioma associated; Hh – Hedgehog.

---

[17] It's also sometimes called the Californian corn lily.

Cyclopamine fits into a channel in the Smoothened protein. Other Smoothened inhibitors (such as vismodegib and sonidegib) fit into other pockets and grooves in Smoothened [146].

4.5.3 Smoothened Inhibitors as Treatments for Basal Cell Carcinoma and Medulloblastoma

Mutations that activate the Hedgehog pathway are extremely common in two cancer types: basal cell carcinoma skin cancer (BCC) and medulloblastoma.

BCC is the most common type of skin cancer. BCCs tend to be slow growing and can usually be surgically removed before they have spread; as a result, they cause few deaths. However, if BCC does spread, or if it's in a location where surgery isn't possible, such as on someone's face, then it can be much harder to treat [147]. Around 90% of BCCs have mutations in either the gene for Patched or that for Smoothened [148]. Smoothened inhibitors such as vismodegib and sonidegib have both proved to be helpful treatments for BCC in large clinical trials and are licensed both in the United States and in Europe (including the United Kingdom). However, drug resistance and side effects are a problem for many patients. The immune checkpoint inhibitor (see Chapter 5 on checkpoint inhibitors), cemiplimab, has become an important treatment option for people with BCC, especially if they can't have a Smoothened inhibitor, or if they've already had one and their cancer has spread [149].

Medulloblastomas are rare brain tumors that tend to be aggressive and fast growing; they affect more children than adults. Around 70%–75% of children are cured with standard treatments, but at the expense of many long-term side effects [150]. Around 25%–30% of medulloblastomas contain mutations affecting the Hedgehog pathway and are known as the SHH-subtype [151]. Hedgehog inhibitors have been put through trials involving children and adults with SHH-subtype medulloblastomas. Although patients' tumors do shrink to begin with, they quickly become resistant [150]. Another problem is the drugs' inability to efficiently cross the blood-brain barrier and penetrate the tumor tissue [152].

4.5.4 Broadening the Uses of Hedgehog Inhibitors

Hedgehog inhibitors are being explored as treatments for various cancer types for a number of different reasons:[142]

1. As described earlier, Hedgehog pathway inhibitors can help people with BCC or medulloblastoma whose cancers are driven by mutations affecting the Hedgehog pathway. This includes being helpful for people with basal cell nevus syndrome (also called Gorlin-Goltz syndrome), which is caused by an inherited mutation[18] in the gene for Patched [153]. People with Gorlin-Goltz syndrome tend to develop lots of BCCs and other tumors. Trials in these patients (patients with mutations affecting the Hedgehog pathway) have given the best results achieved with Hedgehog pathway inhibitors so far.

2. In other cancers, the Hedgehog pathway is overactive despite there being no mutation affecting the pathway. Sometimes this is because there is autocrine activation of the Hedgehog pathway. "Autocrine activation" means that the same cell both produces a

[18] The mutation might be inherited from an affected parent, or the mutation might have taken place in a single egg or sperm, or in a newly fertilized embryo.

ligand and has the receptors to respond to it. For example, in some bowel cancers, the cancer cells overproduce Hedgehog proteins, and they have Patched and Smoothened receptors, which enable them to respond to it.

3. More commonly, there is paracrine activation of the Hedgehog pathway. "Paracrine activation" means that one cell produces the ligand, but a different, nearby cell responds to it. For example, in pancreatic cancer, the cancer cells produce lots of Hedgehog proteins but don't have Patched or Smoothened receptors. In this instance, Hedgehog activates the Hedgehog pathway in nearby, non-cancer cells, such as epithelial cells, fibroblasts, and white blood cells. Scientists have found paracrine Hedgehog signaling in small cell lung cancer, pancreatic cancer, bowel cancer, metastatic prostate cancer, melanomas, and glioblastoma [148]. However, trials of Hedgehog pathway inhibitors in these cancers have been disappointing so far.

4. The final reason to block the Hedgehog pathway is because it is active in cancer stem cells. Writing anything about cancer stem cells is fraught with problems because no one can agree what a "cancer stem cell" is [154]. However, as I mentioned in Chapter 1, some cancers seem to contain a population of cells that have some of the properties of healthy stem cells, can survive chemotherapy and radiotherapy, and cause a cancer to regrow even if most of its cells have been killed. One cancer in which this theory seems to hold weight is acute myeloid leukemia (AML). Hedgehog signaling is active in leukemic stem cells, and in 2018 glasdegib (a Smoothened inhibitor) was approved by the US FDA as a treatment for some patients with AML in combination with chemotherapy [155].

Because the Hedgehog pathway is active in many different types of cancer, scientists and doctors initially hoped that inhibitors of this pathway would turn out to be useful treatments for lots of people. But, as with many treatments developed in the past, the reality seems to be that they only work against a few cancer types where there is a clear reason for strong activation of the pathway. And, as ever, side effects and treatment resistance limit their uses [156].

4.6 TARGETING EPIGENETIC ENZYMES

Licensed drugs mentioned in this section:		
Treatment class	**Drugs**	**Given to some people with:**
DNA methyltransferase inhibitors	Low dose azacitidine or decitabine	• Acute myeloid leukemia • Myelodysplastic syndromes[a]
EZH2 inhibitors	Tazemetostat	• Epithelioid sarcoma • Follicular non-Hodgkin lymphoma
Isocitrate dehydrogenase (IDH) inhibitors	Ivosidenib, enasidenib, and olutasidenib	• Acute myeloid leukemia • Cholangiocarcinoma • Myelodysplastic syndromes
Histone deacetylase inhibitors	Belinostat, vorinostat, panobinostat, and romidepsin	• Peripheral T cell lymphomas • Cutaneous T cell lymphomas • Myeloma

[a] There are an enormous number of different blood cancers and other diseases caused by faulty blood cells. If you want to learn more about them, I suggest taking a look at the Blood Cancer UK website: bloodcancer.org.uk.

Back in Chapter 1, I started explaining epigenetics. I said that the term refers to chemical additions to the surface of the DNA double helix and to histone proteins. These changes control how tightly packed DNA is, and how accessible its information is to the cell [157].

It's useful to remember that there's around two meters of DNA inside every cell in our body. That DNA must be packaged up to make it manageable for the cell. The first layer of packaging is that the DNA strand is wrapped around histone proteins. A length of DNA wrapped around a set of eight histone proteins is called a nucleosome.[19] Nucleosomes are then coiled, stacked, and looped together to form chromosomes [158].

4.6.1 Epigenetic Control of Our Genes

Genes contain crucial information telling cells how to make proteins. If a gene's DNA is tightly packed, the cell can't access its information, and it can't make the corresponding protein (or proteins). But if a gene is loosely packaged, with the nucleosomes nicely spaced out, the gene's information is far more accessible.

Proteins called epigenetic regulators control the packaging of DNA by making tiny chemical (epigenetic) changes to DNA and to various histone proteins.

When the DNA, and the histone proteins it's wrapped around, have methyl chemical groups attached to them, the nucleosomes pack tightly together (Figure 4.22a). If these methyl groups are removed and acetyl groups are added instead, the structure relaxes (Figure 4.22b). These changes control whether genes in the area are active or inactive (i.e., whether they can be used to make proteins or not) [159].

4.6.2 Epigenetics and Cancer

This might sound relatively straightforward, and yet it's not! Over 700 epigenetic regulators control when, where, why, and what small chemical groups (methyl, acetyl, and many others) get attached to DNA and

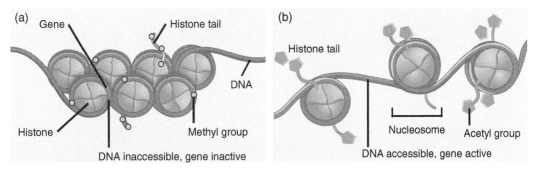

Figure 4.22 **Epigenetic modifications to DNA and histone proteins alter the activity of genes**. **(a)** The addition of methyl groups to DNA and histone proteins causes nucleosomes to pack tightly together. This makes the DNA inaccessible to transcription factors, and the genes in the region cannot be used to make proteins. **(b)** The addition of acetyl groups (acetylation) of histone proteins loosens the packing of nucleosomes and allows them to spread out along the DNA. The DNA in the area is now accessible to transcription factors, which trigger gene transcription and translation, leading to the production of proteins. *Source:* Creative Commons Attribution License (by 4.0) Authors: OpenStax, Copyright Holders: Rice University https://commons.wikimedia.org/wiki/File:Figure_16_03_02.png.

---

[19] For an incredible animated video on how nucleosomes come together and are then packaged into chromosomes, see https://www.youtube.com/watch?v=gbSIBhFwQ4s.

histone proteins, and when they are removed. Mutations affecting virtually all these proteins have been found in cancer cells [160].

Of course, the impact of any change in activity of an epigenetic enzyme is going to depend on which genes become active, or inactive, as a result. Epigenetic enzymes affect every aspect of cell behavior because they affect every gene. There is also an interplay between the genetic mutations and epigenetic alterations found in cancer cells (see Figure 4.23a & b) [161, 162].

One aspect of epigenetics that excites scientists is that epigenetic changes are reversible (depicted by turquoise arrows in Figure 4.23a, f & g). Methyl groups can be removed as well

as added, as can acetyl groups, and other epigenetic modifications to DNA and histone proteins. This is in stark contrast to gene mutations – once a C has been changed to a G, or a chromosome has broken and been wrongly repaired, there's no going back (Figure 4.23c & d).

This reversibility of epigenetic changes paved the way for scientists to create drugs that alter the activity of epigenetic enzymes. Their reasoning being that, for example, if an overactive methylator is preventing the transcription of tumor suppressor genes, then a suitable inhibitor could reverse this (Figure 4.23e).

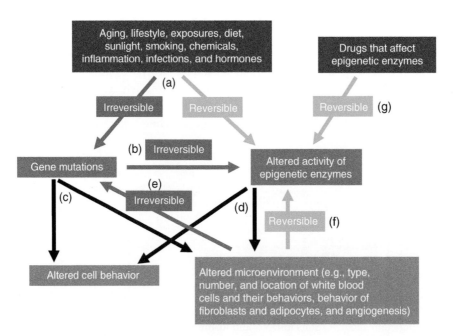

Figure 4.23 The relationship between gene mutations and epigenetic alterations in cancer. (a) Many factors, such as aging processes, exposures, and lifestyle, can cause gene mutations and epigenetic changes. In the case of gene mutations, these changes are irreversible. However, epigenetic changes are temporary and potentially reversible. (b) Sometimes a gene mutation affects the gene for an epigenetic enzyme, permanently altering the activity of the corresponding protein. (c) Gene mutations affect the cell's behavior and impact its microenvironment, as do (d) the altered activity of epigenetic enzymes. (e) Molecules released in the microenvironment, such as oxygen free radicals produced by white blood cells, can increase the rate of mutations in cells. (f) The behaviors of cells such as fibroblasts, and the presence of various proteins, nutrients, and oxygen levels, all (reversibly) alter the activity of epigenetic enzymes in cells. (g) Scientists have developed drugs that block the activity of some epigenetic enzymes, such as DNA methyl transferase (DNMT) and histone deacetylase (HDAC) inhibitors.

4.6.3 Treatments that Target Epigenetic Enzymes

Despite the complexities of epigenetics and the myriad of ways it is defective in cancer cells, we do have some licensed treatments that work by blocking some of the enzymes involved (see Table 4.8 for details). But, as with treatments that target nuclear transport (see Section 4.9), it is virtually impossible to know exactly why any of these treatments works.

DNA Methyltransferase Inhibitors

DNA methyltransferase (DNMT) inhibitors include azacitidine and decitabine. These drugs mimic cytosine (a DNA base) and become incorporated into the cell's DNA and RNA. Once there, the drugs chemically bond with DNMT enzymes, trapping them in place and preventing them from methylating (i.e., adding methyl groups to) DNA and RNA. These drugs are therefore referred to as "hypomethylating agents" (because they prevent methylation, the cell's DNA and RNA become under-[hypo-]methylated). However, the attachment of a protein (in this case DNMT) to DNA is also incredibly toxic to cells; it

leads to double-strand DNA breaks that can trigger cell death [164].

DNMT inhibitors are licensed as treatments for AML. There's lots of evidence to suggest that faulty epigenetic enzymes are important in AML and that these faults happen early in the disease's development. For example, mutations in genes for various epigenetic enzymes are common in AML cells (e.g., mutations affecting *IDH1*, *IDH2*, *DNMT3A*, *ASXL1*, and *TET2*) [160, 165].

The fact that DNMT inhibitors such as azacitidine and decitabine are helpful treatments for AML may be due to the faults in epigenetic enzymes found in this disease. But, as with other treatments that affect epigenetic enzymes, it's hard to know exactly what's going on [160]

EZH2 Inhibitors

The EZH2 protein is the enzyme part of a larger protein called PRC2, which is a histone methyltransferase. PRC2 adds methyl groups to a histone protein, leading to the suppression of various genes. The cells of NHLs such as follicular lymphoma and diffuse large B cell

Table 4.8 Commonly altered epigenetic enzymes in cancer cells and some of the drugs that target them.

Target	Drugs	Stage of development (in the United States and/or Europe/the United Kingdom)
DNMT1, 3A, and 3B: These enzymes attach methyl groups to cytosines in DNA	Azacitidine and decitabine ("hypomethylators")	Approved for AML and myelodysplastic syndromes
EZH2: Attaches methyl groups to lysine 27 in the histone-3 protein	Tazemetostat	Approved for follicular lymphoma with *EZH2* mutations and for epithelioid sarcoma
IDH1 and IDH2: When mutated, these enzymes create 2-HG, which cause increased DNA and histone methylation	Ivosidenib, enasidenib, vorasidenib, and olutasidenib	AML, myelodysplastic syndrome, or cholangiocarcinoma containing an *IDH1* or *IDH2* (AML only) gene mutation
HDAC enzymes: Remove acetyl groups from histones and from various cytoplasmic proteins	Vorinostat, belinostat, panobinostat, entinostat, mocetinostat, and romidepsin	Myeloma, peripheral T cell lymphomas, and cutaneous T cell lymphomas

Source: Adapted from [159, 160, 163].
Abbreviations: AML – acute myeloid leukemia; DNMT – DNA methyltransferase; EZH2 – enhancer of zeste homolog 2; HDAC – histone deacetylase; IDH – isocitrate dehydrogenase; TET2 – tet methylcytosine dioxygenase 2.

lymphoma sometimes contain an *EZH2* gene mutation. These mutations increase PRC2 activity and heighten the suppression of genes. Tazemetostat is an EZH2 inhibitor approved for people with follicular lymphomas that contain *EZH2* mutations [166].

IDH1 and IDH2 Inhibitors

One set of epigenetic modifiers whose mechanism of action is (slightly) easier to understand is the isocitrate dehydrogenase -1 (IDH1) and IDH2 inhibitors, which include ivosidenib and olutasidenib (which block IDH1), enasidenib (which blocks IDH2), and vorasidenib (which blocks IDH1 and IDH2 and has better brain penetration [167]).

These treatments seem most effective against cancers that contain mutations in the *IDH1* or *IDH2* genes (see below for details). The IDH1 and IDH2 proteins made from these genes are enzymes that indirectly reduce DNA and histone methylation. When they're mutated, their actions change, and they increase methylation. After that, their mechanism of action once again gets hazy, as the consequences of methylation are diverse and context dependent. Also, IDH1 and IDH2 enzymes affect cell metabolism as well as methylation, making the impact of IDH inhibitors even harder to unpick [160, 168, 169].

Cancers with *IDH2* or *IDH2* mutations include the following: [169, 170]
- 80% of low-grade gliomas (slow-growing brain tumors)
- 15%–20% of AML and myelodysplastic syndrome
- 15%–20% of intrahepatic cholangiocarcinomas (occur within bile ducts in the liver)
- 50%–90% of chondrosarcomas (bone cancers that develop from faulty cells in the cartilage)

So far, IDH inhibitors are approved treatments for people with *IDH1*- or *IDH2*-mutated AML, myelodysplastic syndrome, or cholangiocarcinoma. Whether it's helpful to target IDH enzymes in people with chondrosarcoma is still unclear [169]. Vorasidenib, an IDH1 and

IDH2 inhibitor able to penetrate brain tissue, looks promising as a treatment for people with *IDH*-mutated, low-grade glioma [171].

HDAC Inhibitors

Histone deacetylase (HDAC) inhibitors (such as panobinostat, belinostat, vorinostat, and romidepsin) prevent acetyl groups from being removed from histone proteins. The idea is that when the histones' acetyl groups are intact, the DNA is relaxed, and genes for tumor suppressor proteins are active. These proteins are then thought to do helpful things like preventing further cell growth and encouraging cells to specialize rather than multiply. But no one actually knows if this is why HDAC inhibitors work.

There are 11 different HDAC enzymes in our cells, and they remove acetyl groups from many proteins in the cell cytoplasm as well as from histones in the nucleus. So, no one can say whether HDAC inhibitors' effects on tumor suppressor genes are responsible for their impact. It might be their impact on cytoplasmic proteins that is responsible for their effects [160].

Despite all the complexity I have outlined earlier, epigenetic enzymes are still promising as targets for new cancer treatments. But it's important to remember how complicated the system is: the vast number of epigenetic regulators, the many different influences on them, and the many ways in which they impact cell behavior. This makes the results from each trial difficult to interpret or improve on.

4.7 TARGETING CELL SURVIVAL

Licensed drugs mentioned in this section:		
Treatment class	**Drugs**	**Given to some people with:**
Bcl-2 inhibitors	Venetoclax	• Chronic lymphocytic leukemia • Acute myeloid leukemia

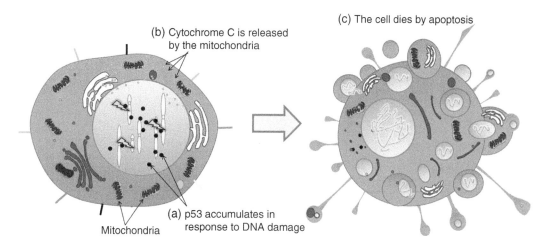

Figure 4.24 **Cells can trigger their own death using a process called apoptosis. (a)** If a cell sustains irreparable DNA damage (depicted by yellow lightning bolts), this leads levels of p53 to increase. When levels of p53 rise, it triggers the production of apoptosis-causing proteins such as PUMA and NOXA. **(b)** PUMA, NOXA, and other proteins cause the cell's mitochondria to release their stores of cytochrome C. **(c)** Cytochrome C activates caspase enzymes, which chop up all the cell's proteins and internal structures. The cell fragments and dies.

One of the things that normally protects us from cancer is that our cells have an inbuilt ability to trigger their own death if things go wrong. The main mechanism through which cells self-destruct is called apoptosis, or programmed cell death (Figure 4.24). But, as I described in Chapter 1, cancer cells' apoptosis machinery is faulty. This means they stay alive despite having numerous problems, like a lack of oxygen, containing lots of DNA damage, and receiving negative messages from their neighbors, such as "don't multiply" or "please die."

Apoptosis, like the cell cycle, is a step-by-step series of orderly events. Only, at the end of it, the cell dies rather than multiplies. Controlling the process of apoptosis are the Bcl-2 family of proteins. There are numerous family members, some of which prevent apoptosis and some of which cause it (see Table 4.9) [172, 173].

Confusingly, there are at least 16 different members of the Bcl-2 family of proteins in human cells. It's taken scientists several decades to work out the details of them and to use this knowledge to create cancer treatments.

Table 4.9 Some Bcl-2 family members cause apoptosis, while others protect against it.

Bcl-2 family member	Function
Bcl-2, Mcl-1, Bcl-X$_L$, and Bcl-W	**Inhibit apoptosis**
BAX and BAK	Cause apoptosis
BIM, BID, and PUMA	Cause apoptosis by activating BAX and BAK. Sometimes referred to as "Activator BH3-only proteins".
BAD, NOXA, BMF, BIK, and HRK	Cause apoptosis by inhibiting Bcl-2, Mcl-1, Bcl-X$_L$, and Bcl-W Sometimes referred to as "Sensitizer BH3-only proteins".

Source: Adapted from [172, 173].

4.7.1 Bcl-2 Protects Cancer Cells from Apoptosis

One of the most common ways that cancer cells avoid death is by producing high levels of apoptosis-suppressing proteins like Bcl-2 and/or its close relatives Mcl-1 and Bcl-X$_L$. These proteins prevent apoptosis by blocking BAX and BAD and preventing cytochrome C release (Figure 4.25) [174].

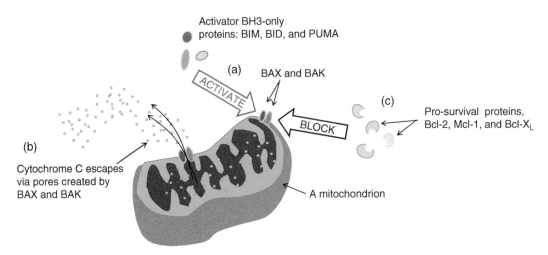

Figure 4.25 Bcl-2 protects cells from apoptosis. **(a)** BAX and BAK cause apoptosis. They are activated by BIM, BID, and PUMA. When activated, BAX and BAK come together and form pores in the outer surface of the cell's mitochondria. **(b)** Cytochrome C exits the mitochondria through the pores and triggers apoptosis. **(c)** Pro-survival proteins such as Bcl-2 prevent BAX and BAK from forming pores and so prevent apoptosis.

Bcl-2 was first discovered in the cells of people with follicular lymphoma (a type of B cell NHL). In this cancer, a chromosome translocation causes massive overproduction of Bcl-2 [175]. The cells of chronic lymphocytic leukemia (CLL), myeloma, diffuse large B cell lymphoma (DLBCL), mantle cell lymphoma, acute lymphoblastic leukemia, and some solid tumors also contain high levels of Bcl-2 [175–177]. In some cancers, it is not Bcl-2 that protects the cancer cells from apoptosis but another protein such as Mcl-1, or there's a lack of BAX or BAK [175].

4.7.2 Mechanism of Action of Bcl-2 Inhibitors

Scientists have tried various approaches to block Bcl-2. The approach that has so far proved most useful is to create drugs that directly interact with Bcl-2 and prevent it from blocking apoptosis. These drugs are known as "BH3 mimetics" because they mimic the BH3 domain[20] found in naturally occurring, BH3-only proteins (Figure 4.26).

The first Bcl-2 inhibitor to become an approved cancer treatment is a drug called venetoclax. This treatment was approved for people with CLL in 2016, and for people with AML in 2021. A quick search on clinicaltrials.gov (the vast trials database) reveals well over a hundred ongoing clinical trials with venetoclax. These include various treatment combinations for patients with CLL or AML, as well as numerous trials involving patients with diseases such as myeloma, chronic myeloid leukemia, or mantle cell lymphoma.

Various other Bcl-2 inhibitors are in trials, including a related compound called navitoclax [178]. There are also drugs that target other Bcl-2 family members that protect against apoptosis, such as Bcl-X_L and Mcl-1 [179]. All of these treatments appear to be much less effective against solid tumors compared to their impact on hematological cancers [180].

---

[20] Its full name is the Bcl-2 homology domain-3.

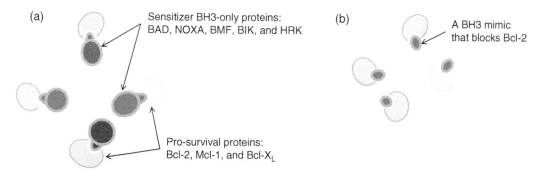

Figure 4.26 Bcl-2 inhibitors mimic the BH3-only domain. (a) Some BH3-only proteins encourage damaged cells to undergo apoptosis by blocking the actions of survival proteins such as Bcl-2. (b) Bcl-2 inhibitors do the same by mimicking the shape of the BH3-only domain.

4.7.3 How Else Can We Trigger Apoptosis?

Death Receptor Agonists

Cells undergo apoptosis when they contain too much, or too severe, DNA damage. But they also undergo apoptosis when told to do so by other cells, or in response to other triggers. To facilitate this, our cells have so-called "death receptors" on their surface. Treatments that trigger these receptors (called death receptor agonists) include monoclonal antibodies that activate death receptor-4 (DR4) and DR5 [181].

p53-targeted Treatments

TP53 (the gene for making p53 protein on chromosome 17) is mutated in at least half of all human cancers [182]. It normally helps our cells respond appropriately to DNA damage – by either provoking cells to repair the damage or die. In cancer cells, either the p53 protein is missing, or a mutated p53 protein is present. Instead of triggering apoptosis, the mutant protein is distorted and protects against cell death rather than causing it.

Normally, we only have small amounts of p53 in our cells because it's constantly being destroyed thanks to a protein called MDM2.

But, when the cell's DNA is damaged, p53 levels rise.

There are two main strategies being explored to raise levels of normal p53 protein in cancer cells to a point where they trigger apoptosis:[182]
- Prevent p53 from being destroyed by creating MDM2 inhibitors
- Create drugs that attach to distorted versions of p53 and restore them to their proper shape

Treatments in both categories are in clinical trials.

"Inhibitor of Apoptosis Protein" Antagonists

Inhibitor of apoptosis proteins (IAPs) are a group of proteins that share a part of their structure called the baculovirus IAP repeat (BIR) domain. As you might guess from their name, these proteins can block apoptosis and they're overproduced by a range of different cancers [183]. Treatments that block IAPs generally work by mimicking the shape of another protein called Smac.[21] However, IAP inhibitors don't appear to be able to help cancer patients if given on their own. Instead, it looks like they could be useful if given in combination with another treatment such as

---

[21] To confuse matters, Smac's other name is DIABLO – direct inhibitor of apoptosis-binding protein with low pI.

chemotherapy, radiotherapy, or a combination of the two – chemoradiotherapy. A treatment called xevinapant is the furthest along in trials. Most of the ongoing trials are investigating it as a treatment for people with head and neck cancer [184].

4.8 TARGETING B CELL RECEPTOR SIGNALING

Licensed drugs mentioned in this section:		
Treatment class	**Drugs**	**Given to some people with:**
Irreversible BTK inhibitors	Ibrutinib, acalabrutinib, and zanubrutinib	• Chronic lymphocytic leukemia • Mantle cell lymphoma • Waldenstrom macroglobulinemia • Marginal zone lymphoma
Reversible BTK inhibitors	Pirtobrutinib	• Mantle cell lymphoma • Chronic lymphocytic leukemia
PI3K-delta inhibitors	Idelalisib, copanlisib, and duvelisib	• Chronic lymphocytic leukemia • Follicular lymphoma
CD79b-targeted antibody-drug conjugate	Polatuzumab vedotin	• Diffuse large B cell lymphoma

In Section 2.2 (and Figure 2.4), I introduced you to antibodies and to B cell receptors (BCRs). I said that each B cell generally has around 100,000 copies of a unique BCR sticking out from its surface. Figure 4.27 shows the structure of a single BCR. Each BCR is made up of an antibody, which is tethered to the B cell's surface by two proteins called CD79a and CD79b. To be clear, what we refer to as "the BCR" is actually a group of three proteins, one of which is an antibody.

4.8.1 The Normal Function of BCRs
To understand why drugs that block BCR-controlled signaling pathways are used as cancer treatments, it's useful to know a bit more about them:[185, 186]

• When a B cell's BCRs connect with an antigen (often something found on the surface of a bacteria or virus), they cluster together and trigger various signaling pathways inside the cell that involve many different kinases (Figure 4.28).

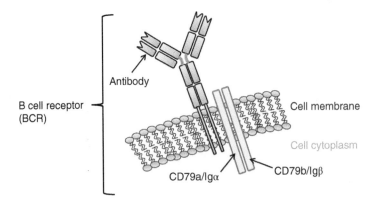

Figure 4.27 **The B cell receptor (BCR).** The BCR is made up of an antibody (also known as an immunoglobulin – Ig), tethered to the surface of the B cell by two proteins known as CD79a and CD79b (also known as Igα and Igβ) that span the cell membrane.

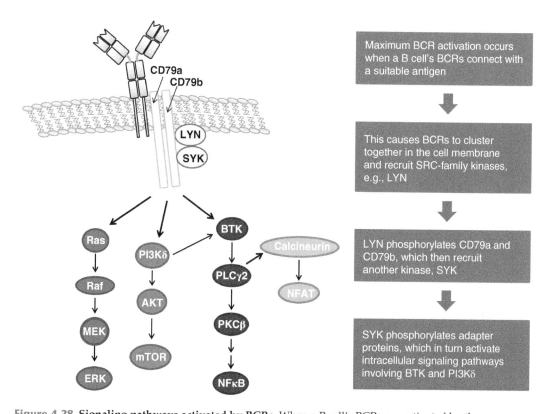

Figure 4.28 Signaling pathways activated by BCRs. When a B cell's BCRs are activated by the presence of an antigen, they trigger the activation of various signaling pathways inside the cell. This activation is mediated via kinases (such as LYN and SYK) that associate with CD79a and CD79b. In addition to being activated by antigens, low-level (tonic) activity of the BCR is necessary for cell survival.

Abbreviations: BCR – B cell receptor; BTK – Bruton tyrosine kinase; ERK – extracellular signal-regulated kinase; mTOR – mechanistic target of rapamycin; NFAT – nuclear factor of activated T cells; NFκB – nuclear factor-kappa-B; PI3K – phosphoinositide 3-kinase; PKCβ – protein kinase C-beta; PLCγ – phospholipase C-gamma; SFK – SRC family kinase.

- Like the signaling pathways controlled by growth factor receptors, these signaling pathways can cause B cells to grow, multiply, stay alive, and specialize (among other things).
- BCR-controlled signaling pathways involve many of the same proteins that cause cell growth, survival, and proliferation in solid tumors, such as Ras, Raf, MEK, AKT, mTOR, and NFκB.
- BCRs also activate proteins that are vitally important only to white blood cells, such as BTK and the δ (delta) form of PI3K

(in solid tumors, it's more likely to be PI3Kα or PI3Kβ that is overactive).
- All our B cells (not just ones activated by an antigen) need a bit of tonic (i.e., low-level) BCR signaling to keep them alive.
- Many of the proteins controlled by BCRs (including BTK, PI3Kδ, and SYK) are also activated by various other cell surface receptors.
- Unlike the growth factor receptors mentioned in Chapter 3, BCRs aren't kinases, so you can't block them with a kinase inhibitor.

- In many cancers that develop from faulty B cells, the cancer cells still depend on BCR-controlled signaling to keep them alive.

4.8.2 How BCR Signaling Goes Wrong in Cancer Cells

In addition to being essential for the survival and activation of healthy B cells, the BCR is also essential for the survival of many B cell leukemias and lymphomas. Sometimes, BCR signaling is overactive because of mutations in the cells' DNA. For example, the cancer cells of a type of NHL called "activated B cell-like diffuse large B cell lymphoma" (ABC DLBCL) often contain mutations in the genes for CD79a or CD79b. In other cancers (such as CLL), the BCRs on the surface of the person's cancer cells are essentially normal. However, the BCRs have mistakenly been activated by normal proteins on the surface of nearby cells (these proteins are generally referred to as autoantigens, and they don't normally activate BCRs) [185, 186].

What scientists have now realized is that in each type and subtype of B cell cancer, the BCR seems to play a slightly different role. For example, ABC DLBCL cells rely on BCR signaling for their survival. But in a different type of DLBCL – germinal center B cell-like DLBCL (GCB DLBCL) – only a very low level of BCR signaling takes place, and blocking BCR signaling generally has no effect [185, 186]. Table 4.10 briefly summarizes what we know about BCR signaling in various B cell cancers.

Table 4.10   BCR signaling in various B cell cancers.

Cancer type	Subtype	Level of BCR signaling in cancer cells
Non-Hodgkin lymphoma (NHL)	ABC DLBCL	• High level of BCR signaling • BCRs are often mistakenly responding to an autoantigen • Mutations affecting CD79b or CD79a also amplify signals generated by activated BCRs
	GCB DLBCL	• Cancer cells rely on tonic, low-level activity of BCRs, which primarily activates the PI3K-AKT-mTOR pathway but not BTK • BCRs have not responded to antigen and are not clustered together on the cell surface
	Burkitt's lymphoma	• Cells may rely on tonic signaling for survival (similar to GCB DLBCL)
	Follicular lymphoma	• High level of BCR signaling • The cells' BCRs are often mistakenly responding to an autoantigen on the surface of neighboring cells, or to a protein found in the cells' environment
	Mantle cell lymphoma	• High level of BCR signaling • BCRs are often mistakenly responding to an autoantigen
	Marginal zone lymphoma	• The cells' BCRs are often mistakenly responding to an autoantigen and/or an infection (viral or bacterial) in the cells' environment
Chronic lymphocytic leukemia (CLL)		• High level of BCR signaling • BCRs are often mistakenly responding to one, or commonly to more than one, autoantigen – these are often proteins or other complex molecules found on the surface of macrophages or on cells undergoing apoptosis • BCRs may be responding to antigens from bacteria, viruses, or fungi
Hodgkin lymphoma		• No BCR signaling
Myeloma		• BCR is not present; no BCR signaling
Waldenstrom macroglobulinemia		• Mutations affecting BCR signaling are common • BCR signaling is important

Source: Adapted from [185, 186].
Abbreviations: ABC – activated B cell-like; BCR – B cell receptor; BTK – Bruton tyrosine kinase; DLBCL – diffuse large B cell lymphoma; GCB – germinal center B cell-like.

4.8.3 The Effects of Blocking BCR-Controlled Signaling

Drugs that block signaling pathways controlled by BCRs have two main effects: [186]

1. They can cause cancer cells to stop multiplying or die. This is a direct effect of blocking BCR signaling. The impact that the drug has will depend on how dependent the cancer cells were on their BCRs for survival.

2. They cause cancer cells to detach from the cells around them and move into the blood, where they die off. This is an indirect effect of these drugs. Kinases such as BTK, PI3Kδ, and SYK are activated by many different types of receptors found on white blood cells, including ones that control cell movement and adhesion.

4.8.4 BTK Inhibitors

Ibrutinib was the first BTK inhibitor developed. It is an irreversible inhibitor that chemically binds to an amino acid (a cysteine at position 481 in the BTK protein). This cysteine sits inside BTK's ATP-binding pocket (remember that BTK is a kinase, and it therefore needs ATP to phosphorylate its targets).

Ibrutinib has proven to be a very useful treatment, but it isn't very selective. In addition to blocking BTK, it also blocks at least nine other kinases, including ITK, TEC, BLK, JAK3, EGFR, and HER2. Some of this inhibition is responsible for side effects such as bleeding, rash, diarrhea, and atrial fibrillation [187].

Since the development of ibrutinib, many other BTK inhibitors have been developed and many of them are more selective for BTK (see Table 4.11 for information on just some of them). Some, like acalabrutinib, are similar to ibrutinib in that they are irreversible inhibitors that connect with cysteine 481. Others, such as pirtobrutinib, are reversible inhibitors that don't need cysteine 481 to be present to work [187].

BTK inhibitors are licensed treatments for some people with CLL, and for several forms of NHL (including Waldenström macroglobulinemia) (Table 4.12).

Resistance to BTK Inhibitors

Not everyone who is given a BTK inhibitor is helped by it. Also, some people whose cancer initially responds will later develop

Table 4.11 A comparison of BTK inhibitors.

	Type of inhibition	Potency against BTK	Selectivity for BTK	Can it overcome resistance mechanisms to ibrutinib?	
				Blocks C481S mutant?	Blocks PLCγ₂ signaling?
Ibrutinib	Irreversible; covalent	0.5 nM	Low	No	No
Acalabrutinib	Irreversible; covalent	5.1 nM	High	No	No
Spebrutinib	Irreversible; covalent	<0.5 nM	Low	No	No
Tirabrutinib	Irreversible; covalent	5.6 nM	High	No	No
Zanubrutinib	Irreversible; covalent	0.5 nM	Moderate	No	No
Nemtabrutinib	Reversible; non-covalent	0.85 nM	Low	Yes	Yes, indirectly
Pirtobrutinib	Reversible; non-covalent	0.85 nM	High	Yes	?
Vecabrutinib	Reversible; non-covalent	24 nM	Moderate	Yes	?

Source: Adapted from [187–192].
NB. Potency is given in terms of each drug's IC50; the lower the number, the more potent the drug. The mutation that creates a serine at position 481 (called the C481S mutation) is a common reason for resistance to ibrutinib, as are mutations that lead to overactivity of PLCγ₂.

Table 4.12 Licensed BTK inhibitors.

Drug	Licensed in the United States and/or Europe for:
Ibrutinib	CLL, mantle cell lymphoma, and Waldenström macroglubulinemia
Acalabrutinib	CLL and mantle cell lymphoma
Zanubrutinib	CLL, mantle cell lymphoma, marginal zone lymphoma, follicular lymphoma, and Waldenström macroglobulinemia
Pirtobrutinib	CLL and mantle cell lymphoma

Source: Adapted from [193, 194].
Abbreviations: CLL – chronic lymphocytic leukemia (also including small lymphocytic lymphoma).

resistance. Scientists have concluded that there are a variety of reasons for drug resistance, including the following: [185, 187, 191, 192]

1. Mutations affecting BTK. These often affect the cysteine at position 481 (C481) that ibrutinib and other covalent inhibitors attach to, turning it into a serine or other amino acid instead.
2. Mutations affecting PLCγ (a kinase activated by BTK): The mutations cause PLCγ to be active despite BTK being blocked.
3. Overactive PI3K-AKT signaling pathway.
4. Increased NFκB activity that is no longer dependent on BTK. NFκB is a powerful protein that promotes cell survival.
5. Increased activity of other signaling pathways that compensate for BTK being blocked.

Thankfully, the reversible, non-covalent BTK inhibitors (such as pirtobrutinib) can block some of the mutated forms of BTK that are resistant to ibrutinib and other covalent inhibitors.

4.8.5 PI3Kδ Inhibitors

I have already introduced PI3K and PI3K inhibitors in Section 3.8.3, but now I want to say more about PI3K inhibitors as treatments for people with hematological cancers.

About PI3Kδ

PI3Kδ (PI3K-delta) is activated by BCRs (see Figure 4.27). It is found in normal B cells, T cells, and NK cells, and it's also found in cancer-causing B cells [195]. The tonic, low-level activity of BCR signaling that keeps healthy B cells alive depends on PI3Kδ. It is also activated when BCRs respond to an antigen [196]. In addition to being activated by the BCR, PI3Kδ is also activated by other receptors found on the surface of white blood cells, such as chemokine receptors.

When it is activated, PI3Kδ (like other forms of PI3K) converts phosphatidylinositol 4,5-bisphosphate $(PIP_2)^{22}$ into phosphatidylinositol 3,4,5-triphosphate (PIP_3). PIP_3 then activates AKT.

PI3Kδ Inhibitors

As with BTK inhibitors, PI3Kδ inhibitors can block BCR signaling, and they interfere with the cancer cells' ability to home to lymph nodes, causing them to move into the blood [197]. These effects cause cancer cells to die.

Idelalisib was the first selective PI3Kδ inhibitor to be licensed as a treatment for people with CLL and B cell NHL. This was followed by copanlisib (a dual PI3Kα and PI3Kδ inhibitor), duvelisib (a dual PI3Kγ and PI3Kδ inhibitor), and umbralisib (a dual PI3Kδ and CK1ε inhibitor).

Since these approvals, problems with severe side effects and a high risk of infections have come to light. This has led to a series of warnings and withdrawals of drug approvals [198].

---

[22] PIP_2 is a small lipid molecule found in the cell membrane.

As a result, BTK inhibitors are given to many more people than PI3Kδ inhibitors.

4.8.6 Treatments that Target CD79b or Other Cell Surface Proteins

BTK and PI3Kδ are both intracellular proteins. To block them, you need a drug that easily enters cells and that can block intracellular targets. In contrast, CD79b, which is part of the BCR, is on the cell surface and is therefore accessible to antibody-based treatments. Another useful property of CD79b is that when antibody-based treatments attach to it, the cell membrane folds inward and both CD79b and the therapeutic antibody end up inside the cell [199, 200]. This is perfect for ADCs, as you want the ADC to end up inside the cell and release its chemotherapy payload.

So far, only one ADC targeting CD79b is licensed – called polatuzumab vedotin. It is a treatment for people with DLBCL (an aggressive form of B cell NHL) [201]. However, other ADCs are in trials, such as one currently called DCDS0780A [202]. There are also T cell engagers being developed that target both CD79b and CD3 (see Chapter 6 for more about T cell engagers) [203].

4.9 NUCLEAR TRANSPORT INHIBITORS

Licensed drugs mentioned in this section:		
Treatment class	Drugs	Given to some people with:
Exportin-1 inhibitors	Selinexor	• Myleoma

Cells make thousands of different proteins, and they're constantly moving them around. All proteins are manufactured by ribosomes in the cell cytoplasm, but some are needed in the nucleus, and others get transferred to the cell surface. Our cells therefore contain proteins that exist to transport other proteins to where they're needed, including taking them in and out of the nucleus.

4.9.1 Nuclear Transport and Cancer

The cell's nucleus, which contains its chromosomes, is separated from the rest of the cell by a "nuclear envelope." Embedded in this envelope are pores, which allow various things – proteins, amino acids, mRNAs, etc., to travel between the nucleus and the cytoplasm. Some things travel in and out by simple diffusion, but many are carried as cargo by proteins called "importins" and "exportins."

Sometimes the cargo being carried in or out of the nucleus is a tumor suppressor protein, or an oncogenic (cancer causing) protein. Depending on where in the cell the protein ends up, it is likely to have a different impact on the cell's behavior. For example, if a transcription factor (a protein that binds to DNA and switches genes on and off) ends up in the cytoplasm, it won't be able to do its job.

One of the most important exportins (a protein that transports cargo out of the nucleus) in our cells is a protein called Exportin-1 (it sometimes also gets called CRM1 – chromosomal region maintenance-1) (see Figure 4.29). This exportin possibly transports up to a thousand different proteins (including various tumor suppressor proteins and oncogenic proteins) and various types of RNA (ribosomal RNA, small nunclear RNA, messenger RNA, micro RNA, and transfer RNA) out of the nucleus and into the cytoplasm [204, 205].

Exportin-1 is overproduced by the cancer cells of many different cancer types and seems particularly important to hematological cancers [204]. Also, because it's an enzyme, scientists have been able to create small chemical compounds that block it. It has therefore been investigated as a potentially useful treatment target.

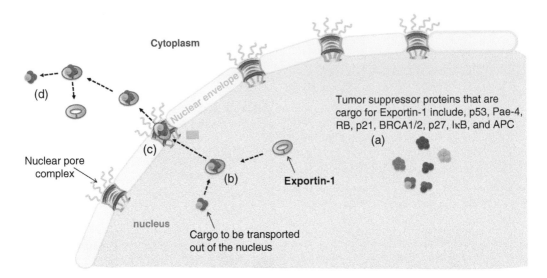

Cytoplasm

(d)

Nuclear envelope

(c)

Nuclear pore
complex

(b)

Exportin-1

nucleus

Cargo to be transported
out of the nucleus

Tumor suppressor proteins that are
cargo for Exportin-1 include, p53, Pae-4,
RB, p21, BRCA1/2, p27, IκB, and APC

(a)

Figure 4.29 Exportin-1 transports cargo proteins out of the nucleus via the nuclear pore complex.
(a) Cargo for Exportin-1 includes many proteins that are implicated in cancer, such as various tumor
suppressor proteins. **(b)** Cargo proteins are loaded onto Exportin-1 in the nucleus. **(c)** Exportin 1 carries
its cargo out of the nucleus and into the cytoplasm through the nuclear pore complex. **(d)** The cargo is
released in the cell cytoplasm.
Abbreviations: APC – adenomatous polyposis coli; BRCA – breast cancer associated; RB – retinoblastoma
protein.

4.9.2 Exportin-1 Inhibitors

Numerous Exportin-1 inhibitors have been
created [206]. But as of 2024, only one,
selinexor, had been licensed as a cancer treatment. The idea behind its use as a cancer
treatment is that by inhibiting Exportin-1, it
reactivates tumor suppressor proteins by
trapping them in the nucleus. But, seeing as
Exportin-1 probably transports over 1,000 proteins and large molecules out of the nucleus,
it's very difficult to say exactly why it has any
selectivity for killing cancer cells [204].

Clinical trials to investigate selinexor as a
treatment for solid tumors have mostly given
disappointing results, although there are some
signs of it being useful as a treatment for endometrial cancer [207]. However, it is an approved
treatment for people with myeloma – a cancer
of antibody-producing B cells – and for some
people with DLBCL. It's also being explored
as a treatment for people with some other
hematological cancers [205].

4.10 PROTEASOME INHIBITORS

Licensed drugs mentioned in this section:		
Treatment class	Drugs	Given to some people with:
Proteasome inhibitors	Bortezomib, carfilzomib, and ixazomib	• Myeloma • Mantle cell lymphoma

Proteasome inhibitors are primarily used as
treatments for people with myeloma, a cancer
of antibody-producing B cells called plasma
cells. Myeloma is very much a disease of older
age; the peak incidence rate is in people aged
85–89 years [208].

It is worth noting that proteasome inhibitors weren't deliberately created as cancer
treatments. In fact, prior to being tested for
cancer, bortezomib was first explored as a
treatment to prevent muscle wasting, and
later as an anti-inflammatory [209]. So, what

we know now about proteasome inhibitors' mechanisms of action has been pieced together after clinical trials proved them to be effective.

4.10.1 About the Proteasome

Proteasomes are hollow, cylindrical structures built from many separate proteins. They are found in the nucleus and cytoplasm of human cells. Their purpose is to break down proteins that have worn out, that haven't been made properly, or that the cell doesn't want [210].

One particularly mind-boggling fact that underlines the importance of proteasomes is that there's roughly a million of them inside each cell in our body [211].

Cells use their proteasomes to recycle unwanted and broken proteins, as their buildup is highly toxic. Proteasomes are also responsible for the orderly and precise destruction of proteins such as cyclins during the cell cycle. This is essential to ensure that the cell grows and splits into two healthy "daughter" cells [210]. In fact, our cells' proteasomes are vital for the day-to-day functioning of our cells,

and they have a role to play in virtually every process and change in behavior. They act as our cells' recycling units, breaking up old proteins and releasing their amino acids ready to make new ones [212] (Figure 4.30).

When a cell wants to destroy a protein, it first attaches multiple copies of a small protein called ubiquitin to it (this is a complicated process involving a variety of enzymes). The ubiquitin attached to the protein acts as a signal telling the proteasome that the protein needs destroying. When it has taken hold of a protein, the proteasome then unravels the protein and feeds it through its cylindrical core. This core has many enzyme sites, which chop up the protein and release its amino acids for reuse (see Figure 4.31).

4.10.2 The Actions of Proteasome Inhibitors

Proteasome inhibitors such as bortezomib, carfilzomib, ixazomib, marizomib, and oprozomib all work by blocking some of the proteasome's internal enzyme sites [212, 213]. Bortezomib, the first proteasome inhibitor ever

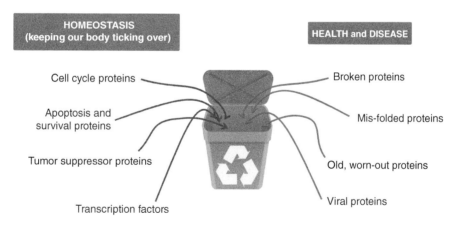

Figure 4.30 Proteasomes are our cells' recycling units. Proteasomes play a crucial role in helping our cells behave in an orderly and regulated fashion. At each junction in a cell's life – whether it wants to multiply, die, move, or simply stay alive – some proteins need to be destroyed (by proteasomes), and others made. Also, old, unwanted, damaged, and misfolded proteins need recycling. Additionally, if the cell should be infected by a virus, its proteasomes will chop up virus proteins as a means of self-protection. *Source:* Recycling bin image from Pixabay.

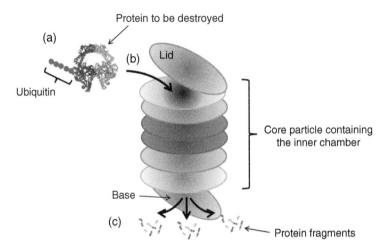

Figure 4.31 Protein destruction by a proteasome. **(a)** Proteasomes destroy proteins that have been labeled with multiple copies of a protein called ubiquitin. **(b)** The labeled protein attaches to the proteasome's lid. The proteasome then unfolds the protein and feeds it through its hollow, cylindrical core. Within this core are enzyme sites that chop up the protein. **(c)** Finally, tiny protein fragments (peptides) exit the proteasome from its base.

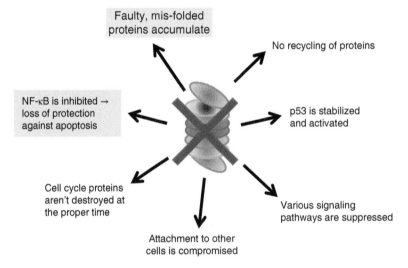

Figure 4.32 Possible reasons why proteasome inhibitors kill cancer cells. The relative importance and impact of each of these mechanisms is still unknown. The two mechanisms thought to be most important in the treatment of people with myeloma are highlighted in blue.
Abbreviation: NFκB – nuclear factor-kappa-B.

tested in clinical trials, is a reversible inhibitor, as is ixazomib. Carfilzomib and oprozomib are irreversible inhibitors.

The precise reason why proteasome inhibitors kill cancer cells is still controversial. However, they are known to have a variety of impacts on cells (summarized in Figure 4.32). One of the earliest mechanisms discovered was that proteasome inhibitors indirectly inhibit NFκB [213]. NFκB protects cells (particularly cancer cells) against apoptosis, so proteasome inhibitors encourage them to die.

Other potential mechanisms of action of proteasome inhibitors include the following: [213, 214]

• Causing the toxic accumulation of misfolded and broken proteins
• Causing the accumulation of cyclins at inappropriate stages of the cell cycle
• Causing the accumulation of p53, a powerful tumor suppressor protein able to trigger apoptosis (cell death)
• Activating the JNK cell signaling pathway, which also triggers cell death

Bortezomib was the first proteasome inhibitor to become a licensed treatment, and others have followed. I provide a summary of some of their properties in Table 4.13 [213].

As of 2024, bortezomib, carfilzomib, and ixazomib were licensed treatments (but not oprozomib, marizomib, or delanzomib).

4.10.3 Proteasome Inhibitors as Treatments for Myeloma

Proteasome inhibitors are often given to people with myeloma, usually as part of a combination with other treatments. Myeloma develops from plasma cells: antibody-producing B lymphocytes (B cells) of the immune system. Plasma cells are B cells that have undergone many adaptations that allow them to churn out thousands of copies of an antibody protein per second. Myeloma cells do the same. However, this constant production of antibody protein seems to overload the cell's proteasomes, which need to quickly recycle misfolded and broken antibodies to keep the cell alive. Proteasome inhibition, which leads to the rapid accumulation of misfolded antibody protein, can push the cells toward death [215].

4.10.4 Proteasome Inhibitors as Treatments for Other Cancers

In addition to being much used as a treatment for people with myeloma, bortezomib is also an approved treatment for people with mantle cell lymphoma, an aggressive type of non-Hodgkin lymphoma. As with myeloma, the precise mechanism of action and reasons why mantle cell lymphoma is sensitive to bortezomib aren't clear [216].

Table 4.13 A summary of the chemical and pharmacological properties of various proteasome inhibitors.

Drug	Chemistry and type of inhibition	Route of administration	Potency (IC50 in nM)	Half-life (minutes)
Bortezomib	A boronic acid drug; **reversible inhibitor**	IV, subcutaneous	5.7	110
Carfilzomib	An epoxyketone; **irreversible inhibitor**	IV	5	<30
Ixazomib	A boronic acid drug; **reversible inhibitor**	Oral	5.9	18
Oprozomib	An epoxyketone; **irreversible inhibitor**	Oral	6–12	30–90
Marizomib	A salinospore; **irreversible inhibitor**	IV	9.1	10–15
Delanzomib	A boronic acid drug; **reversible inhibitor**	Oral	5.6	62 hours

N.B. the precise mechanism of action of a boronic acid versus an epoxyketone is not what's important (at least, not for the purposes of this book). However, I did want to illustrate that some of these treatments are more closely related than others.
Abbreviation: IV – intravenous.

Proteasome inhibitors have also been explored as possible treatments for a wide variety of other types of cancer, including bone cancers, prostate cancer, ovarian cancer, acute lymphoblastic leukemia, and bladder cancer. However, although it's relatively easy to come up with logical reasons as to why proteasome inhibitors might be effective against any cancer type, the results of trials have often been disappointing [217].

4.11 FINAL THOUGHTS

In this chapter, I have discussed treatments that have various different targets and mechanisms of action.

First, we looked at angiogenesis inhibitors that block VEGF signaling. These drugs were first developed in the late 1990s, and the optimism surrounding them has waxed and waned. Since their creation, hundreds of clinical trials with angiogenesis inhibitors have taken place around the world. The cancer in which they work best is clear cell renal carcinoma (the most common type of kidney cancer). In this cancer, *VHL* mutations renders tumours particularly sensitive to angiogenesis inhibitors. However, outside of kidney cancer, the benefits of angiogenesis inhibitors tend to be more modest. Occasionally they are given alone, but they're more often given in combination with other treatments, such as chemotherapy, or immunotherapy.

Second, we looked at ADCs. This group of treatments is currently creating a huge amount of excitement and hopeful anticipation among scientists and doctors. There are hundreds of ADCs in trials, and an enormous amount of progress has been made in the past decade in improving various aspects of their design. These improvements include technical advances in linker design, and the inclusion of different forms of chemotherapy. Numerous successful trials involving the

HER2-targeted ADC, trastuzumab deruxtecan, have added to the general air of excitement that currently surrounds ADCs. However, we should always remember that HER2 is a powerful protein that forces cells to multiply and survive. It might therefore be an outlier in terms of the effectiveness of ADCs that target it. ADCs that target proteins that are not necessary for cell survival are likely to be less potent cancer treatments. In addition, if an ADC target is present on a lot of healthy cells, side effects may limit its use. Lastly, we must always bear in mind that only a tiny percentage of any ADC given to patients ends up in their cancer cells.

Next, we looked at PARP inhibitors. These treatments were created with one particular group of patients in mind: people with inherited *BRCA* gene defects who have developed breast or ovarian cancer. However, it now seems that PARP inhibitors might benefit a wider group of people with ovarian cancer: those whose tumors have responded to treatment with platinum-based chemotherapy and therefore presumably have some defect in the homologous recombination process of DNA repair. The very fact that their cancer has shrunk in response to platinum-based chemotherapy predicts a likelihood of benefit from a PARP inhibitor as well. More recently, PARP inhibitors have been approved as treatments for some people with prostate cancer or pancreatic cancer, and they are being explored in other cancer types.

I then turned to CDK inhibitors, and specifically the drugs that block CDK4 and CDK6 (CDK4/6). Optimism around these drugs was initially sky-high. But, as with all new treatments, initial optimism has been replaced with a more realistic and pragmatic view of what they can deliver. Currently they are only given to people with hormone receptor-positive breast cancer in combination with hormone therapy. Their effectiveness against hormone receptor-positive breast cancer is thought to be because of the interplay between cyclin D and hormone receptors: Hormone receptors trigger the production of cyclin D (which activates CDK4/6), and, in return, cyclin D enhances the activation of hormone receptors.

Hedgehog (Hh) pathway inhibitors are another group of treatments where initial excitement has later subsided into something more muted. This pathway is crucial in embryonic development, and in adult stem cells. There are many reasons why the Hh pathway is active in cancer cells. Yet only people whose cancers contain a mutation directly affecting the pathway seem to derive a reasonable level of benefit from a Hh pathway inhibitor. The cancers most likely to contain a mutation affecting the Hh pathway are basal cell carcinoma (BCC) skin cancer and medulloblastoma. However, BCC is generally cured very easily with surgery, and medulloblastoma is very rare.

Epigenetic enzyme inhibitors – These treatments affect many different processes in the cell by influencing the production of an untold number of proteins. Often, their mechanism of action is unknown. They are mostly given to people with some types of leukemia or lymphoma.

Treatments that target cell survival proteins – The Bcl-2 inhibitor venetoclax is the most widely used. It appears to be most effective against cancers that produce high levels of Bcl-2, which protects them from apoptosis. These cancers include chronic lymphocytic leukemia, acute myeloid leukemia, and some myelomas. More Bcl-2 inhibitors are being developed, as are treatments that target its close relative, Mcl-1, and other cell survival proteins. One potentially exciting group of treatments are those that reinstate p53 activity, either by increasing its stability or restoring mutant p53 protein to its proper shape.

Targeting B cell receptor (BCR)-controlled signaling pathways. BCRs are found on B cells, and they are important for the survival of various different cancers that develop from faulty B cells, such as B cell leukemias and lymphomas. BTK inhibitors have been the most successful so far, and they are extensively used in the treatment of people with chronic lymphocytic leukemia.

Nuclear transport inhibitors affect the level of an enormous range of proteins in the cell nucleus and cytoplasm, and their precise mechanism of action is unclear. They are currently given to some people with myeloma or non-Hodgkin lymphoma.

Proteasome inhibitors. Again, these treatments affect an enormous range of proteins and processes in our cells. They are most effective against myeloma cells. This might be because these cells are dependent on their proteasomes to protect them against the toxic effects of misfolded proteins.

REFERENCES

1 Pezzella F (2019). Mechanisms of resistance to anti-angiogenic treatments. *Cancer Drug Resist.* **2**(3). doi: 10.20517/cdr.2019.39.

2 Jayson GC *et al.* (2016). Antiangiogenic therapy in oncology: Current status and future directions. *Lancet* **388**(10043). doi: 10.1016/S0140-6736(15)01088-0.

3 Sherwood LM, Parris EE, Folkman J (1971). Tumor angiogenesis: Therapeutic implications. *N. Engl. J. Med.* **285**(21). doi: 10.1056/nejm197111182852108.

4 NIH Definition of drug – NCI dictionary of cancer terms. National Cancer Institute.

5 NCI NCI – drugs approved for different types of cancer. [Online] Available: https://www.cancer.gov/about-cancer/treatment/drugs/cancer-type [Accessed March, 21 2024].

6 MHRA products website. [Online] Available: https://products.mhra.gov.uk/ [Accessed July 20, 2022].

7 European medicines agency. [Online] Available: https://www.ema.europa.eu/en [Accessed: July 20, 2022].

8 Escudier B *et al.* (2019). Renal cell carcinoma: ESMO clinical practice guidelines for diagnosis, treatment and follow-up. *Ann. Oncol.* **30**(5). doi: 10.1093/annonc/mdz056.

9 Kasherman L *et al.* (2022). Angiogenesis inhibitors and immunomodulation in renal cell cancers: The past, present, and future. *Cancers (Basel)* **14**(6). doi: 10.3390/cancers14061406.

10 Weis SM, Cheresh DA (2011). Tumor angiogenesis: Molecular pathways and therapeutic targets. *Nat. Med.* **17**(11). doi: 10.1038/nm.2537.

11 Siemann DW, Horsman MR (2015). Modulation of the tumor vasculature and oxygenation to improve therapy. *Pharmacol. Ther.* **153**. doi: 10.1016/j.pharmthera.2015.06.006.

12 Niu G, Chen X (2010). Vascular endothelial growth factor as an anti-angiogenic target for cancer therapy. *Curr. Drug Targets* **11**(8). doi: 10.2174/138945010791591395.

13 Lopes-Coelho F *et al.* (2021). Anti-angiogenic therapy: Current challenges and future perspectives. *Int. J. Mol. Sci.* **22**(7). doi: 10.3390/ijms22073765.

14 Byrne AM, Bouchier-Hayes DJ, Harmey JH (2005). Angiogenic and cell survival functions of Vascular Endothelial Growth Factor (VEGF). *J. Cell. Mol. Med.* **9**(4). doi: 10.1016/S0001-2092(06)60356-6.

15 Ellis LM, Hicklin DJ (2008). VEGF-targeted therapy: Mechanisms of anti-tumour activity. *Nat. Rev. Cancer* **8**(8). doi: 10.1038/nrc2403.

16 Ferrara N *et al.* (2004). Discovery and development of bevacizumab, an anti-VEGF antibody for treating cancer. *Nat. Rev. Drug Discov.* **3**(5). doi: 10.1038/nrd1381.

17 Holash J *et al.* (2002). VEGF-Trap: A VEGF blocker with potent antitumor effects. *Proc. Natl. Acad. Sci. USA* **99**(17). doi: 10.1073/pnas.172398299.

18 Chiron M *et al.* (2014). Differential antitumor activity of aflibercept and bevacizumab in patient-derived xenograft models of colorectal cancer. *Mol. Cancer Ther.* **13**(6). doi: 10.1158/1535-7163.MCT-13-0753.

19 Zhang J *et al.* (2015). Bevacizumab, Aflibercept or Ramucirmab combined with chemotherapy as second-line treatment for metastatic colorectal cancer following progression with Bevacizumab in first-line therapy: A systematic review and indirect comparison. *J. Clin. Oncol.* **33**(15_suppl). doi: 10.1200/jco.2015.33.15_suppl.e14601.

20 Aprile G *et al.* (2014). Ramucirumab: Preclinical research and clinical development. *Onco. Targets Ther.* **7**. doi: 10.2147/OTT.S61132.

21 Gotink KJ, Verheul HMW (2010). Anti-angiogenic tyrosine kinase inhibitors: What is their mechanism of action? *Angiogenesis* **13**(1). doi: 10.1007/s10456-009-9160-6.

22 McLellan B, Kerr H (2011). Cutaneous toxicities of the multikinase inhibitors sorafenib and sunitinib. *Dermatol. Ther.* **24**(4). doi: 10.1111/j.1529-8019.2011.01435.x.

23 Tan Q *et al.* (2015). Therapeutic effects and associated adverse events of multikinase inhibitors in metastatic renal cell carcinoma: A meta-analysis. *Exp Ther Med* **9**(6). doi: 10.3892/etm.2015.2427.

24 Roskoski R, Sadeghi-Nejad A (2018). Role of RET protein-tyrosine kinase inhibitors in the treatment RET-driven thyroid and lung cancers. *Pharmacol. Res.* **128**. doi: 10.1016/j.phrs.2017.12.021.

25 Stjepanovic N, Capdevila J (2014). Multikinase inhibitors in the treatment of thyroid cancer: Specific role of lenvatinib. *Biol.: Targets Ther.* **8**. doi: 10.2147/BTT.S39381.

26 Viola D *et al.* (2016). Treatment of advanced thyroid cancer with targeted therapies: Ten years of experience. *Endocr. Relat. Cancer* **23**(4). doi: 10.1530/ERC-15-0555.

27 del Bufalo D *et al.* (2006). Antiangiogenic potential of the mammalian target of rapamycin inhibitor temsirolimus. *Cancer Res.* **66**(11). doi: 10.1158/0008-5472.CAN-05-2825.

28 Lin T *et al.* (2016). Mammalian target of rapamycin (mTOR) inhibitors in solid tumours. *Clin. Pharm.* **8**(3). doi: 10.1211/CP.2016.20200813.

29 Bui TO *et al.* (2022). Genomics of clear-cell renal cell carcinoma: A systematic review and meta-analysis. *Eur. Urol.* **81**(4). doi: 10.1016/j.eururo.2021.12.010.

30 Gossage L, Eisen T, Maher ER (2015). VHL, the story of a tumour suppressor gene. *Nat. Rev. Cancer* **15**(1). doi: 10.1038/nrc3844.

31 Haase VH (2006). The VHL/HIF oxygen-sensing pathway and its relevance to kidney disease. *Kidney Int.* **69**(8). doi: 10.1038/sj.ki.5000221.

32 Qian CN *et al.* (2009). Complexity of tumor vasculature in clear cell renal cell carcinoma. *Cancer.* doi: 10.1002/cncr.24238.

33 Jonasch E *et al.* (2021). Belzutifan for renal cell carcinoma in von Hippel–Lindau disease. *N. Engl. J. Med.* **385**(22). doi: 10.1056/nejmoa 2103425.

34 Goodstein T *et al.* (2023). Two is company, is three a crowd? Triplet therapy, novel molecular targets, and updates on the management of advanced renal cell carcinoma. *Curr. Opin. Oncol.* **35**(3): 206–217. doi: 10.1097/CCO. 0000000000000939.

35 Suárez C *et al.* (2023). Selective HIF2A inhibitors in the management of clear cell renal cancer and von Hippel–Lindau-Disease-Associated Tumors. *Med. Sci.* **11**(3): 46. doi: 10.3390/medsci 11030046.

36 Jain RK (2014). Antiangiogenesis strategies revisited: From starving tumors to alleviating hypoxia. *Cancer Cell* **26**(5). doi: 10.1016/j.ccell.2014.10.006.

37 Bergers G, Hanahan D (2008). Modes of resistance to anti-angiogenic therapy. *Nat. Rev. Cancer* **8**(8). doi: 10.1038/nrc2442.

38 Lee WS *et al.* (2020). Combination of anti-angiogenic therapy and immune checkpoint blockade normalizes vascular-immune crosstalk to potentiate cancer immunity. *Exp. Mol. Med.* **52**(9). doi: 10.1038/s12276-020-00500-y.

39 Palmer AC *et al.* (2022). Predictable clinical benefits without evidence of synergy in trials of combination therapies with immune-checkpoint inhibitors. *Clin. Cancer Res.* **28**(2). doi: 10.1158/1078-0432.CCR-21-2275.

40 Tarantino P *et al.* (2023). Optimizing the safety of antibody–drug conjugates for patients with solid tumours. *Nat. Rev. Clin. Oncol.* **20**(8): 558–576. doi: 10.1038/s41571-023-00783-w.

41 Fu Z *et al.* (2022). Antibody drug conjugate: The "biological missile" for targeted cancer therapy. *Signal Transduction Targeted Ther.* **7**(1): 93. doi: 10.1038/s41392-022-00947-7.

42 Conilh L *et al.* (2023). Payload diversification: A key step in the development of antibody–drug conjugates. *J. Hematol. Oncol.* **16**(1): 3. doi: 10.1186/s13045-022-01397-y.

43 Chau CH, Steeg PS, Figg WD (2019). Antibody–drug conjugates for cancer. *Lancet* **394**(10200): 793–804. doi: 10.1016/S0140-6736(19)31774-X.

44 Thomas A, Teicher BA, Hassan R (2016). Antibody–drug conjugates for cancer therapy. *Lancet Oncol.* **17**(6): e254–e262. doi: 10.1016/S1470-2045(16)30030-4.

45 Su Z *et al.* (2021). Antibody–drug conjugates: Recent advances in linker chemistry. *Acta Pharm. Sin. B* **11**(12). doi: 10.1016/j.apsb.2021.03.042.

46 Beck A *et al.* (2017). Strategies and challenges for the next generation of antibody-drug conjugates. *Nat. Rev. Drug Discov.* **16**(5). doi: 10.1038/nrd.2016.268.

47 Eiger D *et al.* (2021). The exciting new field of HER2-low breast cancer treatment. *Cancers (Basel)* **13**(5): 1015. doi: 10.3390/cancers13051015.

48 Rassy E, Rached L, Pistilli B (2022). Antibody drug conjugates targeting HER2: Clinical development in metastatic breast cancer. *Breast* **66**: 217–226. doi: 10.1016/j.breast.2022.10.016.

49 Indini A, Rijavec E, Grossi F (2021). Trastuzumab deruxtecan: Changing the destiny of her2 expressing solid tumors. *Int. J. Mol. Sci.* **22**(9). doi: 10.3390/ijms22094774.

50 Díaz-Rodríguez E *et al.* (2021). Novel ADCs and strategies to overcome resistance to anti-HER2 ADCs. *Cancers (Basel)* **14**(1): 154. doi: 10.3390/cancers14010154.

51 Cortés J *et al.* (2021). LBA1 Trastuzumab deruxtecan (T-DXd) vs trastuzumab emtansine (T-DM1) in patients (Pts) with HER2+ metastatic breast cancer (mBC): Results of the randomized phase III DESTINY-Breast03 study. *Ann. Oncol.* **32**. doi: 10.1016/j.annonc.2021.08.2087.

52 Criscitiello C, Morganti S, Curigliano G (2021). Antibody–drug conjugates in solid tumors: A look into novel targets. *J. Hematol. Oncol.* **14**(1): 20. doi: 10.1186/s13045-021-01035-z.

53 Petrillo A, Smyth EC, van Laarhoven HWM (2023). Emerging targets in gastroesophageal adenocarcinoma: What the future looks like. *Ther. Adv. Med. Oncol.* **15**: 175883592311731. doi: 10.1177/17588359231173177.

54 Cortinovis DL *et al.* (2022). Harnessing DLL3 inhibition: From old promises to new therapeutic horizons. *Front. Med. (Lausanne)* **9**. doi: 10.3389/fmed.2022.989405.

55 Chu Y, Zhou X, Wang X (2021). Antibody-drug conjugates for the treatment of lymphoma: Clinical advances and latest progress. *J. Hematol. Oncol.* **14**(1): 88. doi: 10.1186/s13045-021-01097-z.

56 Gogia P *et al.* (2023). Antibody–drug conjugates: A review of approved drugs and their clinical level of evidence. *Cancers (Basel)* **15**(15): 3886. doi: 10.3390/cancers15153886.

57 Corti C *et al.* (2023). Future potential targets of antibody-drug conjugates in breast cancer. *Breast* **69**: 312–322. doi: 10.1016/j.breast.2023.03.007.

58 Klümper N *et al.* (2023). Membranous NECTIN-4 expression frequently decreases during metastatic spread of urothelial carcinoma and is associated with enfortumab vedotin resistance. *Clin. Cancer Res.* **29**(8): 1496–1505. doi: 10.1158/1078-0432.CCR-22-1764.

59 Gonzalez-Ochoa E, Veneziani AC, Oza AM (2023). Mirvetuximab soravtansine in platinum-resistant ovarian cancer. *Clin. Med. Insights Oncol.* **17**. doi: 10.1177/11795549231187264.

60 Dilawari A *et al.* (2023). FDA approval summary: Mirvetuximab soravtansine-Gynx for FRα-positive, platinum-resistant ovarian cancer. *Clin. Cancer Res.* **29**(19): 3835–3840. doi: 10.1158/1078-0432.CCR-23-0991.

61 Matulonis UA *et al.* (2023). Efficacy and safety of Mirvetuximab soravtansine in patients with platinum-resistant ovarian cancer with high folate receptor alpha expression: Results from the SORAYA study. *J. Clin. Oncol.* **41**(13): 2436–2445. doi: 10.1200/JCO.22.01900.

62 Tolcher A, Hamilton E, Coleman RL (2023). The evolving landscape of antibody-drug conjugates in gynecologic cancers. *Cancer Treat. Rev.* **116**: 102546. doi: 10.1016/j.ctrv.2023.102546.

63 Nguyen TD, Bordeau BM, Balthasar JP (2023). Mechanisms of ADC toxicity and strategies to increase ADC tolerability. *Cancers (Basel)* **15**(3): 713. doi: 10.3390/cancers15030713.

64 Richardson DL (2023). Ocular toxicity and mitigation strategies for antibody drug conjugates in gynecologic oncology. *Gynecol. Oncol. Rep.* **46**: 101148. doi: 10.1016/j.gore.2023.101148.

65 Parakh S *et al.* (2022). Radiolabeled antibodies for cancer imaging and therapy. *Cancers (Basel)* **14**(6): 1454. doi: 10.3390/cancers14061454.

66 Sgouros G *et al.* (2020). Radiopharmaceutical therapy in cancer: Clinical advances and challenges. *Nat. Rev. Drug Discov.* **19**(9): 589–608. doi: 10.1038/s41573-020-0073-9.

67 Czerwińska M *et al.* (2020). Targeted radionuclide therapy of prostate cancer – from basic research to clinical perspectives. *Molecules* **25**(7): 1743. doi: 10.3390/molecules25071743.

68 Illidge TM (2010). Radioimmunotherapy of lymphoma: A treatment approach ahead of its time or past its sell-by date? *J. Clin. Oncol.* **28**(18): 2944–2946. doi: 10.1200/JCO.2009.26.8748.

69 Larson SM *et al.* (2015). Radioimmunotherapy of human tumours. *Nat. Rev. Cancer* **15**(6): 347–360. doi: 10.1038/nrc3925.

70 Gong L *et al.* (2023). Research advances in peptide–drug conjugates. *Acta Pharm. Sin. B* **13**(9): 3659–3677. doi: 10.1016/j.apsb.2023.02.013.

71 Nhàn NTT, Yamada T, Yamada KH (2023). Peptide-based agents for cancer treatment: Current applications and future directions. *Int. J. Mol. Sci.* **24**(16): 12931. doi: 10.3390/ijms241612931.

72 Alamdari-palangi V *et al.* (2023). Recent advances and applications of peptide–agent conjugates for targeting tumor cells. *J. Cancer Res. Clin. Oncol.* **149**(16): 15249–15273. doi: 10.1007/s00432-023-05144-9.

73 Chavda VP *et al.* (2022). Peptide-drug conjugates: A new hope for cancer management. *Molecules* **27**(21): 7232. doi: 10.3390/molecules27217232.

74 Dhillon S (2018). Moxetumomab pasudotox: First global approval. *Drugs* **78**(16): 1763–1767. doi: 10.1007/s40265-018-1000-9.

75 Rosa R (2023). FDA issues complete response letter to denileukin diftitox for R/R cutaneous T-cell lymphoma. OncLive. https://www.onclive.com/view/fda-issues-complete-response-letter-to-denileukin-diftitox-for-r-r-cutaneous-t-cell-lymphoma [Accessed March 21, 2024].

76 Pemmaraju N *et al.* (2022). Long-term benefits of tagraxofusp for patients with blastic plasmacytoid dendritic cell neoplasm. *J. Clin. Oncol.* **40**(26): 3032–3036. doi: 10.1200/JCO.22.00034.

77 Li M *et al.* (2022). Strategies to mitigate the on- and off-target toxicities of recombinant immunotoxins: An antibody engineering perspective. *Antib. Ther.* **5**(3): 164–176. doi: 10.1093/abt/tbac014.

78 Konecny GE, Kristeleit RS (2016). PARP inhibitors for BRCA1/2-mutated and sporadic

ovarian cancer: Current practice and future directions. *Br. J. Cancer* **115**(10). doi: 10.1038/bjc.2016.311.

79 Plummer R (2011). Poly(ADP-ribose) polymerase inhibition: A new direction for BRCA and triple-negative breast cancer? *Breast Cancer Res.* **13**(4). doi: 10.1186/bcr2877.

80 Sullivan LB, Chandel NS (2014). Mitochondrial reactive oxygen species and cancer. *Cancer Metab* **2**(17). doi: 10.1186/2049-3002-2-17.

81 Zheng F *et al.* (2020). Mechanism and current progress of Poly ADP-ribose polymerase (PARP) inhibitors in the treatment of ovarian cancer. *Biomed. Pharmacother.* **123**. doi: 10.1016/j.biopha.2019.109661.

82 Rose M *et al.* (2020). PARP inhibitors: Clinical relevance, mechanisms of action and tumor resistance. *Front. Cell Dev. Biol.* **8**. doi: 10.3389/fcell.2020.564601.

83 Verdin E (2015). NAD+ in aging, metabolism, and neurodegeneration. *Science (1979)* **350**(6265): 1208–1213. doi: 10.1126/science.aac4854.

84 Wright WD, Shah SS, Heyer WD (2018). Homologous recombination and the repair of DNA double-strand breaks. *J. Biol. Chem.* **293**(27). doi: 10.1074/jbc.TM118.000372.

85 Cancer Research UK (2021). Inherited genes and cancer types. [Online] Available: https://www.cancerresearchuk.org/about-cancer/causes-of-cancer/inherited-cancer-genes-and-increased-cancer-risk/inherited-genes-and-cancer-types [Accessed July 28, 2022].

86 Vietri MT *et al.* (2013). Double heterozygosity in the *BRCA1* and *BRCA2* genes in Italian family. *Clin. Chem. Lab. Med.* **51**(12): 2319–2324. doi: 10.1515/cclm-2013-0263.

87 Roy R, Chun J, Powell SN (2012). BRCA1 and BRCA2: Different roles in a common pathway of genome protection. *Nat. Rev. Cancer* **12**(1). doi: 10.1038/nrc3181.

88 Jolie A (2013). My medical choice. The New York Times. [Online] Available: https://www.nytimes.com/2013/05/14/opinion/my-medical-choice.html [Accessed July 28, 2022].

89 Jolie Pitt A (2015). Angelina Jolie Pitt: Diary of a surgery. The New York Times. [Online] Available: https://www.nytimes.com/2015/03/24/opinion/angelina-jolie-pitt-diary-of-a-surgery.html [Accessed July 28, 2022].

90 Scowcroft H (2013). Angelina Jolie, inherited breast cancer and the BRCA1 gene. Science blog, Cancer Research UK. [Online] Available: https://news.cancerresearchuk.org/2013/05/14/angelina-jolie-inherited-breast-cancer-and-the-brca1-gene/ [Accessed July 28, 2022].

91 Lord CJ, Ashworth A (2012). The DNA damage response and cancer therapy. *Nature* **481**(7381). doi: 10.1038/nature10760.

92 Deng CX, Scott F (2000). Role of the tumor suppressor gene Brca1 in genetic stability and mammary gland tumor formation. *Oncogene* **19**(8). doi: 10.1038/sj.onc.1203269.

93 National Cancer Institute Genetics of breast and gynecologic cancers (PDQ®)–health professional version. [Online] Available: https://www.cancer.gov/types/breast/hp/breast-ovarian-genetics-pdq#_117 [Accessed July 28, 2022].

94 Ibrahim M *et al.* (2018). Male BRCA mutation carriers: Clinical characteristics and cancer spectrum. *BMC Cancer* **18**(1): 179. doi: 10.1186/s12885-018-4098-y.

95 Singh AK, Yu X (2020). Tissue-specific carcinogens as soil to seed BRCA1/2-mutant hereditary cancers. *Trends Cancer* **6**(7). doi: 10.1016/j.trecan.2020.03.004.

96 Godet I, Gilkes DM (2017). BRCA1 and BRCA2 mutations and treatment strategies for breast cancer. *Integr. Cancer Sci. Ther.* **4**(1). doi: 10.15761/icst.1000228.

97 Konstantinopoulos PA *et al.* (2015). Homologous recombination deficiency: Exploiting the fundamental vulnerability of ovarian cancer. *Cancer Discov.* **5**(11). doi: 10.1158/2159-8290.CD-15-0714.

98 Cancer Genome Atlas Research Network (2011). Integrated genomic analyses of ovarian carcinoma. *Nature* **474**(7353): 609–615. doi: 10.1038/nature10166.

99 Moore K *et al.* (2018). Maintenance Olaparib in patients with newly diagnosed advanced ovarian cancer. *N. Engl. J. Med.* **379**(26). doi: 10.1056/nejmoa1810858.

100 Ray-Coquard I *et al.* (2019). Olaparib plus bev-acizumab as first-line maintenance in ovarian cancer. *N. Engl. J. Med.* **381**(25). doi: 10.1056/nejmoa1911361.

101 González-Martín A *et al.* (2019). Niraparib in patients with newly diagnosed advanced ovarian cancer. *N. Engl. J. Med.* **381**(25). doi: 10.1056/nejmoa1910962.

102 McMullen M *et al.* (2020). Overcoming platinum and parp-inhibitor resistance in ovarian cancer. *Cancers* **12**(6). doi: 10.3390/cancers 12061607.

103 Wicks AJ *et al.* (2022). Opinion: PARP inhibitors in cancer – what do we still need to know? *Open Biol.* **12**(7). doi: 10.1098/rsob.220118.

104 Abdel-Rahman Abdelsalam O, Salem M (2021). Incorporating PARP inhibitors into the pancreatic cancer treatment armamentarium. ASCO Daily News. [Online] Available: https://dailynews.ascopubs.org/do/10.1200/ADN.21.200507/full/ [Accessed August 1, 2022].

105 NCI Staff (2020). With two FDA approvals, prostate cancer treatment enters the PARP era. National Cancer Institute. [Online] Available: https://www.cancer.gov/news-events/cancer-currents-blog/2020/fda-olaparib-rucaparib-prostate-cancer [Accessed August 1, 2022].

106 Deluce JE *et al.* (2022). Emerging biomarker-guided therapies in prostate cancer. *Curr. Oncol.* **29**(7): 5054–5076. doi: 10.3390/curroncol29070400.

107 Lord CJ, Ashworth A (2017). PARP inhibitors: The first synthetic lethal targeted therapy. *Science* **355**(6330).

108 Ghiorzo P (2014). Genetic predisposition to pancreatic cancer. *World J. Gastroenterol.* **20**(31). doi: 10.3748/wjg.v20.i31.10778.

109 Robinson D *et al.* (2015). Integrative clinical genomics of advanced prostate cancer. *Cell* **161**(5). doi: 10.1016/j.cell.2015.05.001.

110 DiSilvestro P *et al.* (2023). Overall survival with maintenance Olaparib at a 7-year follow-up in patients with newly diagnosed advanced ovarian cancer and a BRCA mutation: The SOLO1/GOG 3004 trial. *J. Clin. Oncol.* **41**(3): 609–617. doi: 10.1200/JCO.22.01549.

111 Miller RE, El-Shakankery KH, Lee JY (2022). PARP inhibitors in ovarian cancer: Overcoming resistance with combination strategies. *J. Gynecol. Oncol.* **33**(3). doi: 10.3802/jgo.2022.33.e44.

112 Scitable by Nature Education How do cells know when to divide?[Online] Available: https://www.nature.com/scitable/ebooks/essentials-of-cell-biology-14749010/how-do-cells-know-when-to-divide-14751793/ [Accessed August 02, 2022].

113 Chen E (2016). Pharmacology of Anticancer Drugs. In Tannock I *et al.* (eds) *The Basic Science of Oncology.* 5th ed. McGraw Hill.

114 Payne S, Miles D (2008). Mechanisms of Anticancer Drugs. In Gleeson M (ed.) *Scott-Brown's Otorhinolaryngology: Head and Neck Surgery.* 7th ed. CRC Press.

115 Malumbres M (2014). Cyclin-dependent kinases. *Genome Biol.* **15**(6): 122. doi: 10.1186/gb4184.

116 Asghar U *et al.* (2015). The history and future of targeting cyclin-dependent kinases in cancer therapy. *Nat. Rev. Drug Discov.* **14**(2): 130–146. doi: 10.1038/nrd4504.

117 Magadum S *et al.* (2013). Gene duplication as a major force in evolution. *J. Genet.* **92**(1): 155–161. doi: 10.1007/s12041-013-0212-8.

118 Musgrove EA *et al.* (2011). Cyclin D as a therapeutic target in cancer. *Nat. Rev. Cancer* **11**(8). doi: 10.1038/nrc3090.

119 O'Leary B, Finn RS, Turner NC (2016). Treating cancer with selective CDK4/6 inhibitors. *Nat. Rev. Clin. Oncol.* **13**(7). doi: 10.1038/nrclinonc.2016.26.

120 Finn RS, Aleshin A, Slamon DJ (2016). Targeting the cyclin-dependent kinases (CDK) 4/6 in estrogen receptor-positive breast cancers. *Breast Cancer Res.* **18**(1). doi: 10.1186/s13058-015-0661-5.

121 Fassl A, Geng Y, Sicinski P (2022). CDK4 and CDK6 kinases: From basic science to cancer therapy. *Science* **375**(6577). doi: 10.1126/science.abc1495.

122 Álvarez-Fernández M, Malumbres M (2020). Mechanisms of sensitivity and resistance to CDK4/6 inhibition. *Cancer Cell* **37**(4). doi: 10.1016/j.ccell.2020.03.010.

123 Suski JM *et al.* (2021). Targeting cell-cycle machinery in cancer. *Cancer Cell* **39**(6). doi: 10.1016/j.ccell.2021.03.010.

124 Welboren WJ *et al.* (2007). Identifying estrogen receptor target genes. *Mol. Oncol.* **1**(2). doi: 10.1016/j.molonc.2007.04.001.

125 Manavathi B *et al.* (2013). Derailed estrogen signaling and breast cancer: An authentic couple. *Endocr. Rev.* **34**(1). doi: 10.1210/er.2011-1057.

126 Preusser M *et al.* (2018). CDK4/6 inhibitors in the treatment of patients with breast cancer: Summary of a multidisciplinary round-table discussion. *ESMO Open* **3**(5). doi: 10.1136/esmoopen-2018-000368.

127 Ferrarotto R *et al.* (2021). Trilaciclib prior to chemotherapy reduces the usage of supportive care interventions for chemotherapy-induced myelosuppression in patients with small cell lung cancer: Pooled analysis of three randomized phase 2 trials. *Cancer Med.* **10**(17). doi: 10.1002/cam4.4089.

128 Powell K, Prasad V (2021). Concerning FDA approval of trilaciclib (Cosela) in extensive-stage small-cell lung cancer. *Transl. Oncol.* **14**(11). doi: 10.1016/j.tranon.2021.101206.

129 Sava J (2023). PRESERVE 1 trial of Trilaciclib in mCRC ended due to efficacy results. Targeted Oncology. [Online] Available: https://www.targetedonc.com/view/preserve-1-trial-of-trilaciclib-in-mcrc-ended-due-to-efficacy-results [Accessed November 8, 2023].

130 Spring LM *et al.* (2020). Cyclin-dependent kinase 4 and 6 inhibitors for hormone receptor-positive breast cancer: Past, present, and future. *Lancet* **395**(10226). doi: 10.1016/S0140-6736(20)30165-3.

131 Bavetsias V, Linardopoulos S (2015). Aurora kinase inhibitors: Current status and outlook. *Front. Oncol.* **5**(DEC). doi: 10.3389/fonc.2015.00278.

132 Rampioni Vinciguerra GL *et al.* (2022). CDK4/6 inhibitors in combination therapies: Better in company than alone: A mini review. *Front. Oncol.* **12**. doi: 10.3389/fonc.2022.891580.

133 Otto T, Sicinski P (2017). Cell cycle proteins as promising targets in cancer therapy. *Nat. Rev. Cancer* **17**(2). doi: 10.1038/nrc.2016.138.

134 Sørensen CS, Syljuåsen RG (2012). Safeguarding genome integrity: The checkpoint kinases ATR, CHK1 and WEE1 restrain CDK activity during normal DNA replication. *Nucleic Acids Res.* **40**(2). doi: 10.1093/nar/gkr697.

135 Kim C-H *et al.* (2022). Mitotic protein kinase-driven crosstalk of machineries for mitosis and metastasis. *Exp. Mol. Med.* **54**(4): 414–425. doi: 10.1038/s12276-022-00750-y.

136 Yano K, Shiotani B (2023). Emerging strategies for cancer therapy by ATR inhibitors. *Cancer Sci.* **114**(7): 2709–2721. doi: 10.1111/cas.15845.

137 Machado CB *et al.* (2021). The relevance of aurora kinase inhibition in hematological malignancies. *Cancer Diagn. Progn.* **1**(3). doi: 10.21873/cdp.10016.

138 Gutteridge REA *et al.* (2016). Plk1 inhibitors in cancer therapy: From laboratory to clinics. *Mol. Cancer Ther.* **15**(7). doi: 10.1158/1535-7163.MCT-15-0897.

139 Bukhari AB, Chan GK, Gamper AM (2022). Targeting the DNA damage response for cancer therapy by inhibiting the kinase wee1. *Front. Oncol.* **12**. doi: 10.3389/fonc.2022.828684.

140 Varjosalo M, Taipale J (2008). Hedgehog: Functions and mechanisms. *Genes Dev.* **22**(18). doi: 10.1101/gad.1693608.

141 Petrova R, Joyner AL (2014). Roles for Hedgehog signaling in adult organ homeostasis and repair. *Development (Cambridge)* **141**(18). doi: 10.1242/dev.083691.

142 Amakye D, Jagani Z, Dorsch M (2013). Unraveling the therapeutic potential of the Hedgehog pathway in cancer. *Nat. Med.* **19**(11). doi: 10.1038/nm.3389.

143 Xie H *et al.* (2019). Recent advances in the clinical targeting of hedgehog/GLI signaling in cancer. *Cells* **8**(5). doi: 10.3390/cells8050394.

144 Rubin LL, de Sauvage FJ (2006). Targeting the Hedgehog pathway in cancer. *Nat. Rev. Drug Discov.* **5**(12): 1026–1033. doi: 10.1038/nrd2086.

145 Heretsch P, Tzagkaroulaki L, Giannis A (2010). Cyclopamine and hedgehog signaling: Chemistry, biology, medical perspectives. *Angew. Chem. Int. Ed.* **49**(20). doi: 10.1002/anie.200906967.

146 Sharpe HJ *et al.* (2015). Regulation of the oncoprotein Smoothened by small molecules. *Nat. Chem. Biol.* **11**(4). doi: 10.1038/nchembio.1776.

147 Lear JT *et al.* (2014). Challenges and new horizons in the management of advanced basal cell

carcinoma: A UK perspective. *Br. J. Cancer* **111**(8). doi: 10.1038/bjc.2014.270.

148 McMillan R, Matsui W (2012). Molecular pathways: The hedgehog signaling pathway in cancer. *Clin. Cancer Res.* **18**(18). doi: 10.1158/1078-0432.CCR-11-2509.

149 Davis CM, Lewis KD (2022). Brief overview: Cemiplimab for the treatment of advanced basal cell carcinoma: PD-1 strikes again. *Ther. Adv. Med. Oncol.* **14**: 175883592110661. doi: 10.1177/17588359211066147.

150 Gajjar AJ, Robinson GW (2014). Medulloblastoma – translating discoveries from the bench to the bedside. *Nat. Rev. Clin. Oncol.* **11**(12). doi: 10.1038/nrclinonc.2014.181.

151 Fang FY *et al.* (2022). New developments in the pathogenesis, therapeutic targeting, and treatment of pediatric medulloblastoma. *Cancers (Basel)* **14**(9): 2285. doi: 10.3390/cancers14092285.

152 Caimano M *et al.* (2021). Drug delivery systems for hedgehog inhibitors in the treatment of SHH-medulloblastoma. *Front. Chem.* **9**. doi: 10.3389/fchem.2021.688108.

153 Fernández LT *et al.* (2021). Basal cell nevus syndrome: An update on clinical findings. *Int. J. Dermatol.* doi: 10.1111/ijd.15884.

154 Hung KF, Yang T, Kao SY (2019). Cancer stem cell theory: Are we moving past the mist? *J. Chin. Med. Assoc.* **82**(11). doi: 10.1097/JCMA.0000000000000186.

155 Lainez-González D, Serrano-López J, Alonso-Domínguez JM (2021). Understanding the hedgehog signaling pathway in acute myeloid leukemia stem cells: A necessary step toward a cure. *Biology* **10**(4). doi: 10.3390/biology10040255.

156 de Lartigue J (2020). Targeting the Hedgehog pathway holds promises and pitfalls. OncologyLive. [Online] Available: https://www.onclive.com/view/targeting-the-hedgehog-pathway-holds-promises-and-pitfalls [Accessed August 1, 2022].

157 CDC Centers for Disease Control and Prevention, "What is Epigenetics?," Genomics and Precision Health. Accessed: Aug. 08, 2022. [Online]. Available: https://www.cdc.gov/genomics/disease/epigenetics.htm

158 Annunziato A, "DNA Packaging: Nucleosomes and Chromatin," Nature Education. Accessed: Aug. 08, 2022. [Online]. Available: https://www.nature.com/scitable/topicpage/dna-packaging-nucleosomes-and-chromatin-310/

159 Cheng Y *et al.* (2019). Targeting epigenetic regulators for cancer therapy: Mechanisms and advances in clinical trials. *Signal Transduction Targeted Ther.* **4**(1). doi: 10.1038/s41392-019-0095-0.

160 Bates SE (2020). Epigenetic therapies for cancer. *N. Engl. J. Med.* **383**(7). doi: 10.1056/nejmra1805035.

161 You JS, Jones PA (2012). Cancer genetics and epigenetics: Two sides of the same coin? *Cancer Cell* **22**(1). doi: 10.1016/j.ccr.2012.06.008.

162 Takeshima H, Ushijima T (2019). Accumulation of genetic and epigenetic alterations in normal cells and cancer risk. *npj Precis. Oncol.* **3**(1). doi: 10.1038/s41698-019-0079-0.

163 Duan R, Du W, Guo W (2020). EZH2: A novel target for cancer treatment. *J. Hematol. Oncol.* **13**(1). doi: 10.1186/s13045-020-00937-8.

164 Aumer T *et al.* (2022). Comprehensive comparison between azacytidine and decitabine treatment in an acute myeloid leukemia cell line. *Clin. Epigenetics* **14**(1): 113. doi: 10.1186/s13148-022-01329-0.

165 Papaemmanuil E *et al.* (2016). Genomic classification and prognosis in acute myeloid leukemia. *N. Engl. J. Med.* **374**(23): 2209–2221. doi: 10.1056/NEJMoa1516192.

166 Straining PR, Eighmy PW (2022). Tazemetostat: EZH2 inhibitor. *J. Adv. Pract. Oncol.* **13**(2): 158–163. doi: 10.6004/jadpro.2022.13.2.7.

167 Konteatis Z *et al.* (2020). Vorasidenib (AG-881): A first-in-class, brain-penetrant dual inhibitor of mutant IDH1 and 2 for treatment of glioma. *ACS Med. Chem. Lett.* **11**(2). doi: 10.1021/acsmedchemlett.9b00509.

168 Raineri S, Mellor J (2018). IDH1: Linking metabolism and epigenetics. *Front. Genet.* **9**. doi: 10.3389/fgene.2018.00493.

169 Venneker S, Bovée JVMG (2023). IDH mutations in chondrosarcoma: Case closed or not? *Cancers (Basel)* **15**(14): 3603. doi: 10.3390/cancers15143603.

170 Cojocaru E *et al.* (2020). Is the IDH mutation a good target for chondrosarcoma treatment? *Curr. Mol. Biol. Rep.* **6**(1). doi: 10.1007/s40610-020-00126-z.

171 Tucker N (2023). Vorasidenib delays disease progression or death in IDH+ low-grade glioma. Targeted Oncology. [Online] Available: https://www.targetedonc.com/view/vorasidenib-delays-disease-progression-or-death-in-idh-low-grade-glioma [Accessed November 10, 2023].

172 Pandey MK *et al.* (2016). Targeting cell survival proteins for cancer cell death. *Pharmaceuticals* **9**(1). doi: 10.3390/ph9010011.

173 Perini GF *et al.* (2018). BCL-2 as therapeutic target for hematological malignancies. *J. Hematol. Oncol.* **11**(1). doi: 10.1186/s13045-018-0608-2.

174 Czabotar PE *et al.* (2014). Control of apoptosis by the BCL-2 protein family: Implications for physiology and therapy. *Nat. Rev. Mol. Cell Biol.* **15**(1). doi: 10.1038/nrm3722.

175 Delbridge ARD, Strasser A (2015). The BCL-2 protein family, BH3-mimetics and cancer therapy. *Cell Death Differ.* **22**(7). doi: 10.1038/cdd.2015.50.

176 Anderson MA, Huang D, Roberts A (2014). Targeting BCL2 for the treatment of lymphoid malignancies. *Semin. Hematol.* **51**(3). doi: 10.1053/j.seminhematol.2014.05.008.

177 Delbridge ARD *et al.* (2016). Thirty years of BCL-2: Translating cell death discoveries into novel cancer therapies. *Nat. Rev. Cancer* **16**(2). doi: 10.1038/nrc.2015.17.

178 Pemmaraju N *et al.* (2023). New era for myelofibrosis treatment with novel agents beyond Janus kinase-inhibitor monotherapy: Focus on clinical development of BCL-X$_L$/BCL-2 inhibition with navitoclax. *Cancer* **129**(22): 3535–3545. doi: 10.1002/cncr.34986.

179 Wang H *et al.* (2021). Targeting MCL-1 in cancer: Current status and perspectives. *J. Hematol. Oncol.* **14**(1): 67. doi: 10.1186/s13045-021-01079-1.

180 Ploumaki I *et al.* (2023). Bcl-2 pathway inhibition in solid tumors: A review of clinical trials. *Clin. Transl. Oncol.* **25**(6): 1554–1578. doi: 10.1007/s12094-022-03070-9.

181 Carneiro BA, El-Deiry WS (2020). Targeting apoptosis in cancer therapy. *Nat. Rev. Clin. Oncol.* **17**(7). doi: 10.1038/s41571-020-0341-y.

182 Hu J *et al.* (2021). Targeting mutant p53 for cancer therapy: Direct and indirect strategies. *J. Hematol. Oncol.* **14**(1). doi: 10.1186/s13045-021-01169-0.

183 Cetraro P *et al.* (2022). A review of the current impact of inhibitors of apoptosis proteins and their repression in cancer. *Cancers* **14**(7). doi: 10.3390/cancers14071671.

184 Bourhis J *et al.* (2022). Xevinapant or placebo plus chemoradiotherapy in locally advanced squamous cell carcinoma of the head and neck: TrilynX phase III study design. *Future Oncol.* **18**(14). doi: 10.2217/fon-2021-1634.

185 Efremov DG, Turkalj S, Laurenti L (2020). Mechanisms of B cell receptor activation and responses to B cell receptor inhibitors in B cell malignancies. *Cancers (Basel)* **12**(6): 1396. doi: 10.3390/cancers12061396.

186 Burger JA, Wiestner A (2018). Targeting B cell receptor signalling in cancer: Preclinical and clinical advances. *Nat. Rev. Cancer* **18**(3): 148–167. doi: 10.1038/nrc.2017.121.

187 Robak T, Witkowska M, Smolewski P (2022). The role of Bruton's kinase inhibitors in chronic lymphocytic leukemia: Current status and future directions. *Cancers (Basel)* **14**(3): 771. doi: 10.3390/cancers14030771.

188 Woyach JA *et al.* (2022). Efficacy and safety of nemtabrutinib, a wild-type and C481S-mutated bruton tyrosine kinase inhibitor for B-cell malignancies: Updated analysis of the open-label phase 1/2 dose-expansion bellwave-001 study. *Blood* **140**(Supplement 1): 7004–7006. doi: 10.1182/blood-2022-163596.

189 Jebaraj BMC *et al.* (2022). Evaluation of vecabrutinib as a model for noncovalent BTK/ITK inhibition for treatment of chronic lymphocytic leukemia. *Blood* **139**(6): 859–875. doi: 10.1182/blood.2021011516.

190 Jensen JL *et al.* (2022). The potential of pirtobrutinib in multiple B-cell malignancies. *Ther. Adv. Hematol.* **13**: 204062072211016. doi: 10.1177/20406207221101697.

191 Bond DA, Woyach JA (2019). Targeting BTK in CLL: Beyond Ibrutinib. *Curr. Hematol.*

Malig. Rep. **14**(3): 197–205. doi: 10.1007/s11899-019-00512-0.

192 Kaptein A *et al.* (2018). Potency and selectivity of BTK inhibitors in clinical development for B-cell malignancies. *Blood* **132**(Supplement 1): 1871–1871. doi: 10.1182/blood-2018-99-109973.

193 Medicines. European Medicines Agency. [Online] Available: https://www.ema.europa.eu/en/medicines [Accessed August 18, 2023].

194 A to Z List of Cancer Drugs. National Cancer Institute. [Online] Available: https://www.cancer.gov/about-cancer/treatment/drugs [Accessed August 18, 2023].

195 Maffei R *et al.* (2015). Targeting neoplastic B cells and harnessing microenvironment: The "double face" of ibrutinib and idelalisib. *J. Hematol. Oncol.* **8**(1): 60. doi: 10.1186/s13045-015-0157-x.

196 Young RM, Staudt LM (2013). Targeting pathological B cell receptor signalling in lymphoid malignancies. *Nat. Rev. Drug Discov.* **12**(3): 229–243. doi: 10.1038/nrd3937.

197 Blunt MD, Steele AJ (2015). Pharmacological targeting of PI3K isoforms as a therapeutic strategy in chronic lymphocytic leukaemia. *Leuk. Res. Rep.* **4**(2): 60–63. doi: 10.1016/j.lrr.2015.09.001.

198 Bou Zeid N, Yazbeck V (2023). PI3k inhibitors in NHL and CLL: An unfulfilled promise. *Blood Lymphat Cancer* **13**: 1–12. doi: 10.2147/BLCTT.S309171.

199 Polson AG *et al.* (2007). Antibody-drug conjugates targeted to CD79 for the treatment of non-Hodgkin lymphoma. *Blood* **110**(2): 616–623. doi: 10.1182/blood-2007-01-066704.

200 Zheng B *et al.* (2009). In vivo effects of targeting CD79b with antibodies and antibody-drug conjugates. *Mol. Cancer Ther.* **8**(10): 2937–2946. doi: 10.1158/1535-7163.MCT-09-0369.

201 Hill BT, Kahl B (2022). Upfront therapy for diffuse large B-cell lymphoma: Looking beyond R-CHOP. *Expert Rev. Hematol.* **15**(9): 805–812. doi: 10.1080/17474086.2022.2124156.

202 Herrera AF *et al.* (2022). Anti-CD79B antibody–drug conjugate DCDS0780A in patients with B-cell non-hodgkin lymphoma: Phase 1 dose-escalation study. *Clin. Cancer Res.* **28**(7): 1294–1301. doi: 10.1158/1078-0432.CCR-21-3261.

203 Wang J *et al.* (2023). Characterization of anti-CD79b/CD3 bispecific antibody, a potential therapy for B cell malignancies. *Cancer Immunol. Immunother.* **72**(2): 493–507. doi: 10.1007/s00262-022-03267-5.

204 Azizian NG *et al.* (2020). XPO1-dependent nuclear export as a target for cancer therapy. *J. Hematol. Oncol.* **13**(1). doi: 10.1186/s13045-020-00903-4.

205 Balasubramanian SK, Azmi AS, Maciejewski J (2022). Selective inhibition of nuclear export: A promising approach in the shifting treatment paradigms for hematological neoplasms. *Leukemia* **36**(3). doi: 10.1038/s41375-021-01483-z.

206 Kosyna FK, Depping R (2018). Controlling the gatekeeper: Therapeutic targeting of nuclear transport. *Cells* 7(11). doi: 10.3390/cells7110221.

207 Helwick C (2022). Selinexor improves progression-free survival in endometrial cancer. The ASCO Post. [Online] Available: https://ascopost.com/issues/april-25-2022/selinexor-improves-progression-free-survival-in-endometrial-cancer/ [Accessed August 5, 2022].

208 Cancer Research UK. Myeloma incidence statistics. [Online] Available: https://www.cancerresearchuk.org/health-professional/cancer-statistics/statistics-by-cancer-type/myeloma/incidence [Accessed November 10, 2023].

209 Sánchez-Serrano I (2006). Success in translational research: Lessons from the development of bortezomib. *Nat. Rev. Drug Discov.* **5**(2). doi: 10.1038/nrd1959.

210 Navon A, Ciechanover A (2009). The 26 S proteasome: From basic mechanisms to drug targeting. *J. Biol. Chem.* **284**(49). doi: 10.1074/jbc.R109.018481.

211 Harper JW, Bennett EJ (2016). Proteome complexity and the forces that drive proteome imbalance. *Nature* **537**(7620). doi: 10.1038/nature19947.

212 Thibaudeau TA, Smith DM (2019). A practical review of proteasome pharmacology. *Pharmacol. Rev.* **71**(2). doi: 10.1124/pr.117.015370.

213 Ito S (2020). Proteasome inhibitors for the treatment of multiple myeloma. *Cancers* **12**(2). doi: 10.3390/cancers12020265.

214 Crawford LJ, Walker B, Irvine AE (2011). Proteasome inhibitors in cancer therapy. *J. Cell Commun. Signaling* **5**(2). doi: 10.1007/s12079-011-0121-7.

215 Saavedra-García P, Martini F, Auner HW (2020). Proteasome inhibition in multiple myeloma: Lessons for other cancers. *Am. J. Physiol. Cell Physiol.* **318**(3). doi: 10.1152/ajpcell.00286.2019.

216 Arkwright R *et al.* (2017). The preclinical discovery and development of bortezomib for the treatment of mantle cell lymphoma. *Expert Opin. Drug Discov.* **12**(2): 225–235. doi: 10.1080/17460441.2017.1268596.

217 Huang Z *et al.* (2014). Efficacy of therapy with bortezomib in solid tumors: A review based on 32 clinical trials. *Future Oncol.* **10**(10): 1795–1807. doi: 10.2217/fon.14.30.

CHAPTER 5

Immunotherapy with Checkpoint Inhibitors

IN BRIEF

Immunotherapies – treatments that use the immune system to destroy cancer – have existed for over a century. Despite this, they have only become a standard way of treating many types of cancer in the last 10 years or so.

In this chapter and the next, I describe many types of immunotherapy. First, in this chapter, I discuss the immune checkpoint inhibitors. Then, in Chapter 6, I look at other forms of immunotherapy, such as immune modulators, CAR T cells, vaccine-based treatments, and T cell engagers.

The immune checkpoint inhibitors work by boosting the activity of the patient's T cells. Before I get into the details of these treatments, I'll explain more about T cells and why they're such an important target of immunotherapy. I'll then turn my attention to the checkpoint proteins on the surface of T cells and the mechanisms of action of various checkpoint inhibitors.

The first checkpoint inhibitor to become a licensed cancer treatment was ipilimumab. It targets a checkpoint protein called CTLA-4. Since then, more checkpoint inhibitors have arrived on the scene, many targeting a checkpoint protein called PD-1 or one of its ligands,[1] PD-L1. LAG-3 targeted checkpoint inhibitors are an even more recent development.

An essential fact about checkpoint inhibitors is that they can only boost T cells that already exist in the person's body before treatment. They can't alert a person's immune system to the presence of cancer or persuade dendritic cells to carry cancer debris to T cells in lymph nodes. The fact that they can create beneficial, long-lasting immune responses, at least for some people, is a welcome finding that runs counter to initial expectations.

In this chapter, I look at what we have learned from the hundreds of clinical trials that have since taken place to investigate checkpoint inhibitors. These treatments have now been given to people with virtually every type of cancer, so there's a lot to try and summarize. I have attempted to pick out general themes and draw conclusions. I hope that by the end, you understand both the promise and limitations of these treatments.

---

[1] A ligand is anything (e.g., a hormone, peptide, protein, or drug) that can attach to a receptor.

5.1 THE IMPORTANCE OF T CELLS

5.1.1 The Importance of T Cells as a Target for Immunotherapy

In Chapter 1, I explained how our immune system responds to cancer, including describing several white blood cell types that can kill cancer cells, such as NK (natural killer) cells, macrophages, and T cells. Scientists even think that white blood cells involved in inflammation, like neutrophils, eosinophils, mast cells, basophils, and other cell types, can kill cancer cells if the circumstances are right [1].

So why is there so much emphasis placed on T cells? Well, there are a few crucial features of T cells that make them an attractive target when it comes to developing immunotherapies for cancer [2, 3]:

- They are powerful. Activated T cells are rapid and efficient killers of cancer cells. They can move from one cancer cell to the next, killing each cancer cell in turn.
- They are precise. Each T cell has thousands of copies of a unique version of the T cell receptor (TCR) on its surface. Each T cell's TCRs respond to a single antigen. When cancer-killing T cells recognize an antigen on the surface of cancer cells, they will kill cancer cells without harming other cells or tissues.
- They have the potential to give long-lasting protection. If you can persuade some memory T cells to get involved, they might offer durable protection and prevent the person's cancer from ever returning.
- T cells can eradicate cancer from a person's body and effectively cure them of their disease. It's difficult to know whether this is

possible across all cancer types, but at least in melanoma skin cancer, we can point to many thousands of people alive today thanks to T cell-directed immunotherapies.

5.1.2 How Do the Various T Cell-Directed Immunotherapies Work?

The Cancer-Immunity Cycle is a good starting point to explain how T cell-directed immunotherapies work. I described the Cancer-Immunity Cycle in Section 1.5.2 and Figure 1.15. The cycle describes how T cells become active, stay active, and destroy cancer cells. The main stages of the cycle are as follows [4]:

1. Various white blood cells detect the presence of cancer cells and raise the alarm.
2. Dendritic cells ingest debris from the cancer environment. They then move to nearby lymph nodes or tertiary lymphoid structures (TLSs), where they show peptide antigens taken from the debris to T cells using their MHC proteins (I mentioned TLSs in Section 1.6.4 and Figure 1.20; MHC proteins are described in Box 1.3).
3. Any T cell whose TCR matches the shape of one of the antigens displayed by a dendritic cell may become active.[2] Activated T cells multiply, leave the lymph node or TLS, and move into the tumor.
4. The T cells (hopefully) stay active in the tumor despite the many forces arrayed against them.
5. Finally, active, cancer-specific T cells react to their target antigen on the surface of cancer cells. They destroy thousands of cancer cells and possibly wipe out the cancer altogether.

As I mentioned in Chapter 1, there are many reasons why the cancer-immunity cycle might never happen or why the cycle occurs in a

---

[2] A peptide that leads to the activation of T cells is often referred to as a "peptide antigen" or as a "tumor antigen" or sometimes as an "antigenic peptide," as it has led to an immune response.

way that is insufficient to destroy or control the person's cancer.

In Figure 5.1, I have categorized treatments that boost T cell-mediated immune responses according to which part of the tumor-immunity cycle they are designed to help with. Treatments highlighted in blue are those I will say more about in this chapter.

For the rest of this chapter, I will focus on the checkpoint inhibitor group of immunotherapies – those that target either a checkpoint protein or one of its ligands.

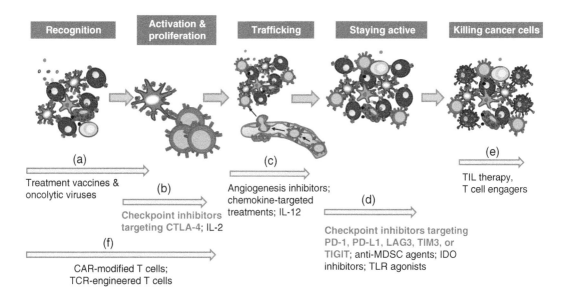

Figure 5.1 Immunotherapies that create or boost cancer-fighting T cells. **(a)** The purpose of vaccine-based treatments and oncolytic viruses is to help the person's immune system recognize and react to their cancer. **(b)** CTLA-4 antibodies and IL-2 increase the number of active T cells produced in lymph nodes or TLSs. **(c)** For T cells to destroy cancer cells, the T cells must first move to where the cancer cells are located. This is called trafficking. There are various ideas as to how T cell trafficking might be improved, such as changing the properties of tumor blood vessels with angiogenesis inhibitors or targeting signaling proteins, such as chemokines or interferon-gamma (IFNγ). **(d)** The environment inside tumors is often hostile and causes the suppression, exclusion, exhaustion, or death of cancer-fighting T cells. Numerous treatments aim to boost T cells and prevent their suppression. **(e)** One way to increase the number of active T cells is to take T cells from a tumor (or blood), activate and multiply them in a laboratory setting, and then give them back to the patient – so-called tumor-infiltrating lymphocyte – TIL – therapy. T cell engagers attach to both cancer cells and to available T cells, redirecting the T cells so that they destroy cancer cells. **(f)** With new technologies, we can now genetically alter some of the person's T cells so that they track down and destroy cancer cells without help from dendritic cells. These are called CAR T cell therapies or TCR-engineered T cell therapies.

Abbreviations: CAR – chimeric antigen receptor; CTLA-4 – cytotoxic T lymphocyte-associated antigen; IDO – indoleamine-2,3-dioxygenase; IFNγ – interferon-gamma; IL – interleukin; LAG3 – lymphocyte activating 3; MDSC – myeloid-derived suppressor cell; PD-1 – programmed death protein 1; PD-L1 – PD-1 ligand 1; TCR – T cell receptor; TIGIT – T cell immunoreceptor with Ig and ITIM domains; TIM3 – T cell immunoglobulin and mucin domain 3; TLR – Toll-like receptor; TLS – tertiary lymphoid structure.

5.2 AN INTRODUCTION TO IMMUNE CHECKPOINT INHIBITORS

Licensed drugs mentioned in this section:

Treatment class	Drugs	Given to some people with:
Checkpoint inhibitors targeting CTLA-4	Ipilimumab, tremelimumab	• Bowel cancer, esophageal cancer, primary liver cancer, mesothelioma, melanoma skin cancer, NSCLC, and kidney cancer
Checkpoint inhibitors targeting PD-1	Camrelizumab, cemiplimab, dostarlimab, nivolumab, pembrolizumab, sintilimab, tislelizumab, toripalimab, retifanlimab	• Melanoma skin cancer, biliary tract cancer, breast cancer, cervical cancer, Hodgkin lymphoma, squamous cell or basal cell carcinoma skin cancer, endometrial (uterine) cancer, esophageal and gastroesophageal junction cancer, stomach cancer, primary liver cancer, NSCLC, primary mediastinal large cell lymphoma, kidney cancer, head and neck cancer, and bladder cancer • Any solid tumor that is MSI, dMMR, or has a high mutation burden
Checkpoint inhibitors targeting PD-L1	Atezolizumab, avelumab, durvalumab	• NSCLC, small cell lung cancer, bladder cancer, Merkel cell skin cancer, alveolar soft part sarcoma, primary liver cancer, melanoma skin cancer, kidney cancer, and biliary tract cancer
Checkpoint inhibitors targeting LAG-3	Relatlimab	• Melanoma skin cancer

Abbreviations: dMMR – deficient in mismatch repair; MSI – microsatellite instability; NSCLC – non-small cell lung cancer.

Immunotherapy with checkpoint inhibitors (often referred to as "immune checkpoint inhibitors," "immune checkpoint blockade," or "checkpoint inhibitors") refers to a group of treatments that prevent (or reverse) the suppression of T cells. Doctors sometimes describe them as treatments that "release the brakes of the immune system" [5]. Checkpoint inhibitors achieve this by attaching to checkpoint proteins on the surface of T cells (such as PD-1) or attaching to a ligand for one of these receptors (such as PD-L1). Either way, they interfere with the connection between a checkpoint protein and one of its ligands.

To understand this group of treatments, I'll talk you through a few concepts:
• The normal role of checkpoint proteins and where they're found.
• The role that checkpoint proteins and their ligands play in suppressing cancer-fighting T cells.
• How current checkpoint inhibitors work – I'll split this into CTLA-4 targeted antibodies, PD-1 and PD-L1-targeted antibodies, and other checkpoint inhibitors.

5.2.1 The Normal Role of Checkpoint Proteins

Cytotoxic T cells (also called cytotoxic T lymphocytes – CTLs) are fantastic at killing other cells. Once activated by dendritic cells, they move to sites of infection or disease and kill virus-infected cells. They also kill damaged and faulty cells, such as cancer cells. However, to avoid chronic inflammation and autoimmune problems, their activities must be tightly controlled so that they only become active under the right circumstances and for the appropriate length of time. The body therefore needs a mechanism to reverse T cell activation and suppress them or tell them to die. For this reason, CTLs have proteins on their surface, known as checkpoint proteins, through which the body can control their activity [6, 7].

Some checkpoint proteins on CTLs help them become fully active. These are the

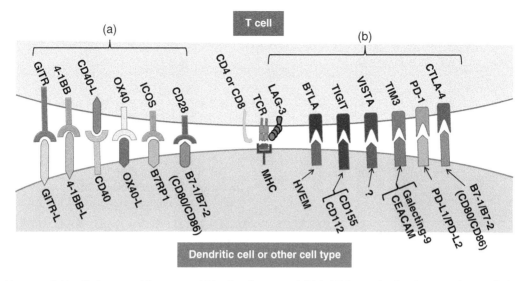

Figure 5.2 T cells have a wide range of (a) stimulatory and (b) inhibitory checkpoint proteins on their surface. Shown in the middle of the diagram is a T cell's T cell receptor (TCR) connecting with a peptide antigen presented by an MHC protein on the surface of an antigen-presenting cell, such as a dendritic cell. CD4 (if it's a helper T cell) or CD8 (if it's a cytotoxic T cell) participate in this interaction. An additional inhibitory protein known as LAG3 also connects with MHC and inhibits T cell activity. For abbreviations, see [7]. *Source:* Adapted from [7].

activating checkpoint proteins (Figure 5.2a). For example, you might remember from Section 1.5.1 that two things must happen for a T cell to become fully active. First, the cell's TCR must recognize and connect to a peptide antigen presented to it by a dendritic cell. Second, an activating checkpoint protein on the T cell called CD28 has to interact with a protein on the dendritic cell called B7. If these two interactions occur, the CTL might become active (although it often also needs encouragement from other cells) (Figure 1.14).

CTLs also have inhibitory checkpoint proteins on their surface (Figure 5.2b). These proteins limit the activity of T cells and make sure that they do not remain active after a threat has passed. They also prevent the activation of T cells that might attack and destroy healthy tissues.

5.2.2 Checkpoint Proteins Sometimes Suppress Cancer-Fighting T Cells

The two most famous inhibitory checkpoint proteins on T cells are CTLA-4 and PD-1. So, before I turn to the mechanism of action of checkpoint inhibitors, I'll say a little more about these two proteins.

The Function of CTLA-4

The function of CTLA-4[3] varies amongst the different types of T cells. This variation is summarized in Table 5.1 and Figure 5.3b [6, 8, 9].

Inhibition of CTLs by CTLA-4 can be extremely helpful:

1. It prevents the activation of T cells that are surplus to requirements. If these T cells became fully active, they might cause inflammation and tissue damage.

---

[3] CTLA-4 stands for Cytotoxic T Lymphocyte-Associated Molecule-4.

Table 5.1 The location and role of CTLA-4 depend on the T cell type.

	Helper T cell or cytotoxic T cell	Regulatory T cell
Ligand for CTLA-4	B7 proteins	B7 proteins
Normal location of CTLA-4	Inside the cell	On the cell surface
Location of CTLA-4 during/after activation of the T cell by a dendritic cell	On the cell surface	On the cell surface
What happens when CTLA-4 connects with a ligand?	The T cell shuts down	The T cell becomes more active
What happens when CTLA-4 is blocked by a CTLA-4-targeted antibody?	The T cell is more likely to become fully activated.	The T cell is suppressed and possibly dies.

2. It prevents the activation of T cells whose TCRs recognize peptides found in healthy cells, and that would otherwise cause autoimmune disease.

In contrast, the suppression of CTLs and helper T cells that recognize antigens on cancer cells is deeply unhelpful. By blocking them, the body unintentionally deprives itself of cancer-fighting T cells that might be highly useful.

The Function of PD-1 (and PD-L1)

PD-1 (programmed cell death protein-1[4]) is another inhibitory checkpoint protein. Whereas CTLA-4 can prevent T cells from becoming active, PD-1 is only found on T cells that have already become active. T cells with PD-1 on their surface are often found at the site of an infection or inside a tumor (sometimes simply referred to as being "in peripheral tissues"). Wherever they are,

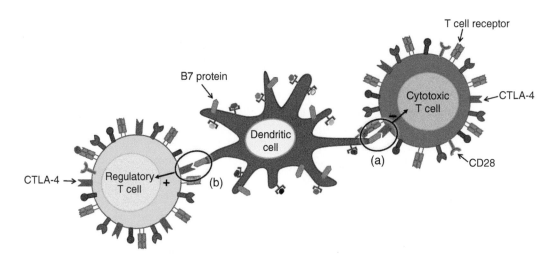

Figure 5.3 CTLA-4 has opposite effects on different types of T cells. (a) When a B7 protein on a dendritic cell connects with CTLA-4 on a cytotoxic T cell (CTL) or a Helper T cell, that T cell never becomes fully active. **(b)** When a B7 protein connects with CTLA-4 on the surface of a regulatory T cell (Treg), the Treg's activity increases. If the Treg is inside a tumor, it might start suppressing any cancer-fighting CTLs in that environment.
Abbreviation: CTLA-4 – cytotoxic T lymphocyte-associated protein 4.

---

[4] Don't read too much into this name. Proteins are often named according to their first known function, but this function might be revised or added to later.

they're in a location where they're repeatedly encountering cells displaying their target antigen. The normal, healthy purpose of PD-1 is to give the body the means to shut down T cells once whatever battle they are fighting has been won. This prevents overzealous T cells from causing tissue damage and helps to prevent autoimmune diseases [6, 10].

There are two ligands for PD-1: PD-L1 and PD-L2 (programmed death ligands 1 and 2). When either of these proteins connects with PD-1, a negative signal is sent into the cell, suppressing its activity and making it less likely to survive.

What should happen is this [8]:

1. CTLs are activated by dendritic cells displaying peptide antigens from an infection (or cancer cells). Only CTLs whose TCR matches the shape of one of these antigens become active.
2. Activated CTLs move to the infected/tumor tissue and kill cells with their target antigen on their surface. Activated CTLs make PD-1 and display it on their surface.

3. Finally, the CTLs' job is done. Other cells use PD-L1 or PD-L2 to trigger PD-1 on the surface of CTLs. This tells CTLs that the threat has passed, and it's time to shut down or even die.

The cells that usually have PD-L1 and PD-L2 on their surface are macrophages and dendritic cells (Figure 5.4a). However, the mere presence of activated CTLs in a tissue also causes nearby cells (white blood cells or any other cell in that tissue) to put PD-L1 on their surface.

To make that clear: PD-L1 is something that cells put on their surface in response to the presence of activated CTLs. Inside tumors, you often find cancer cells with PD-L1 on their surface. This is a sign that activated CTLs are present and that the person's immune system has recognized and reacted to their cancer cells. But it's also a sign that the CTLs generated by their immune system are being suppressed (Figure 5.4b).

In addition, some mutations, overactive pathways, and other defects in cancer cells force them to put PD-L1 on their surface [11].

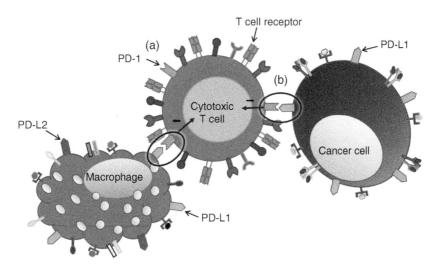

Figure 5.4 Cytotoxic T cells (CTLs) are suppressed and more likely to die when PD-1 proteins on their surface are triggered. (a) Activated CTLs place PD-1 on their surface. Then, when their job fighting an infection or fighting cancer is complete, other white blood cells (such as macrophages) trigger PD-1 using PD-L1 or PD-L2. **(b)** Inside tumors, cancer cells often have PD-L1 on their surface. They use it to suppress CTLs and thereby avoid being destroyed by the immune system.

They use this PD-L1 to protect themselves from destruction by CTLs.

This means that the presence of PD-L1 in a person's tumor doesn't always mean that immunotherapy with a checkpoint inhibitor will help them.

Are There Other Checkpoint Proteins?

The answer to that question is yes; I've already illustrated some of them in Figure 5.2. However, checkpoint proteins aren't limited to T cells. Macrophages, NK cells, and other types of white blood cells also have checkpoint proteins on their surface [12]. I'll mention a few of them later in this chapter.

5.3 HOW CHECKPOINT INHIBITORS WORK

As of now, all the licensed checkpoint inhibitors given to cancer patients are monoclonal antibodies. Most of them target CTLA-4, PD-1, or PD-L1.

CTLA-4-targeted antibodies prevent CTLA-4 from being triggered. This has two effects: it boosts the number of activated CTLs in the body, and it blocks the actions of regulatory T cells (Tregs) (Figure 5.5) [8].

PD-1- and PD-L1-targeted antibodies prevent the connection between PD-1 and PD-L1, which prevents PD-1 from being triggered. This increases the activity of CTLs in peripheral tissues and hopefully reverses the suppression of cancer-fighting CTLs inside tumors (Figure 5.6).

The different ways that CTLA-4, PD-1, and PD-L1 affect white blood cells presumably account for many of the differences seen with these antibodies in clinical trials.

5.3.1 Licensed Checkpoint Inhibitors

CTLA-4-, PD-1-, and PD-L1-targeted antibodies have been approved as cancer treatments (Table 5.2). These are standard treatment options for people with a wide range of cancer

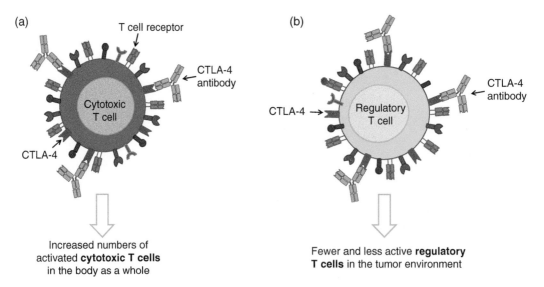

Figure 5.5 CTLA-4 targeted antibodies affect both CTLs and regulatory T cells. (a) CTLA-4 targeted antibodies encourage CTLs trapped in lymph nodes to become fully active and proliferate. Thus, higher numbers of CTLs are made. **(b)** CTLA-4 antibodies also attach to CTLA-4 on Tregs. This reduces their activity and causes their destruction by macrophages and NK cells. As a result, Treg numbers reduce and those that exist are less active.
Abbreviations: CTL – cytotoxic T cell; NK – Natural Killer; Treg – regulatory T cell.

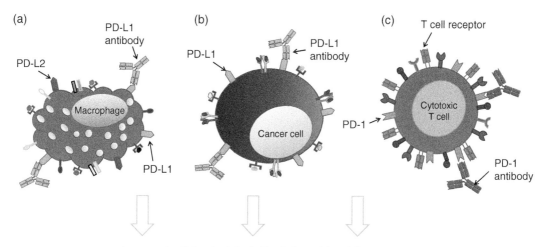

Figure 5.6 PD-1 and PD-L1 antibodies increase the activity of CTLs in peripheral tissues, including inside tumors. PD-L1-targeted antibodies attach to PD-L1 on the surface of various cell types, including macrophages **(a)** and cancer cells **(b)**. This prevents PD-L1 from interacting with PD-1 on CTLs. Thus, CTL suppression by PD-1 is prevented or reversed. **(c)** PD-1-targeted antibodies bind directly to PD-1 on T cells and block any interaction between PD-1 and its ligands, PD-L1 and PD-L2.
Abbreviation: CTL – cytotoxic T cell.

Table 5.2 Approved CTLA-4, PD-1, and PD-L1-targeted antibodies.

Targets	Antibody names
CTLA-4	Ipilimumab Tremelimumab
PD-1	Camrelizumab Cemiplimab Dostarlimab Nivolumab Pembrolizumab Retinfanlimab Sintilimab Tislelizumab Toripalimab
PD-L1	Atezolizumab Avelumab Durvalumab

types, including melanoma skin cancer, non-small cell lung cancer (NSCLC), kidney cancer, bladder cancer, head and neck cancer, and many others. A LAG-3-targeted antibody called relatlimab has also been approved for melanoma skin cancer. By the time this book is published there may well be more to add to the list.

5.4 LESSONS LEARNED FROM CHECKPOINT INHIBITOR TRIALS

The first checkpoint inhibitor (ipilimumab) was approved in 2011 as a treatment for melanoma skin cancer. Since then, thousands of people have been involved in hundreds of clinical trials testing out checkpoint inhibitors as treatments for different types of cancer. In addition, tens of thousands more people have been treated with marketed checkpoint inhibitors since their approval.

It's incredibly hard to make broad generalizations about the results of those trials, but I think it's important to try! So, on the following pages is a list of some of the important lessons we have learned along the way.

In this section, my focus is on checkpoint inhibitor monotherapy (when the inhibitor is given on its own rather than combined with another treatment) and where the patients haven't been selected based on a biomarker test. I'll be coming to combinations and bio-markers later in Sections 5.6 and 5.7.

5.4.1 Some Patients with Advanced Cancer Can Effectively Be Cured

I think the reason why checkpoint inhibitor therapy has created so much excitement and optimism in recent years is because it can offer many years of additional life to some people with advanced cancer. But this isn't what happens for most people. It's important to remember that the first trials involved people with melanoma skin cancer, one of the most immunotherapy-sensitive cancers out there. Just because a new immunotherapy looks good against melanoma skin cancer doesn't mean it's going to work as well for people with other cancers.

Below is a summary of three clinical trials involving people with advanced melanoma skin cancer for which long-term survival data have been published.

As you can see in Table 5.3, roughly half (52%) of the people involved in the CheckMate-067 trial who received ipilimumab plus nivolumab (a CTLA-4 antibody plus a PD-1 antibody) were alive five years after starting treatment. Of these people, 74% of them were not receiving any checkpoint inhibitor or other treatment for cancer at the five-year time point and are likely to have been cured [15]. This contrasts with the people who took part in the CA184-024 trial (this was one of the earliest checkpoint inhibitor trials and began in 2011, two years before the CheckMate 067 trial). In the CA184-024 trial, only 9% of the people who received chemotherapy and 18% of the people given chemotherapy plus ipilimumab were alive five years later.

The results from melanoma trials show that it is possible to cure people with advanced melanoma skin cancer through checkpoint inhibitor therapy. In trials involving people with other cancers, long-term survival is also a possibility, but for a smaller proportion of people. For example, in the CA209-003 trial, in which 270 patients with advanced cancer (melanoma skin cancer, renal cell carcinoma,[5] or NSCLC) were treated with nivolumab, the five-year survival rates were 34% for patients with melanoma, 28% for patients with kidney cancer, and 16% for people with NSCLC [18].

Table 5.3 A summary of survival rates in checkpoint inhibitor clinical trials in people with advanced melanoma skin cancer.

	CA184-024 [13]		CheckMate 067 [14, 15]			KEYNOTE- 001 [16, 17]
	Chemo	Ipi + Chemo	Ipi	Nivo	Ipi + Nivo	Pembro
1-Year survival	36%	48				66
2-Year survival	18%	29%	45%	59%	64%	49–52%
3-Year survival	12%	21%	34%	52%	58%	40%
4-Year survival	10%	19%	30%	46%	53%	38%
5-Year survival	9%	18%	26%	44%	52%	34%

Abbreviations: Chemo – chemotherapy with dacarbazine; Ipi – ipilimumab; Nivo – nivolumab; Pembro – pembrolizumab.

---

[5] Renal cell carcinoma accounts for roughly 80% of kidney cancers, so I'll just call it kidney cancer from now on [source – Cancer Research UK].

5.4.2 Responders to Checkpoint Inhibitor Monotherapy Are Usually in a Minority

Most of the time, when a checkpoint inhibitor is given as monotherapy to someone with advanced cancer, it doesn't help them. Now, there are lots of ways you can define "help," but I'm first going to compare response rates. That is, in what proportion of patients did their tumor (or tumors) shrink in size by at least 30% as measured on scans (this is the usual definition of what a "response" is [19]).

In Table 5.4, I've compared response rates for checkpoint inhibitors when given as a stand-alone treatment for various types of advanced cancer. In every trial, the people involved had already received one or more prior courses of treatment and their disease had nonetheless returned or progressed.

When looking at this table you might want to bear in mind that the response rate to checkpoint inhibitor monotherapy in people with advanced melanoma skin cancer is around 30–40% [17]. It's also good to remember that when patients benefit from checkpoint inhibitor monotherapy, that benefit often lasts a long time. This is very different from other treatments (e.g., chemotherapy), where any benefit is likely to be much shorter-lasting.

It's important to note that these days (as a result of trials such as those in Table 5.4), checkpoint inhibitors are often given as part of a combination and/or they're given at an earlier point in a patient's treatment when they're more likely to help.

You can see from this table that there is a wide variation in the proportion of patients with different cancers who benefit from

Table 5.4 Examples of clinical trials in which checkpoint inhibitor monotherapy has been given to previously treated patients with a variety of advanced cancer types.

Disease; clinical trial name; treatments compared	Response rate
Recurrent NSCLC; summary of data from numerous trials involving nivolumab, pembrolizumab, atezolizumab, or avelumab monotherapy [20]	**14–20%**
Recurrent head and neck cancer: CheckMate 141; nivolumab vs. chemotherapy/cetuximab [21]	**13%** vs. 6%
Recurrent head and neck cancer: KEYNOTE-040; pembrolizumab vs. chemotherapy/cetuximab [22]	**15%** vs. 10%
Recurrent kidney cancer: CheckMate 025; nivolumab vs. everolimus [23]	**25%** vs. 5%
Recurrent bladder cancer: KEYNOTE-045; pembrolizumab vs. doctor's choice of chemotherapy [24]	**21%** vs. 11%
Recurrent bladder cancer: CheckMate 275; nivolumab single-arm [25]	**20%**
Recurrent primary liver cancer: KEYNOTE-224; pembrolizumab single-arm [26]	**17%**
Recurrent bowel cancer; IMblaze370; atezolizumab vs. atezolizumab + cobimetinib vs. regorafenib [27]	**2%** vs. **3%** vs. 2%
Recurrent ovarian cancer; KEYNOTE-100; pembrolizumab single-arm [28]	**8%**
Recurrent cervical cancer; KEYNOTE-158; pembrolizumab single-arm [29]	**12%**
Recurrent prostate cancer; KEYNOTE-199; pembrolizumab given to patients with PD-L1 negative or PD-L1 positive disease [30]	**3% or 5%**
Recurrent triple-negative breast cancer; KEYNOTE-086; pembrolizumab monotherapy [31]	**5%**
Recurrent gastric or gastroesophageal cancer; KEYNOTE-059; pembrolizumab monotherapy [32]	**13%**

checkpoint inhibitor monotherapy. This lack of benefit for most people has fueled the desire to:

1. Identify features that can be measured and used to identify people likely to benefit the most – the search for biomarkers (Section 5.6)
2. Come up with treatment combinations that provide more benefit to a greater proportion of patients they are given to – the search for effective treatment combinations (Section 5.7)
3. Create new immunotherapies that work for more people, or that can be combined with existing checkpoint inhibitors – the search for new immunotherapies (Section 5.8 and Chapter 6)

5.4.3 The Earlier You Can Give the Checkpoint Inhibitor the Better

An observation that holds true across many trials is that people with advanced cancer who haven't already received prior treatment are more likely to benefit from checkpoint inhibitor therapy than people who have received previous treatment (see Table 5.5).

There could be a few reasons for this difference, such as: [37–40]

1. Cancers (and any metastases) that have recurred and/or spread after previous treatments have a more immune-suppressing microenvironment than newly diagnosed cancers.
2. The person's previous treatment killed the more vulnerable cancer cells, and now the cells that have caused their cancer to regrow are more resilient and/or more protected or hidden from their immune system.
3. A person whose cancer has returned is likely to be in worse overall health and more frail than they were when they were first diagnosed. This might affect their chance of benefiting from treatment, and it might mean that they are taking other medicines (e.g., antibiotics/steroids) that also negatively affect their likelihood of benefit.

Because of data such as those shown in Table 5.5, checkpoint inhibitors are often given as the first course of treatment to people with advanced cancer rather than waiting until later.

Table 5.5 Previously untreated patients with advanced cancer derive more benefit from checkpoint inhibitors than people who have received previous treatment.

	Response rate	Median overall survival
KEYNOTE-086 Phase 2 trial, pembrolizumab given to patients with advanced triple-negative breast cancer [31, 33]		
Previously treated patients	5%	9 months
Previously untreated patients	21%	18 months
Phase 1 trial, atezolizumab given to patients with advanced triple-negative breast cancer [34]		
Previously treated patients	6%	7 months
Previously untreated patients	24%	18 months
KEYNOTE-001 Phase 1b trial, pembrolizumab given to people with advanced NSCLC [35, 36]		
Previously treated patients	23%	11 months
Previously untreated patients	42%	22 months

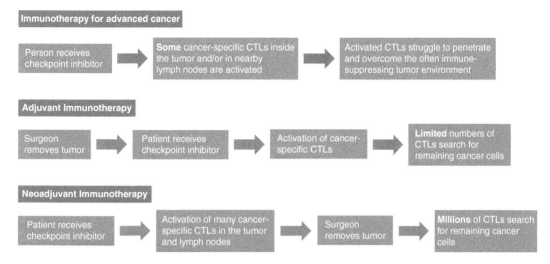

Immunotherapy for advanced cancer

Person receives checkpoint inhibitor → **Some** cancer-specific CTLs inside the tumor and/or in nearby lymph nodes are activated → Activated CTLs struggle to penetrate and overcome the often immune-suppressing tumor environment

Adjuvant Immunotherapy

Surgeon removes tumor → Patient receives checkpoint inhibitor → Activation of cancer-specific CTLs → **Limited** numbers of CTLs search for remaining cancer cells

Neoadjuvant Immunotherapy

Patient receives checkpoint inhibitor → Activation of many cancer-specific CTLs in the tumor and lymph nodes → Surgeon removes tumor → **Millions** of CTLs search for remaining cancer cells

Figure 5.7 The number and activity of cancer-specific cytotoxic T cells (CTLs) activated by checkpoint inhibitor immunotherapy differs depending on when the treatment is given.

Trials involving people with early stage, operable cancer have also provided evidence that giving checkpoint inhibitors before surgery (as a neoadjuvant) is better than afterward (as an adjuvant).

In Figure 5.7, I have outlined the rationale for giving checkpoint inhibitors as a neoadjuvant therapy.

The possible advantage of giving a checkpoint inhibitor before surgery is that, at this point in time, both the tumor and associated lymph vessels and lymph nodes are intact. As a result, many more CTLs will hopefully be activated by the checkpoint inhibitor compared to when it's given as an adjuvant treatment (when the tumor has been removed) or as a treatment for advanced disease (when the tumor environment is likely to be highly immune suppressing) [41, 42].

A clinical trial that highlights the advantages of giving a checkpoint inhibitor as a neoadjuvant rather than as an adjuvant treatment is the SWOG S1801 trial outlined in Figure 5.8 (although the actual comparison was adjuvant vs. neoadjuvant and adjuvant checkpoint inhibitor) [42].

Neoadjuvant checkpoint inhibitor therapy is also approved (in combination with chemotherapy) for people with NSCLC or triple-negative breast cancer. Promising results have also been reported in other cancer types [43–46].

5.4.4 There's Very Little Relationship Between Dose and Response

With chemotherapy, the more treatment you give, the better it is likely to work. Doctors try to find a balance whereby they give as much treatment as possible without making life unbearable for the patient due to side effects. This dose is called the maximum tolerated dose.

In contrast, checkpoint inhibitors (at least with those targeting PD-1 or PD-L1) have no dose–response relationship in terms of their effectiveness or side effects [47–50]. Sometimes, a single dose of a checkpoint inhibitor will cure someone of their disease. But, for many people, no matter how much of the treatment you give them, it has no effect on their cancer.

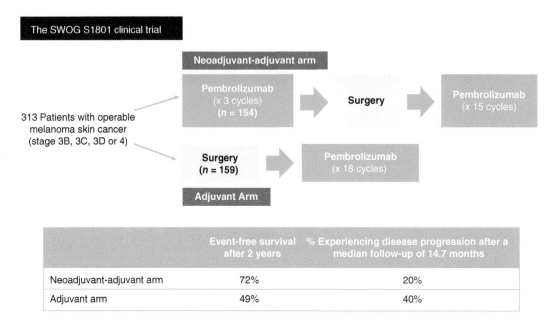

Figure 5.8 **An outline of the design and results of the SWOG S1801 clinical trial**. The trial involved 313 people with operable melanoma skin cancer who were randomized to receive checkpoint inhibitor therapy (pembrolizumab) after surgery or both before and after surgery. The total dose of immunotherapy was the same in both arms. Event-free survival at two years is the proportion of people who were free of any sign of their disease after two years. (To be more precise, the "events" encompassed by "event-free survival" included a patient being unable to commence adjuvant therapy for various reasons, including surgical complications, so technically, a patient could have been free of disease but still have had an event [42].)

When you think back to the science of how checkpoint inhibitors work, I think this does make sense. If someone's cancer has gone undetected by their immune system or is protected by mechanisms unrelated to checkpoint proteins on T cells, then a checkpoint inhibitor won't help them, no matter how much treatment you give. In the opposite scenario, when a person's cancer is highly visible to their immune system, a single dose of a checkpoint inhibitor may activate enough CTLs to bring their cancer under control.

This lack of a dose–response relationship has led to questions such as:

- Can we give patients lower doses and achieve the same impact as with higher doses? If so, this could be better for patients and make these treatments more affordable for healthcare providers.

- If people respond well early on, can they safely stop treatment? If so, how might we decide when it's safe for them to stop treatment?

I'll come back to the second question in Section 5.4.6.

5.4.5 Side Effects Are Unpredictable and Can Be Life Long

Our body uses CTLA-4 and PD-1 on T cells to prevent unwanted T cells from becoming active and to limit the length of time that T cells remain active.

When either CTLA-4 or PD-1 is blocked by a checkpoint inhibitor, this increases the activity of <u>any</u> T cells in the body that are being suppressed via these proteins. This activation of unwanted CTLs is what causes the severe inflammatory reactions called immune-related adverse events (irAEs) [51].

Some irAEs are short-lived and usually easily managed. These include inflammation in the gut, lungs, and skin [51, 52]. However, sometimes irAEs are more severe, more difficult to control, and can cause life-long problems. For example, the activation of T cells that react to healthy cells in the thyroid or pituitary gland can result in the destruction of these glands. If the gland is destroyed, then the person will require life-long hormone replacement treatment [51]. In rare occasions, side effects can be fatal, especially those affecting the bowel, lungs, liver, heart, or brain [53].

Another aspect of irAEs that differs from the side effects of other treatments is their timing. For example, irAEs affecting the skin and bowel tend to build in the first few weeks. In contrast, if it occurs, inflammation of the pituitary gland has a median time of onset of eight weeks after treatment starts (see [54] for detailed information on the timing of various irAEs). Some people even experience irAEs long after treatment has stopped [55].

5.4.6 There Are Various Possible Patterns of Response

The way a person's cancer reacts to checkpoint inhibitor therapy varies widely from patient to patient. It can also differ between the primary tumor and any metastases. The different trajectories depicted in Figure 5.9 are stylized and can only reflect some of the many possible outcomes [56–60].

For example, for some people given checkpoint inhibitor therapy, their tumor(s) shrink and never regrow (they have a durable complete or partial response). For other people, the treatment doesn't reduce the size of their cancer at all, but their disease stabilizes, and this may continue for many months or years (durable, stable disease). But, for some people, their cancer seems unaffected by treatment and carries on growing as before (called progression or primary resistance).

There are also some strange patterns of response. For example, there's pseudoprogression, where white blood cells move into the tumor causing it to initially increase in size but then, as the white blood cells kill cancer cells, the size reduces. There's also a rare phenomenon called hyperprogression, where

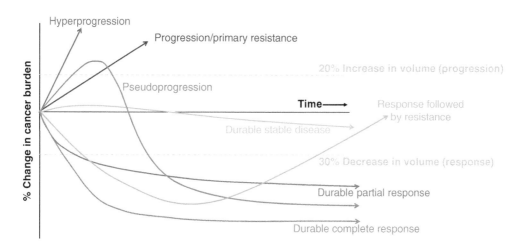

Figure 5.9 There are many different patterns of response and resistance to checkpoint inhibitor immunotherapy.

immunotherapy seems to cause the person's disease to accelerate and worsen much more quickly than it would have done otherwise (although this is very hard to measure or prove) [56, 57].

Response followed by resistance (also called secondary resistance) is also a possibility. This is where the person's cancer shrinks initially, but eventually, cancer cells that are resistant or protected in some way cause the cancer to regrow.

This range of responses is wider and more varied than those seen with chemotherapy or targeted therapy.

The fact that long-lasting responses are possible offers up the question of whether some patients can safely stop treatment. The answer to this is probably yes, at least for people with advanced melanoma skin cancer who experience a durable response [61]. Various clinical trials are underway to define exactly which patients can safely stop treatment and when they can do it without compromising their chances of long-term survival. These include the DANTE trial [62], the STOP-GAP trial [63], PET-Stop [64], and the Safe Stop Trial [65]. (No doubt the results of these trials will be published long before I next update this book, so you might want to Google the trial names and find out what they found.)

5.4.7 Response Rates Are Highest in Tumors With *PD-L1/2* Gene Mutations

One of the anomalies with checkpoint inhibitor therapy is the very high response rate (sometimes over 80%) seen in people with Hodgkin lymphoma and a handful of other, rarer lymphomas [66–71].

The reason behind this is that the cells that cause most Hodgkin lymphomas (called

Reed Sternberg – RS – cells) have extra copies of a segment of chromosome 9 (specifically 9p24.1). The amplified segment contains the genes for PD-L1 and PD-L2, causing RS cells to have large amounts of both proteins on their surface [67, 72]. Perhaps not surprisingly, response rates to checkpoint inhibitors in Hodgkin lymphoma are similar to those seen when you match a mutation in an oncogene to a suitable targeted therapy.

The same amplification is also found in a high proportion of people with some rare forms of large B cell lymphoma, such as primary mediastinal B cell lymphoma, gray zone lymphoma, primary testicular lymphoma, and primary central nervous system lymphoma [69–71].

In contrast, the amplification is present in just 0.7–1.2% of people with solid tumors [73, 74]. Although this percentage is small, it is similar to the prevalence of some of the mutations we now seek out and match with targeted treatments in diseases, such as NSCLC. The data so far suggest that testing for amplification of the *PD-L1* gene might be worth doing, although it doesn't always go together with high levels of PD-L1 protein [75].

5.4.8 Early Data From Immunotherapy Trials Can Be Misleading

The final general point I want to make about experiences from checkpoint inhibitor trials is that the early trial data from these trials often underestimate the long-lasting benefits that checkpoint inhibitors can bring [76–78].

When a drug company (or other organization) sets up a clinical trial, one of its aims is to find out the result of that trial as quickly as possible. This keeps costs down and avoids problems such as patients being lost to follow-up.[6]

---

[6] This is when the team running the trial loses all contact with a person in the trial, and they don't know what happened to them.

One of the earliest pieces of trial data that can be collected is the objective response rate (ORR), i.e., what proportion of patients' tumors shrank? [19, 79] (see Box 5.1 for a brief summary of various measures of success used in clinical trials). Another early piece of data is the median progression-free survival (median PFS), which is how long it takes for half the people in the study to have experienced tumor progression or to have died from any cause.[7]

However, there are problems with ORR and median PFS when it comes to assessing the benefits or otherwise of immunotherapy [19, 82]. For example, let's look back at Figure 5.9. We can see that some people given a checkpoint inhibitor experience long-lasting benefits from treatment despite their disease not meeting the threshold of a "response."

I find the best way to explain the limitations of median PFS is to describe an imaginary clinical trial. In this fictitious trial, a group of 30 patients with advanced cancer have been randomly assigned to receive a checkpoint inhibitor or chemotherapy. Each patient has been followed up for a minimum of a year (Figure 5.10).

The median PFS is calculated by placing the PFS for each patient in ascending numerical order. The point in time when half the patients have experienced disease progression is the median PFS for that arm of the trial. In the imagined trial, the PFS for people in the chemotherapy arm is six months, whereas for the people given the checkpoint inhibitor, it's four months. The problem is that the median PFS figure tells you nothing about what happened to the people whose disease hadn't worsened when the PFS timepoint was reached. For the chemotherapy arm, there's just one person whose disease hasn't progressed (NR stands for not reached), but in the checkpoint inhibitor arm, it's four. So, quite clearly, your chance of experiencing a long-lasting benefit from the checkpoint inhibitor is higher than that for chemotherapy.

A more informative measure might be the one-year PFS rate. In the chemotherapy group, this is 7% (1 out of 15), but in the immunotherapy group, it is 33% (5 out of 15). Although, of course, to calculate this, you'd need to wait much longer than the wait to calculate the median PFS.

In Table 5.6, I've summarized the data from five clinical trials involving people with advanced NSCLC whose disease had progressed after their initial treatment. Now, response rates with subsequent chemotherapy (docetaxel) are pretty low (they range from 9% to 13%), but even so, the median PFS data are better for the chemotherapy arm in most trials. So, if you'd stopped these trials after collecting the PFS data, the checkpoint inhibitor arm of each trial would look pretty unimpressive. However, the real difference comes when you look at the median duration of response (DoR) data and the survival rates at two or three years.

The pattern you see from clinical trials with checkpoint inhibitors reflects two realities: (1) the proportion of patients helped by the treatment is likely to be relatively small, but (2) it's possible that some people will experience long-term benefits and still be alive many years later.

The upshot is that we need to be cautious in interpreting early trial data from checkpoint inhibitor clinical trials[8] [84].

---

[7] The official definition of "PFS" is the time from random assignment (to an arm of a clinical trial) to disease progression or death from any cause. Whereas "disease progression" generally refers to the person's tumor (or tumors) having increased in diameter by at least 20%. If you want to learn more about the definition of disease progression (and the difficulties with this as a measure), there's a great article about it by a doctor called Lynne Elridge [80].

[8] If you want more advice on how to interpret the results of cancer clinical trials, see Vinay Prasad's online article [83].

Box 5.1   What does "good" look like in the world of clinical trials? [79]

When researchers design a clinical trial to test out a new treatment, one of the most important questions they must ask themselves is, "What does good look like?" That is, what are they hoping the new treatment will achieve for patients, how are they going to measure it, how often, and for how long?

Hopefully, they'll pick measures – called **endpoints** – that give an accurate idea of how good the new treatment is and that reflect what matters most to patients. But picking endpoints is a tricky decision to make, as they must balance out cost, practicality, what patients want, and what regulators want too.

The organization or company paying for the trial may also have in mind the financial rewards that come when treatment is approved for use. This might persuade them to look for measures that have the best chance of making their treatment look good, and these might not necessarily align with the priorities of patients [81].

Various common endpoints include:

Overall survival (OS). The length of time from when the patient is randomized (randomly allocated to be in one arm of the trial or another), or from when they entered the trial, to their death.

Progression-free survival (PFS). The length of time from when the patient is randomized, or from when they entered the trial, to the first signs of their disease progressing or them dying. This is a similar measure to **Time to progression.**

Objective response rate. The proportion of patients whose tumor(s) disappear altogether (a complete response) or shrink by at least 30% (a partial response); for a fuller description of these terms, see [79].

Duration of response (DoR). The length of time from when a person has a complete or partial response to when that person's disease progresses. Because this can only be assessed in people who experience a complete or partial response to treatment, the data only reflect what happens to people whose tumor(s) shrink by at least 30% in response to treatment.

Disease-free survival. The length of time from that the person continues to be free of any sign of their cancer after their randomization. It is typically used as a measure of success in trials of adjuvant treatments (treatments given after surgery), where the aim is to prevent or delay the cancer's return.

PFS or OS rate. The proportion of people progression-free (PFS) or still alive (OS) after a certain amount of time since their randomization. For example, it might be PFS rate at one year or two years. These are sometimes called milestones.

Median PFS, OS, DoR, etc. The median value is **the middle value** in a set of numbers. You calculate it by arranging a set of numbers from smallest to largest; the median value is then the number in the middle of the list. In terms of a clinical trial, you can think of it as the length of time it took for half the people in the study to experience whatever it is you're measuring. For example, the median OS is the time it took for half the patients in the study to die.

Censoring. This is when data relating to people in a clinical trial are deliberately excluded. For example, if the trial team loses all contact with someone in a trial, then any data relating to that person might be omitted.

Please note, these definitions assume that the trial in question is a randomized trial – one in which patients have been randomly assigned to receive the treatment under investigation or not. However, not every trial is randomized. Non-randomized trials often include small, early-phase trials, and those involving patients with very rare diseases.

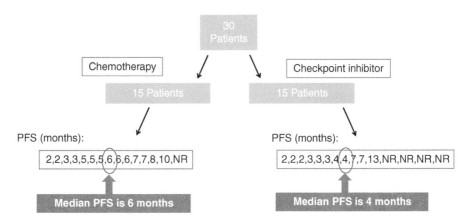

Figure 5.10 Results from an imaginary trial in which 30 people with advanced cancer are randomized to receive either a checkpoint inhibitor or chemotherapy and then followed up for a minimum of a year.
Abbreviations: NR – not reached; PFS – progression-free survival.

5.5 WHY SOME PATIENTS BENEFIT FROM CHECKPOINT INHIBITORS AND OTHERS DON'T

I find it helpful to sort the factors that affect the helpfulness (or otherwise) of checkpoint inhibitors into three classes:

1. Those that operate at the level of the person's cancer cells
2. Those that operate at the level of the tumor microenvironment
3. Those that operate at the level of the person as a whole

5.5.1 The Impact of Cancer Cells

How well a checkpoint inhibitor works partly depends on how "visible" the person's cancer cells are to their immune system, sometimes referred to as a cancer's immunogenicity. (Look back at Figure 1.13 and Section 1.5.1 for a refresher.)

In Figure 5.11, I've summarized some factors affecting whether a person's cancer cells will be visible to their immune system. Visible (immunogenic) cancers are more likely to contain active, cancer-fighting CTLs that can be boosted with checkpoint inhibitors [4, 85–88].

Table 5.6 Data from five trials in which a PD-1- or PD-L1-targeted checkpoint inhibitor was compared to docetaxel in people with advanced NSCLC whose disease had progressed after their initial treatment.

Trial name	KEYNOTE-010	CheckMate017	CheckMate057	OAK	JAVELIN Lung 200
Population	PD-L1 ≥1%[a]; mNSCLC	Squamous mNSCLC	Non-squamous mNSCLC	mNSCLC	PD-L1 ≥1%; mNSCLC
Treatment comparison	Pembrolizumab vs. docetaxel	Nivolumab vs. docetaxel	Nivolumab vs. docetaxel	Atezolizumab vs. docetaxel	Avelumab vs. docetaxel
Objective response rate	18% vs. 9%	20% vs. 9%	19% vs. 12%	14% vs. 13%	19% vs. 12%
Median DoR	17.2 vs. 5.6 months	25.2 vs. 8.4 months	17.2 vs. 5.6 months	16.3 vs. 6.2 months	19.1 vs. 5.7 months
Median PFS	3.9–4.0 vs. 4.0 months	3.5 vs. 2.8 months	2.3 vs. 4.2 months	2.8 vs. 4.0 months	3.4 vs. 4.1 months
Median OS	10.4–12.7 vs. 8.5 months	9.2 vs. 6 months	12.2 vs. 9.4 months	13.8 vs. 9.6 months	11.4 vs. 10.3 months
Milestone OS rate at 2 or 3 years	3-year OS rate: 23% vs. 11%	3-year OS rate: 16% vs. 6%	3-year OS rate: 18% vs. 9%	3-year OS rate: 21% vs. 12.4%	2-year OS rate: 29.9% vs. 20.5%

Abbreviations: mNSCLC – metastatic non-small cell lung cancer; DoR – duration of response; PFS – progression-free survival; OS – overall survival.
[a] In the KEYNOTE-010 and JAVELIN Lung 200 trials, patients could only enter the trial if at least 1% of their tumor cells had PD-L1 on their surface, thus enriching the trial population with people more likely to benefit from checkpoint inhibitor immunotherapy.
Source: Adapted from [20].

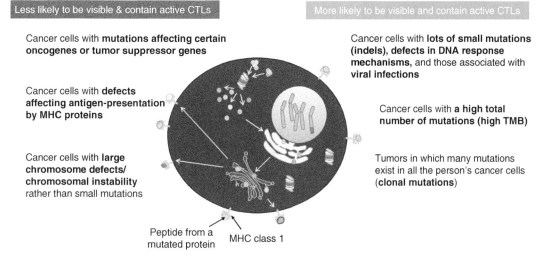

Less likely to be visible & contain active CTLs

Cancer cells with **mutations affecting certain oncogenes or tumor suppressor genes**

Cancer cells with **defects affecting antigen-presentation by MHC proteins**

Cancer cells with **large chromosome defects/ chromosomal instability** rather than small mutations

More likely to be visible and contain active CTLs

Cancer cells with **lots of small mutations (indels), defects in DNA response mechanisms,** and those associated with **viral infections**

Cancer cells with **a high total number of mutations (high TMB)**

Tumors in which many mutations exist in all the person's cancer cells (**clonal mutations**)

Peptide from a mutated protein   MHC class 1

Figure 5.11 Mutations and other defects in cancer cells affect whether the person's cancer is visible to their immune system or not.
Abbreviations: indels – insertions and deletions; MHC – major histocompatibility complex; TMB – tumor mutation burden.

5.5.2 The Impact of the Tumor Microenvironment

Scientists categorize tumors as being "hot," "cold," "immune-suppressed," or "immune-excluded" [4, 87] (all four categories are depicted in Figure 5.12). It's worth remembering, though, that these categories aren't black and white, and there are lots of variations. Nor is a person's tumor always going to be all one thing. For example, one part of a tumor can be "hot" and another part "cold." Or the person might have a "hot" primary tumor but with "immune-suppressed" metastases.

Which Cancers are the Hottest? [89]

The hottest tumors are often those:
- With the highest numbers of mutations – such as those with DNA repair defects.
- Caused by external factors – such as those linked to viral infections, such as the human papillomavirus.
- That exhibit both factors above – such as melanoma skin cancers caused by UV light or NSCLCs in people with a history of smoking.

Which Cancers Are the Coldest? [89]

The coldest tumors tend to be those:
- With the lowest numbers of mutations, e.g., neuroblastoma, glioblastoma, and prostate cancer.
- Driven by mutations that create an immune-suppressing microenvironment, e.g., small cell lung cancer, oncogene-driven NSCLCs in never smokers.
- That exhibit both factors above, e.g., pancreatic cancers tend to have a low number of mutations and 92% contain powerful oncogene mutations that drive immune suppression.

5.5.3 The Patient as a Whole

The Person's Inherited Genetic Makeup

One example of this is the *HLA* genes we inherit from our parents. There are thousands of different versions of these genes, and each of us inherits a set of *HLA* genes from our mother and another set from our father [90]. These genes dictate the shape of the MHC protein "cups" that sit on the surface of our cells and

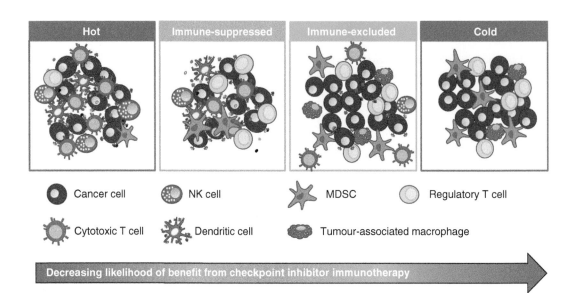

Figure 5.12 Tumors can be categorized according to the white blood cells found within them.
"HOT" tumors contain lots of cytotoxic T cells (CTLs), which are likely to recognize peptides found on the surface of the person's cancer cells. NK cells and mature dendritic cells are also present. There are high levels of PD-L1 on the surface of various cell types. "IMMUNE-SUPPRESSED" tumors contain fewer CTLs and higher numbers of immune-suppressing MDSCs, regulatory T cells, and tumor-associated macrophages. "IMMUNE-EXCLUDED" tumors contain many immune-suppressing white blood cells. Any CTLs present are found in the outer fringes of the tumor. "COLD" tumors contain little or no sign of any past or present immune response. If PD-L1 is present, it is a consequence of mutated oncogenes, and cancer cells are using it to create an immune-suppressing environment.
Abbreviations: CTL – cytotoxic T lymphocyte; MDSC – myeloid-derived suppressor cell; NK – natural killer; PD-L1- programmed death ligand-1.

display peptides to passing white blood cells (see Section 1.5.1 and Box 1.3 for a description). Some people's MHC proteins are more diverse than other people's. The more diverse the range of MHC proteins, the greater the range of peptides our cells can show to our immune system. High diversity correlates with a greater chance of our immune system creating cancer-fighting CTLs and a greater chance of benefiting from checkpoint inhibitors [91].

The Range of Bacteria in Their Digestive Tract

The gut microbiome – the range of bacteria found in our digestive tract – has an enormous impact on our immune system. Imbalances in the bacterial communities in our gut

(called dysbiosis) can be caused by things such as illness, antibiotics, or a poor diet. Dysbiosis increases our risk of chronic inflammation, immune-related illnesses, and cancer. When a tumor has formed, a healthy gut microbiome and dysbiosis have opposing influences on the microenvironment within that tumor. People with a healthy gut microbiome benefit more from immunotherapy with checkpoint inhibitors than people with dysbiosis [92].

This link between the gut microbiome and the degree of benefit from checkpoint inhibitors raises the question of how we can help patients to prepare for immunotherapy. Some of the studies looking at this have given conflicting or confusing results. What does appear to be good for our microbiome is to have a diet rich in fiber, whole grains, fish, nuts, fruit, legumes, and vegetables (often called a Mediterranean diet) [93–95].

What Other Medicines They are Taking

Many people with cancer are taking medicines for a variety of other health conditions, as well as to manage the symptoms of their disease. The medicines that appear to influence the sensitivity of a person's cancer to checkpoint inhibitors also seem to be ones that impact the gut microbiome. For example, broad-spectrum antibiotics, corticosteroids, paracetamol (acetaminophen), opioids, and proton pump inhibitors have all been linked to a lower likelihood of benefiting from checkpoint inhibitors [96–100]. The impact seems to be greatest if these medicines are taken within a few weeks before or after starting checkpoint inhibitor therapy [101].

5.6 BIOMARKERS OF RESPONSE TO CHECKPOINT INHIBITORS

As I've said several times, in many situations, only a relatively small proportion of people given checkpoint inhibitors benefit from them [102]. It would therefore be ideal to be able to predict who these people will be in advance. That way, people who wouldn't be helped could avoid receiving unnecessary treatment.

To identify people who are the most (or least) likely to benefit from checkpoint inhibitors, it is essential to identify biomarkers of response and/or resistance (see Box 5.2

Box 5.2   Biomarkers

So, what's a biomarker? You might feel that you know the answer to this question already, in which case ignore me and read on! Or, you might want a quick refresher, in which case:

A biomarker is:

- Something biological – maybe a gene or a protein,
- That you can objectively, accurately, and reliably measure,
- And that, once measured, provides you with some useful information.

For example, a **predictive biomarker** might help you predict whether a treatment is likely to work for a patient. Whereas a **prognostic biomarker** might give an indication of how aggressive the person's cancer is likely to be and how long they might live.

Biomarkers can include things such as:

- **The presence of a specific gene mutation in the person's cancer cells** – for this, you need to extract DNA from the person's cancer cells (or from their blood – called circulating tumor DNA) and perform a **genetic test**.
- **The presence or absence of a protein** – for this, you need intact cancer cells from a biopsy, aspirate, or tumor block. Protein levels are often measured using **immunohisto-chemistry** and given a numerical score according to the intensity and/or proportion of cells that contain the protein.
- **The person's age, sex, general fitness, and performance status** (their ability to go about their daily life or whether they're unable to get out of bed) [105]; these things are often measured and scored using **a questionnaire**.

Source: Adapted from [105].

about biomarkers). Scientists and doctors have measured and recorded lots and lots of different information about cancer patients and their diseases in the hopes of identifying suitable biomarkers. However, most of their efforts haven't resulted in useful biomarkers that can be widely implemented. There are various reasons for this: [103, 104]

- Sometimes, the biomarker isn't sensitive enough, and it fails to identify everyone who would benefit from treatment.
- Sometimes, it's not specific enough – and the test fails to rule out people who won't benefit.
- Sometimes, there's no obvious cut-off – it's impossible to draw a line that separates the people who do benefit from those who don't.[9]
- Sometimes, you'd like to implement several biomarker tests because they're all partly effective, and together, they'd be more accurate, but you can't afford to do it, or you're unlikely to have large enough tumor samples to run multiple tests.
- Some biomarker tests would be too involved, technical, and time-consuming to implement for every patient, so they're impractical.
- Sometimes, a biomarker is too rare, and you'd have to test thousands of people to find just a handful who have the biomarker you're looking for.

Before I go into any detail, I'll first give you an idea of the sorts of biomarkers that have been explored as ways of predicting response to checkpoint inhibitor immunotherapy (summarized in Table 5.7). These are things in the person's cancer cells, the environment within their tumor(s), or the person as a whole.

I'm not going to go through all the potential biomarkers listed in Table 5.7 in detail. Instead,

I'll focus on the ones that are currently used to select people to receive checkpoint inhibitor therapy.

5.6.1 MSI and dMMR

One of the most clearcut biomarkers is the presence of MSI[10] or dMMR (I'll come to what these terms mean in a second). What I mean by "clearcut" is that people whose tumors exhibit MSI are much more likely to benefit from checkpoint inhibitor therapy than people whose tumors do not.

For example, about 5% of advanced bowel cancers are MSI. The response rate to checkpoint inhibitor therapy in people with MSI advanced bowel cancer is 30%–65%, depending on the people and the treatment [112, 113]. In contrast, in the IMblaze307 study, which involved people with MSS advanced bowel cancer (MSS is the opposite of MSI), the response rate to a checkpoint inhibitor was just 2% [114]. Now, I'm not pretending that these data are directly comparable, as they're from trials involving patients with different characteristics, but the results are worlds apart. A similar pattern has been seen in other cancers [115, 116].

What is MSI?

MSI stands for microsatellite instability. The opposite, MSS, stands for microsatellite stable. MSI is a pattern of DNA damage in a cell's chromosomes that develops when that cell is unable to perform a type of DNA repair called mismatch repair (MMR). Hence, MSI cancers are also sometimes called dMMR – MMR deficient.

Cells that are dMMR tend to accumulate mutations very quickly. Many of these mutations are in the cells' microsatellites (short, repetitive areas of DNA scattered throughout

[9] No biomarker is perfect, so you're not aiming for that, but you do want to identify a test result that can separate out people into those most or least likely to benefit.
[10] MSI cancers are also sometimes called MSI-High or MSI-H, but I'm just going to use the term MSI.

Table 5.7 Examples of biomarkers that could be used to predict benefit from checkpoint inhibitor immunotherapy [103, 106–111].

The cancer cells	The tumor environment	The person
The presence or absence of PD-L1 protein on the surface of the person's cancer cells	The presence or absence of **PD-L1 protein** on the surface of WBCs in the tumor	The health and composition of their **gut microbiome**
The total number of mutations in the person's cancer cells – tumor mutation burden	The presence or absence of T cells in the tumor, their location, and whether they exhibit signs of exhaustion	Whether they have recently taken a course of **broad-spectrum antibiotics**, opioids, or various other medicines
The presence or absence of a pattern of mutations (called MSI) caused by a defect in a DNA repair process called mismatch repair (MMR)	The presence of **tertiary lymphoid structures** in the tumor	The **ratio of lymphocytes to neutrophils** in the person's blood
A high number of mutations being shared by all cancer cells (high degree of mutation clonality)	The **overall immune makeup** of the tumor – is it hot, cold, immune-suppressed, or immune-excluded?	Whether or not they have a **history of smoking** (if they have lung cancer)
The presence or absence of specific mutations	The presence or absence of **specific types of WBCs**, such as Tregs, TAMs, or MDSCs	The presence/absence and clonality of **cancer-specific T cells in the person's blood**
The presence or absence of tumor antigens displayed by MHC proteins		**The level of diversity among the person's** HLA genes[b]

Abbreviations: dMMR – defective mismatch repair; HLA – human leukocyte antigen; MDSCs – myeloid-derived suppressor cells; MHC – major histocompatibility complex; MSI – microsatellite instability; TAMs – tumor-associated macrophages; Tregs – regulatory T cells; WBCs – white blood cells.
[a] Tumor antigens (sometimes called neoantigens) refer to small fragments (peptides) from proteins that are unique to the person's cancer cells and not displayed by cells in the rest of their body.
[b] Rather confusingly, the HLA genes contain the instructions for making MHC proteins.

our chromosomes that are prone to mutations). Defects in MMR also lead to the accumulation of small defects (mis-paired DNA bases and small insertions and deletions – indels) throughout the chromosomes [117].

What causes MSI?

MSI can be caused by: [117, 118]

• An inherited defect in one of the genes necessary for MMR. The most important genes responsible for MMR are *MLH1*, *MSH2*, *MSH6*, and *PMS2*. People who inherit a defect in one of these genes have Lynch syndrome. Because of this, they have a high risk of various cancers, including bowel, endometrial, ovarian, and stomach cancer.

• A sporadic (not inherited) defect in an MMR gene that is present in the person's cancer cells.

• Epigenetic alterations[11] to an MMR gene, which have led to its suppression. The most common situation is that the promotor for the *MLH1* gene[12] has been chemically

---

[11] I said a little bit about epigenetics in Section 1.2.1.
[12] Promotors are a bit like switches in that they control genes and determine whether a gene's information is accessed and used to make a protein or not. If a gene's information is being used to make a protein, we say that it is "active," "switched on," or "expressed." If it's not, we say that the gene is "switched off" or "not expressed."

changed and the gene is permanently switched off. Without the production of MLH1 protein, the cell can't perform MMR and the cell becomes MSI.

Why Are MSI Cancers Unusually Sensitive to Checkpoint Inhibitors?

MSI cancer cells contain thousands of small mutations in their DNA. This, in turn, forces the cell to make many mutated proteins. If the cell's MHC system is working properly,[13] then the MHC class 1 cups on its surface will display many fragments of these mutated proteins to passing cytotoxic T cells (CTLs). So, cells that are MSI-High due to defective MMR should be very visible to the immune system [117].

Of course, just because a person's tumor is MSI doesn't necessarily mean that they will benefit from checkpoint inhibitor therapy – it just makes it much more likely. I was about to

say that you never see 100% of people benefiting, but then I remembered a trial involving 12 people with dMMR rectal cancer, where the response rate was, in fact, 100% [119].

How Can We Test for the Presence of MSI?

There are two main ways of testing a person's tumor for the presence of MSI. The first is to use immunohistochemistry to check for the presence of all four of the main MMR proteins. The second option is to use genetic testing to look for patterns of DNA damage caused by dMMR [117].

Which Cancers Are Most Likely to Be MSI?

The cancers most likely to be MSI are endometrial cancer, bowel cancer, and stomach cancer (Figure 5.13) [120]. Smaller proportions of

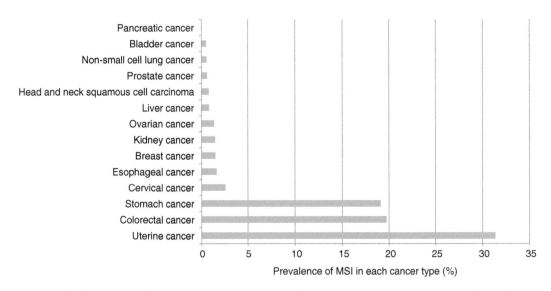

Figure 5.13 Prevalence of MSI in various cancer types. The data are taken from a study conducted by Russell Bonneville et al. in which the researchers analyzed over 11,000 tumor samples from people with 27 cancer types [120]. Uterine cancer is the same thing as endometrial cancer, and colorectal cancer is another term for bowel cancer.
Abbreviation: MSI – microsatellite instability. *Source:* Adapted from [120].

---

[13] Do look back at Section 1.5.1 if you want to remind yourself how the MHC system is meant to work.

other cancers are also MSI. The proportion of cancers that are MSI differs not just from cancer-type to cancer-type, but also with ethnicity, age, stage of disease, and exposure to prior treatments [117].

5.6.2 PD-L1 Protein Levels

PD-L1 protein is found in the following places (depicted in Figure 5.14):
- On the surface of some types of white blood cells.
- On the surface of cells that are reacting to activated CTLs in their vicinity.
- On the surface of cancer cells that contain gene mutations linked to immune suppression.

The presence of PD-L1 can therefore be a signpost saying "activated CTLs are here," indicating that the person is likely to benefit from checkpoint inhibitor immunotherapy.

The opposite can also be true, as the presence of PD-L1 can be a sign that the person's cancer cells are embedded in a highly immune-suppressing microenvironment and unlikely to respond to immunotherapy.

The ambiguity over what the presence or absence of PD-L1 means is borne out in the results of clinical trials. In some cancers and some trials, the presence of PD-L1 has predicted a greater likelihood of benefit from checkpoint inhibitors. In other trials, there was no relationship between the two [110].

This and other problems with using PD-L1 levels to predict the likelihood of response to checkpoint inhibitors can be summarized as follows [110]:
- There is no obvious cut-off – even people with no PD-L1 in their tumor may be helped by checkpoint inhibitors.

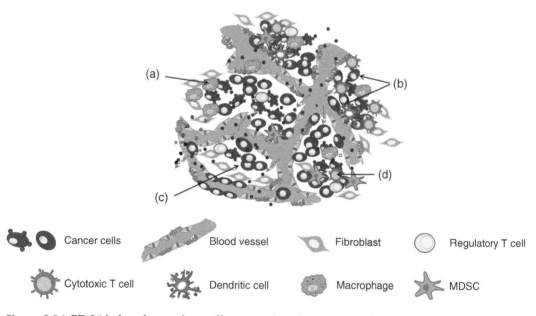

Figure 5.14 PD-L1 is found on various cell types and can be present or absent from tumors. (a) PD-L1 is found on the surface of macrophages and other white blood cells. **(b)** PD-L1 is also found in cells that have been influenced by activated CTLs. **(c)** Parts of the tumor may completely lack any PD-L1; PD-L1 also comes and goes over time and can appear or disappear in response to treatment. **(d)** CTLs can be suppressed via mechanisms that have nothing to do with the checkpoint proteins on their surface. **Abbreviation:** MDSC – myeloid-derived suppressor cell.

- There is no agreed single standard test – there are several tests in use, some of which measure PD-L1 just on cancer cells and some of which look for PD-L1 on both cancer cells and infiltrating white blood cells.
- There is no agreed definition of what is or isn't a positive or negative PD-L1 test result; different tests and trials use different cut-offs.
- PD-L1 levels vary over time and in different parts of a tumor; it can also be present in one part of a tumor but be absent in another.
- The presence or absence of PD-L1 can be different between a primary tumor and any metastases.
- The size of the tumor sample matters – you're more likely to miss PD-L1 in a smaller sample.
- You're more likely to find it in a fresh rather than an archived tumor sample.
- PD-L1 levels seem to predict the benefit of checkpoint inhibitors in some cancers and in some situations but not in others.

Because of these mixed results, regulators have had difficulty in deciding when to mandate PD-L1 testing and when not to. At the moment, we have a mixed bag of approvals. For example, in NSCLC, triple-negative breast cancer, cervical cancer, and a handful of other cancer types, patients can only receive checkpoint inhibitor therapy if their tumor is tested for PD-L1 and the levels meet a certain threshold. However, for people with kidney cancer and several other cancers, no PD-L1 testing is required [121].

5.6.3 Tumor Mutation Burden

Tumor mutation burden (TMB) is defined as the number of non-synonymous mutations per megabase of DNA tested. Just to explain, a non-synonymous mutation is a mutation affecting a gene in a way that affects the production of a protein (mutations outside of genes therefore don't count). A megabase is a stretch of DNA that is a million base pairs long [122].

But, just as with PD-L1 measurements, TMB calculations are not consistent and can be difficult to standardize. The answer you get depends on what bits of DNA you search for mutations, how you do it, and how you interpret what you find [123].

Despite the inconsistencies between TMB calculations, high TMB does often correlate with benefit from checkpoint inhibitor immunotherapy. A tumor that has a very high TMB is often one with some sort of defect in a DNA repair process (such as MMR) or one that has been caused by a very powerful mutator of DNA (such as UV light or tobacco smoke). As I said back in Section 5.5.2, the "hottest" tumors often contain a very high number of mutations.

As with MSI, the theory is that tumors with a high TMB are manufacturing more mutated proteins. Fragments of these proteins end up displayed by the cancer cells' MHC class 1 proteins and are detected by passing TILs. Hence, cancers with a high TMB are likely to be detected by TILs, and the checkpoint inhibitor gives the TILs an added boost.

But, as with PD-L1 levels, there is no universally agreed definition as to what a "high TMB" means. The value picked varies enormously from study to study.

To add to the confusion, PD-L1 levels and TMB don't appear to be related [124]. Tumors that have high PD-L1 levels are not necessarily those with a high TMB, and cancer with a high TMB can be positive or negative for the presence of PD-L1 (see Figure 5.15). If you used a PD-L1 cut-off to select patients to receive checkpoint inhibitor therapy, you would be selecting a different, mostly non-overlapping group of people than if you used TMB as your biomarker.

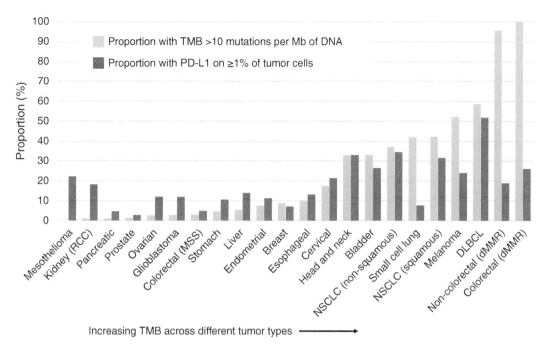

Figure 5.15 There is no correlation between TMB and PD-L1 levels in a tumor. From left to right, tumors are arranged according to the proportion of that tumor type with a high TMB (defined as a TMB of greater than ten mutations per megabase of DNA, shown in turquoise). Thus, dMMR colorectal cancers, at the far right, are the most likely to exhibit a high TMB. Next to the data for TMB, the red bars are the proportion of each cancer type that has PD-L1 on at least 1% of tumor cells. The cancers with the highest PD-L1 levels are not necessarily those with a high TMB. Data taken from [124].
Abbreviations: DLBCL – diffuse large B cell lymphoma; dMMR – defective mismatch repair; Mb – megabase; MSS – microsatellite stable; NSCLC – non-small cell lung cancer; RCC – renal cell carcinoma; TMB – tumor mutation burden.

5.6.4 The Presence or Absence of Specific Mutations

In Section 5.5.1, I mentioned that some mutations found in cancer cells seem to go hand-in-hand with an immune-suppressing microenvironment. Now, different mutations might do different things in different cancer types. However, in NSCLC, scientists are building up a picture of what different mutations mean in terms of response to checkpoint inhibitors.

They have found that cancers that contain mutations linked to a history of smoking (such as *KRAS* mutations) often have a high TMB and high PD-L1, and patients with these cancers often respond to checkpoint inhibitors. In contrast, mutations that are more often found in the cancer cells of non-smokers (such as *EGFR*, *ALK*, *ROS1*, *RET*, and *BRAF* V600E) predict a lack of response [125]. It seems that, even if PD-L1 levels are high in cancers with these mutations, checkpoint inhibitor monotherapy isn't a good strategy.

5.6.5 The Immunoscore

Another biomarker that looks promising is called the "Immunoscore". The Immunoscore is calculated by staining a tumor sample so that the number and location of CTLs and PD-L1-positive cells can be clearly seen. A computer then counts how many CTLs and PD-L1-positive cells are present and the distances between them and calculates an Immunoscore ranging from 0 to 4. For example, a tumor that contains lots of CTLs close to PD-L1-positive cells would be Immunoscore 4. Whereas a tumor with a low number of CTLs, situated far from any tumor cells, would have an Immunoscore of 0 [126].

The Immunoscore could be a useful way of predicting the benefit from checkpoint inhibitor immunotherapy in patients with NSCLC and non-MSI bowel cancer, and it may prove useful in other cancer types [127].

5.6.6 Other Biomarkers

The presence of MSI, PD-L1 levels, and TMB are the only biomarkers that are routinely used to select patients to receive checkpoint inhibitors. Even then, as I've explained, they have varying degrees of usefulness. Other potential biomarkers, such as many of those listed in Table 5.7, are also being explored [103, 111, 128, 129].

5.7 CHECKPOINT INHIBITOR COMBINATIONS

Because response rates to checkpoint inhibitors are low, doctors are keen to combine them with other treatments in the hopes of bringing their benefits to a wider range of patients (Figure 5.16).

The purpose of the second treatment is often to somehow "heat up" a tumor. The hope is to turn a cold, immune-suppressed, or immune-excluded tumor into a "hot" tumor full of CTLs that can be activated with a checkpoint inhibitor. This is a lot harder than it might seem, as the CTLs inside tumors are likely to be exhausted and impossible to reinvigorate [130]. There are also many reasons why CTLs might be absent, excluded, or suppressed, making it hard to know what combination to pick.

Common combinations used in clinical practice and being investigated in trials include [131]:

1. Using chemotherapy and/or radiotherapy to reduce the number of immune-suppressing cells in the cancer microenvironment and to create lots of debris for dendritic cells to use to activate CTLs.
2. Combining two or more checkpoint inhibitors to overcome the suppression mediated by more than one checkpoint protein on CTLs.
3. Adding in an angiogenesis inhibitor to increase the movement of CTLs into the tumor.
4. Adding a targeted agent, such as a kinase inhibitor that reverses the effects of an immune-suppressing mutation.
5. Adding an antibody–drug conjugate that will deliver chemotherapy selectively to cancer cells.

Of course, an enormous number of other strategies are being explored, but these six are the most common (counting chemotherapy and radiotherapy as separate approaches), so I'll stick with them.

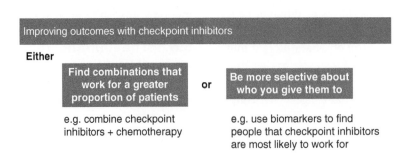

Figure 5.16 The two main strategies to improve outcomes with checkpoint inhibitors.

5.7.1 Combinations with Chemotherapy

Why Do It?

Many research studies have suggested that various forms of chemotherapy can kill cancer cells and affect the tumor environment in ways that help the immune system. The two main things that chemotherapies can do are:

1. Cause immunogenic cell death – i.e., they can kill cancer cells in a way that creates debris and sends signals to the immune system, making it more likely that dendritic cells will pick up the debris and use it to activate CTLs.

2. Reshape the tumor microenvironment – i.e., they can help get rid of CTL-suppressing white blood cells like MDSCs and Tregs, giving CTLs a better chance of staying active and killing cancer cells.

The idea is that giving someone chemotherapy as well as a checkpoint inhibitor will increase the benefits the person derives from the checkpoint inhibitor.

What's the Issue?

The term "chemotherapy" refers to an enormous number of drugs that are toxic to multiplying cells, such as cancer cells. These drugs are given to people in numerous combinations, doses, and schedules that have been refined over many years.

Chemotherapy regimens have been chosen not because of their effects on T cells or the tumor microenvironment, but because they kill cancer cells and shrink tumors (of course, they will kill plenty of healthy, multiplying cells too, accounting for their side effects). Just because a chemotherapy regimen is approved for a type of cancer, that doesn't mean it will work well in combination with a checkpoint inhibitor [132].

Does It Work?

I find this a really difficult question to answer! There are definitely situations where a combination of chemotherapy and checkpoint inhibitor therapy is a person's best option. The problem is that it can be difficult to know this for sure because, in most trials, chemotherapy has been compared to a combination of chemotherapy with a checkpoint inhibitor, i.e., there isn't a third arm in which patients have been given the checkpoint inhibitor alone. This means that the trial's results tell you whether the checkpoint inhibitor adds to the effects of a chemotherapy regimen but not if the chemotherapy adds to the effectiveness of the checkpoint inhibitor.

What Are the Implications?

Again, I think this is hard to say. There are so many chemotherapy agents and possible ways of altering their dose, timing, and ways of combining them that it's virtually impossible to make any generalizations. Plus, every tumor type and sub-type is different in terms of its mutation burden, PD-L1 levels, etc. So, something that works well in one set of patients won't necessarily work well for another.

Maybe the only thing I can say is that we can't take anything for granted. Sometimes a combination will work, but sometimes it won't. Also, if a tumor type is inherently "cold," then it might be that there's no combination of chemotherapy plus checkpoint inhibitor that's going to work (for example, there's a long list of combinations that have been tried and failed in MSS bowel cancer [133]).

5.7.2 Combinations with Radiotherapy

Why Do It?

As with chemotherapy, combining radiotherapy with checkpoint inhibitors seems, at least superficially, like a great combination. The central idea is that radiotherapy will kill cancer cells and reshape the immune microenvironment in tumors, and this will make checkpoint inhibitor therapy more effective [134, 135].

What's the Issue?

The actual situation is much more complicated than this, and the impact of radiotherapy on the immune system is much more varied [134].

One of the potential obstacles in the way of getting the best result with this combination is that the cancer fighting CTLs most likely to be activated by checkpoint inhibitors are those in nearby lymph nodes. This means that if the radiotherapy field includes these lymph nodes, then you will destroy the very T cells you are trying to activate [134–136].

Does It Work?

Many clinical trials in which the combination has been tested have failed to improve survival times for patients [136]. It seems that, as well as considering factors such as cancer type, stage, dose, fractionation, and timing, it's also essential to carefully choose the extent of the radiation field.

5.7.3 Combinations of Multiple Checkpoint Inhibitors

Why Do It?

Each checkpoint inhibitor can boost CTLs that are being suppressed by one specific checkpoint protein on its surface. It therefore makes sense that if you combine checkpoint inhibitors that block different checkpoint proteins, then you'll activate more CTLs than if you just gave one.

What's the Issue?

The main problems with checkpoint inhibitor combinations:

- They don't always work – there are so many different reasons for an inadequate cancer-fighting CTL response, meaning that only targeting checkpoint proteins is often not enough to help people.
- You see extra toxicities – for example, in the CheckMate 067 trial in people with advanced melanoma skin cancer, severe

side effects were reported in 59% of patients given nivolumab plus ipilimumab, 24% of people given nivolumab only, and 28% of people given ipilimumab only.

Does It Work?

Yes, but not all the time. In inherently "hot" tumors like melanoma skin cancer, a combination of checkpoint inhibitors does seem to result in more benefit for a greater proportion of people. For example, if you look back at Table 5.3, you can see that more people were alive five years later if they were given nivolumab plus ipilimumab compared to people given either treatment on its own. A combination of a PD-1 or PD-L1-targeted antibody plus a CTLA-4 antibody is also approved for people with some other cancer types, such as kidney cancer, liver cancer, and MSI bowel cancer.

On the other hand, there are plenty of examples of trials in which a combination hasn't turned out to be helpful (at least in terms of commonly-used trial endpoints).

For example, the MYSTIC trial investigated durvalumab (which targets PD-L1) with or without tremelimumab (which targets CTLA-4) vs. chemotherapy for people with advanced NSCLC with PD-L1 on ≥25% of tumor cells. Median overall survival was 16.3 months with durvalumab, 11.9 months with durvalumab + tremelimumab, and 12.9 months with chemotherapy. However, the addition of tremelimumab did seem helpful for people whose tumors had a very high TMB (defined as ≥20 mutations per megabase of DNA) [137].

Novel checkpoint inhibitors with other targets have also been investigated in combination with PD-1 or PD-L1 antibodies. I'll say more about these checkpoint inhibitors in Section 5.8.

The most well-studied of these novel antibodies is relatlimab. This antibody targets a checkpoint protein called LAG-3, and it has been investigated in several trials in combination with the PD-1 antibody nivolumab. For example, in the RELATIVITY-047 trial, the nivolumab plus relatlimab combination was compared to nivolumab alone, and the combination was better [138].

5.7.4 Combinations with Angiogenesis Inhibitors

Why Do It?

As with other combinations, there's plenty of logic to underpin the idea of using a combination of a checkpoint inhibitor with an angiogenesis inhibitor (see Section 4.1 for a description of angiogenesis inhibitors) [139].

VEGF is a powerful growth factor that causes angiogenesis and affects the tumor microenvironment. For example, it stops T cells from getting into tumors, prevents dendritic cells from maturing, and causes CTL-suppressing white blood cells like MDSCs to proliferate [139, 140].

The idea with the combination is that the VEGF-targeted treatment (either an antibody that targets VEGF or an antibody or kinase inhibitor that targets VEGF receptors) modifies the tumor microenvironment. This hopefully then gives CTLs a better chance of (1) being activated, (2) getting into tumors, and (3) staying active once they've gotten there.

Another way of combining anti-VEGF therapy and a checkpoint inhibitor is to create a single treatment that does both. For example, ivonescimab is a dual-targeted antibody with four attachment sites. It targets both PD-1 and VEGF [141].

What's the Issue?

As with other combinations, the main issues are:

- That it doesn't always work.
- It can be hard to know how much added benefit the angiogenesis inhibitor is

providing due to the design of the trials in which it has been tested.

- That the kinase inhibitor group of angiogenesis inhibitors often blocks many kinases. This makes it impossible to know whether the angiogenesis inhibitor aspect of the drug's activity is helpful (it could be their ability to block other kinases that has the greater impact).
- That this approach is the most effective against cancers where angiogenesis inhibitors and checkpoint inhibitors have already independently proven their worth. It's therefore hard to know if the angiogenesis inhibitor is working together with the checkpoint inhibitor or if they're going about their business separately, i.e., are you seeing a synergistic or purely additive effect?

Does It Work?

The cancer type in which we have the most experience with angiogenesis inhibitor plus checkpoint inhibitor combinations is advanced kidney cancer (renal cell carcinoma). This cancer is relatively insensitive to chemotherapy, and angiogenesis inhibitors have been a standard treatment option for many years. In Table 5.8, I've given a summary of five clinical trials involving people with previously untreated advanced kidney cancer. Four trials investigated a combination of an angiogenesis inhibitor and a checkpoint inhibitor. The fifth, CheckMate 214, explored a combination of two checkpoint inhibitors.

In all five trials, the combination was compared to sunitinib, an angiogenesis inhibitor. You can't compare the data between the trials as they all involved different groups of patients. What you can say is that, in each trial, the people given the combination were better off than those given sunitinib alone.

What these trials don't tell you is whether the angiogenesis inhibitor is enhancing the effects of the checkpoint inhibitor or whether

Table 5.8   Data from five clinical trials in advanced kidney cancer [142–147].

Treatments and trial	Response rate	Median PFS (months)	Median OS (months)	Median DoR (months)	3-Year survival rate
Pembrolizumab + axitinib vs. sunitinib (KEYNOTE-426)	59.3% vs. 35.7%	15.7 vs. 11.1	45.7 vs. 40.1	23.5 vs. 15.9	63% vs. 54%
Avelumab + axitinib vs. sunitinib (JAVELIN Renal 101)	52.5% vs. 27.3%	13.8 vs. 7.0	NR vs. 37.8	18.5 vs. NE	Not reported
Nivolumab + cabozantinib vs. sunitinib (CheckMate-9ER)	55.7% vs. 28.4%	16.6 vs. 8.4	49.5 vs. 35.5	23.1 vs. 15.2	58.7% vs. 49.5%
Pembrolizumab + lenvatinib vs. sunitinib (CLEAR)	71% vs. 36.1%	23.9 vs. 9.2	NR vs. NR	25.8 vs. 14.6	65.5% vs. 61.8%
Nivolumab + ipilimumab vs. sunitinib (CheckMate 214)	39.3% vs. 32.4%	12.3 vs. 12.3	55.7 vs. 38.4	NR vs. 24.8	53.4% vs. 43.3% (four-year data)

[a] Data for PD-L1 – positive tumors (≥1% of immune cells staining positive; 63% of tested patients).
Abbreviations: DoR – duration of response; NE – not estimable; NR – not reached; OS – overall survival; PFS – progression-free survival.

the two treatments are working independently of each other.

Primary liver cancer and endometrial cancer are two other cancers in which a combination of an angiogenesis inhibitor and a checkpoint inhibitor has proven helpful in some trials.

5.7.5 Combinations with Targeted Therapies

These combine a checkpoint inhibitor with a targeted therapy that aims to overcome the immune-suppressing microenvironment created by some powerful mutations.

Why Do It?

As with other combinations, there's plenty of logic to underpin this combination. In theory, a suitable targeted therapy could reverse some mutations' impact on the tumor immune microenvironment. This might then improve the effectiveness of a checkpoint inhibitor.

What's the Issue?

The problem is that what sounds logical and like it should work often doesn't match reality. Also, researchers must always be pragmatic and realistic, and you can't compromise patient safety.

At the moment, the main issues are:

1. Some combinations seem to be particularly toxic. For example, various studies investigating combinations of EGFR inhibitors plus checkpoint inhibitors for people with *EGFR*-mutated NSCLC had problems with toxicity, and some had to be stopped early [148].

2. These combinations often don't work. For example, there was much fanfare around a Phase 3 trial investigating the combination of a MEK inhibitor (cobimetinib) with a checkpoint inhibitor (atezolizumab) in people with MSS bowel cancer (i.e., bowel cancers that aren't MSI). However, the response rates were 3% with the addition of cobimetinib vs. 2% without [114].

Can It Work?

Perhaps the combination where the evidence of activity is most robust is in melanoma skin cancer, where both targeted therapy (with B-Raf + MEK inhibitors) and checkpoint inhibitors are effective. Combination trials involving all three treatments have shown improvements in some measures of success, such as median DoR and median PFS (although this is not necessarily synergy). However, the combination does cause more toxicity, and many doctors seem unconvinced that the triple combination is better than the sequential [149].

5.7.6 Combinations with Antibody–Drug Conjugates

As I said in Chapter 2 and in Chapter 4.2, antibody–drug conjugates (ADCs) are an up-and-coming approach to treating cancer. More and more of them enter clinical trials all the time. Many of the newer ones have cleavable linkers, more copies of drugs per antibody, and better drugs (in terms of potency and permeability) [150].

As it's still early days for ADCs, there aren't many examples of trials where they've been combined with checkpoint inhibitors. However, as with standard chemotherapy, the hope is that causing cancer cell death will lead to greater activation of CTLs by dendritic cells. In addition, because the antibody part of ADCs can also engage some types of white blood cells directly, there's also the possibility of greater synergy [151].

At the end of 2023, one combination, that of enfortumab vedotin (an ADC targeting the nectin-4 protein) with pembrolizumab, was approved for people with advanced bladder cancer [152].

5.7.7 My Conclusions on Combinations

A few concluding thoughts about combinations of checkpoint inhibitors with other treatments:

- In all situations, the details really do matter. None of these combinations look like they will be effective against every cancer type in every situation.
- Just because a combination is based on solid scientific theories with lots of evidence to back it up doesn't mean it will work in practice.
- When designing clinical trials, researchers are practical and pragmatic. This means that the details of a combination usually depend on what was already licensed for a particular cancer type rather than being put together based on scientific evidence.
- Even when a combination does turn out to be helpful, you won't know if the theory behind it is what made it work – you might be seeing something entirely different that you didn't predict.
- The word "synergy" is used far too much – it's generally impossible to know if the second treatment is enhancing and synergizing with the checkpoint inhibitor or if the two treatments are working independently of each other.
- We are edging our way forward in the dark – it's impossible to predict accurately what will or won't work for each cancer type and disease stage. There are hundreds of clinical trials going on, some of which will be successful and some of which won't.

5.8 NOVEL CHECKPOINT INHIBITORS AND ACTIVATORS

In Figure 5.2, I depicted not just PD-1 and CTLA-4 but also a wide range of different checkpoint proteins found on the surface of T cells. Some of these are being explored as targets of either checkpoint protein inhibitors (if the checkpoint protein in question has a negative effect on CTL activity) or checkpoint protein activators (if the protein has a positive impact).

In Figures 5.17 and 5.18, I have depicted some of these other checkpoint proteins and the antibodies being developed [153]. Many of these proteins, and the antibodies that target them, are still in very early stages of development, and I won't say any more about them. I will, however, single out a few as being the targets of approved treatments or because they look particularly promising.

LAG-3

LAG-3 (Lymphocyte-Activation Gene 3), like CTLA-4 and PD-1, is found on the surface of exhausted CTLs. These CTLs may once have had the capacity to kill cancer cells. However, with chronic exposure to their target antigen the CTLs have become over worked, over-stimulated, and dysfunctional [153].

LAG-3 looks a lot like CD4, an important protein found on the surface of helper T cells.

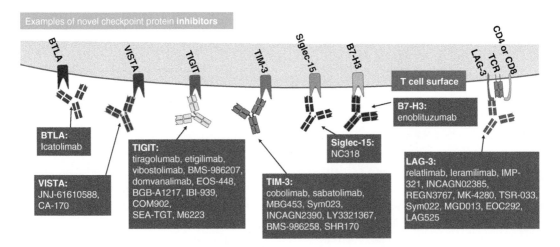

Figure 5.17 Examples of antibodies that block a range of inhibitory checkpoint proteins found on the surface of T cells.
Abbreviation: TCR – T cell receptor.

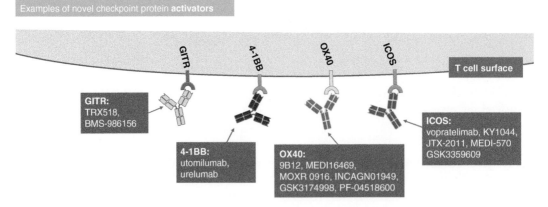

Figure 5.18 Examples of antibodies that act as activators (agonists) for a range of stimulatory checkpoint proteins found on the surface of T cells.

Like CD4, LAG-3 reaches around the TCR and makes connections with MHC class 2 proteins. When CD4 proteins connect with MHC class 2, the T cell becomes active. In contrast, when LAG-3 reaches round and connects with MHC class 2, the T cell shuts down [153].

There are big gaps in our understanding of exactly what LAG-3 does. Despite this, scientists have developed LAG-3 antibodies in the hopes that they, like PD-1 and PD-L1 antibodies, will reverse the suppression and exhaustion of CTLs in tumors.

Of the many LAG-3 antibodies developed, one of them, relatlimab, has been approved in combination with nivolumab as a treatment for people with advanced melanoma skin cancer. This approval was based on the results of the RELATIVITY-047 Phase 3 trial [138].

TIGIT

TIGIT[14] is another inhibitory protein found on activated and exhausted T cells (CTLs and helper T cells) and on natural killer (NK) cells [154].

TIGIT antibodies include tiragolumab, which has reached Phase 3 trials in patients with lung cancer (both small cell and non-small cell). As of February 2024, tiragolumab's future still looks uncertain [155].

TIM-3

TIM-3 (T cell immunoglobulin domain and mucin domain 3) is found on a variety of white blood cells, including CTLs, NK cells, dendritic cells, and some myeloid white blood cells. It's also sometimes found on the cells of acute myeloid leukemia (AML), myelodysplastic syndromes (MDS), and myeloproliferative neoplasms (MPNs) [156]. A handful of large

clinical trials are underway that involve TIM-3-targeted antibodies, but there are no results to report.

CD47

CD47 isn't featured in Figure 5.17 as it's not a T cell checkpoint protein. Instead, it's found on the surface of virtually all healthy cells. Our cells use it to transmit a "don't eat me" signal to macrophages. It does this by connecting to an inhibitory checkpoint protein on macrophages called SIRPα (Signal Regulatory Protein Alpha) [157, 158].

Due to internal damage, many cancer cells have proteins on their surface that say "eat me" to macrophages (as do old red blood cells). Cancer cells also have high levels of CD47, so they avoid destruction. The purpose of CD47-targeted antibodies is to block CD47, allowing macrophages to respond to cancer cells' "eat me" signals and destroy them.

One example of these antibodies is magrolimab, which is being explored as a treatment for various hematological cancers, including AML. Other CD47-targeted treatments are being developed, including a range of bi-specific antibodies and other treatments that target either CD47 or SIRPα [159].

Agonists of Stimulatory Checkpoint Proteins

Stimulatory checkpoint proteins are found on T cells and many other types of white blood cells. When they're triggered by a suitable partner protein (a ligand), they increase T cell activity and cause T cell proliferation. Examples include GITR, OX40, 4-1BB, and ICOS [153].

As with antibodies targeting inhibitory checkpoint proteins, an enormous number of

---

[14] If you really want to know, its full name is "anti-T-cell immunoreceptor with immunoglobulin (Ig) and immunoreceptor tyrosine-based inhibitory motif domains."

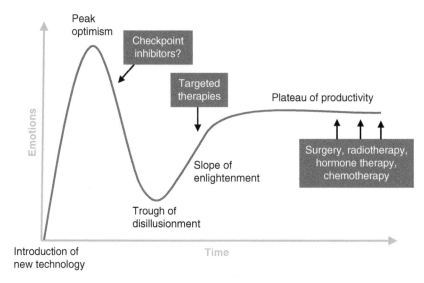

Figure 5.19 My interpretation of the Gartner Hype Cycle and its relevance for the introduction of a new cancer treatment. When a new form of cancer treatment (or other technology) is introduced, it captures people's interest and imagination. Optimism increases, and it initially outstrips what the technology can achieve. When the limitations of the new technology become apparent, optimism wanes, and disillusionment sets in. Gradually, as time passes, a more realistic and balanced set of expectations emerges. Finally, we reach the plateau of productivity, where our expectations and reality match up. *Source:* Adapted from [160].

antibodies are being developed that act as activators of stimulatory checkpoint proteins. These treatments are all still in the early stages of clinical trials.

5.9 FINAL THOUGHTS

I hope that by the end of this chapter, you will feel you have a better idea of why checkpoint inhibitors have caused so much excitement in recent years. However, I also hope this is tempered by understanding these treatments' limitations.

I am often struck by the almost uniformly positive language that is used to describe checkpoint inhibitors. I think, in part, this is because it's so appealing to think of them as being able to harness the power of our immune system and turn it against cancer.

Going back to the late 1990s and early 2000s, the scientific and medical world was enthralled by the progress being made with targeted therapies. This optimism continued for perhaps ten years or so before being tempered by experience. Gradually, it became clear that resistance to these treatments is almost always inevitable if the person has metastatic disease. Even now, we're still learning how to get the most out of these treatments, create better ones, and give them at the right dose and time for each patient.

The development of checkpoint inhibitors seems to be following a similar trajectory: initial optimism, followed by a tempering of expectations and perhaps finally a realistic understanding of when and how to use them (see Figure 5.19 for how this trajectory fits with the theoretical model of the Gartner Hype Cycle).

The first clinical trials with checkpoint inhibitor treatments largely involved people with melanoma skin cancer or other highly immunogenic cancers,[15] such as NSCLC (mostly in smokers and ex-smokers) and kidney cancer. Perhaps our experience in these cancers sets our expectations too high, with people expecting the same level of success in other (perhaps even all?) cancer types.

I wonder if we've now passed the peak of expectations (at least in the scientific community). The goal now is to figure out when to use these treatments and how to get the best from them using biomarkers and combinations.

Hopefully, as time passes, we will develop combinations that can overcome many of the obstacles that stand in the way of cancer-fighting T cells. Perhaps, as you read through the next chapter on other forms of immunotherapy, you will imagine combinations where checkpoint inhibitors are combined with vaccines or other forms of immunotherapy. I hope that we will start putting together approaches that combine and harness what we have learned. For example, it's tantalizing to imagine a multi-pronged approach that combines:

- Preparing the patient by improving their microbiome and reducing inflammation.
- A treatment vaccine to alert their immune system and generate cancer-fighting CTLs.
- A checkpoint inhibitor to boost those CTLs.
- An additional treatment to reduce or suppress MDSCs, Tregs, and other T cell suppressors in the cancer microenvironment.

However, no treatment is ever totally free of side effects. As much as it's tempting to put together such strategies, it may not be safe to implement them.

In addition, it's very likely that for some people with cold or immune-suppressed cancers, no immunotherapy-based combination will ever be enough to cure them of their disease. So, in addition to exploring new immunotherapies and combinations, it will also be important to identify people who would be better served by a different treatment approach.

REFERENCES

1 Liu Y, Zeng G (2012). Cancer and innate immune system interactions: Translational potentials for cancer immunotherapy. *J Immunother* **35**(4). doi: 10.1097/CJI.0b013e3182518e83.

2 Waldman AD, Fritz JM, Lenardo MJ (2020). A guide to cancer immunotherapy: From T cell basic science to clinical practice. *Nat Rev Immunol* **20**(11). doi: 10.1038/s41577-020-0306-5.

3 Weigelin B *et al.* (2021). Cytotoxic T cells are able to efficiently eliminate cancer cells by additive cytotoxicity. *Nat Commun* **12**(1). doi: 10.1038/s41467-021-25282-3.

4 Chen DS, Mellman I (2013). Oncology meets immunology: The cancer-immunity cycle. *Immunity* **39**(1). doi: 10.1016/j.immuni.2013.07.012.

5 E. Berthold and Australian Academy of Science (2023) Releasing the immune system's brakes to fight cancer. [Online] Available at: https://www.science.org.au/curious/people-medicine/releasing-immune-systems-brakes-fight-cancer [Accessed December 21, 2023].

6 Pardoll DM (2012). The blockade of immune checkpoints in cancer immunotherapy. *Nat Rev Cancer* **12**(4). doi: 10.1038/nrc3239.

7 Melero I *et al.* (2015). Evolving synergistic combinations of targeted immunotherapies to combat cancer. *Nat Rev Cancer* **15**(8): 457–472. doi: 10.1038/nrc3973.

8 Buchbinder EI, Desai A (2016). CTLA-4 and PD-1 pathways. *Am J Clin Oncol* **39**(1): 98–106. doi: 10.1097/COC.0000000000000239.

---

[15] A term similar to "hot," which is sometimes used to denote a cancer where the cells are full of the sorts of mutations or other features that make them likely to trigger an immune response.

9 Hong MMY, Maleki Vareki S (2022). Addressing the elephant in the immunotherapy room: Effector T-cell priming versus depletion of regulatory T-cells by anti-CTLA-4 therapy. *Cancers (Basel)* **14**(6): 1580. doi: 10.3390/cancers14061580.

10 Simon S, Labarriere N (2018). PD-1 expression on tumor-specific T cells: Friend or foe for immunotherapy? *Onco Targets Ther* **7**(1): e1364828. doi: 10.1080/2162402X.2017.1364828.

11 Glorieux C, Xia X, Huang P (2021). The role of oncogenes and redox signaling in the regulation of PD-L1 in cancer. *Cancers (Basel)* **13**(17): 4426. doi: 10.3390/cancers13174426.

12 Guo Z et al. (2023). Diversity of immune checkpoints in cancer immunotherapy. *Front Immunol* **14**. doi: 10.3389/fimmu.2023.1121285.

13 Maio M et al. (2015). Five-year survival rates for treatment-naive patients with advanced melanoma who received ipilimumab plus dacarbazine in a phase III trial. *J Clin Oncol* **33**(10): 1191–1196. doi: 10.1200/JCO.2014.56.6018.

14 Wolchok JD et al. (2017). Overall survival with combined nivolumab and ipilimumab in advanced melanoma. *N Engl J Med* **377**(14): 1345–1356. doi: 10.1056/NEJMoa1709684.

15 Larkin J et al. (2019). Five-year survival with combined nivolumab and ipilimumab in advanced melanoma. *N Engl J Med* **381**(16): 1535–1546. doi: 10.1056/NEJMoa1910836.

16 Robert C et al. (2016). Three-year overall survival for patients with advanced melanoma treated with pembrolizumab in KEYNOTE-001. *J Clin Oncol* **34**(15_suppl): 9503–9503. doi: 10.1200/JCO.2016.34.15_suppl.9503.

17 Hamid O et al. (2018). 5-year survival outcomes in patients (pts) with advanced melanoma treated with pembrolizumab (pembro) in KEYNOTE-001. *J Clin Oncol* **36**(15_suppl): 9516–9516. doi: 10.1200/JCO.2018.36.15_suppl.9516.

18 Topalian SL et al. (2019). Five-year survival and correlates among patients with advanced melanoma, renal cell carcinoma, or non–small cell lung cancer treated with nivolumab. *JAMA Oncol* **5**(10): 1411. doi: 10.1001/jamaoncol.2019.2187.

19 Aykan NF, Özatlı T (2020). Objective response rate assessment in oncology: Current situation and future expectations. *World J Clin Oncol* **11**(2): 53–73. doi: 10.5306/wjco.v11.i2.53.

20 Camidge DR, Doebele RC, Kerr KM (2019). Comparing and contrasting predictive biomarkers for immunotherapy and targeted therapy of NSCLC. *Nat Rev Clin Oncol* **16**(6): 341–355. doi: 10.1038/s41571-019-0173-9.

21 Ferris RL et al. (2016). Nivolumab for recurrent squamous-cell carcinoma of the head and neck. *N Engl J Med* **375**(19): 1856–1867. doi: 10.1056/NEJMoa1602252.

22 Cohen EEW et al. (2019). Pembrolizumab versus methotrexate, docetaxel, or cetuximab for recurrent or metastatic head-and-neck squamous cell carcinoma (KEYNOTE-040): A randomised, open-label, phase 3 study. *Lancet* **393**(10167): 156–167. doi: 10.1016/S0140-6736(18)31999-8.

23 Motzer RJ et al. (2015). Nivolumab versus everolimus in advanced renal-cell carcinoma. *N Engl J Med* **373**(19): 1803–1813. doi: 10.1056/NEJMoa1510665.

24 Bellmunt J et al. (2017). Pembrolizumab as second-line therapy for advanced urothelial carcinoma. *N Engl J Med* **376**(11): 1015–1026. doi: 10.1056/NEJMoa1613683.

25 Sharma P et al. (2017). Nivolumab in metastatic urothelial carcinoma after platinum therapy (CheckMate 275): A multicentre, single-arm, phase 2 trial. *Lancet Oncol* **18**(3): 312–322. doi: 10.1016/S1470-2045(17)30065-7.

26 Zhu AX et al. (2018). Pembrolizumab in patients with advanced hepatocellular carcinoma previously treated with sorafenib (KEYNOTE-224): A non-randomised, open-label phase 2 trial. *Lancet Oncol* **19**(7): 940–952. doi: 10.1016/S1470-2045(18)30351-6.

27 Eng C et al. (2019). Atezolizumab with or without cobimetinib versus regorafenib in previously treated metastatic colorectal cancer (IMblaze370): A multicentre, open-label, phase 3, randomised, controlled trial. *Lancet Oncol* **20**(6): 849–861. doi: 10.1016/S1470-2045(19)30027-0.

28 Matulonis UA et al. (2019). Antitumor activity and safety of pembrolizumab in patients with advanced recurrent ovarian cancer: Results from the phase II KEYNOTE-100 study. *Ann Oncol* **30**(7): 1080–1087. doi: 10.1093/annonc/mdz135.

29 Chung HC *et al*. (2019). Efficacy and safety of pembrolizumab in previously treated advanced cervical cancer: Results from the phase II KEYNOTE-158 study. *J Clin Oncol* **37**(17): 1470–1478. doi: 10.1200/JCO.18.01265.

30 Antonarakis ES *et al*. (2020). Pembrolizumab for treatment-refractory metastatic castration-resistant prostate cancer: Multicohort, open-label phase II KEYNOTE-199 study. *J Clin Oncol* **38**(5): 395–405. doi: 10.1200/JCO.19.01638.

31 Adams S *et al*. (2019). Pembrolizumab mono-therapy for previously treated metastatic triple-negative breast cancer: Cohort A of the phase II KEYNOTE-086 study. *Ann Oncol* **30**(3): 397–404. doi: 10.1093/annonc/mdy517.

32 Fashoyin-Aje L *et al*. (2019). FDA approval summary: Pembrolizumab for recurrent locally advanced or metastatic gastric or gastroesophageal junction adenocarcinoma expressing PD-L1. *Oncologist* **24**(1): 103–109. doi: 10.1634/theoncologist.2018-0221.

33 Adams S *et al*. (2019). Pembrolizumab monotherapy for previously untreated, PD-L1-positive, metastatic triple-negative breast cancer: Cohort B of the phase II KEYNOTE-086 study. *Ann Oncol* **30**(3): 405–411. doi: 10.1093/annonc/mdy518.

34 Emens LA *et al*. (2019). Long-term clinical outcomes and biomarker analyses of atezolizumab therapy for patients with metastatic triple-negative breast cancer. *JAMA Oncol* **5**(1): 74. doi: 10.1001/jamaoncol.2018.4224.

35 Garon EB *et al*. (2015). Pembrolizumab for the treatment of non–small-cell lung cancer. *N Engl J Med* **372**(21): 2018–2028. doi: 10.1056/NEJMoa1501824.

36 Garon EB *et al*. (2019). Five-year overall survival for patients with advanced non–small-cell lung cancer treated with pembrolizumab: Results from the phase I KEYNOTE-001 study. *J Clin Oncol* **37**(28): 2518–2527. doi: 10.1200/JCO.19.00934.

37 Bailey C *et al*. (2021). Tracking cancer evolution through the disease course. *Cancer Discov* **11**(4): 916–932. doi: 10.1158/2159-8290.CD-20-1559.

38 Ojalvo LS *et al*. (2018). Tumor-associated macrophages and the tumor immune microenvironment of primary and recurrent epithelial ovarian cancer. *Hum Pathol* **74**: 135–147. doi: 10.1016/j.humpath.2017.12.010.

39 Thol K, Pawlik P, McGranahan N (2022). Therapy sculpts the complex interplay between cancer and the immune system during tumour evolution. *Genome Med* **14**(1): 137. doi: 10.1186/s13073-022-01138-3.

40 Venkatesan S *et al*. (2017). Treatment-induced mutagenesis and selective pressures sculpt cancer evolution. *Cold Spring Harb Perspect Med* **7**(8): a026617. doi: 10.1101/cshperspect.a026617.

41 Fransen MF, van Hall T, Ossendorp F (2021). Immune checkpoint therapy: Tumor draining lymph nodes in the spotlights. *Int J Mol Sci* **22**(17): 9401. doi: 10.3390/ijms22179401.

42 Patel SP *et al*. (2023). Neoadjuvant–adjuvant or adjuvant-only pembrolizumab in advanced melanoma. *N Engl J Med* **388**(9): 813–823. doi: 10.1056/NEJMoa2211437.

43 Versluis JM, Long GV, Blank CU (2020). Learning from clinical trials of neoadjuvant checkpoint blockade. *Nat Med* **26**(4): 475–484. doi: 10.1038/s41591-020-0829-0.

44 Rizzo A *et al*. (2022). KEYNOTE-522, IMpassion031 and GeparNUEVO: Changing the paradigm of neoadjuvant immune checkpoint inhibitors in early triple-negative breast cancer. *Future Oncol* **18**(18): 2301–2309. doi: 10.2217/fon-2021-1647.

45 Sahin IH *et al*. (2023). Neoadjuvant immune checkpoint inhibitor therapy for patients with microsatellite instability-high colorectal cancer: Shedding light on the future. *JCO Oncol Pract* **19**(5): 251–259. doi: 10.1200/OP.22.00762.

46 Conroy MR, Dennehy C, Forde PM (2023). Neoadjuvant immune checkpoint inhibitor therapy in resectable non-small cell lung cancer. *Lung Cancer* **183**: 107314. doi: 10.1016/j.lungcan.2023.107314.

47 Agrawal S *et al*. (2016). Nivolumab dose selection: Challenges, opportunities, and lessons learned for cancer immunotherapy. *J Immunother Cancer* **4**(1): 72. doi: 10.1186/s40425-016-0177-2.

48 Renner A, Burotto M, Rojas C (2019). Immune checkpoint inhibitor dosing: Can we go lower without compromising clinical efficacy? *J Glob Oncol* **5**: 1–5. doi: 10.1200/JGO.19.00142.

49 Maritaz C *et al.* (2022). Immune checkpoint-targeted antibodies: A room for dose and schedule optimization? *J Hematol Oncol* **15**(1): 6. doi: 10.1186/s13045-021-01182-3.

50 Shulgin B *et al.* (2020). Dose dependence of treatment-related adverse events for immune checkpoint inhibitor therapies: A model-based meta-analysis. *Onco Targets Ther* **9**(1). doi: 10.1080/2162402X.2020.1748982.

51 Choi J, Lee SY (2020). Clinical characteristics and treatment of immune-related adverse events of immune checkpoint inhibitors. *Immune Netw* **20**(1). doi: 10.4110/in.2020.20.e9.

52 Haanen J *et al.* (2022). Management of toxicities from immunotherapy: ESMO clinical practice guideline for diagnosis, treatment and follow-up. *Ann Oncol* **33**(12): 1217–1238. doi: 10.1016/j.annonc.2022.10.001.

53 Wang DY *et al.* (2018). Fatal toxic effects associated with immune checkpoint inhibitors. *JAMA Oncol* **4**(12): 1721. doi: 10.1001/jamaoncol.2018.3923.

54 Martins F *et al.* (2019). Adverse effects of immune-checkpoint inhibitors: Epidemiology, management and surveillance. *Nat Rev Clin Oncol* **16**(9): 563–580. doi: 10.1038/s41571-019-0218-0.

55 Couey MA *et al.* (2019). Delayed immune-related events (DIRE) after discontinuation of immunotherapy: Diagnostic hazard of autoimmunity at a distance. *J Immunother Cancer* **7**(1): 165. doi: 10.1186/s40425-019-0645-6.

56 Borcoman E *et al.* (2018). Patterns of response and progression to immunotherapy. *Am Soc Clin Oncol Educ Book* **38**: 169–178. doi: 10.1200/EDBK_200643.

57 Frelaut M, Le Tourneau C, Borcoman E (2019). Hyperprogression under Immunotherapy. *Int J Mol Sci* **20**(11): 2674. doi: 10.3390/ijms20112674.

58 Dercle L *et al.* (2018). 18 F-FDG PET and CT scans detect new imaging patterns of response and progression in patients with Hodgkin lymphoma treated by anti-programmed death 1 immune checkpoint inhibitor. *J Nucl Med* **59**(1): 15–24. doi: 10.2967/jnumed.117.193011.

59 Baxter MA *et al.* (2021). Resistance to immune checkpoint inhibitors in advanced gastro-oesophageal cancers. *Br J Cancer* **125**(8): 1068–1079. doi: 10.1038/s41416-021-01425-7.

60 Borcoman E *et al.* (2019). Novel patterns of response under immunotherapy. *Ann Oncol* **30**(3): 385–396. doi: 10.1093/annonc/mdz003.

61 Marron TU *et al.* (2021). Considerations for treatment duration in responders to immune checkpoint inhibitors. *J Immunother Cancer* **9**(3): e001901. doi: 10.1136/jitc-2020-001901.

62 Coen O *et al.* (2021). The DANTE trial protocol: A randomised phase III trial to evaluate the Duration of ANti-PD-1 monoclonal antibody Treatment in patients with metastatic mElanoma. *BMC Cancer* **21**(1): 761. doi: 10.1186/s12885-021-08509-w.

63 Baetz TD *et al.* (2018). A randomized phase III study of duration of anti-PD-1 therapy in metastatic melanoma (STOP-GAP): Canadian Clinical Trials Group study (CCTG) ME.13. *J Clin Oncol* **36**(15_suppl): TPS9600–TPS9600. doi: 10.1200/JCO.2018.36.15_suppl.TPS9600.

64 Gibney GT *et al.* (2022). A phase II study of biomarker-driven early discontinuation of anti–PD-1 therapy in patients with advanced melanoma (PET-Stop): ECOG-ACRIN EA6192. *J Clin Oncol* **40**(16_suppl): TPS9591–TPS9591. doi: 10.1200/JCO.2022.40.16_suppl.TPS9591.

65 Mulder EEAP *et al.* (2021). Early discontinuation of PD-1 blockade upon achieving a complete or partial response in patients with advanced melanoma: The multicentre prospective Safe Stop trial. *BMC Cancer* **21**(1): 323. doi: 10.1186/s12885-021-08018-w.

66 Armand P *et al.* (2016). Programmed death-1 blockade with pembrolizumab in patients with classical Hodgkin lymphoma after brentuximab vedotin failure. *J Clin Oncol* **34**(31): 3733–3739. doi: 10.1200/JCO.2016.67.3467.

67 Green MR *et al.* (2010). Integrative analysis reveals selective 9p24.1 amplification, increased PD-1 ligand expression, and further induction via JAK2 in nodular sclerosing Hodgkin lymphoma and primary mediastinal large B-cell lymphoma. *Blood* **116**(17): 3268–3277. doi: 10.1182/blood-2010-05-282780.

68 Ansell SM *et al.* (2015). PD-1 blockade with nivolumab in relapsed or refractory Hodgkin's lymphoma. *N Engl J Med* **372**(4): 311–319. doi: 10.1056/NEJMoa1411087.

69 Melani C *et al*. (2017). PD-1 blockade in mediastinal gray-zone lymphoma. *N Engl J Med* **377**(1): 89–91. doi: 10.1056/NEJMc1704767.

70 Lees C *et al*. (2019). Biology and therapy of primary mediastinal B-cell lymphoma: Current status and future directions. *Br J Haematol* **185**(1): 25–41. doi: 10.1111/bjh.15778.

71 Chapuy B *et al*. (2016). Targetable genetic features of primary testicular and primary central nervous system lymphomas. *Blood* **127**(7): 869–881. doi: 10.1182/blood-2015-10-673236.

72 Roemer MGM *et al*. (2016). PD-L1 and PD-L2 genetic alterations define classical Hodgkin lymphoma and predict outcome. *J Clin Oncol* **34**(23): 2690–2697. doi: 10.1200/JCO.2016.66.4482.

73 Goodman AM *et al*. (2018). Prevalence of PDL1 amplification and preliminary response to immune checkpoint blockade in solid tumors. *JAMA Oncol* **4**(9): 1237. doi: 10.1001/jamaoncol.2018.1701.

74 Jardim DL *et al*. (2023). PD-L1 gene amplification and focality: Relationship with protein expression. *J Immunother Cancer* **11**(2): e006311. doi: 10.1136/jitc-2022-006311.

75 Goldmann T *et al*. (2021). PD-L1 amplification is associated with an immune cell rich phenotype in squamous cell cancer of the lung. *Cancer Immunol Immunother* **70**(9): 2577–2587. doi: 10.1007/s00262-020-02825-z.

76 Buyse M, Burzykowski T, Saad ED (2018). The search for surrogate endpoints for immunotherapy trials. *Ann Transl Med* **6**(11): 231–231. doi: 10.21037/atm.2018.05.16.

77 Harper K (2017). Checkpoint inhibitors spur changes in trial design. *Cancer Discov* **7**(11): 1209–1210. doi: 10.1158/2159-8290.CD-ND2017-006.

78 Blumenthal GM *et al*. (2017). Milestone analyses of immune checkpoint inhibitors, targeted therapy, and conventional therapy in metastatic non–small cell lung cancer trials. *JAMA Oncol* **3**(8): e171029. doi: 10.1001/jamaoncol.2017.1029.

79 Delgado A, Guddati AK (2021). Clinical endpoints in oncology – A primer. *Am J Cancer Res* **11**(4): 1121–1131.

80 L. Elridge. Progressive disease and cancer. verywellhealth website. [Online] Available at: https://www.verywellhealth.com/definition-of-progressive-disease-2249171 [Accessed April 20, 2023].

81 Heneghan C, Goldacre B, Mahtani KR (2017). Why clinical trial outcomes fail to translate into benefits for patients. *Trials* **18**(1): 122. doi: 10.1186/s13063-017-1870-2.

82 Hegde PS, Chen DS (2020). Top 10 challenges in cancer immunotherapy. *Immunity* **52**(1): 17–35. doi: 10.1016/j.immuni.2019.12.011.

83 V. Prasad. How to read and interpret a cancer clinical trial. Drug Development Letter. [Online] Available at: https://developdrugs.substack.com/p/how-to-read-and-interpret-a-cancer [Accessed May 1, 2023].

84 Robert C (2020). A decade of immune-checkpoint inhibitors in cancer therapy. *Nat Commun* **11**(1): 3801. doi: 10.1038/s41467-020-17670-y.

85 Fares CM *et al*. (2019). Mechanisms of resistance to immune checkpoint blockade: Why does checkpoint inhibitor immunotherapy not work for all patients? *Am Soc Clin Oncol Educ Book* **39**: 147–164. doi: 10.1200/EDBK_240837.

86 Galon J, Bruni D (2019). Approaches to treat immune hot, altered and cold tumours with combination immunotherapies. *Nat Rev Drug Discov* **18**(3): 197–218. doi: 10.1038/s41573-018-0007-y.

87 Chen DS, Mellman I (2017). Elements of cancer immunity and the cancer–immune set point. *Nature* **541**(7637): 321–330. doi: 10.1038/nature21349.

88 van Weverwijk A, de Visser KE (2023). Mechanisms driving the immunoregulatory function of cancer cells. *Nat Rev Cancer* **23**(4): 193–215. doi: 10.1038/s41568-022-00544-4.

89 Maleki Vareki S (2018). High and low mutational burden tumors versus immunologically hot and cold tumors and response to immune checkpoint inhibitors. *J Immunother Cancer* **6**(1): 157. doi: 10.1186/s40425-018-0479-7.

90 Janeway C *et al*. (2001). The major histocompatibility complex and its functions. In *Immunobiology: The Immune System in Health and Disease*. 5th ed. New York: Garland Science.

91 Sidaway P (2018). HLA-1 genotype influences response to checkpoint inhibitors. *Nat Rev Clin Oncol* **15**(2): 66–66. doi: 10.1038/nrclinonc.2017.210.

92 Li X *et al.* (2022). Gut microbiome in modulating immune checkpoint inhibitors. *EBioMedicine* **82**: 104163. doi: 10.1016/j.ebiom.2022.104163.

93 Mediterranean diet benefits patients with advanced Melanoma. King's College London. [Online] Available at: https://www.kcl.ac.uk/news/mediterranean-diet-benefits-patients-with-advanced-melanoma [Accessed April 25, 2023].

94 Szczyrek M *et al.* (2021). Diet, microbiome, and cancer immunotherapy—A comprehensive review. *Nutrients* **13**(7): 2217. doi: 10.3390/nu13072217.

95 Bolte LA *et al.* (2023). Association of a mediterranean diet with outcomes for patients treated with immune checkpoint blockade for advanced melanoma. *JAMA Oncol.* doi: 10.1001/jamaoncol.2022.7753.

96 Bessede A *et al.* (2022). Impact of acetaminophen on the efficacy of immunotherapy in patients with cancer. *J Clin Oncol* **40**(16_suppl): 12000–12000. doi: 10.1200/JCO.2022.40.16_suppl.12000.

97 Cani M *et al.* (2022). Immune checkpoint inhibitors and opioids in patients with solid tumours: Is their association safe? A systematic literature review. *Healthcare* **11**(1): 116. doi: 10.3390/healthcare11010116.

98 Li Y *et al.* (2022). Analysis of interactions of immune checkpoint inhibitors with antibiotics in cancer therapy. *Front Med* **16**(3): 307–321. doi: 10.1007/s11684-022-0927-0.

99 Cortellini A *et al.* (2021). Differential influence of antibiotic therapy and other medications on oncological outcomes of patients with non-small cell lung cancer treated with first-line pembrolizumab versus cytotoxic chemotherapy. *J Immunother Cancer* **9**(4): e002421. doi: 10.1136/jitc-2021-002421.

100 Hussain N, Naeem M, Pinato DJ (2021). Concomitant medications and immune checkpoint inhibitor therapy for cancer: Causation or association? *Hum Vaccin Immunother* **17**(1): 55–61. doi: 10.1080/21645515.2020.1769398.

101 Colard-Thomas J, Thomas QD, Viala M (2023). Comedications with immune checkpoint inhibitors: Involvement of the microbiota, impact on efficacy and practical implications.

Cancers (Basel) **15**(8): 2276. doi: 10.3390/cancers15082276.

102 Haslam A, Prasad V (2019). Estimation of the percentage of US patients with cancer who are eligible for and respond to checkpoint inhibitor immunotherapy drugs. *JAMA Netw Open* **2**(5): e192535. doi: 10.1001/jamanetworkopen.2019.2535.

103 Lei Y *et al.* (2021). Progress and challenges of predictive biomarkers for immune checkpoint blockade. *Front Oncol* **11**. doi: 10.3389/fonc.2021.617335.

104 McKean WB *et al.* (2020). Biomarkers in precision cancer immunotherapy: Promise and challenges. *Am Soc Clin Oncol Educ Book* **40**: e275–e291. doi: 10.1200/EDBK_280571.

105 (Jack) West H, Jin JO (2015). Performance status in patients with cancer. *JAMA Oncol* **1**(7): 998. doi: 10.1001/jamaoncol.2015.3113.

106 Lagos GG, Izar B, Rizvi NA (2020). Beyond tumor PD-L1: Emerging genomic biomarkers for checkpoint inhibitor immunotherapy. *Am Soc Clin Oncol Educ Book* **40**: e47–e57. doi: 10.1200/EDBK_289967.

107 Havel JJ, Chowell D, Chan TA (2019). The evolving landscape of biomarkers for checkpoint inhibitor immunotherapy. *Nat Rev Cancer* **19**(3): 133–150. doi: 10.1038/s41568-019-0116-x.

108 Wang C, Wang H, Wang L (2022). Biomarkers for predicting the efficacy of immune checkpoint inhibitors. *J Cancer* **13**(2): 481–495. doi: 10.7150/jca.65012.

109 Bai R *et al.* (2020). Predictive biomarkers for cancer immunotherapy with immune checkpoint inhibitors. *Biomark Res* **8**(1): 34. doi: 10.1186/s40364-020-00209-0.

110 Doroshow DB *et al.* (2021). PD-L1 as a biomarker of response to immune-checkpoint inhibitors. *Nat Rev Clin Oncol* **18**(6): 345–362. doi: 10.1038/s41571-021-00473-5.

111 Keenan TE, Burke KP, Van Allen EM (2019). Genomic correlates of response to immune checkpoint blockade. *Nat Med* **25**(3): 389–402. doi: 10.1038/s41591-019-0382-x.

112 Diaz LA *et al.* (2022). Pembrolizumab versus chemotherapy for microsatellite instability-high or mismatch repair-deficient metastatic

colorectal cancer (KEYNOTE-177): Final analysis of a randomised, open-label, phase 3 study. *Lancet Oncol* **23**(5): 659–670. doi: 10.1016/S1470-2045(22)00197-8.

113 André T *et al.* (2022). Nivolumab plus low-dose ipilimumab in previously treated patients with microsatellite instability-high/mismatch repair-deficient metastatic colorectal cancer: 4-year follow-up from CheckMate 142. *Ann Oncol* **33**(10): 1052–1060. doi: 10.1016/j.annonc.2022.06.008.

114 McGregor M, Price TJ (2019). IMblaze 370: Lessons learned and future strategies in colorectal cancer treatment. *Ann Transl Med* **7**(21): 602–602. doi: 10.21037/atm.2019.08.119.

115 Le DT *et al.* (2015). PD-1 blockade in tumors with mismatch-repair deficiency. *N Engl J Med* **372**(26): 2509–2520. doi: 10.1056/NEJMoa1500596.

116 Le DT *et al.* (2017). Mismatch repair deficiency predicts response of solid tumors to PD-1 blockade. *Science (1979)* **357**(6349): 409–413. doi: 10.1126/science.aan6733.

117 Lee V *et al.* (2016). Mismatch repair deficiency and response to immune checkpoint blockade. *Oncologist* **21**(10): 1200–1211. doi: 10.1634/theoncologist.2016-0046.

118 Lynch HT *et al.* (2015). Milestones of lynch syndrome: 1895–2015. *Nat Rev Cancer* **15**(3): 181–194. doi: 10.1038/nrc3878.

119 Cercek A *et al.* (2022). PD-1 blockade in mismatch repair–deficient, locally advanced rectal cancer. *N Engl J Med* **386**(25): 2363–2376. doi: 10.1056/NEJMoa2201445.

120 Bonneville R *et al.* (2017). Landscape of microsatellite instability across 39 cancer types. *JCO Precis Oncol* **1**: 1–15. doi: 10.1200/PO.17.00073.

121 Marletta S *et al.* (2022). Atlas of PD-L1 for pathologists: Indications, scores, diagnostic platforms and reporting systems. *J Pers Med* **12**(7): 1073. doi: 10.3390/jpm12071073.

122 Sha D *et al.* (2020). Tumor mutational burden as a predictive biomarker in solid tumors. *Cancer Discov* **10**(12): 1808–1825. doi: 10.1158/2159-8290.CD-20-0522.

123 Makrooni MA, O'Sullivan B, Seoighe C (2022). Bias and inconsistency in the estimation of tumour mutation burden. *BMC Cancer* **22**(1): 840. doi: 10.1186/s12885-022-09897-3.

124 Yarchoan M *et al.* (2019). PD-L1 expression and tumor mutational burden are independent biomarkers in most cancers. *JCI Insight* **4**(6). doi: 10.1172/jci.insight.126908.

125 Otano I *et al.* (2023). At the crossroads of immunotherapy for oncogene-addicted subsets of NSCLC. *Nat Rev Clin Oncol* **20**(3): 143–159. doi: 10.1038/s41571-022-00718-x.

126 Ghiringhelli F *et al.* (2023). Immunoscore immune checkpoint using spatial quantitative analysis of CD8 and PD-L1 markers is predictive of the efficacy of anti- PD1/PD-L1 immunotherapy in non-small cell lung cancer. *EBioMedicine* **92**: 104633. doi: 10.1016/j.ebiom.2023.104633.

127 Hijazi A *et al.* (2023). Light on life: Immunoscore immune-checkpoint, a predictor of immunotherapy response. *Onco Targets Ther* **12**(1). doi: 10.1080/2162402X.2023.2243169.

128 Li H, van der Merwe PA, Sivakumar S (2022). Biomarkers of response to PD-1 pathway blockade. *Br J Cancer* **126**(12): 1663–1675. doi: 10.1038/s41416-022-01743-4.

129 Burdett N, Desai J (2020). New biomarkers for checkpoint inhibitor therapy. *ESMO Open* **5**: e000597. doi: 10.1136/esmoopen-2019-000597.

130 Chow A *et al.* (2022). Clinical implications of T cell exhaustion for cancer immunotherapy. *Nat Rev Clin Oncol* **19**(12): 775–790. doi: 10.1038/s41571-022-00689-z.

131 Tang J, Shalabi A, Hubbard-Lucey VM (2018). Comprehensive analysis of the clinical immuno-oncology landscape. *Ann Oncol* **29**(1): 84–91. doi: 10.1093/annonc/mdx755.

132 Kwon M *et al.* (2021). The right timing, right combination, right sequence, and right delivery for cancer immunotherapy. *J Control Release* **331**: 321–334. doi: 10.1016/j.jconrel.2021.01.009.

133 Lote H *et al.* (2022). Advances in immunotherapy for MMR proficient colorectal cancer. *Cancer Treat Rev* **111**: 102480. doi: 10.1016/j.ctrv.2022.102480.

134 Colton M *et al.* (2020). Reprogramming the tumour microenvironment by radiotherapy: Implications for radiotherapy and

immunotherapy combinations. *Radiat Oncol* **15**(1): 254. doi: 10.1186/s13014-020-01678-1.

135 Galluzzi L *et al.* (2023). Emerging evidence for adapting radiotherapy to immunotherapy. *Nat Rev Clin Oncol* **20**(8): 543–557. doi: 10.1038/s41571-023-00782-x.

136 Qian JM, Schoenfeld JD (2021). Radiotherapy and immunotherapy for head and neck cancer: Current evidence and challenges. *Front Oncol* **10**. doi: 10.3389/fonc.2020.608772.

137 Rizvi NA *et al.* (2020). Durvalumab with or without tremelimumab vs standard chemotherapy in first-line treatment of metastatic non–small cell lung cancer. *JAMA Oncol* **6**(5): 661. doi: 10.1001/jamaoncol.2020.0237.

138 Tawbi HA *et al.* (2022). Relatlimab and nivolumab versus nivolumab in untreated advanced melanoma. *N Engl J Med* **386**(1): 24–34. doi: 10.1056/NEJMoa2109970.

139 Morganti S, Curigliano G (2020). Combinations using checkpoint blockade to overcome resistance. *Ecancermedicalscience* **14**. doi: 10.3332/ecancer.2020.1148.

140 Ohm JE, Carbone DP (2001). VEGF as a mediator of tumor-associated immunodeficiency. *Immunol Res* **23**(2–3): 263–272. doi: 10.1385/IR:23:2-3:263.

141 Wang L *et al.* (2023). A phase Ib study of ivonescimab, a PD-1/VEGF bispecific antibody, as first- or second-line therapy for advanced or metastatic immunotherapy naïve non-small-cell lung cancer. *J Thorac Oncol.* doi: 10.1016/j.jtho.2023.10.014.

142 Rini BI *et al.* (2019). Pembrolizumab plus axitinib versus sunitinib for advanced renal-cell carcinoma. *N Engl J Med* **380**(12): 1116–1127. doi: 10.1056/NEJMoa1816714.

143 Motzer RJ *et al.* (2019). Avelumab plus axitinib versus sunitinib for advanced renal-cell carcinoma. *N Engl J Med* **380**(12): 1103–1115. doi: 10.1056/NEJMoa1816047.

144 Burotto M *et al.* (2023). Nivolumab plus cabozantinib vs sunitinib for first-line treatment of advanced renal cell carcinoma (aRCC): 3-year follow-up from the phase 3 CheckMate 9ER trial. *J Clin Oncol* **41**(6_suppl): 603–603. doi: 10.1200/JCO.2023.41.6_suppl.603.

145 Choueiri TK *et al.* (2021). Nivolumab plus cabozantinib versus sunitinib for advanced renal-cell carcinoma. *N Engl J Med* **384**(9): 829–841. doi: 10.1056/NEJMoa2026982.

146 Motzer RJ *et al.* (2022). Conditional survival and long-term efficacy with nivolumab plus ipilimumab versus sunitinib in patients with advanced renal cell carcinoma. *Cancer* **128**(11): 2085–2097. doi: 10.1002/cncr.34180.

147 Choueiri TK *et al.* (2023). Lenvatinib plus pembrolizumab versus sunitinib as first-line treatment of patients with advanced renal cell carcinoma (CLEAR): Extended follow-up from the phase 3, randomised, open-label study. *Lancet Oncol* **24**(3): 228–238. doi: 10.1016/S1470-2045(23)00049-9.

148 Wiest N *et al.* (2021). Role of immune checkpoint inhibitor therapy in advanced EGFR-mutant non-small cell lung cancer. *Front Oncol* **11**. doi: 10.3389/fonc.2021.751209.

149 C. Helwick. Are triplets necessary for BRAF-mutated melanoma? Available at: https://ascopost.com/issues/september-10-2021/are-triplets-necessary-for-braf-mutated-melanoma/ [Accessed May 2 2023].

150 Drago JZ, Modi S, Chandarlapaty S (2021). Unlocking the potential of antibody–drug conjugates for cancer therapy. *Nat Rev Clin Oncol* **18**(6): 327–344. doi: 10.1038/s41571-021-00470-8.

151 Nicolò E *et al.* (2022). Combining antibody-drug conjugates with immunotherapy in solid tumors: Current landscape and future perspectives. *Cancer Treat Rev* **106**: 102395. doi: 10.1016/j.ctrv.2022.102395.

152 FDA. FDA approves enfortumab vedotin-ejfv with pembrolizumab for locally advanced or metastatic urothelial cancer. [Online] Available at: https://www.fda.gov/drugs/resources-information-approved-drugs/fda-approves-enfortumab-vedotin-ejfv-pembrolizumab-locally-advanced-or-metastatic-urothelial-cancer [Accessed December 19, 2023].

153 Kraehenbuehl L *et al.* (2022). Enhancing immunotherapy in cancer by targeting emerging immunomodulatory pathways. *Nat Rev Clin Oncol* **19**(1): 37–50. doi: 10.1038/s41571-021-00552-7.

154 Rousseau A, Parisi C, Barlesi F (2023). Anti-TIGIT therapies for solid tumors: A systematic review. *ESMO Open* **8**(2): 101184. doi: 10.1016/j.esmoop.2023.101184.

155 OncLive. Tiragolumab plus atezolizumab falls short in unexpected OS analysis in PD-L1–high NSCLC. [Online] Available at: https://www.onclive.com/view/tiragolumab-plus-atezolizumab-falls-short-in-unexpected-os-analysis-in-pd-l1-high-nsclc [Accessed December 19, 2023].

156 Zeidan AM, Komrokji RS, Brunner AM (2021). TIM-3 pathway dysregulation and targeting in cancer. *Expert Rev Anticancer Ther* **21**(5): 523–534. doi: 10.1080/14737140.2021.1865814.

157 Bian H-T *et al.* (2022). CD47: Beyond an immune checkpoint in cancer treatment. *Biochim Biophys Acta Rev Cancer*, vol. 1877 (5): 188771. doi: 10.1016/j.bbcan.2022.188771.

158 van Duijn A, Van der Burg SH, Scheeren FA (2022). CD47/SIRPα axis: Bridging innate and adaptive immunity. *J Immunother Cancer* **10**(7): e004589. doi: 10.1136/jitc-2022-004589.

159 Maute R, Xu J, Weissman IL (2022). CD47–SIRPα-targeted therapeutics: Status and prospects. *Immuno-Oncol Technol* **13**: 100070. doi: 10.1016/j.iotech.2022.100070.

160 Gartner Hype Cycle. Gartner.co.uk. [Online] Available at: https://www.gartner.co.uk/en/methodologies/gartner-hype-cycle [Accessed May 5, 2023].

Other Forms of Immunotherapy

CHAPTER 6

IN BRIEF

In this chapter, I turn my attention to immunotherapies other than checkpoint inhibitors. These treatments take various forms: antibodies, small molecules, whole cells, modified proteins, and even DNA or mRNA molecules.

In Sections 6.2 and 6.3, I begin with treatments that have been around for over 20 years – naked antibody therapies and immunomodulators (IMiDs).

Naked antibody therapies attach to cancer cells and recruit natural killer (NK) cells, macrophages, and complement proteins. The oldest of these, rituximab, was licensed by the FDA in 1997 and is still very much in use.

The second group of treatments, the IMiDs, took years for scientists to unpick and understand. But, now that we have a detailed understanding of their target – a protein called cereblon – an increasing number are being developed. These treatments play a central role as myeloma treatments.

The other treatments described in this chapter – adoptive cell therapies (ACTs), T cell engagers, and treatment vaccines – all share a common goal: to generate a powerful cancer-fighting immune response mediated by T cells.

When living T cells are given as the person's treatment, this is called adoptive cell therapy (ACT) (or it might be referred to as effector T cell therapy). One of these treatments, CAR (chimeric antigen receptor) T cell therapy, has become an important treatment option for some patients with B cell hematological cancers such as B cell acute lymphoblastic leukemia, some B cell non-Hodgkin lymphomas, or myeloma. I also explain other ACTs, such as TILs (tumor-infiltrating lymphocytes) and T cell receptor (TCR)-engineered T cells, which might be more effective against solid tumors.

Another option is to recruit and activate the person's T cells in vivo, i.e., leveraging the T cells that already exist in the person's body without modifying them in any way. This can be done using antibody-based treatments that have two (or occasionally three) targets called T cell engagers. T cell engagers are off-the-shelf treatments that are relatively easy to make

A Beginner's Guide to Targeted Cancer Treatments and Cancer Immunotherapy, Second Edition. Elaine Vickers.
© 2025 John Wiley & Sons Ltd. Published 2025 by John Wiley & Sons Ltd.

(compared to an ACT), and that can be given to multiple patients. As you'll find out, there are enormous numbers of T cell engagers in trials, and many different designs are being tested.

Lastly, I look at vaccine-based treatments. The aim here is to educate the person's immune system and alert it to the presence of an existing cancer. Scientists hope to create vaccines that teach the immune system (particularly T cells) what cancer cells look like and persuade the T cells to attack. Currently, there are two main stumbling blocks that hold back vaccine-based approaches. The first is that the treatment can't tell the immune system where the person's cancer cells are located. The second is that a vaccine alone can't overcome the immune-suppressing environment inside tumors. Thus, the key will be to combine vaccines with other treatments that overcome these limitations.

By the end of this chapter, I hope you will be both wowed by the science involved and optimistic about the benefits these treatments might bring to people with cancer.

6.1 INTRODUCTION

In Chapter 5, I focused all my attention on immune checkpoint inhibitors such as nivolumab and pembrolizumab. In this chapter, I again wish to build on the foundational knowledge I provided in Chapter 1, but instead of focusing on checkpoint inhibitors, I'll describe various other forms of immunotherapy. Many of these aim to create a T cell response against a person's cancer (outlined in Figure 5.1).

This chapter feels like it contains rather a mixed bag of immunotherapy approaches. For example, it includes some treatments that have been around for several decades alongside those that are still in their infancy.

The development of immunotherapy as a way of treating cancer actually began in earnest in the late 1800s and early 1900s. An American doctor called William Coley experimented with injecting bacteria into patients with various sarcomas to trigger cancer-fighting immune reactions; by the end of his career, he had treated almost 900 patients [1]. But, even up until the dawn of checkpoint inhibitors (the first was approved in 2011), eminent scientists were bemoaning our lack of progress with immunotherapy [2].

Until 2011, you could still count on one hand the number of immunotherapies given to people with cancer:

- First licensed in 1997, the naked monoclonal antibody, rituximab, is used for some people with hematological cancers, where the cancer cells have the CD20 protein on their surface (B cell NHL or CLL).
- First licensed in 1997, thalidomide (famously known for its catastrophic effects when taken during pregnancy) is licensed as a treatment for people with myeloma. The mechanism of action of thalidomide was only cleared up relatively recently, with the identification of its target being discovered by Japanese scientists in 2010 [3]. A second, related treatment, called lenalidomide, was first approved in 2006.
- First licensed in the 1970s the BCG (Bacillus Calmette-Guérin) vaccine for people with bladder cancer – not covered in detail in this book, as the mechanism of action (although it clearly involves immune activation) is still murky [4].
- First licensed in 1992 for kidney cancer, and in 1998 for melanoma skin cancer, interleukin-2 (IL-2) is a signaling protein

(a cytokine) produced by some white blood cells. It has a potent and varied impact on B cells and T cells, and it causes a lot of toxicities. As with the BCG vaccine, I don't cover it in detail in this book. These days, IL-2 is mostly given as an adjuvant – an extra boost – to other immunotherapies such as TILs or CAR T cells [5]. You'll hear more about this in Sections 6.5 and 6.10.

In the decade after the approvals of rituximab and thalidomide, it felt like scientists made little headway. But, since the arrival of the first checkpoint inhibitors, we've also seen a rapid expansion in the range of different types of immunotherapies investigated in trials.

It now feels like (in scientific and in medical circles at least) immunotherapy is the place to be. Billions of dollars, entire research institutes, new journals, and new conferences, have all sprung up to develop and discuss the latest advances. Immunologists, who might once have been on the fringes of cancer research, now take center stage at the world's biggest cancer conferences.

In this chapter, I will describe some of the latest innovations and ideas that are taking the scientific world by storm.

6.2 NAKED ANTIBODIES THAT TRIGGER AN IMMUNE RESPONSE

Licensed drugs mentioned in this section:		
Treatment class	Drugs	Given to some people with:
Naked antibodies targeting CD20	Rituximab, ofatumumab, obinutuzumab	• B cell non-Hodgkin lymphoma • Chronic lymphocytic leukemia • B cell acute lymphoblastic leukemia
Naked antibodies targeting CD38	Daratumumab, isatuximab	• Myeloma
Naked antibodies targeting CD19	Tafasitamab	• B cell non-Hodgkin lymphoma
Naked antibodies targeting CD52	Alemtuzumab	• Chronic lymphocytic leukemia
Naked antibodies targeting CS1/SLAMF7	Elotuzumab	• Myeloma
Naked antibodies targeting CCR4	Mogamulizumab	• Mycosis fungoides or Sezary syndrome (types of cutaneous T cell lymphoma)
Naked antibodies targeting GD2	Dinutuximab, naxitamab	• Neuroblastoma

In Section 2.2.5, I described how a naked antibody that attaches to a protein on the surface of a person's cancer cells can trigger an immune response (Figure 2.14). This response is predominantly down to an antibody's Fc portion (the back end, away from the antigen-binding sites), which connects with Fc receptors on white blood cells such as macrophages and NK cells. The Fc region also acts as an attachment site for a complement protein called C1q.[1]

Naked monoclonal antibodies (this doesn't include checkpoint inhibitors, which have an entirely different mechanism discussed in depth in Chapter 5) can attach to a target on

[1] Complement proteins are a group of proteins found in our blood that work with antibodies and other parts of our immune system to rid us of infections.

cancer cells and trigger three different types of immune response:

1. Antibody-dependent cellular phagocytosis (ADCP) (depicted in Figure 2.14a) is undertaken by macrophages. They attach to the antibody using their Fc receptors, then engulf and destroy the target cell by a process called phagocytosis [6, 7].
2. Antibody-dependent cell-mediated cytotoxicity (ADCC) (depicted in Figure 2.14b) is triggered when NK cells are recruited by an antibody that has attached to a cancer cell. The recruited NK cells release cell-killing enzymes (called perforins and granzymes), other cell-killing proteins (such as Fas ligand), and various signaling proteins that trigger cell death [8, 9].
3. Complement-dependent cytotoxicity (CDC) (depicted in Figure 2.14c). This is triggered when one of the complement proteins found naturally in our blood, called C1q, attaches to the Fc portion of an antibody. C1q recruits further complement proteins, which gradually assemble to form the "membrane attack complex" (MAC). The MAC creates a channel through the cell membrane, and a bit like a burst balloon, the cell dies [10].

Many of the monoclonal antibody therapies given to people with cancer work through a combination of ADCP, ADCC, and CDC (see Table 6.1). However, antibodies don't have to be restricted to doing just one thing. For example, an antibody–drug conjugate (ADC) such as trastuzumab deruxtecan might combine several different mechanisms of action. It is capable of blocking HER2 and triggering cell death, releasing chemotherapy, and activating an immune response.

Most of the naked antibody therapies listed in Table 6.1 are licensed as treatments for people with hematological cancers rather than solid tumors. This is for reasons of safety, effectiveness, and availability of suitable targets [7]:

1. It is relatively safe because we can often survive quite happily despite the destruc-

tion of the hematological cancer cells' healthy counterparts. For example, a CD20-targeted antibody will deplete the body of B cells, but this is rarely life-threatening. It is rare to find safe targets on the surface of cancer cells of solid tumors.
2. The environment in which hematological cancer cells live in is generally less immune suppressing, with more white blood cells coming and going than inside a solid tumor. This means that an approach that involves the recruitment of the patient's healthy white blood cells is generally more effective against a hematological cancer.
3. Compared to cells in other organs and tissues, white blood cells are very accessible and easy to study. Therefore, the scientific community has many decades of experience in discovering, categorizing, and exploring cell surface proteins on white blood cells as targets for cancer treatments.

6.3 IMMUNOMODULATORS AND CELMoDs

Licensed drugs mentioned in this section:		
Treatment class	Drugs	Given to some people with:
Immuno-modulators	Thalidomide, lenalidomide, and pomalidomide	• Myeloma • B cell non-Hodgkin lymphoma • Kaposi sarcoma

Despite the imprecise-sounding name, the term "immunomodulator" (often abbreviated to IMiD) refers to a specific group of treatments. The most well-known of them is thalidomide, the drug famous for causing thousands of women to give birth to children with deformities in the early 1960s.

Thalidomide has come a long way since then, both in terms of our understanding of it and in terms of becoming an established treatment for a

Table 6.1 Licensed monoclonal antibody therapies that trigger a cancer-fighting immune response [6, 7, 11–14].

Antibody name	Target	Indications	Notes
Antibodies that primarily kill cancer cells by triggering an immune response mediated by NK cells, macrophages, and complement proteins			
Rituximab (including rituximab biosimilars)	CD20	B cell NHL, CLL	Causes CDC, ADCC and triggers cancer cell death by apoptosis.
Ofatumumab	CD20	CLL	Causes more CDC and apoptosis than rituximab.
Obinutuzumab	CD20	B cell NHL, CLL	A glycoengineered antibody. Causes more ADCC than rituximab.
Daratumumab	CD38	Myeloma	Causes ADCC, CDC and ADCP, and directly kills myeloma cells.
Isatuximab	CD38	Myeloma	Similar to daratumumab.
Tafasitamab	CD19	B cell NHL	Engineered to enhance ADCC and ADCP.
Alemtuzumab	CD52	T cell prolymphocytic leukemia, T cell cutaneous lymphoma	Mostly causes CDC and ADCC.
Elotuzumab	CS1/ SLAMF7	Myeloma	Not widely used; predominantly activates NK cells.
Mogamulizumab	CCR4	Mycosis fungoides, Sezary syndrome	A glycoengineered antibody; doesn't cause CDC but highly potent at triggering ADCC.
Dinutuximab	GD2	Neuroblastoma	Causes ADCC, ADCP, and CDC.
Naxitamab	GD2	Neuroblastoma	Causes ADCC, ADCP, and CDC.
Zolbetuximab	Claudin 18.2	Stomach cancer	Causes ADCC and CDC.
Antibodies that also directly kill cancer cells			
Trastuzumab, margetuximab, pertuzumab	HER2	Breast cancer, stomach cancer, gastroesophageal junction cancer	These treatments primarily work by killing cancer cells directly.
Cetuximab, panitumumab	EGFR	Bowel cancer	These treatments primarily work by killing cancer cells directly.
Amivantamab	EGFR and MET	NSCLC	A bi-specific antibody that binds both EGFR and MET.
Antibody–drug conjugates	Various	Various	All these treatments retain their ability to trigger an immune response.

Abbreviations: ADC – antibody-dependent cell-mediated cytotoxicity; ADCP – antibody-dependent cellular phagocytosis; CDC – complement-dependent cytotoxicity; CLL – chronic lymphocytic leukemia; NHL – non Hodgkin lymphoma; NSCLC – non-small cell lung cancer.

range of medical conditions, including leprosy. It is also an important treatment for myeloma, a cancer caused by faulty plasma cells (antibody-secreting B cells). Two closely related compounds, lenalidomide and pomalidomide, have also been approved. Pomalidomide is given to some people with Kaposi sarcoma or myeloma; lenalido-mide is a treatment for myeloma and some kinds of B cell non-Hodgkin lymphoma (NHL).

6.3.1 The Mechanisms of Action of IMiDs

The mechanisms of action of IMiDs in the treatment of myeloma are outlined in Table 6.2.

Table 6.2 Summary of the major mechanisms of action of ImiDs in the treatment of myeloma [15, 16].

Mechanism of action	Relative potencies of Thalidomide, Lenalidomide, Pomalidomide		
	T	L	P
Assisting in the activation of cancer-fighting T cells and NK cells	+	++++	+++++
Suppressing regulatory T cells	−	+	+
Enhancing myeloma cell destruction via antibody-dependent cell-mediated cytotoxicity	−	++++	++++
Blocking angiogenesis	++++	+++	+++
Reducing inflammation	+	++++	+++++
Disrupting connections between myeloma cells and other cells in their environment	+	++++	+++++
Protecting bone by inhibiting the maturation and actions of osteoclasts (bone destroyers) and promoting the maturation of osteoblasts (bone creators)	+	++++	+++++
Direct effects on myeloma cells, include blocking cell proliferation and encouraging cell death	+	+++	+++

Despite their range of effects, these treatments all work by interacting with a single protein called cereblon [17]. Scientists now think that all the effects of thalidomide and other IMiDs (including causing birth defects) come down to their ability to change the behaviour of cereblon.

When cereblon was discovered as the primary target of thalidomide, no one knew what it did or what happened when thalidomide binds to it. Subsequently, scientists realized that when an IMiD binds to cereblon, this causes the destruction of two transcription factors[2] called Ikaros and Aiolos by the cell's proteasomes [18, 19]. This process is akin to the destruction of HIF-2α caused by VHL (see Figure 4.5a).

Ikaros and Aiolos are mostly made by white blood cells. They attach to many different genes and control the production of a wide range of proteins. This is presumably why the IMiDs, which only bind to cereblon, exert such a wide range of different effects [18].

6.3.2 Novel Cereblon Modulators

Because we now understand how thalidomide and other IMiDs work, we can create new, more potent cereblon modulators that might work even better. These drugs are generally referred to as cereblon modulators or cereblon E3 ligase modulators (CELMoDs). As of the start of 2024, two CELMoDs, iberdomide and mezigdomide, are in Phase 3 clinical trials involving people with myeloma.

As they are more potent than IMiDs, treatments like iberdomide and mezigdomide might be able to help patients whose disease is resistant to IMiDs. Ikaros and Aiolos are also found in a variety of different types of white blood cells. It's therefore also possible that CELMoDs might have uses outside of the treatment of myeloma.

6.3.3 What Sorts of Side Effects Do They Cause?

IMiDs and CELMoDs all work by impacting cereblon to varying degrees. The range and

[2] I've mentioned transcription factors before. These are specialized proteins that attach to genes and tell the cell whether or not to produce the corresponding proteins. It generally takes a whole bunch of transcription factors and other proteins coming together on a gene to trigger protein production.

severity of their side effects seem to relate to this mechanism of action [16]. Side effects often include low numbers of neutrophils and platelets in the blood, blood clots, and damage to peripheral nerves (peripheral neuropathy – mostly caused by thalidomide).

6.4 INTRODUCTION TO ADOPTIVE CELL THERAPIES

6.4.1 The Bigger Picture

Immunotherapies that aim to create an immune response that is primarily undertaken by T cells broadly fit into one of three categories:

1. Adoptive cell therapies (ACTs): In this group, there are approaches that involve introducing cancer-fighting immune cells into the body. They include tumor-infiltrating lymphocyte (TIL) therapy, CAR T cells, and TCR-engineered T cells. This group also includes NK and macrophage cellular therapies.

2. T cell engagers: These include BiTEs (Bispecific T cell Engagers),[3] bispecific antibodies, ImmTACs[4] (Immune Mobilizing Monoclonal TCRs Against Cancer), and other related strategies that aim to create a physical connection between a person's cancer cells and T cells. As each T cell is engaged, it kills the cancer cell to which it has become attached. They are sometimes referred to as "bispecific T cell engaging antibodies".

3. Treatment vaccines: These aim to alert a person's immune system to the presence of cancer cells and trigger a T cell response. Strategies include introducing DNA, mRNA, or tumor antigens into the body. They also

include incubating dendritic cells with antigens outside the body, or using oncolytic viruses to trigger the release of tumor antigens inside a tumor.

In this section of the chapter, I will focus on ACTs.

6.4.2 ACTs that Use the Patient's Own T Cells

ACT usually refers to treatments in which some of the patient's own white blood cells are removed from their blood (by a process called leukapheresis), deliberately modified (or carefully selected) in the laboratory, allowed to multiply, and then infused back into their blood. Occasionally, white blood cells from a donor (allogeneic) are used in the treatment rather than the patient's own (autologous). However, this runs the risk of the donated cells attacking the patient's body, causing GVHD – graft versus host disease.

One advantage of ACT is that millions of cancer-fighting white blood cells can be created in the laboratory in a highly efficient manner. This is a much more reliable way of increasing the number of activated, cancer-fighting T cells compared to using checkpoint inhibitors. (If you remember from Chapter 5, with checkpoint inhibitors, you just have to hope that there are already cancer-fighting T cells in the patient's body that are being suppressed via the checkpoint protein that you are blocking.)

Another advantage of ACT is that you can prepare the person's body to receive the cells. This is usually done by giving the person a course of chemotherapy to reduce the number of white blood cells in their body.[5] Then, when you introduce the new cells into the body, they aren't

---

[3] BiTE is a registered trademark of Micromet AG (a fully owned subsidiary of Amgen Inc.).
[4] ImmTAC is a registered trademark of Immunocore Ltd.
[5] This is generally referred to as "lymphodepleting" or "non-myeloablative" chemotherapy to differentiate it from the chemotherapy normally given to patients prior to a stem cell transplant. Lymphodepleting/non-myeloablative chemotherapy reduces the number of white blood cells in the person's body but doesn't totally wipe them out.

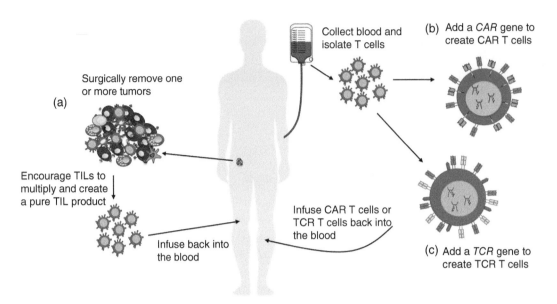

Figure 6.1 Introducing TIL therapy, CAR T cell therapy, and TCR T cell therapy. **(a)** For TIL therapy, a surgeon first removes one or more tumors. These are chopped up and grown in conditions where TILs become the only cell type. These are then infused back into the patient's blood. In contrast, CAR T cell therapy and TCR T cell therapy involve genetically altering T cells taken from the patient's blood. **(b)** For a CAR T cell product, the T cells are modified so that they produce a CAR protein. **(c)** For a TCR-engineered T cell product, the T cells are altered so that they produce and display a new TCR. The altered cells are then returned to the patient.
Abbreviations: CAR – chimeric antigen receptor; TCR – T cell receptor; TIL – tumor-infiltrating lymphocyte.

blocked or destroyed by regulatory T cells, and they're not competing for nutrients or cytokines[6] with the patient's other white blood cells [20, 21].

The types of ACT that I am going to describe in this part of the chapter are TIL therapy, CAR T cells, and TCR-engineered T cells (described in brief in Figure 6.1).

As you'll see when I describe these approaches, each has properties that make it suitable as a treatment for certain cancer types. However, scientists are working hard to expand their usefulness, often by adding modifications or using complex strategies to overcome existing limitations.

As I write this in early 2024, TIL therapy is a licensed treatment for some people with melanoma skin cancer, and CAR T cell therapy is a standard treatment for people with some hematological cancers. TCR-engineered T cell therapy isn't yet an established treatment for any cancer, but it holds promise as a new way of treating solid tumors.

6.5 TUMOR-INFILTRATING LYMPHOCYTE THERAPY

Licensed drugs mentioned in this section:		
Treatment class	**Drugs**	**Given to some people with:**
Tumor-infiltrating lymphocyte (TIL) therapy	Lifileucel	• Melanoma skin cancer

---

[6] You might remember from earlier chapters that cytokines are a family of small proteins that act as signals sent out by white blood cells and other cell types. They include interleukins and interferons.

TILs are naturally occurring lymphocytes (mostly T cells) found inside tumors. The first evidence that TILs could be removed from someone's tumor, multiplied, and put back into their body as a helpful treatment came in 1988 [22]. The approach was pioneered by Dr. Steven Rosenberg, now a legend among the immunotherapy community [23]. The 1988 trial involved 20 patients with advanced melanoma skin cancer,[7] 11 of whom benefited from the therapy – their tumors shrank, and the effect lasted anywhere from 2 to more than 13 months [22].

6.5.1 Why is TIL Therapy Mostly Just for People with Melanoma?

As I said in Section 5.5.1, melanoma skin cancer is one of the most immunogenic cancers out there. By "immunogenic," I mean that (1) melanoma cells often have a high number of DNA mutations, (2) these mutations are generally of a sort that lends themselves to detection by the immune system, and (3) this recognition often leads to a cancer-fighting immune response mediated by cytotoxic T cells that infiltrate the tumor (TILs) [24].

Melanomas tend to contain more TILs than many other types of solid tumor, which creates optimism for the TIL approach [24, 25]. In addition, through years of experience, we know that melanoma skin cancers are often sensitive to immune checkpoint inhibitors and other forms of immunotherapy. All of this has meant that most trials assessing TIL therapy have involved people with melanoma.

6.5.2 How Does TIL Therapy Work?

The goal of the TIL approach, as with checkpoint inhibitors, is to remove the suppressive forces that prevent cancer-fighting lympho-cytes from destroying a patient's cancer cells. Checkpoint inhibitors do this by blocking the activation of inhibitory checkpoint proteins.

With the TIL approach, however, the lymphocytes are physically removed from the suppressive environment, encouraged to grow and multiply in the laboratory, and then returned to the patient's body [20, 22, 26–30]. Hopefully, the TILs then migrate into the tumor and any metastases and mount an attack.

The way that TILs are grown and put back into patients has slowly been improved. However, this evolution and improvement has (at least to my way of thinking) taken a rather unexpected turn. When I wrote the first edition of this book, I included a figure explaining the TIL therapy process. This process, as I explained it, included taking TILs from a patient's tumor and carefully finding the ones that had reacted to their cancer cells. These TILs were grown in a laboratory to massively increase their numbers and then returned to the patient [31].

However, the TIL therapy approach that has become a licensed treatment is simpler than this. It seems that speed is of the essence when creating an effective TIL product. So, instead of spending time finding TILs that have reacted to a person's cancer cells, it has (at least so far) proven more effective to just encourage all the TILs you can find to multiply as quickly as possible [30] (see Figure 6.2 for the series of steps necessary to create a TIL product for a patient). Using this shortened process (although it still takes a few weeks), the TIL product contains "younger" TILs that are more likely to remain active and multiply in the person's body.

What happens to the patient before and after receiving their infusion of TILs is a crucial element of TIL therapy. Beforehand,

---

[7] Melanomas generally develop in the skin (usually exposed to the sun or sunbeds). However, they can arise anywhere that you find melanocytes, which includes in the eyes and on mucous membranes lining the mouth, vagina, anus, and other locations. TILs are a treatment option only for people with melanoma in the skin.

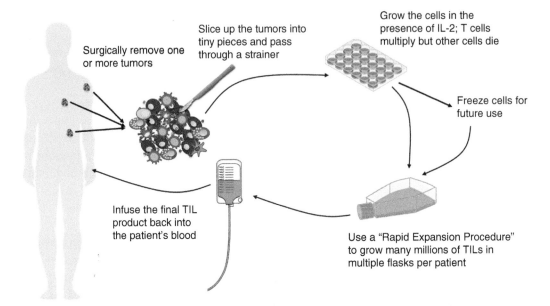

Figure 6.2 Creating an effective TIL therapy product. Using the method illustrated here, a few small surgical samples containing a mixture of T cells, cancer cells, and other cell types can be turned into a pure TIL product containing many millions of TILs. The whole process takes several weeks, including around two weeks for the so-called Rapid Expansion Procedure.
Abbreviations: IL-2 – interleukin-2; TIL – tumor-infiltrating lymphocyte.

the patient receives chemotherapy over the course of a week. This depletes the body (and possibly any tumors) of cells that would suppress TILs, such as MDSCs (myeloid-derived suppressor cells) and Tregs (regulatory T cells). Chemotherapy also seems to encourage white blood cells to generate more signals that encourage TILs to survive and multiply [21]. After their infusion, the patient also receives repeated infusions of IL-2; this gives the TILs important added encouragement.

6.5.3 What Results Do We Have So Far?

Since the TIL trial in 1988, scientists have conducted lots of other smallish studies of TIL therapy [32]. However, it wasn't until 2022

that initial results were published from the first ever Phase 3 trial of TIL therapy [27]. The M14TIL trial involved 168 patients with advanced melanoma, 86% of whom had already received treatment with a PD-1 antibody such as pembrolizumab or nivolumab. Half the patients were treated with TIL therapy, and the other half were given ipilimumab, a CTLA-4 targeted checkpoint inhibitor. For the people who received TIL therapy, their treatment began with surgery to remove one or more metastases (depending on their size), followed by a course of chemotherapy. A week after the chemotherapy, they received an infusion of between 5 billion and 500 billion TILs.[8] After the TIL infusion, each patient received up to 15 doses of IL-2. TIL preparation

---

[8] Where 5 billion is 5000 million, or 5,000,000,000.

Table 6.3 Results from the M14TIL trial, which compared TIL therapy to ipilimumab given to people with advanced melanoma skin cancer.

	TIL therapy (84 patients)	Ipilimumab (84 patients)
Overall response rate	49%	21%
Median progression-free survival	7.2 months	3.1 months
Median overall survival	25.8 months	18.9 months
Proportion of patients whose disease hadn't worsened 6 months after their first scan[a]	52.7%	21.4%
Two-year survival rate	54.3%	44.1%
Proportion who experienced side effects of Grade 3 or higher	100%	57%

[a] The TIL group had their first scan six weeks after their TIL infusion. The ipilimumab group had theirs 12 weeks after the first dose of ipilimumab. This meant that everyone had their first scan at roughly the same time.
Source: Data from [27].

generally took about five weeks for each patient. The people who were randomly allocated to the ipilimumab arm of the trial received up to four doses of ipilimumab, which was given every three weeks. Table 6.3 contains a summary of the results.

These results have generated lots of enthusiasm and excitement around TIL therapy, and it became a licensed treatment in the United States in March 2024.

6.5.4 What Sorts of Side Effects Does TIL Therapy Cause?

This question is actually quite difficult to answer, as most of the side effects of TIL therapy are not caused by the TILs but by the pre-infusion course of chemotherapy and post-infusion IL-2. For example, in the M14TIL trial, everyone in the TIL arm of the trial experienced Grade 3 or worse side effects, but

these were largely caused by chemotherapy and included problems such as low white blood cell counts [27, 33].

6.5.5 Is It Being Explored as a Treatment for Other Cancers?

Everything I've said about TILs so far relates to people with melanoma skin cancer. But this isn't the only group of patients taking part in TIL therapy trials. Melanoma skin cancer is thought to be particularly visible to a patient's immune system because of the number, and the types, of mutations the cancer cells tend to contain. Other cancer types that also contain TILs and for which TIL therapy trials are underway are non-small cell lung cancer (NSCLC), cervical cancer, colorectal (bowel) cancer, cholangiocarcinoma (bile duct cancer), sarcomas, ovarian cancer, and renal (kidney) cancer [26].

6.5.6 How Is It Being Improved?

Scientists are pursuing various ways of making TIL therapy more effective and useful for a wide range of people with cancer. I've outlined three such strategies below [21, 26].

Enrich TIL products with T cells most likely to react to the patient's cancer cells
TILs that have PD-1 and/or various other checkpoint proteins on their surface are likely to be ones that recognize and can react to a patient's cancer cells. Scientists are using techniques such as FACS (fluorescence-activated cell sorting) to sort through the TILs they find and select just the ones they want. Hopefully, having used this (relatively quick) selection step, the final TIL product will contain a high proportion of cancer-fighting TILs.

Use a selection step so that only TILs that react to the patient's cancer cells are included in the final product
There are various ways of doing this, and some of them are incredibly complicated and

time-consuming (which, when speed appears to be of the essence, may be a limiting factor). For example, one method involves exposing the patient's TILs to neoantigens[9] from their tumor and isolating any TILs that recognize and react to them. This sounds a lot simpler than it actually is!

The most technical part of this is predicting which of the mutations in the person's cancer cells have led to neoantigens that are displayed on their surface. Cancer cells can contain thousands of mutations in their DNA. Only some of these mutations affect proteins. And only some of the mutated proteins they make will result in the creation of neoantigens. In addition, only some of these neoantigens have the potential to cause a cancer-fighting T cell response. Scientists have developed computer models to identify mutations that lead to neoantigens. But this is only useful if (1) their prediction is accurate, (2) it can be done quickly enough that the patient is well enough to receive their TIL product, and (3) the TIL product contains T cells that survive, multiply, and attack cancer cells in the patient's body.

Use biomarkers to find patients most likely to benefit from TIL therapy

There are several possible biomarkers that could be used to identify patients likely to benefit from TIL therapy. For example, you could select patients whose tumors contain a high number of mutations (high mutational burden) or that contain defects in a DNA repair pathway or were caused by viral infections such as the human papillomavirus (HPV). All these things and a high degree of

mutation clonality,[10] create tumors that are more likely to be immunogenic (display lots of neoantigens) and therefore are likely to contain TILs.

6.5.7 What Does the Future of TIL Therapy Look Like?

In March 2024, TIL therapy became a licensed treatment for some people with advanced melanoma skin cancer. However, the problem is always going to be justifying the cost of this approach and developing a TIL product quickly enough to be useful.

6.6 CAR T CELL THERAPY

Licensed drugs mentioned in this section:		
Treatment class	**Drugs**	**Given to some people with:**
CAR T cell therapies targeting CD19	Axicabtagene ciloleucel, brexucabtagene autoleucel, lisocabtagene maraleucel, tisagenlecleucel	• B cell non-Hodgkin lymphoma • B cell acute lymphoblastic leukemia
CAR T cell therapies targeting BCMA	Idecabtagene vicleucel, ciltacabtagene autoleucel	• Myeloma

The mechanism of the CAR T cell approach is different from that of checkpoint inhibitors and TILs. As I've mentioned before, checkpoint inhibitors and TILs aim to overcome or remove things that suppress the activity of T cells. These approaches aim to increase the

---

[9] A neoantigen is a peptide that comes from a mutated protein. Crucially, the peptide includes amino acids that are different from normal because of the mutation. Because a neoantigen has come from a mutated protein, it shouldn't be produced by non-cancer cells. Hopefully, the immune system recognizes the neoantigen as a sign that something is wrong and generates T cells that react to it.

[10] If you look back at Table 5.7, you'll see a list of various biomarkers that predict sensitivity to checkpoint inhibitors and that might also be used to predict which patients are likely to benefit from of TIL therapy.

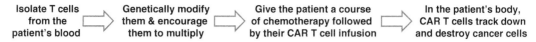

Figure 6.3 **A basic outline of the CAR T cell therapy process.** The goal of CAR T cell therapy is to treat the patient with genetically-modified versions of their own T cells. First, T cells are collected from their blood. The gene for a CAR protein is then introduced into the T cell's chromosomes, forcing the T cell to manufacture thousands of copies of the CAR protein and place them on its surface. The T cells are then given time to multiply. Once back in the patient's body, the CAR protein enables the modified T cells to attach to target cells (hopefully cancer cells) and destroy them.
Abbreviation: CAR – chimeric antigen receptor.

number and activity of cancer-killing T cells that have been generated naturally by the patient's immune system.

The goal of CAR T cells, however, is to create tens of millions of genetically-modified T cells that:

1. Would never naturally exist in a patient's body.
2. All attach to one particular protein on the surface of the person's cancer cells.
3. Become activated when their CAR protein attaches to its target and kills the targeted cell without requiring any further activation signals.
4. Multiply and stay alive long enough to completely eradicate cancer cells from the patient's body.

Figure 6.3 outlines the basic process of CAR T cell therapy. However, for you to get a proper idea of how it works, I'm going to provide some more detail. First, I'll explain CAR T cells and how they're made. Then, I'll discuss their targets and which cancers they're currently being used to treat and why. Finally, I'll look at how it's being improved and which other cancers it might be used for in the future.

6.6.1 What Are CAR T Cells and How Are They Made?

What Is a CAR Protein?

CAR proteins are made from various bits and pieces of antibodies and other proteins (see Figure 6.4a) [34, 35]. The first CAR proteins were designed in the late 1980s and were relatively simple. The early CAR proteins have gradually been improved upon to create CAR proteins with a greater ability to cause T cells to stay alive, multiply, and become active. The idea is that a CAR T cell will use its CAR proteins to lock onto a target on the surface of another cell. This then activates the T cell and causes it to kill the target cell. It also causes the CAR T cell to multiply and create lots more CAR T cells that will do the same.

The outer portion of the CAR protein is the bit that sticks out from the surface of a CAR T cell. This is generally made from an antibody tip (the antigen-binding site). The originating antibody is often a mouse antibody, such as with tisa-cel, liso-cel, axi-cel, brexu-cel, and ide-cel (see Table 6.4 for their full names). However, cilta-cel is a little different in that it has two antigen-binding regions taken from two different camelid antibodies.[11]

---

[11] Camelids include llamas and camels. Instead of our antibodies and those of mice, where the antigen-binding site is made from two separate protein pieces, the antigen-binding site of a camelid antibody is made from a single protein piece and is therefore smaller. This makes it possible to make a CAR protein that contains two binding sites for the target antigen rather than one.

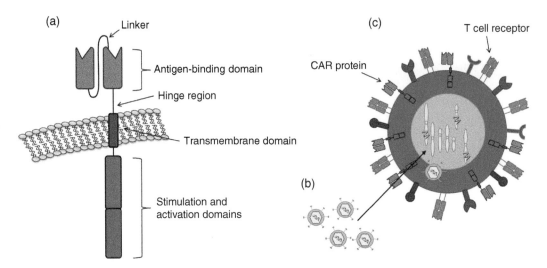

Figure 6.4 CAR proteins and CAR T cells. (a) CAR proteins are constructed from various protein pieces taken from a variety of sources. The external (extracellular) antigen-binding region is the variable region (also called the scFv) of an antibody, which is held together by a linker – a short string of amino acids. This is joined to a hinge region, which provides flexibility. This, in turn, is connected to the transmembrane domain, which spans the outer membrane of a T cell. Inside the cell are usually two (but sometimes more) stimulatory domains. When the CAR protein locks on to its target, these protein segments trigger cell-killing activity. They also give the modified T cell signals to stay alive and multiply. **(b)** CAR T cells are usually created using a modified virus that delivers instructions (in the form of a gene made from DNA) for making the CAR protein into T cells. The *CAR* gene hopefully becomes a permanent part of the cell's chromosomes. **(c)** The *CAR* gene instructs the modified T cell to manufacture thousands of copies of the CAR protein and place them on its surface alongside its T cell receptor and other cell surface proteins. **Abbreviation:** CAR – chimeric antigen receptor.

Another crucial part of a CAR protein is the stimulatory and activation domains. These are responsible for activating the CAR T cell's cell-killing activities and telling the T cell to survive and multiply. CAR proteins always include the activation domain of the CD3ζ (CD3-zeta) protein. They also include either the costimulatory section of the 4-1BB protein or that from the CD28 protein. There's some evidence that when a CAR protein contains the CD28 domain the T cells fire up and multiply more quickly in the patient's body, and reach higher levels, than when the 4-1BB domain is used. CAR proteins containing the CD28 protein have thus been linked to faster patient responses but also to greater toxicities [36, 37].

How Do You Make CAR T Cells?

T cells can be persuaded to manufacture a CAR protein by inserting into their chromosomes the instructions (i.e., the gene,[12] made from DNA) to make such a protein. CAR proteins are an amalgam of different protein pieces. For this reason, the gene telling a T cell how to make a CAR protein consists of a series of gene segments that correspond to each protein part.

The entire man-made gene can be inserted into a T cell's chromosomes using a variety of

---

[12] In case you want a refresher or are new to biology: genes are lengths of DNA that contain the instructions to make proteins. For decades, scientists have been able to insert new genes into cells. This forces them to make proteins that they would never otherwise make.

methods [35]. The most common method is to package up the gene inside a virus capsule (see Figure 6.4b). The virus (which has been emptied of all disease-causing material) enters the cell and inserts the *CAR* gene into the T cell's chromosomes. The T cell then uses the instructions in the *CAR* gene to make thousands of copies of the CAR protein, which it slots into its outer membrane (Figure 6.4c).

Once the T cells have been modified, they are encouraged to multiply until many millions of CAR T cells are ready to be returned to the patient [38].

The whole manufacturing process – from obtaining a patient's T cells, through to modifying them, multiplying them, and finally returning them to their blood – generally takes several weeks.

What Do CAR Proteins Do?

When present on the surface of T cells, CAR proteins allow T cells to directly attach to targets on the surface of cancer cells. This attachment triggers the T cells' cell-killing ability, and they directly destroy cancer cells (and any other cells with the same target on their surface). Hopefully, some of the activated T cells are memory cells, which give long-lasting protection against the cancer returning. A vital property of CAR proteins is that they enable T cells to react to a target without first needing to be activated by a dendritic cell.

What Do CAR Proteins Target?

In Section 1.5, I described how T cells normally respond to cancer cells by using their TCRs. TCRs react to tiny fragments of proteins (called peptide antigens, or simply antigens) that are sat insde MHC protein 'cups', which stick out from our cells' surface.

CAR proteins have different targets because they're made using the tip of an antibody and not the tip of a TCR. Antibodies (unlike TCRs) react to intact proteins and large molecules (Figure 6.5). The precise location on its target where the antibody binds is called an epitope.

So far, most licensed CAR T cell products either target a protein called CD19 or one called BCMA (B cell maturation antigen). Scientists think these proteins fulfill the criteria shown in Figure 6.5 because [35, 39]:

- These proteins are present in high amounts on the cells of the cancers they are used to treat. For example, CD19 is found on the cancer cells of B cell acute lymphoblastic leukemia (ALL) and on most B cell NHLs (such as DLBCL, follicular lymphoma, and

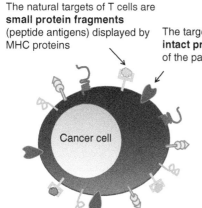

The natural targets of T cells are **small protein fragments** (peptide antigens) displayed by MHC proteins

The target of a CAR protein is an **intact protein** found on the surface of the patient's cancer cells

CAR protein targets:

- Need to be <u>reliably present</u> in <u>large quantities</u> on <u>the surface</u> of the patient's cancer cells

- Need to <u>not disappear</u> from the cell surface (or get nibbled off)

- If they're also found on the surface of healthy cells, then these cells must be <u>expendable</u>

Figure 6.5 Properties of CAR protein targets.
Abbreviations: CAR – chimeric antigen receptor; MHC – major histocompatibility complex.

mantle cell lymphoma). BCMA is found on the cancer cells of myeloma.

- These proteins don't generally get nibbled off by other cells. However, a lack of CD19, or the loss of it from the surface of cancer cells, is a common reason why the treatment doesn't work or why the patient's disease comes back. This seems to be less of a problem with BCMA (summarized in [40]).
- Although CD19 and BCMA are present on some groups of healthy B cells, and these cells are killed by the CAR T cells, this is not life-threatening.

6.6.2 How Do We Know that CAR T Cell Therapy Works?

Most of the largest clinical trials of CD19-targeted CAR T have involved patients who either had ALL or a B cell NHL. The trials with

BCMA-targeted CAR T cells involved patients with myeloma.

Table 6.4 provides a current (as of early 2024) list of approved CAR T cell products. Please note that I haven't provided details on exactly which patients each product is given to. I've kept things brief as eligibility differs between the United States and Europe, and it's also changing rapidly as new trial results become available.

CD19 CAR T Cells for Children and Adults with ALL

CAR T cell therapy is a licensed approach for children and adults with relapsed ALL that is resistant to chemotherapy. This is due to the results of two main trials – ELIANA (which involved children and young adults up to age 25) and ZUMA-3 (which involved older adults). In these trials, the rates of complete response

Table 6.4 Licensed CAR T cell therapies.

Product	Target	Co-stimulation domain	Approvals
Tisagenlecleucel (Tisa-cel)	CD19	4-1BB	• Children and young adults (up to 25 years old) with refractory/relapsed **B cell ALL** • Adults with refractory/relapsed **DLBCL** or **follicular lymphoma**
Axicabtagene ciloleucel (Axi-cel)	CD19	CD28	• Adults with refractory/relapsed **DLBCL** or **PMBCL** • Adults with refractory/relapsed **follicular lymphoma**
Brexucabtagene autoleucel (Brexu-cel)	CD19	CD28	• Adults with refractory/relapsed **mantle cell lymphoma** • **Adults** with refractory/relapsed **B-cell ALL**
Lisocabtagene maraleucel (Liso-cel)	CD19	4-1BB	• Adults with refractory/relapsed **DLBCL, PMBCL, mantle cell lymphoma**, or **follicular lymphoma grade 3B** • Adults with refractory/relapsed **CLL/SLL**
Idecabtagene vicleucel (Ide-cel)	BCMA	4-1BB	• Refractory/relapsed **myeloma**
Ciltacabtagene autoleucel (Cilta-cel)	BCMA	4-1BB	• Refractory/relapsed **myeloma**

Abbreviations: ALL – acute lymphoblastic leukemia; BCMA – B cell maturation antigen; CLL – chronic lymphocytic leukemia; DLBCL – diffuse large B cell lymphoma; PMBCL – primary mediastinal large B cell lymphoma; SLL – small lymphocytic lymphoma.

were around 70%–80%, with many of these patients remaining disease-free years later [40–44]. However, the likelihood of remaining relapse-free appears to be greater in children than in adults [40].

CD19 CAR T Cells for Adults with B Cell NHL

CAR T cell therapy is an established treatment for some people with the most common, aggressive form of NHL (diffuse large B cell lymphoma [DLBCL]) and for the less common form, primary mediastinal large B cell lymphoma (PMBCL). It's given after or instead of a stem cell transplant [45–48]. It's also an option for some people with mantle cell lymphoma or follicular lymphoma [49]. The evidence that CAR T cell therapy is helpful for patients with DLBCL has come from numerous clinical trials, which generally report complete response rates of around 50%–80% depending on the characteristics of the patients involved [48]. Trials involving people with less aggressive lymphomas, such as follicular lymphoma, again report complete response rates of around 60%–80% [50]. For people with any of these cancers, CAR T cell therapy brings the possibility of being cured of their disease [40].

BCMA CAR T Cells for People with Myeloma

BCMA is found on the cancer cells of myeloma, a disease that generally affects much older patients compared to diseases such as ALL or NHL [51]. As with CD19-targeted CAR T cell therapy, BCMA-targeted therapy seems to be effective for a lot of the patients it's given to (many of whom have received multiple other treatments, often given as treatment combinations over the course of several years). Response rates in the region of 70%–100% were recorded in two large trials: CARTITUDE-4 and KarMMa-3 [52, 53].

Again, some of these patients were still disease-free several years later. However, because the trials are more recent and have given more mixed results, the medical community is hesitant to say that any of these people have truly been cured.

6.6.3 Why Doesn't CAR T Cell Therapy Work for Everyone, and Why Do Some People's Cancers Come Back?

Whether or not someone is helped by CAR T cell therapy and whether their disease comes back seems to depend on a few things (some of which are depicted in Figure 6.6) [40, 54–56].

- The depth of the person's initial response – this feels a bit like saying "if it's worked then it's worked," But it's still probably worth pointing out that if the person's disease appears to have disappeared then the treatment is likely to work for longer than if lots of cancer cells are still detectable following treatment.
- How many cancer cells were in the person's body, and where they were located when they received CAR T cell therapy. People with fewer cancer cells in their body (a lower burden of disease) tend to do better and have milder side effects.
- The type of cancer the patient has: people with B cell lymphomas appear to be a bit less likely to experience a complete response to treatment compared to someone with ALL or myeloma. But, if a patient with B cell lymphoma does have a complete response, then it's likely to last longer.
- The health of the patient's T cells that were used to manufacture their CAR T cell product. This will influence how long the CAR T cells live, whether they multiply, and how many cancer cells they kill. Some patients have received a lot of treatments that damage T cells prior to receiving CAR T cell therapy, and cancer cells can also

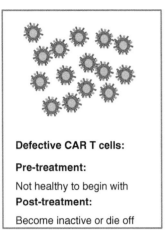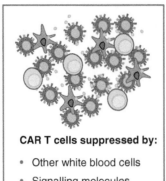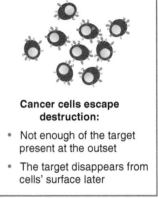

Defective CAR T cells:

Pre-treatment:

Not healthy to begin with

Post-treatment:

Become inactive or die off

CAR T cells suppressed by:

- Other white blood cells
- Signalling molecules
- Checkpoint proteins

Cancer cells escape destruction:

- Not enough of the target present at the outset
- The target disappears from cells' surface later

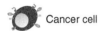 Cancer cell   CAR T cell   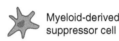 Myeloid-derived suppressor cell   Regulatory T cell

Figure 6.6 Some of the reasons why patients might not benefit from CAR T cell therapy.
Abbreviation: CAR – chimeric antigen receptor.

send out signals and create an environment that suppresses T cells. Perhaps it's not surprising that not everyone's T cells can create a powerful, active, and long-lasting population of CAR T cells.

- The amount of the target protein on the surface of the person's cancer cells and how much variation there is from one cancer cell to the next. CAR T cells need a lot of their target to be present (compared to how much a natural TCR needs) to successfully kill target cells. Cancer cells with low levels of the target protein on their surface are likely to survive and cause the person's cancer to return.
- Whether or not the CAR T cells get suppressed by inhibitory checkpoint proteins (e.g., PD-1), inhibitory cells (e.g., regulatory T cells), or inhibitory signaling proteins (e.g., interleukin-10), and whether they can get to where they're needed.
- Whether and for how long the person's CAR T cells multiply and survive in their body. People whose CAR T cells multiply to higher levels generally fare better than

people whose CAR T cells disappear quickly [57, 58] (see Figure 6.7).

It's also important to remember that not everyone who agrees to try CAR T cell therapy ultimately receives an infusion of cells. In every trial conducted, a proportion of the patients who decided to take part never received an infusion of CAR T cells. Reasons for this include [59]:

- Manufacturing failures, where not enough T cells could be purified from the patient's blood, or they failed to multiply to sufficiently high levels, to create a viable CAR T cell product.
- The person's health deteriorated too quickly for them to be well enough to receive their CAR T cell product.

6.6.4 What Sorts of Side Effects Does CAR T Cell Therapy Cause?

One of the most important and dangerous side effects of CAR T cell therapy is cytokine release syndrome (CRS). A second important toxicity is a range neurological problems

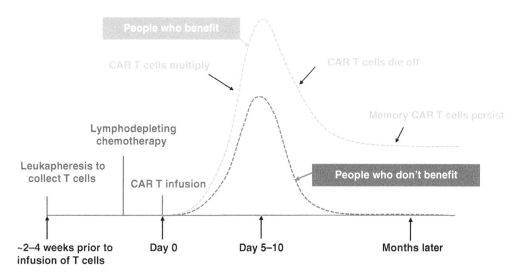

Figure 6.7 CAR T cells tend to multiply to higher levels, and be detectable in the blood for longer, in people who benefit from CAR T cell therapy compared to those who don't.
Abbreviation: CAR – chimeric antigen receptor.

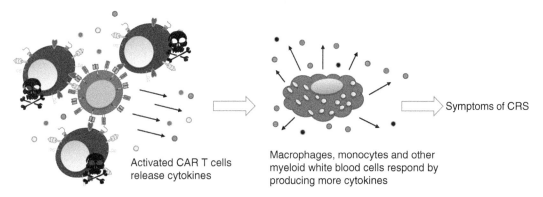

Figure 6.8 **Activated CAR T cells indirectly cause CRS**. Activated CAR T cells release cytokines into their surroundings, such as IFN-γ, TNFα, and GM-CSF. In response, macrophages and other myeloid white blood cells produce cytokines such as IL-6, IL-1, and iNOS. Together, these proteins cause physiological changes that the patient experiences as the symptoms of CRS.
Abbreviations: CAR – chimeric antigen receptor; CRS – cytokine release syndrome; GM-CSF – granulocyte-macrophage colony-stimulating factor; IFN-γ – interferon-gamma; IL-6 – interleukin-6; IL-1 – interleukin-1; iNOS – inducible nitric oxide synthase; TNFα – tumor necrosis factor-alpha.

collectively called immune effector cell-associated neurotoxicity syndrome (ICANS).

CRS includes symptoms such as a high fever, fatigue, headache, joint and muscle pains, nausea, diarrhea, and vomiting. These symptoms are caused by the actions of small signaling proteins (various cytokines) released by myeloid white blood cells such as macrophages. These cells in turn are responding to cytokines released by activated CAR T cells (Figure 6.8) [60–62].

ICANS symptoms include the person being unable to express themselves properly through speech (expressive aphasia) or

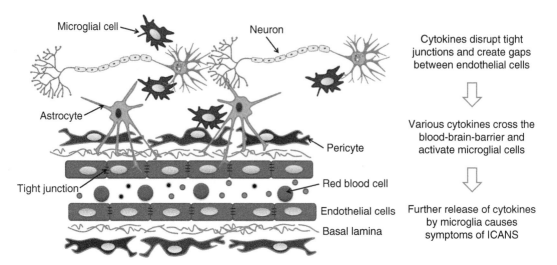

Figure 6.9 Activated CAR T cells indirectly cause ICANS by releasing cytokines that cross the blood-brain-barrier.
Abbreviations: CAR – chimeric antigen receptor; ICANS – immune effector cell-associated neurotoxicity syndrome. *Source:* Sanu N / https://commons.wikimedia.org/wiki/File:Structure_of_Neuron.png / Last accessed on April 05, 2024.

writing (dysgraphia), tremors, and lethargy, as well as seizures and loss of consciousness. These symptoms have a similar foundation to CRS (Figure 6.9). That is, cytokines released by CAR T cells and macrophages pass through the blood-brain-barrier[13] and enter brain tissue. Here, they cause macrophage-like cells called microglia to produce yet more cytokines, which cause brain inflammation and the symptoms of ICANS.

CRS and ICANS are potential problems with all CAR T cell therapies and aren't related to the CAR T cells' target. These side effects can also be caused by other treatments that activate a lot of T cells and kill lots of cancer cells very quickly, such as the T cell engagers that I come to later in this chapter.

Of course, as well as killing the person's cancer cells, CAR T cells will also kill any other cells with the same target on their surface. Hence, one of the side effects of CD19-targeted CAR T cells is hypogammaglobulinemia (their immune system can't create antibodies), which can put the person at risk of dangerous infections.

Hypogammaglobulinemia is a consequence of the person's CAR T cells having killed off their healthy B cells alongside their cancer-causing B cells. For many patients who experience this lack of B cells (and therefore lack of antibody production), the effect lasts for as long as the CAR T cell therapy is working. If B cells (and antibody production) re-emerge, this can be (but isn't always) a sign that the person's cancer is about to return [63].

As I mentioned below, CAR T cells are being created with many targets other than CD19. As with CD19 CAR T cells, each of

---

[13] The blood-brain barrier is a protective layer that lines the inner surfaces of blood vessels inside the brain. All blood vessels are lined with endothelial cells, but in the brain, these cells are much more tightly packed together. Together, the endothelial cells control what gets in and out of brain tissue.

them is likely to cause some toxicities due to the destruction of healthy cells with the CAR protein's target on their surface.

6.6.5 How Is CAR T Cell Therapy for Hematological Cancers Being Improved?

There are so many different strategies being pursued that it can be hard to keep up! China and the United States are the main two countries in which this work is taking place.

In Figure 6.6, I outlined some of the main limitations of CAR T cell therapy. In Figure 6.10, I summarize some of the approaches that scientists are taking to overcome these limitations.

Overcoming a Lack of CAR T Cell Persistence or Activity

Persistence – how long the CAR T cells live – can be influenced by the choice of the co-stimulation domain in the CAR protein. Hence, scientists are exploring different domains or creating CAR proteins that have

more than one. They are also looking at the choice of cells and the manufacturing process [64].

A patient's T cells are often harvested at a time when the patient has already undergone multiple treatments for their disease, and so their cells are already damaged. This affects the survival of the CAR T cells that are produced and hinders their ability to kill cancer cells. A strategy being explored is to create CAR T cells that have been made from healthy donor T cells [65].

Scientists are also hoping to create "universal CAR T cells" (Figure 6.11). In this strategy, the CAR protein on the donor T cells is incomplete and lacks an antigen-binding domain. Instead, a separate targeting protein is used – one end is an antigen-binding region, and the other attaches to the incomplete protein on the donor T cell. When the two are given together (the modified donor T cells and the targeting protein), they create a complete CAR protein that allows the modified T cells to destroy target cells. Many different designs are being

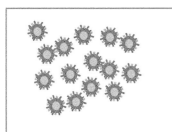

Problem–defective CAR T cells

Solution:

• **Use T cells from a healthy donor to create allogeneic CAR T cell products**

• **Include more memory-like and naïve T cells, change the CAR protein design, or alter the manufacturing process**

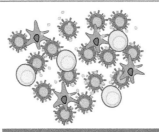

Problem–CAR T cell suppression

Solution:

• **Combinations with other treatments e.g. checkpoint inhibitors, BTK inhibitors**

• **Create "armored" CAR T cells that produce additional proteins e.g., cytokines or BiTEs**

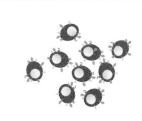

Problem–cancer cell escape

Solution:

• **Create CAR T cells that have more than one target**

Figure 6.10 **Some of the ways CAR T cell therapy is being improved**.
Abbreviations: BiTE – bi-specific T cell engager; BTK – Bruton's tyrosine kinase; CAR – chimeric antigen receptor.

(a)   (b)

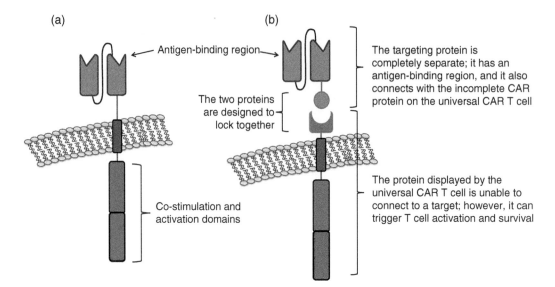

Figure 6.11 Comparing the structure of a conventional CAR protein with a universal CAR protein.
(a) A conventional CAR protein includes an antigen-binding domain and co-stimulation and activation domains. **(b)** In contrast, the CAR protein on a universal CAR T cell only contains the co-stimulation and activation domains. The antigen-binding region is on a separate protein. When the two proteins connect, a complete CAR protein is created.

developed [66, 67]. An advantage of this approach is that you only need a single population of modified donor T cells, which are used no matter what the target is. You simply give the patient the donor T cells along with a targeting protein of your choice.

Overcoming the Problem of CAR T Cell Suppression

There are two main strategies being pursued to overcome this problem.

The first is to create CAR T cells with extra bells and whistles in the form of additional elements that help them recruit other helpful white blood cells or overcome suppressive forces. For example, scientists have made CAR T cells that also manufacture a BiTE – a bispecific T cell engager. BiTEs are double-ended proteins that create a physical connection between a target cell and a T cell. So, in theory, they could help recruit ordinary nearby T cells and encourage them to destroy cancer cells. Other strategies include creating CAR T cells

that produce signaling proteins that activate other types of white blood cells [68].

Another strategy is to combine giving CAR T cell therapy with a second treatment that provides an additional boost to T cells (such as a checkpoint inhibitor). BTK inhibitors, a common treatment for people with chronic lymphocytic leukemia, are also being tested as a way of boosting CAR T cell activity. A different approach is to follow CAR T cell therapy with a stem cell transplant [69, 70].

Overcoming the Problem of Cancer Cell Escape

Cancer cell escape is when cancer cells emerge that no longer have the CAR protein's target on their surface, or where there's not enough of the target to activate CAR T cells. One potential way to get around this is to create CAR T cells with more than one target. This can be done by [71, 72]:

• Creating a single CAR protein that connects to more than one target.

- Creating CAR T cells that produce more than one CAR protein.
- Creating multiple populations of CAR T cells and mixing them together.

These approaches are all being tried out in clinical trials.

6.6.6 What About CAR T Cell Therapy for Other Hematological Cancers?

There are many different proteins being explored as possible targets for CAR T cell therapy for cancers other than ALL and B cell NHL (see Table 6.5 for some examples).

There are various obstacles that stand in the way of creating effective CAR T cell therapies for these other cancers. I'll summarize just a few of those obstacles below.

Chronic Lymphocytic Leukemia (CLL)

Some of the chief problems seem to be that (1) people with CLL tend to have very unhealthy T cells, (2) the cancer cells live in an immune-suppressing microenvironment that quickly shuts down CAR T cells, and (3) cancer cells seem to quickly lose target proteins such as

Table 6.5 Examples of possible CAR T cell targets for other hematological cancers [73–79].

Cancer	Possible CAR T cell targets
Chronic lymphocytic leukemia	CD19, CD20, CD22, ROR-1, Siglec-6
Myeloma	BCMA, SLAMF7, CD38, GPR5D
Acute myeloid leukemia	CD33, CD123, CLL-1, CD13, CD7, NKG2D ligand, CD38, CD70, TIM3, siglec-6, Lewis Y antigen
T cell leukemias and lymphomas	CD7, CD5, TRBC-1, TRBC-2
Hodgkin lymphoma	CD30
Chronic myeloid leukemia	IL1RAP

CD19 from their surface. Most trials so far have been small and with very mixed results [79]. Despite this, a CD19-targeted CAR T cell product was awarded accelerated approval by the FDA (in America) in March 2024.

Acute Myeloid Leukemia (AML)

We've yet to make much progress in creating CAR T cell therapies for people with AML. The biggest problems are [73, 74, 76, 77]:

- A lack of CAR protein targets that are exclusive to leukemia cells. Most AML cell surface proteins are also found on stem cells, immature myeloid white blood cells, and the cells of important organs and tissues. Because of this, CAR T cell therapy for AML is often highly toxic.
- A wide variation in the properties of AML cells between different patients. This makes it impossible to identify targets that are common to every patient's leukemia cells. The consequence of this is that no single CAR protein target will lead to an effective treatment for all AML patients.
- A wide variation in the cancer cells of each individual patient (this is called intratumoral heterogeneity). This means that different populations of cancer cells in the patient's body are driven by different faults and have different combinations of proteins on their surface. This makes it virtually impossible to make a CAR T cell therapy that will be able to cure someone of AML.

T Cell Leukemias and Lymphomas

As with AML, it is impossible to find a CAR T cell target for T cell cancers that isn't also on the surface of healthy T cells. Another problem is that CAR T cells directed towards a target found on T cells are likely to kill one another (called CAR T cell fratricide). However, various gene editing techniques, such as Base Editing, TALEN, and CRISPR/Cas9, are having some success [73–75].

Chronic Myeloid Leukemia and Hodgkin Lymphoma

One of the main obstacles holding back the creation of CAR T cell therapies for these cancers is that we already have so many different effective treatments. In fact, most people newly diagnosed with chronic myeloid leukemia (CML) will have a next-to-normal life span [80]. It is therefore difficult to identify what incentive (economic or medical) there would be for creating CAR T cell therapy for CML.

The case for developing CAR T cell therapy for Hodgkin lymphoma (HL) is perhaps stronger – it is a more common disease that carries a greater risk of life-threatening treatment resistance or relapse. The most common CAR protein target being explored for HL is CD30, the same target as for brentuximab vedotin, an ADC [81]. Some promising results with CAR T cell therapy have been reported [81–83].

6.6.7 Can CAR T Cells Be Used as a Treatment for Solid Tumors?

To explain why it's so difficult to create an effective CAR T cell therapy for someone with a solid tumor, I first want to underline why this approach is successful against hematological cancers. It is for four main reasons listed in Table 6.6.

In contrast, none of the properties outlined in Table 6.4 are true for solid tumors. Instead, there are many problems (Table 6.7).

In response to these problems, scientists are testing out many possible solutions (Table 6.8).

From what I can see, there are three main sets of solid tumors for which many CAR T cell therapy strategies are being pursued and for which clinical trials are underway [84, 88, 89]:

1. Cancers for which immunotherapy-based strategies have already proven to be effective, and therefore there is a reasonable chance of CAR T cell therapy also being

Table 6.6 Why CAR T cell therapy is effective against hematological cancers.

AVAILABLE TARGETS	• The cancer cells of hematological cancers have on their surface the same proteins as their healthy counterparts (e.g., CD19) • So long as these counterparts are expendable, you can afford to target and destroy them (although this will inevitably cause some side effects) • There's therefore no need to find cancer-specific targets for many hematological cancers (e.g., ALL, B cell NHL)
ABUNDANT TARGETS	• If you pick a naturally abundant protein, there will be plenty of it on the cancer cells for CAR T cells to attach to and become activated by
ACCESSIBLE CANCER CELLS	• Cancer cells are naturally in the blood, lymph nodes, lymph tissues, bone marrow … all the same places that CAR T cells will naturally visit
AGREEABLE NEIGHBORS	• Cancer cells are surrounded by other cell types; some may be hostile to CAR T cells, but many are not

Abbreviations: ALL – acute lymphoblastic leukemia; CAR – chimeric antigen receptor; NHL – non-Hodgkin lymphoma.

effective. Examples include NSCLC and virus-associated cancers, such as HPV-positive cervical and head and neck cancers.

2. Cancers for which very few effective treatment options are available, and therefore survival times are particularly poor. For these cancers, any treatment that looks at all helpful will be looked on favorably by patients, doctors, and regulators. Examples include pancreatic cancer (specifically pancreatic ductal adenocarcinoma [PDAC]), ovarian cancer, and glioblastoma.

3. Cancers that display a protein believed to be a particularly promising CAR T cell target. For example, high levels of the mesothelin protein are found on the cancer

Table 6.7 Obstacles to the creation of CAR T cell therapy for solid tumors [84–87].

LACK OF SAFE TARGETS	• Proteins on cancer cells are often the same as on healthy cells in organs and tissues that you can't afford to destroy • Finding completely cancer-specific targets is impossible; therefore, toxicity is a continual problem – sometimes a lethal one
PATCHY TARGETS	• Targets are often only present at low levels, with patchy presence due to heterogeneity amongst cancer cells • Therefore, efficacy is a problem – CAR T cells need a lot of their target to be present to become active
INACCESSIBLE CANCER CELLS	• CAR T cells won't naturally make their way into tumors • Even if they get there, abnormal tumor blood vessels and a fibrous protein network often trap T cells and prevent them from accessing cancer cells
DISAGREEABLE NEIGHBORS	• Cancer cells live in a highly immune-suppressing environment, full of Tregs, MDSCs, and TAMs, and low in oxygen and nutrients • CAR T cells quickly become suppressed, exhausted or die out

Abbreviations: CAR – chimeric antigen receptor; MDSC – myeloid suppressor cell; TAMs – tumor-associated macrophages; Treg – regulatory T cell.

Table 6.8 Strategies to create safe and effective CAR T cell therapies for solid tumors [84–87].

LACK OF SAFE TARGETS	• Create CAR T cells that can be turned on and off or that can be told to self-destruct, thus reducing the harm to essential healthy cells that also have the CAR T cells' target on their surface. • Continue searching for suitable targets on cancer cells
PATCHY TARGETS	• Create CAR T cells that attach to multiple targets so that they're not reliant on the presence of just one
INACCESSIBLE CANCER CELLS	• Administer via injection directly into tumors • Modify CAR T cells so that they also produce cytokines that help them move into tumors
DISAGREEABLE NEIGHBORS	• Modify CAR T cells so that they also secrete cytokines/proteins that help CAR T cells remain active and/or that activate other T cells in their environment • Remove checkpoint proteins from the surface of CAR T cells so they're less likely to become suppressed or exhausted • Deplete the tumor of Tregs and MDSCs prior to administering the CAR T cell infusion

cells of mesothelioma, ovarian cancer, PDAC, stomach cancer, and several other solid tumors. It also appears to be a relatively safe target. A second protein, called Claudin 18.2 (CLDN18.2), is another possibly safe target, this time for various cancers of the digestive system.

6.6.8 Final Comments on CAR T Cells

CAR T cell therapy is an effective treatment for people with some hematological cancers. However, it doesn't work for every cancer type. Also, many patients who receive it aren't helped, and for many who are helped their disease later comes back. As a result, work on this approach continues, with enormous efforts being made to expand the range of cancers and patients for which it is effective.

Some early concerns around CAR T cell therapy still stand – largely around cost, safety, and keeping patients stable while they wait for their CAR T cells to be manufactured. However, the exciting results obtained during clinical trials do seem to be being replicated in the real world [90–93]. The main caveat to this is that in some of these trials, patients who were:

• in poorer general health to begin with (i.e., people who had difficulties going about their daily lives due to their illness and/or who also had other medical conditions)

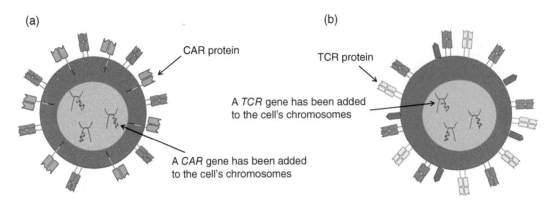

Figure 6.12 Comparing a CAR T cell with a TCR T cell. (a) A CAR T cell has the gene for making a CAR protein inserted into its chromosomes. It uses this gene to make thousands of copies of a cell surface CAR protein. **(b)** A TCR T cell is modified with the gene for a new TCR protein rather than a CAR protein. Again, the modified T cell makes thousands of copies of this new TCR and places them on its surface. **Abbreviations:** CAR – chimeric antigen receptor; TCR – T cell receptor.

• and/or had a greater burden of cancer in their body

• and/or had received more prior treatments tended to have a lower chance of benefiting from CAR T cell therapy and were at a greater risk of relapse if they did initially benefit [90, 91].

Outside of hematological cancers, CAR T cell therapy has yet to make an impact. The obstacles that stand in the way of effective CAR T cell therapy for people with solid tumors have so far proven to be too great to overcome. However, one of these barriers – a lack of targets – is much less of a problem with the closely related approach of TCR-engineered T cell therapy, and I'll turn my attention to this now.

6.7 TCR-ENGINEERED T CELL THERAPY

The basic idea behind TCR-engineered T cell therapy (TCR T cell therapy for short) is very similar to that of CAR T cell therapy. Again, T cells are removed from a person's blood,

purified, genetically modified, and then returned. The main differences are:

1. The person's T cells are being forced to make thousands of copies of a new TCR protein rather than a CAR protein.

2. The antigen-binding site of the new TCR (the bit of the protein that directs the modified T cells to their target) is the tip of a TCR rather than the tip of an antibody (as in CAR T cell therapy) (Figure 6.12); this changes what the modified T cells can target (more on this below).

3. The treatment may need to be HLA-matched to the patient, whereas there is no need for HLA matching with CAR T cell therapy (again, I've written more about this below).

6.7.1 What Do TCR T Cells Target?

Because TCR T cells use their new TCR to detect cancer cells, their target must be a protein fragment (a peptide antigen) sitting inside an MHC protein 'cup' [94–96]. This contrasts with the sorts of cell surface proteins (such as CD19 or BCMA) targeted by a

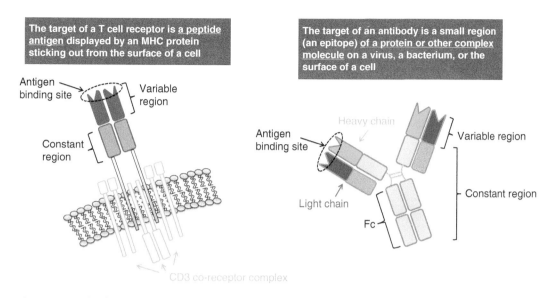

The target of a T cell receptor is <u>a peptide antigen</u> displayed by an MHC protein sticking out from the surface of a cell

The target of an antibody is a small region (an epitope) <u>of a protein or other complex molecule</u> on a virus, a bacterium, or the surface of a cell

Antigen binding site — Variable region

Constant region

CD3 co-receptor complex

Antigen binding site — Heavy chain — Variable region

Light chain — Constant region

Fc

Figure 6.13 Similarities and differences between an antibody (right) and a T cell receptor (TCR) (left). Both antibodies and TCRs have a constant region and a variable region. At the tip of the variable region is the antigen-binding site. However, TCRs and antibodies differ in terms of their target antigen. T cells use their TCRs to react to small peptide antigens presented to them by MHC proteins. Antibodies react to a small portion of a whole protein found on a pathogen or on the surface of cells.

Abbreviations: Fc – the name given to the back portion of an antibody; MHC – major histocompatibility complex; TCR – T cell receptor.

CAR protein. Their different targets reflect the contrasting properties of TCRs and antibodies (Figure 6.13).

Over the past decade, scientists have explored many different potential targets for TCR T cells. They have been searching for proteins that fulfill the following criteria [97]:

- Whatever protein it is, cancer cells must end up with small fragments of it (peptide antigens) displayed by some of their MHC proteins (Figure 6.14).
- The chosen peptide antigen must be reliably displayed by all the patient's cancer cells (TCR T cells won't recognize or kill cells unless they are displaying their target).
- The chosen peptide antigen must also be absent from healthy cells in important organs and tissues (otherwise, the person will experience toxicities caused by TCR T cells attacking these tissues).

- Ideally, the peptide antigen is not unique to one patient, so that time isn't spent identifying a new target for each patient.
- The chosen peptide antigen must be one that can elicit an immune response from T cells – there's no point picking a peptide that TCR T cells are going to ignore.

The main sources of potential targets are [96, 97]:

- Peptide fragments from mutated proteins that the cell makes due to mutations in the corresponding genes – these are usually referred to as neoantigens. These are usually unique to each patient's cancer.
- Peptide fragments from proteins that cancer cells make a lot of but that healthy cells make less of – known as tumor-associated antigens. These are not unique to each patient (which is useful), but they are often also made by healthy cells (which is a problem).

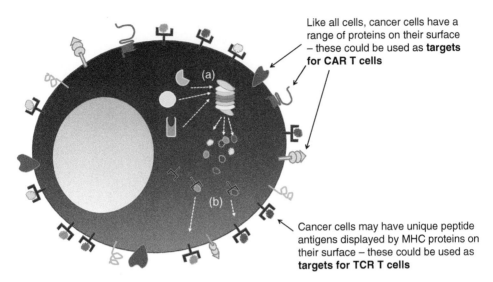

Like all cells, cancer cells have a range of proteins on their surface – these could be used as **targets for CAR T cells**

Cancer cells may have unique peptide antigens displayed by MHC proteins on their surface – these could be used as **targets for TCR T cells**

Figure 6.14 Targets for TCR T cells are peptide antigens displayed by MHC proteins. (a) Cells contain thousands of proteins that they recycle by digesting them into small fragments. **(b)** Some of these fragments are loaded onto MHC proteins and transferred to the cell's surface.
Abbreviations: CAR – chimeric antigen receptor; MHC – major histocompatibility complex; TCR – T cell receptor.

- Peptide fragments from virus proteins that the cell is making due to infection by a virus (e.g., Epstein–Barr virus, HPVs, or hepatitis viruses) – these are called viral antigens.
- Cancer-testis antigens (also called cancer germline antigens) – are usually not present in adult cells, or they're only present in cells that don't have MHC proteins, such as cells in the testes. However, cancer cells sometimes produce and display them on their MHC proteins.

6.7.2 How are TCR T Cells Made?
Many of the later steps for creating a TCR T cell therapy for a patient are the same as for a CAR T cell therapy (I gave a rough outline in Figure 6.3, with more detail in Figure 6.4b & c). However, for CAR T cell therapy, the new gene that is put into the person's T cells is the gene for a CAR protein (Figure 6.4a), whereas for TCR T cell therapy, the new gene is for a new TCR. The person's T cells put this TCR onto their surface alongside their original TCR

(Figure 6.12b). So, that leaves us with the question of where this new *TCR* gene comes from.

There's no single answer to this question. TCR T cell therapy is still new, and scientists are working out how to find the best TCR for a chosen target [96, 97]. Most strategies involve exposing antigen-presenting cells (such as dendritic cells) to a chosen antigen before mixing them with T cells (perhaps from a patient or perhaps from a healthy donor). Scientists then isolate any T cells that have become activated. Finally, a single T cell is selected, and its *TCR* gene is sequenced. This gene is inserted into a virus, which is used to transport the new gene into a patient's T cells.

6.7.3 Why Might You Need to Perform HLA Matching for TCR T Cell Therapy?
So far, I've said that TCR T cell therapy involves modifying a person's T cells so that they produce a new TCR. With this new

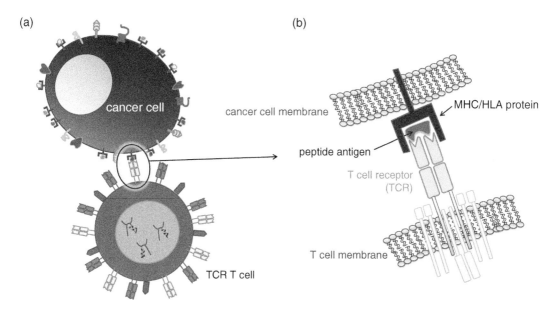

Figure 6.15 A TCR will only connect with its target antigen if it is displayed by an MHC protein.
(a) The TCR T cell connects to its target antigen using its new TCRs. **(b)** The antigen is nestled inside an MHC protein found on the person's cancer cells. (In my imaging, I think of MHC proteins as little cups sticking out from the surface of our cells. Nestled within each cup is a tiny antigen being held out for passing T cells to look at using their TCRs).
Abbreviations: HLA – human leukocyte antigen; MHC – major histocompatibility complex; TCR – T cell receptor; TCR T cell – TCR-engineered T cell.

TCR, the modified T cells interact with a peptide antigen displayed by an MHC class 1 protein on the person's cancer cells. If this interaction takes place, the TCR T cells kill the cancer cells.

However, an important caveat is that each MHC protein 'cup' can only display peptide antigens of certain sizes and shapes.

This is important because each of us inherits a set of genes from each biological parent that determines the range of different-shaped MHC class 1 proteins our cells make. We inherit three MHC class 1 genes from our mother, and three more from our father. So, our cells have a maximum of 6 different-shaped MHC class 1 cups on their surface[14]. In the human population, there are thousands of different versions of MHC cups [98].

The upshot is that before modifying a person's T cells with a new *TCR* gene, you must understand what MHC cups their cells make. This is done through a process of "HLA matching" (MHC is the term used to talking about the MHC system in general, whereas the term HLA – human leukocyte antigen – relates just to the MHC system in humans). Using HLA matching you find out whether the person's MHC proteins are capable of displaying the antigen targeted by the new TCR.

---

[14] Some peoples' cells make a smaller number than this because it's possible to inherit an overlapping set of genes from our mother and father.

If not, then the TCR T cells will be targeting an antigen that doesn't exist on the surface of the patient's cancer cells and the treatment won't work.

6.7.4 What Are the Advantages of TCR T Cell Therapy Over CAR T Cell Therapy?

The fact that TCR T cells use their new TCR to connect with a target on the person's cancer cells comes with a few advantages over CAR T cells [94–97].

1. The target can be an intracellular protein so long as fragments of the protein end up on MHC proteins displayed on the cell's surface – do look back at Figure 1.13 if you'd like a refresher as to how and why this happens. This means there are thousands of potential targets to choose from, creating more opportunities to create TCR T cell therapies for solid tumors.
2. TCRs are highly sensitive – you only need a tiny amount of the target antigen (possibly just a handful of copies) displayed by MHC proteins on the surface of cancer cells for the T cell to be activated (this contrasts with CAR T cell therapy, where much higher amounts of the target need to be present for CAR T cells to become active).
3. The TCR made by the modified T cells is still a natural protein (unlike a CAR protein). When a TCR connects to a target, this creates a more orderly and potentially longer-lasting activation of the T cell compared to a CAR protein.
4. Again, because the new TCR made by the modified cells is still a natural protein, TCR T cell therapy is potentially safer than CAR T cell therapy, with less risk of CRS or neurological toxicity.
5. TCR T cell therapy is potentially more precise than CAR T cell therapy, with less danger of the modified T cells attacking healthy tissues. This is particularly true if the chosen target comes from a mutated protein that is absent from non-cancer cells.

6.7.5 Current Limitations and Problems with TCR T Cell Therapy

The obstacle that TCR T cell therapy overcomes compared to CAR T cell therapy is a lack of suitable targets. Sadly, all the other obstacles remain, including the immune-suppressing environment inside tumors. Thus, for TCR T cell therapy to become an effective treatment for people with solid tumors, there are still other problems to solve.

In addition, there are further concerns that are unique to TCR T cell therapy. One of the chief causes for concern with this treatment is the mispairing of the new TCR and the T cells' own TCR. Figure 6.12b shows a TCR T cell having two kinds of TCRs on its surface, both its original TCRs and the new TCR that it's making because of the introduction of the new *TCR* gene into its DNA. Each TCR is made of two pieces. So, a TCR T cell is making four pieces in total, which won't necessarily pair up in the way you intended. This problem is called TCR mispairing. It can lead TCR T cells to make TCRs with an entirely different target to their original one, or that of the intended TCR. There have been some very rare cases where TCR T cells with mispaired TCRs have caused lethal damage to patients [96].

6.7.6 Where Have We Got with this Approach?

Hundreds of (mostly small) clinical trials are taking place, the majority of which are being carried out in the United States and China. These involve patients with a variety of different solid tumors [94, 96, 97]. However, It is likely to be years before an effective, safe TCR T cell therapy becomes a standard treatment for any common cancer type.

6.8 CELL THERAPY WITH OTHER WHITE BLOOD CELLS

So far, I have spoken only about genetically modified T cells as cancer treatments. But T cells aren't the only white blood cells with the capacity to kill cancer cells. Various white blood cells are being explored as starting points for the creation of novel ACTs. Perhaps the two most interesting and have the greatest potential are natural killer (NK cells) and macrophages.

6.8.1 CAR NK Cells

CAR NK cell therapy is still in the early stages of investigation. Clinical trials are underway, but these trials are very small at the moment. The CAR protein of CAR NK cells is usually very similar or identical to those being developed for CAR T cell therapy [99].

Below, I've provided a brief summary of the key features of NK cells and the pros and cons of CAR NK cells.

Cell type: CAR NK cell	Key points [99, 100]
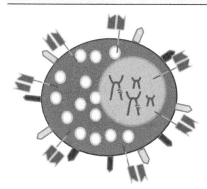	• Like T cells, NK cells can directly kill target cells. • CAR NK cells can be allogeneic (derived from a healthy donor) without the risk of the donated cells attacking the patient – no GVHD (graft versus host disease). • As well as being directed towards cancer cells by their CAR protein, NK cells naturally attack cells that have lost MHC proteins from their surface (this is a common phenomenon amongst cancer cells). • There is a lower risk of CRS and ICANS than with CAR T cells because NK cells produce a different range of cytokines compared to T cells. • BUT, NK cells don't naturally enter tumors and, like CAR T cells, they are quickly suppressed by the hostile environment within tumors. • They also have a short lifespan of about two weeks; therefore, any toxicity they cause is likely to be short-lived but the patient may need repeated infusions.

6.8.2 CAR Macrophages

CAR macrophage therapy is also still very new. I always think of macrophages as being the "Jack of all trades" of the immune system. There are billions of them pretty much everywhere in the body, although sometimes they look a bit different and have specific functions, and names, depending on where they're found. For example, macrophages are called Kupffer cells in the liver and Langerhans cells in the skin.

Macrophages get involved in lots of different aspects of day-to-day life in our tissues [101]. For example, they can engulf and destroy microbes like bacteria and viruses, get rid of debris and dead cells, and coordi-nate and send lots of signals to other white blood cells. One of their functions during an infection is to encourage T cells to keep going. They do this from within an infected tissue by repeatedly showing antigens to T cells using MHC proteins (macrophages are therefore classed as antigen-presenting cells) [102].

A key feature of macrophages that makes them exciting as a prospect for cell-based therapy for solid tumors is that they are naturally found in high numbers inside tumors. Also, unlike CAR T cells and CAR NK cells, they don't seem to become suppressed and inactive inside tumors.

I've summarized some of the key features of CAR macrophage cells below.

Cell type: CAR macrophage	Key points [99]
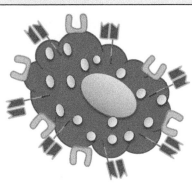	• Macrophages naturally infiltrate tumors and are usually abundant inside them. They often account for up to 50% of the white blood cells in tumors. • They are recruited into tumors by hypoxia-induced cytokines, which are produced by tumor cells. • They are less likely to become exhausted and inactive compared to CAR T cells. • They are efficient at activating other white blood cells (they can act as antigen-presenting cells for T cells). • CAR macrophages require novel CAR protein designs compared to CAR T cells or CAR NK cells.

6.9 T CELL ENGAGERS

Licensed drugs mentioned in this section:		
Treatment class	**Drugs**	**Given to some people with:**
T cell engagers targeting CD19/CD3	Blinatumomab	• B cell acute lymphoblastic leukemia
T cell engagers targeting CD20/CD3	Mosunetuzumab, epcoritamab, glofitamab	• B cell non-Hodgkin lymphoma
T cell engagers targeting BCMA/CD3	Teclistamab, elranatamab	• Myeloma
T cell engagers targeting GPRC5D/CD3	Talquetamab	• Myeloma
T cell engagers targeting Gp100/CD3	Tebentafusp	• Uveal melanoma
T cell engagers targeting DLL3/CD3	Tarlatamab	• Small cell lung cancer

T cell engagers are treatments that create a physical connection between a cancer cell and a T cell. The idea is that this connection activates the T cell and causes it to kill the cancer cell. T cell engagers are mostly made by tethering together the tips (called scFvs[15]) of two different antibodies (Figure 6.16), hence their other name of bispecific antibodies.

The linker holding together the two scFvs is long enough to allow each scFv to rotate and maneuver into place to connect with its target [103]. One target is <u>always</u> CD3, which forms part of the TCR complex on the surface of T cells. Crucially, CD3 is permanently present on the surface of T cells. The other end of the T cell engager attaches to a target found on the surface of cancer cells. In the case of blinatumomab, the first BiTE to become a licensed cancer treatment, the second protein is a cell surface protein called CD19, found on the surface of B cells (Figure 6.17). As you might remember, CD19 is also the target of many CAR T cell therapies.

---

[15] An scFv is the variable region of an antibody. But, because it consists of two pieces of protein (taken from the antibody's heavy chain and light chain), it is held together using a short linker so that it has the same antigen-binding site as the antibody that it came from.

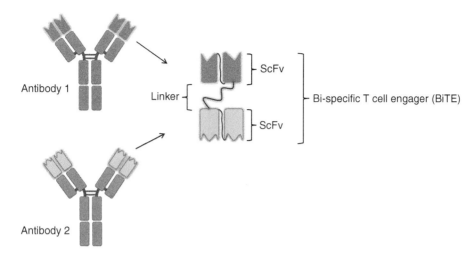

Figure 6.16 A common design for a T cell engager. This layout is called a BiTE – a bi-specific T cell engager. The BiTE is constructed from two scFvs that connect to different targets.

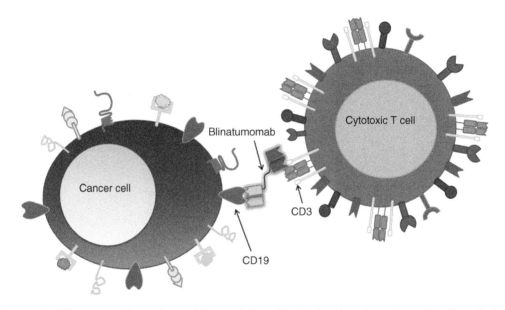

Figure 6.17 Blinatumomab attaches to CD19 and CD3. CD19 is found on the surface of B cells, including B cells that give rise to acute lymphoblastic leukemia (ALL). Blinatumomab brings together B cells and cytotoxic T cells. This forces the T cell to kill the cancer cell.

6.9.1 A Few Notes on Their Design

Initially, the most promising T cell engagers looked to be ones that were very small, such as the BiTEs (Figure 6.18a–c). However, BiTEs have a couple of important features that affect their usefulness in both good and bad ways [103]:

1. BiTEs are very small proteins. This is useful, as it helps them move around the body and penetrate deep into tissues.

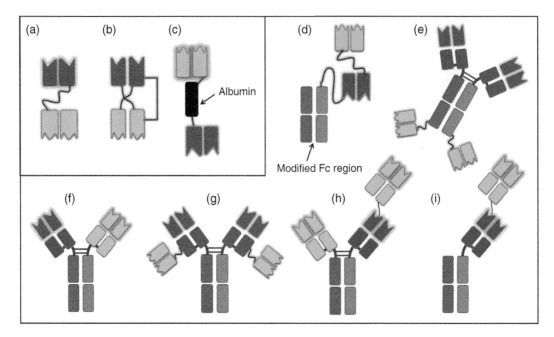

Figure 6.18 A few examples of the enormous number of different T cell engager designs. Some **(a)** are short-lived, but very small proteins. Their longevity can be extended by modifications such as the addition of extra linkers and proteins **(b & c)**. Others **(d–i)** incorporate a modified Fc region. These are larger but much longer lasting in the body.

2. BiTEs have a very short lifespan in the body. If you give someone an infusion of blinatumomab, half of it is gone after just two hours[16] (the kidneys get rid of it very quickly). The consequence of this is that BiTEs are generally administered as a continuous infusion over a period of days. If this wasn't done, the amount of the BiTE in the body wouldn't be high enough for long enough to help the patient.

The short lifespan of BiTEs has led scientists to come up with alternative designs.

For example, one way to extend a BiTE's longevity is to add extra links to the BiTE's structure (Figure 6.18b). Another is to incorporate a protein such as albumin into the structure of the BiTE (Figure 6.18c) [104]. The most popular strategy is to include the "back-end" (called the Fc region) of an antibody in the design. This extends the half-life of the protein dramatically, making it similar to that of a natural antibody [103, 105]. As a result, T cell engagers that incorporate an Fc region (Figure 6.18d–i) can be given to patients as a single infusion every two to three weeks, rather than as a continual infusion, as with blinatumomab.

There are an enormous number of T cell engagers in development whose structure I haven't included in Figure 6.18. There are simply too many of them! For example, there are CiTEs (checkpoint inhibitory T cell engagers), which also block inhibitory checkpoint proteins; SMITEs (simultaneous multiple interaction T cell engagers), where two BiTEs are given together; and TriKEs (trispecific killer engagers), which direct NK cells to cancer cells [103, 106].

What all of them have in common is the basic premise of using a double- (or occasionally triple-) ended protein to create a physical

---

[16] This is referred to as its half-life.

connection between T cells (or occasionally NK cells) and cancer cells.

6.9.2 About Their Targets

An important feature of T cell engagers (including those with an Fc) is that they are created using two scFvs. Like their parent antibodies, scFvs can only attach to intact, cell surface proteins. This limits their range of targets to proteins naturally found on a cancer cell's surface (just like a CAR protein). Common targets of T cell engagers include CD19 and CD20, which are both found on early and mature B cells and many B cell cancers, and BCMA and GPRC5D, which are found on myeloma cells.

As with CAR T cells, we have made much less progress in developing T cell engagers that are effective and safe for people with solid tumors. (Currently, the only T cell engager licensed for a solid tumor, which targets two cell surface proteins, is tarlatamab. It targets CD3 and DLL3.)

When you are limited to targeting cell surface proteins, it's incredibly difficult to identify proteins that are on the surface of cancer cells but absent from other cell types. This limitation of T cell engagers has driven scientists' desire to expand the range of potential targets to include intracellular proteins. One way they've achieved this is by swapping out one of the scFvs and replacing it with a soluble version of a T cell receptor (TCR) (Figure 6.19) [107]. The resulting protein – called an ImmTAC – uses its scFv to attach to CD3 on T cells (like a BiTE). But with its other end, the TCR end, it attaches to a peptide antigen displayed by an MHC protein (like a normal TCR) [107, 108].

The advantage of this design is the vastly increased number of potential targets compared to a design that relies solely on scFvs. It also creates an opportunity to target peptide antigens that are completely absent from healthy cells, which would reduce toxicities. Both these features make ImmTACs an exciting prospect as treatments for solid tumors. But, as with TCR T cells, you have to perform HLA matching. This is to make sure that the person's cancer cells are capable of displaying the antigen that the ImmTAC targets.

As with BiTEs (T cell engagers that lack an Fc region), ImmTACs are relatively short-lived proteins. Tebentafusp, a treatment for people with uveal melanoma (melanoma affecting the eye), was the first ImmTAC to be licensed. It has a half-life of six to eight hours. However, scientists believe the ImmTAC protein stays attached to its target for far longer than it is detectable in the blood. They also believe that you get "epitope spreading," which is when the destruction of cancer cells by engaged T cells leads to an immune response against nearby cancer cells that lack the ImmTAC's target [109]. Because of its predicted prolonged presence and epitope spreading, tebentafusp is given as a series of weekly infusions (rather than as a continuous infusion as with blinatumomab) [110, 111].

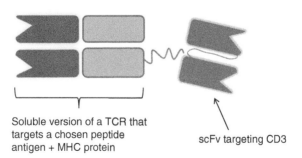

Soluble version of a TCR that targets a chosen peptide antigen + MHC protein

scFv targeting CD3

Figure 6.19 A so-called ImmTAC protein made from a soluble TCR and an scFv.
Abbreviations: ImmTAC – immune-mobilizing monoclonal TCRs against cancer; scFv – single-chain variable fragment; TCR – T cell receptor.

A variation on an ImmTAC is to use just the variable region of a TCR (rather than both the variable and constant region, as shown in Figure 6.19). However, this seems to result in a protein that is less specific and has a lower affinity for its target than if you use the design shown [107]. Yet another option is to create antibodies that recognize peptide antigens (called T cell receptor-like antibodies) [112].

6.9.3 Comparing the Properties Imparted by Different Designs

The various different designs of T cell engager impact the treatments' properties, such as, how much of their target needs to present on the surface of the patients' cancer cells for them to engage, and their possible range of targets. Some of these variations are summarized in Table 6.9.

Table 6.9   Some properties of T cell engagers reflect their different designs [106, 111].

	BiTE (no Fc)	T cell engager (including a modified Fc)	ImmTAC
Design example			
What does it attach to cancer cells with?	The scFv from an antibody that targets a chosen protein		A soluble TCR that targets a chosen peptide antigen
Range of targets?	Limited to cell surface proteins		Can be intracellular or cell surface proteins
Sensitivity to its target	A lot of the target is needed – perhaps 1,000–10,000 copies per cell		Very little of the target needs to be present, perhaps 10 copies per cell
Needs HLA matching?	No	No	Yes
Administration	Repeated treatment cycles; given as a continuous infusion	Repeated treatment cycles; given as infusion every two or three weeks	Repeated treatment cycles; given as a weekly infusion
Useful against hematologic cancers or solid tumors?	One licensed for hematologic cancers with more in trials; a few trials for solid tumors	Several licensed for hematologic cancers and many more in trials; one licensed for a solid tumor: small cell lung cancer	Mostly in trials for solid tumors; one licensed so far
Side effects	Often include CRS, ICANS, and vulnerability to infections		

Abbreviations: BiTE – bi-specific T cell engager; CRS – cytokine release syndrome; HLA – human leukocyte antigen; ICANS – immune effector cell-associated neurotoxicity syndrome; ImmTAC – immune-mobilizing monoclonal TCRs against cancer; scFv – single chain variable region of an antibody; TCR – T cell receptor.

6.9.4 Where Do the Engaged T Cells Come From?

All the T cell engagers I've described incorporate an scFv from a CD3-targeted antibody. This end connects with the CD3 complex on T cells. But where do these T cells come from?

The T cells engaged and activated by T cell engagers are so-called "endogenous T cells." That is, ones that pre-existed in the patient's body and were probably already in the cancer's neighborhood. When activated by a T cell engager, these T cells undertake "serial killing."

One T cell, with BiTEs clinging to its CD3 proteins, connects with the BiTE's other target on multiple cancer cells, killing each one in turn [113].

However, because we're relying on whatever T cells existed in the patient prior to treatment, the effectiveness of the T cell engager will depend on how fit and active these T cells are. As I've said before, immunotherapies tend to be more successful against hematological cancers than solid tumors because the T cells have an easier time getting close to cancer cells and are less likely to be exhausted or suppressed.

As a result, most of the trials and approvals to date are for people with hematological cancers. The only T cell engagers approved for solid tumors (as of May 2024) are tebentafusp and tarlatamab. Tebentafusp is given to some people with a solid tumor called uveal melanoma. It was approved by both the FDA (in the United States) and EMA (in the EU/EEA) in 2022. Tarlatamab was approved by the FDA for some people with small cell lung cancer in May 2024.

6.9.5 Licensed T Cell Engagers

It's always impossible to predict exactly which new treatments will end up being approved for use, and when that might happen. As I write this in early 2024, it feels like we're at the cusp of a lot of approvals for T cell engagers. So, as well as listing those that are already approved, I've also listed in Table 6.10 just some of the ones that are in trials, but not yet approved, at the point this book was published.

Please be aware that this table only includes a tiny fraction of the T cell engagers in trials [114]. There are hundreds of them!

6.9.6 Reasons for Resistance

So far, most of our experience with T cell engagers comes from trials involving people with hematological cancers. As with all treatments, they don't work for everyone, or they work for a time but then the person's cancer worsens again.

Reasons why T cell engagers don't always work include [106, 115]:

- The patient's T cells are exhausted and not up to the task of killing cancer cells.
- The patient's cancer cells (and/or other cells in the vicinity) have PD-L1 on their surface and use it to suppress T cells drawn close by the T cell engager.
- The patient's cancer cells don't have enough of the T cell engager's target on their surface for T cells to be activated, or they start producing less of it.

Similar resistance mechanisms seem to be important when using T cell engagers for solid tumors. The main difference is the level of immune suppression in the tumor microenvironment, plus physical barriers such as defective tumor blood vessels.

The fact that PD-L1 seems to be a common reason for resistance to T cell engagers has led to trials in which they are combined with a PD-1 or PD-L1 antibody (for more on these, see Chapter 5). There are also versions of T cell engagers where there is an additional segment of protein that simultaneously blocks PD-1 [104, 106, 114].

6.9.7 Side Effects of T Cell Engagers

As with CAR T cell therapy and TCR T cell therapy, T cell engagers can cause CRS and neurological toxicities. An increased risk of serious infections also seems to be a danger with these treatments [106, 115, 116].

These treatments will also cause side effects if the T cell engager's target on cancer cells is also present on healthy cells. This is a particular problem when giving a T cell engager to a person with a solid tumor for two main reasons [117]:

1. Because of the physical barriers that stand in the way, a person with a solid tumor tends to need a higher dose of a T cell engager compared to someone with a hematological cancer. With increased dosing comes an increase in side effects.

Table 6.10   A selection of T cell engagers (approved or in trials) that connect to a target protein on cancer cells using an scFv.

Treatment name	Targets	Indication	Design
Treatments for hematological cancers			
Blinatumomab	CD19 and CD3	ALL – **approved**	No Fc; Figure 6.18a
Mosunetuzumab	CD20 and CD3	B cell NHL (FL) – **approved**	Includes Fc; Figure 6.18f
Epcoritamab	CD20 and CD3	B cell NHL (DLBCL) – **approved**	Includes Fc; Figure 6.18f
Glofitamab	CD20 and CD3	B cell NHL (DLBCL) – **approved**	Includes Fc; Figure 6.18h
Odronextamab	CD20 and CD3	B cell NHL (DLBCL & FL)	Includes Fc; Figure 6.18f
Teclistamab	BCMA and CD3	Myeloma – **approved**	Includes Fc; Figure 6.18f
Elranatamab	BCMA and CD3	Myeloma – **approved**	Includes Fc; Figure 6.18f
Alnuctamab	BCMA and CD3	Myeloma	Includes Fc; Figure 6.18h
Linvoseltamab	BCMA and CD3	Myeloma	Includes Fc; Figure 6.18f
Talquetamab	GPRC5D and CD3	Myeloma – **approved**	Includes Fc; Figure 6.18f
Flotetuzumab	CD123 and CD3	AML	No Fc; Figure 6.18a
Treatments for solid tumors			
Tebentafusp	Gp100 and CD3	Uveal melanoma – **approved**	No Fc; Figure 6.19
Tarlatamab	DLL3 and CD3	Small cell lung cancer – **approved**	Includes Fc; Figure 6.18d
HPN328	DLL3 and CD3	Small cell lung cancer	No Fc; Figure 6.18c
Acapatamab	PSMA and CD3	Prostate cancer	Includes Fc; Figure 6.18i

Abbreviations: ALL – acute lymphoblastic leukemia; AML – acute myeloid leukemia; BCMA – B cell maturation antigen; DLBCL – diffuse large B cell lymphoma; DLL – delta-like ligand-3; FL – follicular lymphoma; NHL – non-Hodgkin lymphoma; PSMA – prostate-specific membrane antigen.

2. It is virtually impossible to identify targets on cancer cells that don't exist on healthy cells, too. The T cell engager will attach to its target wherever that might be, leading T cells to attack healthy cells. (Hopefully, this is less of a problem with T cell engagers such as the ImmTAC proteins, which allow a far wider range of potential targets to pick from.)

6.9.8 Comparing T Cell Engagers with CAR T Cells

There are many similarities and differences between CAR T cell therapy, TCR T cell therapy, and the T cell engagers [106, 118]. I have summarized some of them in Table 6.11.

Table 6.11 A comparison of CAR T cells and TCR T cells with T cell engagers.

	CAR T cells and TCR T cells	T cell engagers (constructed using scFvs; with or without an Fc region)
What's the nature of the treatment?	T cells that have been genetically engineered to produce a CAR protein or new TCR	The treatment is a small protein that creates a bridge between the patient's T cells and their cancer cells
Which T cells are activated and kill cancer cells?	CAR/TCR T cells are responsible for killing cancer cells; they will hopefully multiply (expand) when they engage their target	Various endogenous T cells in the patient's body prior to treatment are responsible for killing cancer cells; they are unlikely to multiply when they engage their target
Manufacturing time?	Several weeks – a unique product is made for each patient	None – an "off the shelf" treatment
Administration	Single infusion	Repeated treatment cycles; dose and schedule depends on design; there is often a dose ramp-up phase at the beginning to mitigate side effects
Is conditioning chemotherapy required?	Yes	No, but sometimes an additional treatment is given prior to the T cell engager to mitigate side effects
Can manufacturing fail?	Yes	No
Range of targets?	Limited to cell surface proteins for CAR T cells; could be intracellular targets for TCR T cells	Limited to cell surface proteins
Need HLA matching?	No for CAR T cells Yes for TCR T cells	No
Side effects	Include CRS and ICANS	Include CRS and ICANS
Safety	Expansion and persistence of CAR/TCR T cells means that it is difficult to reverse toxicities	Treatment dose can be lowered or discontinued to reverse/manage side effects
Reasons for resistance	Exhausted, defective, or suppressed CAR/TCR T cells; insufficient or absent target on cancer cells	Exhaustion of endogenous T cells is a reason for resistance, but this is potentially reversible through treatment-free intervals; insufficient or absent target on cancer cells
Response rates	High response rates reported for CAR T cell therapy for hematological cancers	High response rates reported for T cell engagers treating hematological cancers
Cost	High, due to creation of a unique treatment for each patient, preconditioning, hospital stays, managing side effects	Still high due to requirement for repeat treatment cycles, but possibly lower than for CAR/TCR T cells

Abbreviations: CAR T cell – chimeric antigen receptor T cell therapy; CRS – cytokine release syndrome; HLA – human leukocyte antigen; ICANS – immune effector cell-associated neurotoxicity syndrome; scFv – single chain variable region of an antibody; TCR T cell – T cell receptor-engineered T cell therapy.

6.9.9 Final Thoughts on T Cell Engagers

As I've already commented, there are hundreds of T cell engagers in clinical trials. Sometimes they're being given on their own, but often they're being combined with one or more checkpoint inhibitors.

These highly sophisticated proteins are quickly emerging as an important set of treatments for a range of hematological cancers, albeit more for people with B cell cancers (such as types of B cell NHL, ALL, and myeloma) rather than for people with AML or T cell cancers.

The early success of tebentafusp as a treatment for uveal melanoma is creating optimism that T cell engagers (with scFv- or TCR-targeting) might be effective treatments for people with many different types of solid tumors.

T cell engagers, like CAR T cells and TCR T cells, kill cancer cells using T cells. But the source of these T cells differs. T cell engagers are an off-the-shelf treatment that could be made immediately available to patients in poorer overall health who can't wait weeks for manufacturing. They can also be incorporated into existing treatment combinations. This makes these treatments incredibly appealing.

Finally, as I have written this section, I have struggled with inconsistencies in the way people use terminology. For example, for some researchers, "BiTE" purely relates to blinatumomab-like proteins (two scFvs linked back-to-back). For others, "BiTE" can include structures that include an Fc region. For yet other people, the term can extend all the way to include ImmTAC proteins (a soluble TCR linked to an scFv). I think this is simply yet to be ironed out! The current lack of consistency simply reflects the fact that these treatments are still very new, and there are many different iterations with overlapping properties. Hopefully, the way we talk about them will become more coherent over time.

6.10 CANCER TREATMENT VACCINES

Licensed drugs mentioned in this section:		
Treatment class	**Drugs**	**Given to some people with:**
Dendritic cell vaccines	Sipuleucel-T	• Prostate cancer
Oncolytic viruses	Talimogene laherparepvec (T-VEC)	• Melanoma skin cancer
Bacterial vaccines	Bacillus Calmette-Guérin (BCG) vaccine	• Bladder cancer

The goal of cancer treatment vaccines is to alert the patient's immune system to the presence of a cancer that already exists in their body. Hopefully, if you provoke a strong enough reaction with your vaccine, the immune cells that have been activated will seek out and destroy the person's cancer cells. The basic idea of treatment vaccines is outlined in Figure 6.20.

Before we go further, you might want to glance back at Figures 1.14 and 1.15 for a refresher on how dendritic cells activate T cells. You might also find it useful to check back at Figure 5.1 to see how vaccines and oncolytic viruses fit into the bigger picture of immunotherapy. In that diagram, I show vaccines and oncolytic viruses as helping the patient's immune system to recognize cancer cells as a threat.

For decades, I have been reading about clinical trials, sometimes large, Phase 3 trials, involving hundreds of patients in which cancer vaccines have been tested. But, year after year, these trials have failed to help enough people to meet their targets (Reference [119] provides a list of 40 unsuccessful Phase 3 trials). Tantalizingly, most vaccines do seem to elicit a cancer-fighting T cell response. However, it rarely seems to be strong enough or last long enough to be helpful for most patients [119–121].

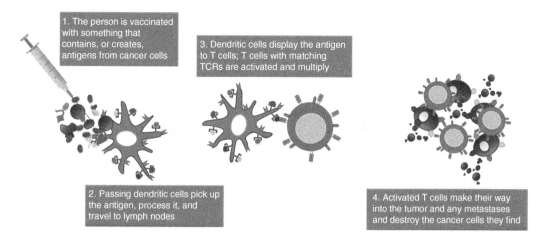

Figure 6.20 The basic idea of most cancer treatment vaccines. The vaccine is introduced into the person's body in the hope that it will generate a T cell response against the person's cancer cells. Dendritic cells are a necessary intermediary, as they activate the person's T cells.
Abbreviation: TCR – T cell receptor. *Source:* Syringe image from Pixabay.

Presumably, the reason for these failures is that vaccines only help with the recognition step of the immune response. They can't enhance T cell activation in lymph nodes, tell T cells where to go, or help T cells overcome immune suppression in the cancer environment. This means that vaccines face an uphill struggle in creating a strong enough T cell response to help people with cancer.

As of early 2024, only three vaccine-based treatments have been approved for use in the United States or the EU/EEA. These are:

- Sipuleucel-T: a dendritic cell vaccine for prostate cancer
- Talimogene laherparepvec (T-VEC): an oncolytic virus for melanoma skin cancer
- BCG vaccine for bladder cancer (the precise mechanism of which is still unclear [122])

However, these approved vaccine treatments are just the tip of the iceberg compared to what's been tried and what's coming. So, I'm going to tell you about more vaccine treatments than simply those three.

6.10.1 Different Types of Treatment Vaccines

There are two main ways that people tend to classify treatment vaccine approaches [123]:

1. According to the physical nature of the vaccine. For example, whether it's made from living cells, dead cells, proteins, peptides, DNA, mRNA, or microbes such as viruses or bacteria.

2. According to whether you know what antigen[17] (or antigens) you're trying to provoke an immune response against. For example, if you vaccinate a person with an oncolytic virus, you won't know exactly what it is that the person's immune system might mount an attack against. But, if you introduce into the

---

[17] In case you want another quick refresher, "antigen" is a term used to refer to things that can provoke immune responses from B cells and T cells. Antigens for B cells are usually proteins or other large, complicated molecules. In contrast, T cells react to "peptide antigens" – small protein fragments – which are presented to them by MHC proteins.

body a handful of carefully chosen peptide antigens, then you know exactly what you want the person's immune system to react to.

I'm going to use the second classification system and split vaccines into two groups according to whether you know what antigens the vaccine is targeted against.

Vaccines that generate an immune response against known antigens:

1. Antigen vaccines: these involve introducing into the patient's body one or more antigens from cancer cells. The hope is that the dendritic cells will pick up the antigen and use it to activate T cells. Hopefully, sufficient T cells are activated to rid the body of cancer. I'll turn my attention to what these antigens might be, shortly.

2. Some dendritic cell vaccines: in which dendritic cells are purified from the patient's blood, incubated with known antigens, and returned to the patient.

Vaccines that generate an immune response against unknown antigens:

1. Oncolytic viruses: these are modified viruses that preferentially multiply inside cancer cells. The virus infects and destroys cancer cells, creating antigen-containing debris for dendritic cells to pick up and take to T cells. Hopefully, activated T cells mount a powerful cancer-fighting immune response. You won't know what antigens those T cells are targeted against.

2. Bacterial vaccines: these use a bacterial species to generate a non-specific immune response – e.g., BCG vaccine for the treatment of bladder cancer. Their precise mechanism is unknown.

3. Some dendritic cell vaccines: in which dendritic cells are purified from the

patient's blood, incubated with unknown antigens, and returned to the patient.

As you can see from these lists, dendritic cell vaccines can be targeted against known or unknown antigens (Figure 6.21). One advantage of dendritic cell vaccines is that once you've removed dendritic cells from the patient's blood, you can activate them in the lab, far away from the immune-suppressing environment found inside tumors [121]. However, there are also lots of difficulties and obstacles to creating effective dendritic cell vaccines. Not least is the massive variation amongst the behaviors and functions of different dendritic cell types and their scarcity in the blood. Only one dendritic cell vaccine has ever been licensed, a treatment for prostate cancer called Sipuleucel-T. This vaccine achieved some success in clinical trials and has been approved for use in the United States. However, its cost and the creation of other new prostate cancer treatments (such as abiraterone, enzalutamide, and radium-223) resulted in it being little used.

6.10.2 Vaccines Directed Against Known Antigens

I first want to look at the antigens that these vaccines are targeted against.

The ideal target for a cancer vaccine is virtually identical to the targets chosen for the creation of TCR T cells. As with these targets, your ideal target would be [120]:

- Something exclusive to the person's cancer cells (i.e., not present on any of their healthy cells)
- Something necessary for cancer cell survival (so that cells can't just get rid of it and carry on as they were)
- Something that is highly immunogenic (i.e., something the immune system takes

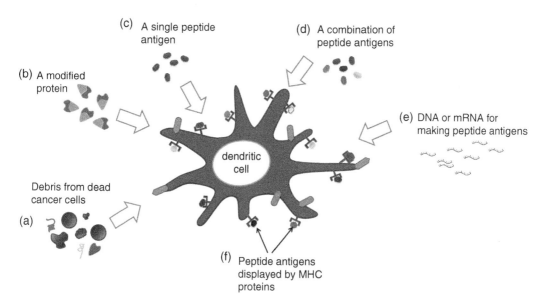

Figure 6.21 Dendritic cell vaccines. To create such a vaccine, dendritic cells taken from a patient might be incubated with (**a**) dead cancer cells from their tumor, (**b**) a modified protein that includes a known antigen, (**c**) a single, purified peptide antigen, (**d**) a combination of antigens, or (**e**) the DNA or mRNA instructions for making one or more antigens. The aim is that (**f**) the dendritic cells will display peptide antigens from the patient's cancer cells to T cells using their MHC class 1 and class 2 proteins. **Abbreviation:** MHC – major histocompatibility complex.

notice of and recognizes as a danger signal rather than as something to ignore[18])
- Something that cancer cells make, break down, and then display fragments of to T cells. (Even if the antigen meets all the criteria above, but not this last one, then the vaccine won't work – the chosen antigen must be displayed by the cancer cells' MHC proteins, or the person's T cells won't react to it.)

Scientists generally split antigens into two groups: tumor-associated antigens and tumor-specific antigens. I've summarized some of their properties in Table 6.12.

Tumor-Associated Antigens [123–125]
- Proteins that are over-expressed (i.e., overproduced) by cancer cells but that are also made by a significant number of healthy cells. For example, HER2 on breast cancer cells. (Because they're made by healthy cells, it isn't always possible to elicit an immune response against these proteins. Their presence on healthy cells also leads to toxicity.)
- Cancer germline antigens (also called cancer testes antigens) or differentiation antigens – these are proteins often made by cancer cells of specific cancer types.

---

[18] Our body goes to great lengths to identify and destroy any B cells or T cells that recognize the body's own proteins and that might cause and auto-immune disease if allowed to survive. So, many of the things displayed by cancer cells either aren't recognized by the immune system at all, or they tell the immune system to leave the cell alone.

Table 6.12 Properties of tumor-associated antigens and tumor-specific antigens for the creation of cancer treatment vaccines [120, 123].

	Tumor-associated antigens		Tumor-specific antigens		
	Normal proteins over-produced by cancer cells	Cancer germline antigens	Virus proteins	Neoantigens[a] common in a particular cancer type	Neoantigens[a] unique to each patient
Is the antigen exclusive to cancer cells?	Varies; probably not	Pretty specific but not perfect	Probably		
How likely is it that the immune system will ignore the antigen?	Very	Possible	Unlikely		
Could the vaccine be useful for lots of patients?	Yes		Yes		No – it would have to be unique for each patient
Examples	p53 in various cancers; HER2 in breast, stomach, ovarian; gp100 in melanoma, PAP in prostate cancer	NY-ESO-1 in melanoma, ovarian, esophageal; MAGE-A3 in melanoma, myeloma, NSCLC	E6 and E7 proteins from HPV; LMP1 and LMP2 proteins from EBV	EGFRvIII in glioblastoma, NSCLC; *BRAF*[V600E] in melanoma	No specific examples – they are as varied as the mutations found in human cancer cells

[a] A neoantigen is a peptide that has come from a mutated protein. Crucially, the peptide includes amino acids that are different from normal because of the mutation.
Abbreviations: EBV – Epstein-Barr virus; EGFRvIII – EGF receptor variant-3; HER2 – Human EGF receptor-2; HPV – human papillomavirus; NSCLC – non-small cell lung cancer; PAP – prostatic acid phosphatase.

Tumor-Specific Antigens [123–125]

- Mutated versions of proteins found in cancer cells (neoantigens). The immune system is unlikely to have come across these before; therefore, it's theoretically easier to target T cells against them. However, because every cancer contains a unique combination of neoantigens, it's difficult to translate this approach into an "off-the-shelf" treatment for multiple patients.
- Virus proteins are commonly found in the cells of cancers linked to viral infections, such as HPV proteins in cervical, vulval, and head and neck cancer cells; EBV proteins in the cancer cells of some lymphomas and nasopharyngeal carcinoma;

and HBV (hepatitis B virus) in liver cancer cells.

- Peptide or neoantigen conjugates – these are proteins or peptides that have been deliberately designed by scientists. They are often made up of various protein pieces thought to trigger a powerful immune response.

As well as picking a suitable antigen (or antigen combination), scientists developing vaccines must also choose [124]:

- what physical form the vaccine will take,
- which patients to give it to,
- a suitable route of administration,
- a suitable adjuvant (something that gives an extra boost to the immune system),
- whether it should be given alone or in combination with another treatment.

The Vaccine's Physical Form

Here, there are various options. Having decided on the vaccine's target, the scientists might decide to introduce it into the body as a peptide antigen. The hope is that passing dendritic cells will pick it up and immediately display the antigen on their surface. Another option is to deliver the instructions for making the peptide antigen to dendritic cells in the form of DNA or mRNA. The dendritic cells will hopefully pick this up and then manufacture the peptides themselves. Whether the vaccine is a peptide, or the DNA or mRNA used to make a peptide, it usually needs parceling up and protecting in some way, often in some kind of nanoparticle [124].

Which Patients to Give Them To

With cancer treatment vaccines, the goal is to provoke sufficient cancer-fighting white blood cells into action so that they destroy an existing tumor. This contrasts with a preventative vaccine, which only needs to activate some memory cells (enough that the immune system is primed to fight off the potential invader). The T cells activated by your vaccine also need to be so active that they can overcome the immune-suppressive cancer microenvironment. So far, vaccines have struggled to do this.

Instead, where treatment vaccines have been more effective (although it's still early days) is in the destruction of cancer cells that remain in a person's body after they have received other treatments (e.g., surgery, radiotherapy, chemotherapy, or hormone therapy). In these situations, any T cells that become active have a better chance of destroying the cancer cells they meet. They are also more likely to kill a high enough proportion of the patient's cancer cells to do them some good.

When it comes to destroying an established metastatic cancer, treatment vaccines have so far been less successful. But scientists are

determined to get this approach to work, and they're making progress all the time.

Route of Administration

Most vaccine treatments are administered via injection into the skin, muscle, blood or lymph nodes, or directly into tumors. Wherever the vaccine is put, the hope is that dendritic cells will find it, take it to lymph nodes, and present it to T cells.

Adjuvants

Dendritic cells and T cells need more than just exposure to an antigen to become fully active. That's why vaccine treatments often rely heavily on adjuvants – mixtures of chemicals, growth factors, or other proteins – that give an extra boost to white blood cells.

Popular adjuvants include GM-CSF, IL-2, Toll-like receptor ligands, and bacterial proteins (or fragments of them) [126]. Another way to include an adjuvant into a vaccine is to use the adjuvant as a delivery device. For example, some DNA or RNA vaccines are delivered inside modified virus particles. The virus particle not only helps the vaccine stick around long enough to get picked up, but it also sends activation signals to the immune system [127].

Combinations

As I said earlier, vaccines can sometimes activate T cells, but they can't tell those activated T cells where to go. They also do nothing to overcome the immune-suppressing environment inside a solid tumor. The purpose of giving a combination is to overcome these limitations.

For example [124]:

1. Combinations with checkpoint inhibitors. The idea is that the vaccine will alert the patient's immune system to the presence of cancer, and the checkpoint inhibitor will prevent the cancer-fighting T cells generated from being suppressed.

2. Combinations with chemotherapy. Chemotherapy kills cancer cells and creates lots of tumor debris. It can also deplete tumors of immune-suppressing white blood cells. Both these things can help the immune system do its work and could synergize with a cancer vaccine.

6.10.3 A Promising Approach: Personalized mRNA Vaccines

The vaccine treatment approach that is perhaps getting the most attention at the moment is that of personalized mRNA vaccines. This approach has been around for years, with some promising results from small studies. However, the COVID-19 pandemic threw a spotlight on the potential of using mRNA vaccines to create powerful immune responses. It also accelerated research into how to manufacture and formulate these treatments at great speed [128].

To make sense of mRNA vaccines, it's vital to understand the relationship between DNA, mRNA, and proteins.[19] In a nutshell (of *tiny* proportions!), mRNA is the intermediary between DNA and proteins. Cells make mRNA as a necessary step when they want to make a protein.[20] Normally, they use the information in their DNA to make a copy in the form of mRNA, and then they use this mRNA as the set of instructions for making a protein. So, if you put a strand of mRNA into a cell, it will immediately make the corresponding protein. It follows that if you put only a short piece of mRNA into a cell, it will make an equally short protein, a peptide.

The Central Idea

In short [129–131]:

1. First, identify mutations in the person's cancer cells that are not found in their healthy cells.
2. Use computer programs to predict which of these mutations leads to the creation of neoantigens[21] displayed by MHC proteins on the cancer cells' surface.
3. Then, create strands of mRNA corresponding to your chosen neoantigens and parcel them up inside some kind of nanoparticle.
4. Inject the personalized mRNA vaccine into the patient.
5. Hopefully, dendritic cells in the vicinity pick up the mRNA and use it to make the various neoantigens that you selected.
6. Dendritic cells travel to lymph nodes and display the neoantigens they've made to T cells using their MHC proteins.
7. T cells with TCRs that match the chosen neoantigens become active.
8. Activated cytotoxic T cells seek out and destroy cancer cells with the same neoantigens displayed on their surface.
9. Hopefully, the cancer cell debris created by these T cells is picked up by more dendritic cells, which go on to activate T cells that recognize a wider range of neoantigens (this is called *epitope spreading*), enhancing the immune response.

I have attempted to depict steps 1–3 in Figure 6.22; steps 4–8 are shown in Figure 6.20.

The trickiest part of this process is the second part: how do you identify mutations in the person's cancer cells that the cells display to the immune system as neoantigens? The key is to compare the mutations found in the person's

---

[19] You might find some of the information on the Khan Academy website useful if you want a refresher: https://www.khanacademy.org/science/ap-biology/gene-expression-and-regulation
[20] There's a great little video called "What is DNA?" here: www.youtube.com/watch? v=zwibgNGe4aY
[21] As I've said before, a neoantigen is a peptide that reflects a mutation in cancer cells' DNA. They are unique to the person's cancer cells and should provoke a reaction from their immune system.

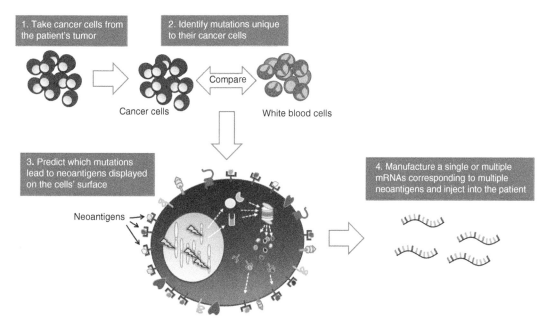

1. Take cancer cells from the patient's tumor

2. Identify mutations unique to their cancer cells

Compare

Cancer cells

White blood cells

3. Predict which mutations lead to neoantigens displayed on the cells' surface

4. Manufacture a single or multiple mRNAs corresponding to multiple neoantigens and inject into the patient

Neoantigens

Figure 6.22 Creating a personalized mRNA treatment vaccine. The process begins when a surgeon removes the patient's tumor. The tumor cells' DNA is sequenced and compared to DNA from healthy white blood cells. Mutations that are unique to the person's cancer cells are identified, and computer modeling is used to identify mutations (depicted as yellow lightning bolts) that lead to neoantigens being displayed on the cell's surface. (The diagram shows the cell making mutated proteins from its damaged DNA. These proteins are broken down by the cell's proteasomes and neoantigens are assembled onto MHC proteins and transported to the cell's surface.) Finally, scientists use the amino acid sequence of the predicted neoantigens to design and manufacture a set of mRNA strands that correspond to their sequence, and that can be injected into the patient as a personalized vaccine.
Abbreviations: mRNA – messenger RNA; mRNA image by Christine I Miller, licensed under the Creative Commons Attribution-Share Alike 4.0 International license.

cancer cells with those from healthy cells (white blood cells are the easiest to get hold of). From the mutations the scientists identify as being exclusive to the person's cancer cells, they then use computer modeling to decide [131]:

- Which of the mutations they've identified is likely to lead to the creation of peptides that will fit inside the patient's MHC proteins. (Over 16,000 different shaped MHC proteins have been found in the human population, and each can only display peptides of a certain shape and size.)
- Which of the peptides that will fit inside their MHC proteins will act as neoantigen.

Obviously, this stuff is not easy, which is why it's so exciting to see some positive results coming out of clinical trials [132, 133]. As with other vaccine trials, most involve combining the vaccine with a checkpoint inhibitor and possibly also chemotherapy.

There's now an enormous number of clinical trials testing out personalized mRNA treatment vaccines [129–131]. One partnership, called the Cancer Vaccine Launch Pad, aims to deliver this technology to 10,000 patients living in the United Kingdom [134]. In most vaccine trials, the patients involved tend to be either: people who have had surgery for their cancer but are at risk of relapse or people with metastatic disease who have exhausted all standard treatment options [131].

Advantages of mRNA Vaccines

- The immune system is primed to react to mRNA as being potentially dangerous. Therefore, mRNA vaccines act as their own adjuvant, boosting immune responses to the peptides they encode.
- mRNA vaccines are quickly destroyed in the body, limiting side effects.
- Manufacture is now rapid and inexpensive compared to what it was in the past.

Related Strategies [129]

As well as personalized mRNA vaccines, there are a wide range of similar vaccine approaches in trials, such as:

- "Off the shelf" combinations of mRNAs corresponding to tumor-associated antigens (such as NY-ESO-1, PSA, PAP) that can be given to many patients with certain cancer types.
- "Off the shelf" combinations of mRNAs corresponding to viral antigens for the treatment of virus-linked cancers (such as cervical cancer or head and neck cancer).
- Personalized dendritic cell vaccines created using the patient's own dendritic cells that have been incubated with mRNAs or neoantigens.
- Personalized neoantigen vaccines using peptides or DNA rather than mRNA.

6.10.4 Vaccines Directed Against Unknown Antigens

Given how clever the vaccines I've already described sound, you might be surprised to know that there's still an enormous number of vaccines being developed where the scientists don't know what the target antigen might be. These might not have the same allure as something like a personalized mRNA vaccine, but it's important to remember how limited and incomplete our understanding of our immune system still is. Many vaccine trials and strategies have failed to make any difference to the quantity or quality of life of people with cancer. So, methods where we don't try to predict what it is about a person's cancer that might provoke their immune system into action are still an active and potentially fruitful way forward. Numerous of these vaccines are in trials [123].

They include approaches such as [123, 124, 135]:

- Creating cancer cell populations that can be grown in the laboratory, altering them so that they secrete cytokines that activate white blood cells, and then killing them and injecting them into patients.
- Taking cancer cells from a patient's tumor, killing them, and mixing them with adjuvants such as cytokines or proteins from bacteria. The mixture is then injected into the patient.
- Purifying dendritic cells from a patient and incubating them with dead cancer cells and various adjuvants before returning them.

In most trials in which these sorts of vaccines have been tested, some patients have been helped by them. Long lists of trials in which they've been tested out can be collated, and in virtually all these trials, you can find patients in which the approach worked. However, these approaches tend to be expensive, laborious, and technically demanding. So, off-the-shelf approaches such as checkpoint inhibitors have been much more widely implemented.

6.10.5 Oncolytic Viruses

Oncolytic viruses are another massive area of vaccine research. An oncolytic virus is a virus that prefers infecting cancer cells (onco) and that can burst them open (lytic). This method doesn't sit very easily in any category of cancer treatments, but it does rely on antigens,

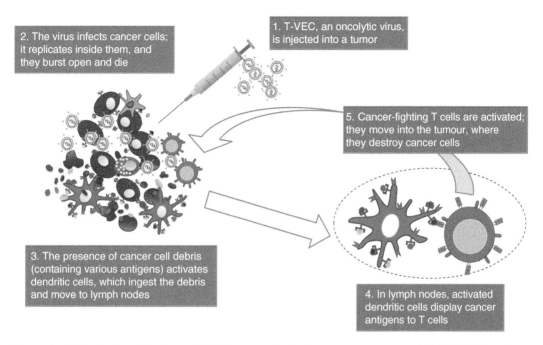

2. The virus infects cancer cells; it replicates inside them, and they burst open and die

1. T-VEC, an oncolytic virus, is injected into a tumor

5. Cancer-fighting T cells are activated; they move into the tumour, where they destroy cancer cells

3. The presence of cancer cell debris (containing various antigens) activates dendritic cells, which ingest the debris and move to lymph nodes

4. In lymph nodes, activated dendritic cells display cancer antigens to T cells

Figure 6.23 Mechanism of action of T-VEC, an oncolytic virus cancer treatment. 1. T-VEC is injected into the patient's tumors. 2. The virus multiplies easily in cancer cells because they contain many mutations and are less able to defend themselves than healthy cells. The virus also forces infected cells to produce GM-CSF, a growth factor that helps to activate white blood cells such as dendritic cells. Some infected cancer cells burst open (they lyse), releasing all their inner proteins and other molecules into their surroundings. 3. Dendritic cells pick up some of the debris and display cancer peptides on their surface with MHC proteins. 4. They leave the tumor and enter lymph nodes, where they activate T cells. 5. Activated T cells leave the lymph node, enter the tumor, and attack cancer cells.
Abbreviations: GM-CSF – granulocyte-macrophage colony-stimulating factor; MHC – major histocompatibility complex. *Source:* Syringe image from Pixabay.

dendritic cells, and T cells, which is why it's often described as a vaccine.

A variety of different viruses have been used as oncolytic virus treatments, such as herpes viruses, influenza viruses, vaccinia viruses, adenoviruses, and many others. Usually, the virus is modified so that [136]:

- It no longer causes disease.
- It multiplies quickly in cancer cells, causing the cells to burst open and release antigens into their surroundings.
- It contains the gene for an adjuvant such as GM-CSF, which helps activate any

dendritic cells that pick up cancer cell debris and increases the likelihood that they will travel to lymph nodes and activate T cells.

The first oncolytic virus to become a licensed cancer treatment is T-VEC (Figure 6.23). T-VEC was licensed as a treatment for some people with advanced melanoma skin cancer back in 2015 but, as yet, no other oncolytic viruses have been approved in the United States or Europe/ the UK. T-VEC uses a modified genetically engineered herpes simplex virus. Many other viruses, methods of delivery, and treatment combinations are being explored.

6.10.6 Final Thoughts on Cancer Treatment Vaccines

Cancer vaccines are constantly making it into the news. However, this isn't necessarily because they are helping lots of people. Instead, they get coverage because they sound clever and sophisticated; because there are endless iterations of them; because they're new; or because they come under the general label of immunotherapy, which is currently generating lots of exciting trial results.

When reading about vaccines, I found endless variety and hundreds of trials. However, almost none of these have led to reliable benefits for a large enough proportion of people to be considered a success.

Right now, the spotlight is firmly on the personalized mRNA vaccines covered in Section 6.10.3. I hope that the amount of time and money being invested in them, and the lives of the thousands of patients involved in trials, will not be wasted. It's tempting to hope that with this amount of effort going into them, we will see significant successes in the years to come.

My hunch is that it will only be by combining vaccines with other immunotherapy approaches, such as T cell engagers and checkpoint inhibitors, that we will substantially improve the outlook for a substantial proportion of patients. Even so, I wonder if some people will never be helped by a vaccine approach. People whose cancers are cold, hidden from their immune system, with few mutations, and full of immune-suppressing white blood cells, perhaps. Because even with vaccine combinations, you still need certain things to be true about a person's cancer to have a chance of success:

- Their cancer cells need to contain mutations that lead to the creation of neoantigens.
- The cancer cells' MHC system needs to be intact, so there's a chance these neoantigens will be displayed on their surface.

- There needs not to be too much variation amongst their cancer cells. Otherwise, you would need an endless number of T cells targeted towards all the neoantigens the cells display.
- Dendritic cells and T cells need to be able to get in and out of their tumor and any metastases.
- T cells in their tumor and any metastases need to not be suppressed by things that are beyond our means to manipulate (e.g., we can block checkpoint proteins, but we find it harder to tackle other causes of T cell suppression and exhaustion).

Even if all the points above are true, there are still so many "ifs," "buts," and "maybes" with vaccine treatments. For example, they work:

- If you can persuade dendritic cells to pick up antigens from cancer cells and think of them as something dangerous rather than something to ignore.
- If those dendritic cells go to lymph nodes and present these antigens to T cells in a way that leads to their activation.
- If they activate sufficient T cells.
- If activated, T cells can get inside tumors and get close enough to cancer cells to "see" what's on their surface.
- If the T cells find the target they're looking for on the cancer cells' MHC proteins.
- If there's enough of the target to trigger the T cells into cell-killing action.
- And, if the T cells stay active long enough to kill sufficient cancer cells to make a difference to the patient.

So many ifs!

I hope that despite the many obstacles arrayed against them, we will see many more approved treatment vaccines in the years to come. The sheer volume of vaccine trials and the number of different approaches makes me hesitant to predict which of them will lead to the greatest success.

6.11 FINAL THOUGHTS

In this chapter, I've described many different immunotherapy approaches. No doubt, by the time this book is published, more of these treatments will have been approved for use. (Of course, the opposite may also be true: some of those I've mentioned may have been deemed ineffective and withdrawn from trials).

This rapid progress that has been made in immunotherapy is testament to several factors:

1. Immunotherapy has been proven to work; therefore, there is massive optimism and a huge appetite from doctors to enter patients into immunotherapy trials.
2. The optimism around immunotherapy expressed in our newspapers and cancer conferences means that people with cancer are willing to enter such trials.
3. The successes so far have whetted the appetite of pharmaceutical companies and are driving investment in drug development and clinical trials.
4. Technologies and manufacturing processes have become better, safer, and (at least somewhat) cheaper, providing even the most technologically demanding vaccines with a potential route to market.
5. Immunotherapies are potentially applicable to many, if not all, types of cancer, meaning that trials are recruiting people with a huge range of different cancer types.
6. Some of the cancers in which immunotherapy seems to work best (e.g., melanoma skin cancer and NSCLC) are relatively common and difficult to cure using other types of treatment.

However, future progress in immunotherapy will depend on scientists and doctors being able to overcome some of the current obstacles, such as:

- Effectiveness for only some cancers. For example, CAR-modified T cell therapy is currently only useful for hematological cancers. Many barriers need to be overcome before they can be used safely and effectively in solid tumors.
- Side effects. Some of the side effects caused by immunotherapies (such as CRS and neurotoxicity) are potentially life-threatening, and we need better ways of managing them or reducing their severity.
- Inability to overcome the immune-suppressing microenvironment of solid tumors. The hostile, T cell-suppressing environment in which cancer cells live (especially in solid tumors) is an enormous obstacle to the effective use of approaches such as cancer treatment vaccines.
- Lack of safe targets. We are still hampered by a lack of suitable, safe targets for many solid tumor types. Clinical trials often report patient deaths due to excessive toxicity to vital organs and tissues.
- Inherently cold tumors. Some cancer types simply do not lend themselves to immunotherapy, especially if the cancer is advanced. You only have to look at the fibrous, compacted, immune-suppressed environment of advanced pancreatic cancers for your heart to sink.
- Excessive heterogeneity. In some cancers (glioblastoma comes to mind), there is enormous variation among a patient's cancer cells. In this circumstance, you would need an equally enormous range of activated T cells to wipe them out.
- Cost. Some immunotherapies, such as ACT, rely on harvesting and modifying the patient's white blood cells. This is incredibly costly and requires specialist resources and highly trained scientists. At the time of writing, this can only be done at specialist hospitals, pharmaceutical company manufacturing facilities, and research institutes.

However, despite these many obstacles, I am enormously optimistic about the future of immunotherapy. Surely this, more than any other approach, has the potential to cure people with advanced cancer.

REFERENCES

1 Parish CR (2003). Cancer immunotherapy: The past, the present and the future. *Immunol Cell Biol* **81**(2). doi: 10.1046/j.0818-9641.2003.01151.x.

2 Lesterhuis WJ, Haanen JBAG, Punt CJA (2011). Cancer immunotherapy – Revisited. *Nat Rev Drug Discov* **10**(8): 591–600. doi: 10.1038/nrd3500.

3 Ito T *et al.* (2010). Identification of a primary target of thalidomide teratogenicity. *Science (1979)* **327**(5971): 1345–1350. doi: 10.1126/science.1177319.

4 Redelman-Sidi G, Glickman MS, Bochner BH (2014). The mechanism of action of BCG therapy for bladder cancer – A current perspective. *Nat Rev Urol* **11**(3): 153–162. doi: 10.1038/nrurol.2014.15.

5 Jiang T, Zhou C, Ren S (2016). Role of IL-2 in cancer immunotherapy. *Onco Targets Ther* **5**(6): e1163462. doi: 10.1080/2162402X.2016.1163462.

6 Zahavi D, Weiner L (2020). Monoclonal antibodies in cancer therapy. *Antibodies* **9**(3): 34. doi: 10.3390/antib9030034.

7 Cuesta-Mateos C *et al.* (2018). Monoclonal antibody therapies for hematological malignancies: Not just lineage-specific targets. *Front Immunol* **8**. doi: 10.3389/fimmu.2017.01936.

8 Lo Nigro C *et al.* (2019). NK-mediated antibody-dependent cell-mediated cytotoxicity in solid tumors: Biological evidence and clinical perspectives. *Ann Transl Med* **7**(5): 105–105. doi: 10.21037/atm.2019.01.42.

9 Campbell KS, Hasegawa J (2013). Natural killer cell biology: An update and future directions. *J Allergy Clin Immunol* **132**(3): 536–544. doi: 10.1016/j.jaci.2013.07.006.

10 Reis ES *et al.* (2018). Complement in cancer: Untangling an intricate relationship. *Nat Rev Immunol* **18**(1): 5–18. doi: 10.1038/nri.2017.97.

11 National Cancer Institute. Drugs Approved for Different Types of Cancer. [Online] Available at: https://www.cancer.gov/about-cancer/treatment/drugs/cancer-type [Accessed October 13, 2023].

12 Shen F, Shen W (2022). Isatuximab in the treatment of multiple myeloma: A review and comparison with daratumumab. *Technol Cancer Res Treat* **21**: 153303382211065. doi: 10.1177/15330338221106563.

13 Düll J, Topp M, Salles G (2021). The use of tafasitamab in diffuse large B-cell lymphoma. *Ther Adv Hematol* **12**: 204062072110274. doi: 10.1177/20406207211027458.

14 Chan GC-F, Chan CM (2022). Anti-GD2 Directed Immunotherapy for High-Risk and Metastatic Neuroblastoma. *Biomolecules* **12**(3): 358. doi: 10.3390/biom12030358.

15 Quach H *et al.* (2010). Mechanism of action of immunomodulatory drugs (IMiDS) in multiple myeloma. *Leukemia* **24**(1): 22–32. doi: 10.1038/leu.2009.236.

16 Costacurta M *et al.* (2021). Molecular mechanisms of cereblon-interacting small molecules in multiple myeloma therapy. *J Pers Med* **11**(11): 1185. doi: 10.3390/jpm11111185.

17 Ito T, Handa H (2020). Molecular mechanisms of thalidomide and its derivatives. *Proc Jpn Acad Ser B* **96**(6): 189–203. doi: 10.2183/pjab.96.016.

18 Cippitelli M *et al.* (2021). Role of aiolos and ikaros in the antitumor and immunomodulatory activity of IMiDs in multiple myeloma: Better to lose than to find them. *Int J Mol Sci* **22**(3): 1103. doi: 10.3390/ijms22031103.

19 Asatsuma-Okumura T, Ito T, Handa H (2019). Molecular mechanisms of cereblon-based drugs. *Pharmacol Ther* **202**: 132–139. doi: 10.1016/j.pharmthera.2019.06.004.

20 Besser MJ *et al.* (2013). Adoptive transfer of tumor-infiltrating lymphocytes in patients with metastatic melanoma: Intent-to-treat analysis and efficacy after failure to prior immunotherapies. *Clin Cancer Res* **19**(17): 4792–4800. doi: 10.1158/1078-0432.CCR-13-0380.

21 Kumar A, Watkins R, Vilgelm AE (2021). Cell therapy with TILs: Training and taming T cells to fight cancer. *Front Immunol* **12**. doi: 10.3389/fimmu.2021.690499.

22 Rosenberg SA *et al.* (1988). Use of tumor-infiltrating lymphocytes and interleukin-2 in the immunotherapy of patients with metastatic

melanoma. *N Engl J Med* **319**(25): 1676–1680. doi: 10.1056/NEJM198812223192527.

23 Rosenberg SA (2021). A journey in Science: Immersion in the search for effective cancer immunotherapies. *Mol Med* **27**(1): 63. doi: 10.1186/s10020-021-00321-3.

24 Ralli M *et al*. (2020). Immunotherapy in the treatment of metastatic melanoma: Current knowledge and future directions. *J Immunol Res* **2020**: 1–12. doi: 10.1155/2020/9235638.

25 Wang P, Chen Y, Wang C (2021). Beyond tumor mutation burden: Tumor neoantigen burden as a biomarker for immunotherapy and other types of therapy. *Front Oncol* **11**. doi: 10.3389/fonc.2021.672677.

26 Zhao Y *et al*. (2022). Tumor infiltrating lymphocyte (TIL) therapy for solid tumor treatment: Progressions and challenges. *Cancers (Basel)* **14**(17): 4160. doi: 10.3390/cancers14174160.

27 Rohaan MW *et al*. (2022). Tumor-infiltrating lymphocyte therapy or ipilimumab in advanced melanoma. *N Engl J Med* **387**(23): 2113–2125. doi: 10.1056/NEJMoa2210233.

28 van den Berg JH *et al*. (2020). Tumor infiltrating lymphocytes (TIL) therapy in metastatic melanoma: Boosting of neoantigen-specific T cell reactivity and long-term follow-up. *J Immunother Cancer* **8**(2): e000848. doi: 10.1136/jitc-2020-000848.

29 Dudley ME *et al*. (2005). Adoptive cell transfer therapy following non-myeloablative but lymphodepleting chemotherapy for the treatment of patients with refractory metastatic melanoma. *J Clin Oncol* **23**(10): 2346–2357. doi: 10.1200/JCO.2005.00.240.

30 Itzhaki O *et al*. (2011). Establishment and large-scale expansion of minimally cultured 'young' tumor infiltrating lymphocytes for adoptive transfer therapy. *J Immunother* **34**(2): 212–220. doi: 10.1097/CJI.0b013e318209c94c.

31 Vickers E (2018). *A Beginner's Guide to Targeted Cancer Treatments*, 1st ed. Wiley-Blackwell.

32 Dafni U *et al*. (2019). Efficacy of adoptive therapy with tumor-infiltrating lymphocytes and recombinant interleukin-2 in advanced cutaneous melanoma: A systematic review and meta-analysis. *Ann Oncol* **30**(12): 1902–1913. doi: 10.1093/annonc/mdz398.

33 Rohaan MW *et al*. (2018). Adoptive transfer of tumor-infiltrating lymphocytes in melanoma: A viable treatment option. *J Immunother Cancer* **6**(1): 102. doi: 10.1186/s40425-018-0391-1.

34 June CH *et al*. (2018). CAR T cell immunotherapy for human cancer. *Science (1979)* **359**(6382): 1361–1365. doi: 10.1126/science.aar6711.

35 Ghorashian S, Pule M, Amrolia P (2015). CD19 chimeric antigen receptor T cell therapy for haematological malignancies. *Br J Haematol* **169**(4): 463–478. doi: 10.1111/bjh.13340.

36 Wu L *et al*. (2023). Difference in efficacy and safety of anti-CD19 chimeric antigen receptor T-cell therapy containing 4-1BB and CD28 Co-stimulatory domains for B-cell acute lymphoblastic leukemia. *Cancers (Basel)* **15**(10): 2767. doi: 10.3390/cancers15102767.

37 Cappell KM, Kochenderfer JN (2021). A comparison of chimeric antigen receptors containing CD28 versus 4-1BB costimulatory domains. *Nat Rev Clin Oncol* **18**(11): 715–727. doi: 10.1038/s41571-021-00530-z.

38 Fesnak A, O'Doherty U (2017). Clinical development and manufacture of chimeric antigen receptor T cells and the role of leukapheresis. *Eur Oncol Haematol* **13**(01): 28. doi: 10.17925/EOH.2017.13.01.28.

39 Wang Z *et al*. (2022). Chimeric antigen receptor T-cell therapy for multiple myeloma. *Front Immunol* **13**. doi: 10.3389/fimmu.2022.1050522.

40 Cappell KM, Kochenderfer JN (2023). Long-term outcomes following CAR T cell therapy: What we know so far. *Nat Rev Clin Oncol* **20**(6): 359–371. doi: 10.1038/s41571-023-00754-1.

41 Shah BD *et al*. (2022). Two-year follow-up of KTE-X19, an anti-CD19 chimeric antigen receptor (CAR) T-cell therapy, in adult patients (Pts) with relapsed/refractory B-cell acute lymphoblastic leukemia (R/R B-ALL) in ZUMA-3. *J Clin Oncol* **40**(16_suppl): 7010–7010. doi: 10.1200/JCO.2022.40.16_suppl.7010.

42 Shah BD *et al*. (2021). KTE-X19 for relapsed or refractory adult B-cell acute lymphoblastic leukaemia: Phase 2 results of the single-arm, open-label, multicentre ZUMA-3 study. *Lancet* **398**(10299): 491–502. doi: 10.1016/S0140-6736(21)01222-8.

43 Laetsch TW *et al*. (2023). Three-year update of tisagenlecleucel in pediatric and young adult

patients with relapsed/refractory acute lymph-oblastic leukemia in the ELIANA trial. *J Clin Oncol* **41**(9): 1664–1669. doi: 10.1200/JCO. 22.00642.

44 Maude SL *et al*. (2018). Tisagenlecleucel in chil-dren and young adults with B-Cell lymphoblas-tic leukemia. *N Engl J Med* **378**(5): 439–448. doi: 10.1056/NEJMoa1709866.

45 Abramson JS *et al*. (2020). Lisocabtagene maraleucel for patients with relapsed or refrac-tory large B-cell lymphomas (TRANSCEND NHL 001): A multicentre seamless design study. *Lancet* **396**(10254): 839–852. doi: 10.1016/S0140-6736(20)31366-0.

46 Schuster SJ *et al*. (2019). Tisagenlecleucel in adult relapsed or refractory diffuse large B-cell lymphoma. *N Engl J Med* **380**(1): 45–56. doi: 10.1056/NEJMoa1804980.

47 Neelapu SS *et al*. (2017). Axicabtagene ciloleucel CAR T-cell therapy in refractory large B-cell lymphoma. *N Engl J Med* **377**(26): 2531–2544. doi: 10.1056/NEJMoa1707447.

48 Albanyan O, Chavez J, Munoz J (2022). The role of CAR-T cell therapy as second line in diffuse large B-cell lymphoma. *Ther Adv Hematol* **13**: 204062072211415. doi: 10.1177/20406207221141511.

49 Mohty R, Kharfan-Dabaja MA (2022). CAR T-cell therapy for follicular lymphoma and mantle cell lymphoma. *Ther Adv Hematol* **13**: 204062072211421. doi: 10.1177/20406207221142133.

50 Denlinger N, Bond D, Jaglowski S (2022). CAR T-cell therapy for B-cell lymphoma. *Curr Probl Cancer* **46**(1): 100826. doi: 10.1016/j.currprobl cancer.2021.100826.

51 Myeloma incidence statistics. Cancer Research UK. [Online] Available at: https://www.cancerresearchuk.org/health-professional/cancer-statistics/statistics-by-cancer-type/myeloma/incidence [Accessed July 24, 2023].

52 Rodriguez-Otero P *et al*. (2023). Ide-cel or stand-ard regimens in relapsed and refractory multi-ple myeloma. *N Engl J Med* **388**(11): 1002–1014. doi: 10.1056/NEJMoa2213614.

53 San-Miguel J *et al*. (2023). Cilta-cel or standard care in lenalidomide-refractory multiple mye-loma. *N Engl J Med*. doi: 10.1056/NEJMoa2303379.

54 Sterner RC, Sterner RM (2021). CAR-T cell therapy: Current limitations and potential strategies. *Blood Cancer J* **11**(4): 69. doi: 10.1038/s41408-021-00459-7.

55 Lemoine J, Ruella M, Houot R (2021). Born to survive: How cancer cells resist CAR T cell therapy. *J Hematol Oncol* **14**(1): 199. doi: 10.1186/s13045-021-01209-9.

56 Pietrobon V *et al*. (2021). Improving CAR T-cell persistence. *Int J Mol Sci* **22**(19): 10828. doi: 10.3390/ijms221910828.

57 Mueller KT *et al*. (2017). Cellular kinetics of CTL019 in relapsed/refractory B-cell acute lymphoblastic leukemia and chronic lympho-cytic leukemia. *Blood* **130**(21): 2317–2325. doi: 10.1182/blood-2017-06-786129.

58 Liu C *et al*. (2021). Model-based cellular kinetic analysis of chimeric antigen receptor-T cells in humans. *Clin Pharmacol Ther* **109**(3): 716–727. doi: 10.1002/cpt.2040.

59 Jo T *et al*. (2023). Risk factors for CAR-T cell manufacturing failure among DLBCL patients: A nationwide survey in Japan. *Br J Haematol* **202**(2): 256–266. doi: 10.1111/bjh.18831.

60 Shimabukuro-Vornhagen A *et al*. (2018). Cytokine release syndrome. *J Immunother Cancer* **6**(1): 56. doi: 10.1186/s40425-018-0343-9.

61 Yáñez L, Sánchez-Escamilla M, Perales M-A (2019). CAR T cell toxicity: Current manage-ment and future directions. *Hemasphere* **3**(2): e186. doi: 10.1097/HS9.0000000000000186.

62 Siegler EL, Kenderian SS (2020). Neurotoxicity and cytokine release syndrome after chimeric antigen receptor T cell therapy: Insights into mechanisms and novel therapies. *Front Immunol* **11**. doi: 10.3389/fimmu.2020.01973.

63 Wat J, Barmettler S (2022). Hypogammaglob-ulinemia after chimeric antigen receptor (CAR) T-cell therapy: Characteristics, management, and future directions. *J Allergy Clin Immunol Pract* **10**(2): 460–466. doi: 10.1016/j.jaip.2021.10.037.

64 López-Cantillo G *et al*. (2022). CAR-T cell perfor-mance: How to improve their persistence? *Front Immunol* **13**. doi: 10.3389/fimmu.2022.878209.

65 Depil S *et al*. (2020). 'Off-the-shelf' allogeneic CAR T cells: Development and challenges. *Nat Rev Drug Discov* **19**(3): 185–199. doi: 10.1038/s41573-019-0051-2.

66 Sutherland AR, Owens MN, Geyer CR (2020). Modular chimeric antigen receptor systems for

universal CAR T cell retargeting. *Int J Mol Sci* **21**(19): 7222. doi: 10.3390/ijms21197222.

67 Qasim W (2023). Genome-edited allogeneic donor 'universal' chimeric antigen receptor T cells. *Blood* **141**(8): 835–845. doi: 10.1182/blood.2022016204.

68 Hawkins ER, D'Souza RR, Klampatsa A (2021). Armored CAR T-cells: The next chapter in T-cell cancer immunotherapy. *Biologics* **15**: 95–105. doi: 10.2147/BTT.S291768.

69 Xiao X *et al.* (2022). Combination strategies to optimize the efficacy of chimeric antigen receptor T cell therapy in haematological malignancies. *Front Immunol* **13**. doi: 10.3389/fimmu.2022.954235.

70 Yang Y *et al.* (2020). Additional possibilities of chimeric antigen receptor T-cells in B-cell lymphoma: Combination therapy. *Transl Cancer Res* **9**(11): 7310–7322. doi: 10.21037/tcr-20-72.

71 van der Schans JJ, van de Donk NWCJ, Mutis T (2020). Dual targeting to overcome current challenges in multiple myeloma CAR T-cell treatment. *Front Oncol* **10**. doi: 10.3389/fonc.2020.01362.

72 Xie B *et al.* (2022). Current status and perspectives of dual-targeting chimeric antigen receptor T-cell therapy for the treatment of hematological malignancies. *Cancers (Basel)* **14**(13): 3230. doi: 10.3390/cancers14133230.

73 Liu J *et al.* (2023). Targeted CD7 CAR T-cells for treatment of T-Lymphocyte leukemia and lymphoma and acute myeloid leukemia: Recent advances. *Front Immunol* **14**. doi: 10.3389/fimmu.2023.1170968.

74 Wei W *et al.* (2022). Chimeric antigen receptor T-cell therapy for T-ALL and AML. *Front Oncol* **12**. doi: 10.3389/fonc.2022.967754.

75 Georgiadis C *et al.* (2021). Base-edited CAR T cells for combinational therapy against T cell malignancies. *Leukemia* **35**(12): 3466–3481. doi: 10.1038/s41375-021-01282-6.

76 Atilla E, Benabdellah K (2023). The black hole: CAR T cell therapy in AML. *Cancers (Basel)* **15**(10): 2713. doi: 10.3390/cancers15102713.

77 Mardiana S, Gill S (2020). CAR T cells for acute myeloid leukemia: State of the art and future directions. *Front Oncol* **10**. doi: 10.3389/fonc.2020.00697.

78 Leick MB, Maus MV (2019). CAR-T cells beyond CD19, UnCAR-Ted territory. *Am J Hematol* **94**(S1): S34–S41. doi: 10.1002/ajh.25398.

79 Heyman BM, Tzachanis D, Kipps TJ (2022). Recent advances in CAR T-cell therapy for patients with chronic lymphocytic leukemia. *Cancers (Basel)* **14**(7): 1715. doi: 10.3390/cancers14071715.

80 Hochhaus A *et al.* (2020). European Leukemia Net 2020 recommendations for treating chronic myeloid leukemia. *Leukemia* **34**(4): 966–984. doi: 10.1038/s41375-020-0776-2.

81 Meier JA, Savoldo B, Grover NS (2022). The emerging role of CAR T cell therapy in relapsed/refractory Hodgkin lymphoma. *J Pers Med* **12**(2): 197. doi: 10.3390/jpm12020197.

82 Othman T, Herrera A, Mei M (2021). Emerging therapies in relapsed and refractory hodgkin lymphoma: What comes next after brentuximab vedotin and PD-1 inhibition? *Curr Hematol Malig Rep* **16**(1): 1–7. doi: 10.1007/s11899-020-00603-3.

83 Maaroufi M (2023). Immunotherapy for Hodgkin lymphoma: From monoclonal antibodies to chimeric antigen receptor T-cell therapy. *Crit Rev Oncol Hematol* **182**: 103923. doi: 10.1016/j.critrevonc.2023.103923.

84 Guzman G *et al.* (2023). CAR-T therapies in solid tumors: Opportunities and challenges. *Curr Oncol Rep* **25**(5): 479–489. doi: 10.1007/s11912-023-01380-x.

85 Rodriguez-Garcia A *et al.* (2020). CAR-T cells hit the tumor microenvironment: Strategies to overcome tumor escape. *Front Immunol* **11**. doi: 10.3389/fimmu.2020.01109.

86 Wang Z *et al.* (2019). A long way to the battlefront: CAR T cell therapy against solid cancers. *J Cancer* **10**(14): 3112–3123. doi: 10.7150/jca.30406.

87 Yong CSM *et al.* (2017). CAR T-cell therapy of solid tumors. *Immunol Cell Biol* **95**(4): 356–363. doi: 10.1038/icb.2016.128.

88 Daei Sorkhabi A *et al.* (2023). The current landscape of CAR T-cell therapy for solid tumors: Mechanisms, research progress, challenges, and counterstrategies. *Front Immunol* **14**. doi: 10.3389/fimmu.2023.1113882.

89 Klobuch S, Seijkens TTP, Haanen JBAG (2023). The emerging role for CAR T cells in solid tumor oncology. *Chin Clin Oncol* **12**(2): 19–19. doi: 10.21037/cco-22-125.

90 Sesques P *et al.* (2020). Commercial anti-CD19 CAR T cell therapy for patients with relapsed/

refractory aggressive B cell lymphoma in a European center. *Am J Hematol* **95**(11): 1324–1333. doi: 10.1002/ajh.25951.

91 Jacobson CA *et al.* (2020). Axicabtagene ciloleucel in the non-trial setting: Outcomes and correlates of response, resistance, and toxicity. *J Clin Oncol* **38**(27): 3095–3106. doi: 10.1200/JCO.19.02103.

92 Bethge WA *et al.* (2022). GLA/DRST real-world outcome analysis of CAR-T cell therapies for large B-cell lymphoma in Germany. *Blood*. doi: 10.1182/blood.2021015209.

93 Casadei B *et al.* (2021). Real world evidence of CAR T-cell therapies for the treatment of relapsed/refractory B-cell non-Hodgkin lymphoma: A monocentric experience. *Cancers (Basel)* **13**(19): 4789. doi: 10.3390/cancers 13194789.

94 Zhang J, Wang L (2019). The emerging world of TCR-T cell trials against cancer: A systematic review. *Technol Cancer Res Treat* **18**: 153303381983106. doi: 10.1177/1533033819831068.

95 He Q *et al.* (2019). Targeting cancers through TCR-peptide/MHC interactions. *J Hematol Oncol* **12**(1): 139. doi: 10.1186/s13045-019-0812-8.

96 Shafer P, Kelly LM, Hoyos V (2022). Cancer therapy with TCR-engineered T cells: Current strategies, challenges, and prospects. *Front Immunol* **13**. doi: 10.3389/fimmu.2022.835762.

97 Sun Y *et al.* (2021). Evolution of CD8+ T cell receptor (TCR) engineered therapies for the treatment of cancer. *Cells* **10**(9): 2379. doi: 10.3390/cells10092379.

98 Delves P *et al.* (2017). Membrane receptors for antigen. In *Roitt's Essential Immunology*. 13th ed. Wiley-Blackwell. pp. 97–138.

99 Pan K *et al.* (2022). CAR race to cancer immunotherapy: From CAR T, CAR NK to CAR macrophage therapy. *J Exp Clin Cancer Res* **41**(1): 119. doi: 10.1186/s13046-022-02327-z.

100 Li H *et al.* (2022). Preclinical and clinical studies of CAR-NK-cell therapies for malignancies. *Front Immunol* **13**. doi: 10.3389/fimmu.2022.992232.

101 Hirayama D, Iida T, Nakase H (2017). The phagocytic function of macrophage-enforcing innate immunity and tissue homeostasis. *Int J Mol Sci* **19**(1): 92. doi: 10.3390/ijms19010092.

102 Guerriero JL (2019). Macrophages: Their untold story in T cell activation and function. *Int Rev Cell Mol Biol*: 73–93. doi: 10.1016/bs. ircmb.2018.07.001.

103 Wang Q *et al.* (2019). Design and production of bispecific antibodies. *Antibodies* **8**(3): 43. doi: 10.3390/antib8030043.

104 Li H, Er Saw P, Song E (2020). Challenges and strategies for next-generation bispecific antibody-based antitumor therapeutics. *Cell Mol Immunol* **17**(5): 451–461. doi: 10.1038/s41423-020-0417-8.

105 Arvedson T *et al.* (2022). Targeting solid tumors with bispecific T cell engager immune therapy. *Annu Rev Cancer Biol* **6**(1): 17–34. doi: 10.1146/annurev-cancerbio-070620-104325.

106 Goebeler M-E, Bargou RC (2020). T cell-engaging therapies – BiTEs and beyond. *Nat Rev Clin Oncol* **17**(7): 418–434. doi: 10.1038/s41571-020-0347-5.

107 Lowe KL *et al.* (2019). Novel TCR-based biologics: Mobilising T cells to warm 'cold' tumours. *Cancer Treat Rev* **77**: 35–43. doi: 10.1016/j.ctrv.2019.06.001.

108 Hickman ES, Lomax ME, Jakobsen BK (2016). Antigen selection for enhanced affinity T-cell receptor–based cancer therapies. *SLAS Discov* **21**(8): 769–785. doi: 10.1177/1087057116637837.

109 Bossi G *et al.* (2014). ImmTAC-redirected tumour cell killing induces and potentiates antigen cross-presentation by dendritic cells. *Cancer Immunol Immunother* **63**(5): 437–448. doi: 10.1007/s00262-014-1525-z.

110 Carvajal RD *et al.* (2022). Phase I study of safety, tolerability, and efficacy of tebentafusp using a step-up dosing regimen and expansion in patients with metastatic uveal melanoma. *J Clin Oncol* **40**(17): 1939–1948. doi: 10.1200/JCO.21.01805.

111 Berman DM, Bell JI (2023). Redirecting polyclonal T cells against cancer with soluble T-cell receptors. *Clin Cancer Res* **29**(4): 697–704. doi: 10.1158/1078-0432.CCR-22-0028.

112 Sergeeva A *et al.* (2011). An anti–PR1/HLA-A2 T-cell receptor–like antibody mediates complement-dependent cytotoxicity against acute myeloid leukemia progenitor cells. *Blood* **117**(16): 4262–4272. doi: 10.1182/blood-2010-07-299248.

113 Hoffmann P *et al.* (2005). Serial killing of tumor cells by cytotoxic T cells redirected with a CD19-/CD3-bispecific single-chain antibody construct. *Int J Cancer* **115**(1): 98–104. doi: 10.1002/ijc.20908.

114 Wei J *et al.* (2022). Current landscape and future directions of bispecific antibodies in cancer immunotherapy. *Front Immunol* **13**. doi: 10.3389/fimmu.2022.1035276.

115 Tian Z *et al.* (2021). Bispecific T cell engagers: An emerging therapy for management of hematologic malignancies. *J Hematol Oncol* **14**(1): 75. doi: 10.1186/s13045-021-01084-4.

116 Shanshal M *et al.* (2023). T-cell engagers in solid cancers – Current landscape and future directions. *Cancers (Basel)* **15**(10): 2824. doi: 10.3390/cancers15102824.

117 Baeuerle PA, Wesche H (2022). T-cell-engaging antibodies for the treatment of solid tumors: Challenges and opportunities. *Curr Opin Oncol* **34**(5): 552–558. doi: 10.1097/CCO.0000000000000869.

118 Subklewe M (2021). BiTEs better than CAR T cells. *Blood Adv* **5**(2): 607–612. doi: 10.1182/bloodadvances.2020001792.

119 Morse MA, Gwin WR, Mitchell DA (2021). Vaccine therapies for cancer: Then and now. *Target Oncol* **16**(2): 121–152. doi: 10.1007/s11523-020-00788-w.

120 Hollingsworth RE, Jansen K (2019). Turning the corner on therapeutic cancer vaccines. *NPJ Vaccines* **4**(1): 7. doi: 10.1038/s41541-019-0103-y.

121 Maeng HM, Berzofsky JA (2019). Strategies for developing and optimizing cancer vaccines. *F1000Res* **8**: 654. doi: 10.12688/f1000research.18693.1.

122 Antonelli AC *et al.* (2020). Bacterial immunotherapy for cancer induces CD4-dependent tumor-specific immunity through tumor-intrinsic interferon-γ signaling. *Proc Natl Acad Sci* **117**(31): 18627–18637. doi: 10.1073/pnas.2004421117.

123 Lin MJ *et al.* (2022). Cancer vaccines: The next immunotherapy frontier. *Nat Can* **3**(8): 911–926. doi: 10.1038/s43018-022-00418-6.

124 Saxena M *et al.* (2021). Therapeutic cancer vaccines. *Nat Rev Cancer* **21**(6): 360–378. doi: 10.1038/s41568-021-00346-0.

125 Butterfield LH (2015). Cancer vaccines. *BMJ* **350**(apr22 14): h988. doi: 10.1136/bmj.h988.

126 Khong H, Overwijk WW (2016). Adjuvants for peptide-based cancer vaccines. *J Immunother Cancer* **4**(1): 56. doi: 10.1186/s40425-016-0160-y.

127 Paston SJ *et al.* (2021). Cancer vaccines, adjuvants, and delivery systems. *Front Immunol* **12**. doi: 10.3389/fimmu.2021.627932.

128 Winstead E. Can mRNA Vaccines Help Treat Cancer? [Online] Available at: https://www.cancer.gov/news-events/cancer-currents-blog/2022/mrna-vaccines-to-treat-cancer [Accessed August 14, 2023].

129 Lorentzen CL *et al.* (2022). Clinical advances and ongoing trials of mRNA vaccines for cancer treatment. *Lancet Oncol* **23**(10): e450–e458. doi: 10.1016/S1470-2045(22)00372-2.

130 Barbier AJ *et al.* (2022). The clinical progress of mRNA vaccines and immunotherapies. *Nat Biotechnol* **40**(6): 840–854. doi: 10.1038/s41587-022-01294-2.

131 Blass E, Ott PA (2021). Advances in the development of personalized neoantigen-based therapeutic cancer vaccines. *Nat Rev Clin Oncol* **18**(4): 215–229. doi: 10.1038/s41571-020-00460-2.

132 Zegarac JP. mRNA vaccines are a promising new tool in the fight against cancer. Here's where they stand. ASCO Daily News. [Online] Available at: https://dailynews.ascopubs.org/do/mrna-vaccines-promising-new-tool-fight-against-cancer-here-s-they-stand [Accessed August 10, 2023].

133 Rojas LA *et al.* (2023). Personalized RNA neoantigen vaccines stimulate T cells in pancreatic cancer. *Nature* **618**(7963): 144–150. doi: 10.1038/s41586-023-06063-y.

134 Department of Health and Social Care and S. T. R. H. M. Barclay. New partnership to boost research into vaccines for cancer. GOV.UK. [Online] Available at: https://www.gov.uk/government/news/new-partnership-to-boost-research-into-vaccines-for-cancer [Accessed August 10, 2023].

135 Fritah H *et al.* (2022). The current clinical landscape of personalized cancer vaccines. *Cancer Treat Rev* **106**: 102383. doi: 10.1016/j.ctrv.2022.102383.

136 Reale A *et al.* (2019). Perspectives on immunotherapy via oncolytic viruses. *Infect Agent Cancer* **14**(1): 5. doi: 10.1186/s13027-018-0218-1.

CHAPTER 7

Treatments Relevant to Individual Cancer Types

IN BRIEF

In this chapter, I briefly outline which targeted therapies and immunotherapies are relevant for individual cancer types. For each cancer, I describe a little of the biology of the disease and summarize the proteins and processes that can be targeted with antibody- and small molecule-based treatments. I also discuss whether immunotherapy is effective for each type of cancer and, if so, which immunotherapies are most relevant. I then provide a table (or multiple tables) telling you where in the rest of the book you can find more information on each treatment.

7.1 INTRODUCTION

Throughout this book, I have described many targeted therapies and immunotherapies. I have categorized them according to what they target and how they work. I have also summarized what we know about why each treatment is effective against specific types of cancer. What I haven't done so far is to group together the treatments that are effective against an individual cancer type. In this chapter, I aim to address this omission.

My hope is that this chapter will be a useful starting point for anyone who wants to know which treatments are relevant to the cancer (or cancers) that they are most interested in. Hence, this chapter contains many tables (53 in all!) in which I have tried to list all the treatment approaches relevant to each disease. My expectation is that, rather than

reading this chapter in one go, you will refer to it as and when you wish to familiarize yourself with a particular cancer type.

What this chapter doesn't include:
- Any information about treatments not described in this book (such as surgery, radiotherapy, or chemotherapy). There is also only a passing mention of hormone therapy.
- Detailed discussion of treatment combinations. A person's treatment often involves several different treatments given together, or one after the other. However, I felt that this information was too complicated to include, as it varies so much depending on the person, their diagnosis, stage of disease, and prior treatment.
- I also don't discuss when in a person's treatment the targeted therapy or immunotherapy might be offered to them, i.e., whether it's at the point of diagnosis or at relapse, or

A Beginner's Guide to Targeted Cancer Treatments and Cancer Immunotherapy, Second Edition. Elaine Vickers.
© 2025 John Wiley & Sons Ltd. Published 2025 by John Wiley & Sons Ltd.

whether the treatment is applicable for people with early stage or advanced disease.

- Information about whether a treatment is an established standard-of-care for a disease, versus still in late phase trials, or only available to small subsets of patients. This is beyond the scope of this book, and I leave you to find out this kind of detail for yourself[1].

- Lastly, this chapter is not a comprehensive list of every possible type of cancer. I do not include many of the rarest cancers. I have also omitted some cancers where there are no licensed targeted therapies or immunotherapies.

This chapter contains lists of targeted therapies and immunotherapies relevant to each cancer type. However, some treatments have been approved as tumor-agnostic treatments. That is, they are (in theory at least) available to anyone whose cancer contains a specific mutation or displays a particular feature. This situation is steadily becoming more common as scientists and doctors identify mutations or features of cancers that respond to a certain treatment approach, regardless of cancer type[2].

Rather than including these treatments in every table, I list some examples in Table 7.1. A recent approval is that of trastuzumab deruxtecan (a HER2-targeted antibody-drug conjugate). This treatment was approved by the FDA in April 2024 as a treatment for anyone whose cancer cells are HER2-positive (where there are very high levels of HER2 on the surface of the person's cancer cells and/or the cells contain extra copies of the *HER2* gene) [3].

A few final points:

I do not say where in the world each treatment is being used. This is because (1) it would get too complicated and (2) it will have changed by the time this book has been published.

I have mostly taken my information for this chapter from the website of the National Cancer Institute (NCI) in the United States (cancer.gov/about-cancer/treatment/drugs/cancer-type). Again, I made this decision for a couple of practical and pragmatic reasons:

Table 7.1 Cancer type-agnostic approvals [1, 2].

Mutation, feature	Treatment approach	Treatment examples	Relevant book sections
Microsatellite instability (MSI) /deficient in mismatch repair (dMMR)	Immune checkpoint inhibitors	Pembrolizumab, dostarlimab	Chapter 5
High tumor mutation burden	Immune checkpoint inhibitors	Pembrolizumab	Chapter 5
BRAF V600E mutation	B-Raf inhibitor plus a MEK inhibitor	Dabrafenib + trametinib	Section 3.7.5
NTRK gene fusions	TRK protein inhibitors	Larotrectinib, entrectinib	Section 3.6.6
RET gene rearrangements	RET inhibitors	Selpercatinib	Section 3.6.4
HER2-positive	Antibody-drug conjugate	Trastuzumab deruxtecan	Section 3.5 and Section 4.2

---

[1] For those of you who are ESMO (European Society of Medical Oncology) members, you might find that the "ESMO Handbook of Targeted Therapies and Precision Oncology" provides you with more detail on approvals: https://oncologypro.esmo.org/education-library/esmo-books/esmo-handbooks/targeted-therapies-and-precision-oncology

[2] Bear in mind that just because a treatment is approved for use against any cancer that exhibits a particular feature (e.g. all MSI cancers, or all *BRAF V600E* cancers), that doesn't mean that it works equally well against all cancers. The details still do matter, and I wonder if some of the tumor-agnostic approvals will yet be amended to be more precise.

(1) the NCI website helpfully lists which drugs are approved for each type of cancer, (2) if a drug is licensed in the United States, it is highly likely to be (or be about to be) licensed in the United Kingdom and the rest of Europe.

When writing this chapter, I often found myself agonizing, and flip-flopping, over whether or not a treatment is "relevant" for a particular cancer type. I can only emphasize that these tables represent my best guess and that the situation is likely to change over time. I think this is especially true for the immune checkpoint inhibitors: just because they haven't worked well for a particular cancer type so far, doesn't mean that we won't find a time (such as neoadjuvant), a cancer stage (early versus advanced) or a combination, that will prove effective in future. If we implement more patient selection using biomarkers, we are also likely to identify subsets of patients with diverse cancers who are likely to benefit from these treatments.

Also, not every drug mentioned in the tables is licensed for use. In some instances, I have included targets and drugs that are looking particularly interesting, or that are in late phase trials.

Finally, as I'm sure you're aware, every month brings news of new approvals of cancer treatments, and sometimes also situations where a treatment is withdrawn. Thus, this chapter is intended as a guide to the most relevant treatment approaches, rather than an exhaustive list.

7.2 TREATMENTS FOR BREAST CANCER

7.2.1 Treatment Targets in Breast Cancer

An important consideration in treating someone with breast cancer is whether their cancer is hormone receptor (HR)-positive and/or HER2-positive.

Around 70%–80% of breast cancers are classed as being HR-positive (they usually contain both estrogen and progesterone receptors and are also referred to as being hormone-sensitive), and 15%–20% are deemed to be HER2-positive (they contain extra copies of the *HER2* gene and/or contain high levels of HER2 protein) [4–6]. Roughly 10%–20% of breast cancers are triple-negative, being neither HER2- nor HR-positive (Figure 7.1) [7, 8].

However, thanks to increasingly powerful HER2-targeted treatments, we also have a new classification of "HER2-low" breast cancer. These cancers don't have enough HER2 on the cancer cells' surface for an older HER2-targeted treatment to be helpful. But a powerful antibody-drug conjugate (ADC) such as trastuzumab deruxtecan can still work. More than 50% of breast cancers are HER2-low, the majority of which are also HR-positive [9, 10]. There are also individuals (e.g., ~3% of breast cancer patients enrolled in the METABRIC study [16]) whose cancer cells contain an activating mutation in the *HER2* gene. These cancers may be sensitive to trastuzumab deruxtecan or other HER2-targeted treatments [17].

Figure 7.1 provides a rough depiction of what proportion of breast cancers fit into each of the main categories, including the prevalence of some mutations and other features.

Figure 7.1 also contains information relevant for treatment selection. For example:

- *BRCA* gene mutations can create sensitivity to PARP inhibitors.
- The presence or absence of PD-L1 is sometimes used to determine which patients with triple-negative breast cancer may benefit from an immune checkpoint inhibitor.
- *PIK3CA* gene mutations (which cause the enzyme PI3Kα to be overactive) increase the sensitivity of the person's cancer cells to a PI3Kα inhibitor.
- Also shown is the proportion of HR-positive and triple-negative cancers that are now classified as "HER2-low," and for which trastuzumab deruxtecan is an approved treatment.

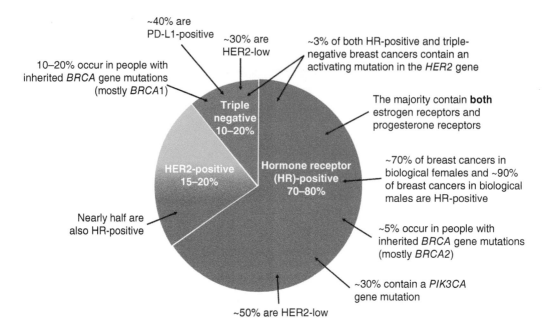

Figure 7.1 Different proportions of breast cancers are HR- or v-positive, or triple-negative [4, 5, 7–15].
Abbreviations: BRCA – breast cancer; HER2 – human epidermal growth factor receptor-2; HR – hormone receptor.

Table 7.2 A summary of treatment approaches relevant to different breast cancer types.

	HR-positive	HER2-positive	Triple-negative
Hormone therapy	Yes	Yes, but only if the cancer is also HR-positive	No
Targeted therapies matched with mutations and/or protein expression	Yes: • CDK4/6 inhibitors • PI3Kα inhibitors • AKT inhibitors • mTOR inhibitors • HER2-targeted therapies if "HER2-low"	Yes: • HER2-targeted therapies	Yes: • PARP inhibitors matched to BRCA gene mutations • HER2-targeted therapies if "HER2-low"
Targeted therapy: antibody-drug conjugates	Yes: targeting TROP2, HER2, HER3	Yes: targeting HER2	Yes: targeting TROP2, HER2
Targeted therapy: angiogenesis inhibitors	No	No	Yes: occasionally combined with chemotherapy
Immunotherapy with checkpoint inhibitors	Could have a role as a neoadjuvant treatment	No	Yes

In addition, Table 7.2 provides an overview of which treatment approaches are relevant for people with HR-positive, HER2-positive, or triple-negative breast cancer. (I have used HER2-positive in its traditional sense, to mean that there are extra copies of the *HER2* gene and/or very high levels of HER2 protein on the cancer cells' surface.)

7.2.2 Treatments for Hormone-Sensitive Breast Cancer

Table 7.3   Targets and treatments for hormone-sensitive breast cancer.

Relevant targets	Treatment approach	Treatment examples	Relevant book sections
Production of estrogen by the aromatase enzyme	Aromatase inhibitors	Exemestane, letrozole, anastrozole	Not covered, see [14–16, 20–24]
Activity of estrogen receptors	Estrogen receptor blockers and estrogen receptor degraders (some do both)	Tamoxifen, raloxifene, toremifene, fulvestrant, elacestrant, camizestrant	
Mutations in the *ESR1* gene in hormone therapy-resistant disease	Novel estrogen receptor-targeted therapies	Elacestrant, camizestrant, amcenestrant, giredestrant, rindodestrant	Not covered, see [20]
Increased Cyclin D production due to hormone receptor activity	Indirect inhibition of Cyclin D using CDK4/6 inhibitors	Palbociclib, ribociclib, abemaciclib	Section 4.4
The PI3K pathway (particularly if *PIK3CA* is mutated) [21]	mTOR inhibitors	Everolimus	Section 3.8
	PI3Kα inhibitors	Alpelisib	
	AKT inhibitors	Capivasertib, ipatasertib	
Cell surface protein: TROP2	ADCs targeting TROP2	Sacituzumab govitecan	Section 4.2
HER2 in "HER2-low" disease	ADCs targeting HER2	Trastuzumab deruxtecan	Sections 3.5 and 4.2

Abbreviation: ADC – antibody-drug conjugate.

7.2.3 Treatments for HER2-Positive Breast Cancer

Table 7.4   Targets and treatments for HER2-positive breast cancer.

Relevant targets/ approaches	Treatment approach	Treatment examples	Relevant book sections
HER2	Naked antibody therapies	Trastuzumab, pertuzumab, margetuximab	
	ADCs	Trastuzumab emtansine, trastuzumab deruxtecan	Section 3.5
	HER2-targeted kinase inhibitors	Lapatinib, neratinib, tucatinib	
In some patients, their cancer is also HR-positive	Hormone therapies	As in Table 7.3	Not covered, see [22–24]

Abbreviation: ADC – antibody-drug conjugate; HR – hormone receptor.

7.2.4 Treatments for Triple-Negative Breast Cancer

Table 7.5 Targets and treatments for triple-negative breast cancer.

Relevant targets	Treatment approach	Treatment examples	Relevant book sections
Immune checkpoint proteins on T cells	Immune checkpoint inhibitors targeting PD-1 or PD-L1[a]	Pembrolizumab, atezolizumab, camrelizumab	Chapter 5
Inherited defects in *BRCA* genes causing genomic instability	PARP inhibitors	Olaparib, talazoparib, niraparib, rucaparib	Section 4.3
The PI3K pathway (particularly if *PIK3CA* is mutated) [21]	PI3Kα inhibitors	Alpelisib	Section 3.8
	AKT inhibitors	Capivasertib, ipatasertib	
HER2 in "HER2-low" disease	ADCs targeting HER2	Trastuzumab deruxtecan	Sections 3.5 and 4.2
Angiogenesis	Angiogenesis inhibitors	Bevacizumab	Section 4.1
Cell surface protein: TROP2	ADCs targeting TROP2	Sacituzumab govitecan	Section 4.2

Abbreviation: ADC – antibody-drug conjugate.
[a] Checkpoint inhibitors are only approved as treatments for specific subsets of patients with triple-negative breast cancer, and they are often combined with chemotherapy [18, 19, 25, 26].

7.3 TREATMENTS FOR BOWEL AND ANAL CANCERS

7.3.1 Treatment Targets in Bowel Cancer

Scientists have proposed many ways of categorizing bowel cancers and have grouped them according to various features. However, many of these classifications don't yet have a practical application.

One feature of bowel cancers that does have a practical application is whether the person's cancer is "MSI" (see Section 5.6.1). That is, do the cancer cells exhibit a pattern of DNA mutations (MSI) that reflects their inability to perform mismatch repair (MMR)? Cells with defective MMR (called dMMR) accumulate thousands of mutations. Occasionally this is due to an inherited condition such as Lynch Syndrome; around 2%–4% of bowel cancers occur in people with this condition [27].

But, in most people, the defect in MMR has occurred in a bowel cell during the person's lifetime and that defective cell has caused their cancer. People with MSI cancers are very likely to benefit from checkpoint inhibitor immunotherapy [28]. If there is a mutation in the DNA polymerase epsilon enzyme (*POLE*) gene, the cancer cells are even more highly mutated. Again, this predicts sensitivity to immune checkpoint inhibitors [29, 30].

If a person's cancer cells can perform MMR, their cancer is described as "microsatellite stable" or MSS. People with these cancers are much less likely to benefit from immunotherapy with checkpoint inhibitors. However, a few people do benefit, and the Immunoscore® classification of bowel cancer could be a way of picking out those patients in advance [31]. The Immunoscore measures the number and location of T cells in a person's tumor, including information such as how close the T cells are to cancer cells. People with a high Immunoscore are most likely to benefit from checkpoint inhibitor therapy. Another possible approach for people with advanced MSS bowel cancer is to combine checkpoint inhibitors with other treatments [32].

As well as wanting to pick out which patients are likely to benefit from immunotherapy, there are a further two (overlapping) groups of patients with advanced bowel cancer whom we want to identify:

1. People whose tumors contain mutations that make them highly unlikely to benefit from an EGFR-targeted antibody such as cetuximab or panitumumab (Section 3.4.1).
2. People whose tumors contain mutations that are known to predict a high likelihood of benefitting from a matching targeted therapy such as a treatment that targets HER2 or B-Raf.

In Figure 7.2. I have depicted what some of these mutations might be (adapted from [33]). I have emphasized mutations (highlighted in turquoise) where there is a treatment approach thought to be suitable for that group of patients (not necessarily licensed). In pink are the mutations for which we have not yet created or identified an effective targeted approach.

You might remember from Section 3.4 that any mutation that activates the MAPK and/or PI3K pathway independently of EGFR will cause resistance to EGFR-targeted antibodies. However, we don't currently test for every possible mutation that is likely to cause resistance. It might be that over time the proportion of patients given an EGFR antibody will shrink further as we implement more testing. For example, two sets of mutations, known as the PRESSING panel and the PRESSING2

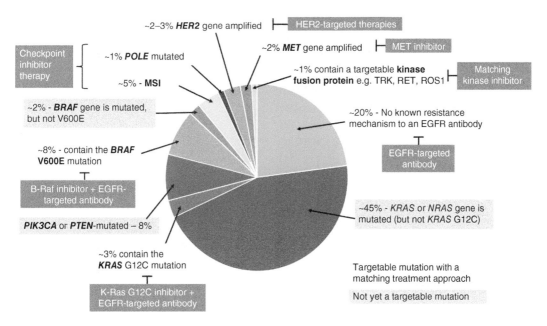

Figure 7.2 Some of the mutations found in the cancer cells of people with advanced bowel cancer. Where the mutation corresponds to a matching treatment approach, the treatment approach is included. Not shown are the hundreds of mutations that don't yet have an impact on treatment selection. Also not shown is where there is overlap between the mutations, i.e., where a person's cancer cells contain more than one driver mutation. *Source:* Adapted from [33].

panel, can be used to find patients with rare, resistance-causing mutations [34, 35].

Be aware that the pie chart does not include mention of angiogenesis inhibitors. This omission is due to our lack of biomarkers to predict response or resistance to this group of treatments [36]. At the current time, angiogenesis inhibitors are generally offered to patients whose tumors are predicted to be resistant to EGFR-targeted antibodies, or where there's no other effective treatment available.

Remember also that there is enormous interest in identifying cell surface proteins that could be targeted with an ADC. Hundreds of these treatments are in trials for virtually every cancer type, including bowel cancer.

Table 7.6   A summary of treatment approaches relevant for people with bowel cancer or anal cancer [28, 29, 33, 36–40].

	MSS bowel cancer	MSI bowel cancer	Anal cancer
Targeted therapies matched with mutations and/or protein expression	Yes: • EGFR-targeted treatments • B-Raf inhibitors • HER2-targeted treatments • K-Ras G12C inhibitors • TRK inhibitors • RET inhibitors	Yes: • B-Raf inhibitors	
Targeted therapy: angiogenesis inhibitors	Yes	Yes	Not yet
Targeted therapy: antibody-drug conjugates	Yes: targeting HER2	Not yet but seems promising	Not yet but seems promising
Immunotherapy with checkpoint inhibitors	No, but there may be some people who would benefit from them Might also add to the benefit derived from chemotherapy	Yes	Yes

7.3.2 Treatments for Bowel Cancer

Table 7.7   Targets and treatments for people with MSS bowel cancer.

Relevant targets	Treatment approach	Treatment examples	Relevant book sections
EGFR	EGFR-targeted antibodies	Cetuximab, panitumumab	Section 3.4.1
BRAF V600E mutation	B-Raf inhibitors + EGFR antibodies	Encorafenib + cetuximab	Section 3.7.5
KRAS G12C mutation	K-Ras G12C inhibitors + EGFR antibodies	Sotorasib + panitumumab, adagrasib + cetuximab	Section 3.7.4
HER2 amplified	HER2-targeted therapies, often two together	Trastuzumab, pertuzumab, lapatinib, tucatinib, trastuzumab deruxtecan	Section 3.5
MET amplified	MET-targeted treatments	Capmatinib, tivantinib	Section 3.6.3

Table 7.7 (Continued)

Kinase fusion proteins including the kinase domain of ALK, ROS1, NTRK1/2/3, or RET proteins	ALK inhibitors	Crizotinib, alectinib, ceritinib	Section 3.6.5
	ROS1 inhibitors	Crizotinib	
	TRKA/B/C inhibitors	Larotrectinib, entrectinib	Section 3.6.6
	RET inhibitors	Selpercatinib	Section 3.6.4
Angiogenesis	Angiogenesis inhibitors	Bevacizumab, regorafenib, lenvatinib, fruquitinib	Section 4.1
Immunotherapy for patients with a high Immunoscore	Immune checkpoint inhibitors targeting PD-1, PD-L1 or CTLA-4	Pembrolizumab, nivolumab, ipilimumab	Chapter 5

Table 7.8 Targets and treatments for MSI or *POLE*-mutant bowel cancer.

Relevant targets	Treatment approach	Treatment examples	Relevant book sections
Sensitivity of MSI or *POLE* mutated bowel cancer to immunotherapy	Immune checkpoint inhibitors targeting PD-1, PD-L1 or CTLA-4	Pembrolizumab, nivolumab, ipilimumab	Chapter 5
20% of MSI bowel cancers also contain the *BRAF* V600E mutation	B-Raf targeting is a potential option [40]	As for MSS bowel cancer	Section 3.7.5

7.3.3 Treatments for Anal Cancer

The most common type of anal cancer is squamous cell carcinoma (SCC), which develops from the cells that line the anal canal and the edge of the anus. The main risk factor is infection with the human papillomavirus (HPV) – usually HPV-16 (a common, cancer-causing version of HPV) [41, 42].

Cancers that are caused by viral infections have features that make immunotherapy an attractive option [42, 43]. For example, the presence of virus proteins is a powerful stimulus to the immune system and can lead to the activation of T cells. Checkpoint inhibitors, such as nivolumab (PD-1), retifanlimab (PD-1), pembrolizumab (PD-1), and ipilimumab (CTLA-4), have all been investigated as possible treatments for anal cancer either alone or combined with other treatments [38, 39].

When used alone, the response rate for checkpoint inhibitor therapy has so far been in the range of 10%–25% [38]. Other types of immunotherapy, such as treatment vaccines and adoptive cell therapies, are also in trials.

7.4 TREATMENTS FOR LUNG CANCER

Lung cancers are divided into two main types: non-small-cell lung cancer (NSCLC) and small cell lung cancer (SCLC). NSCLCs are by far the most common, accounting for around 80%–85% of lung cancers diagnosed in the UK [44].

A much rarer cancer is mesothelioma, which develops in the lining around the lungs rather than the lungs themselves.

7.4.1 Treatment Targets in NSCLC

Within NSCLC, some subdivisions have important implications regarding their sensitivity to various treatments. For example, the two most common types of NSCLC are adenocarcinomas and squamous cell carcinomas (for practical reasons they're often just divided into squamous and non-squamous carcinomas).

Many of the mutations that create targetable, over-active kinases (such as *EGFR* mutations, *ALK* mutations, and *ROS1* mutations) are much more common in people with adenocarcinoma NSCLC than squamous cell NSCLC [45]. Roughly 50% of adenocarcinomas contain a potentially targetable mutation (Figure 7.3) [46–50].

Even when potentially targetable mutations exist in a person with squamous cell NSCLC, matching mutations with targeted treatments hasn't been effective in trials [51].

Another important division in NSCLC is between those that develop in people with a history of smoking (or of using other tobacco products) versus people who have had no, or only a very limited, exposure to tobacco. Lung cancers in people who have never smoked or used tobacco are more likely to be adenocarcinomas and to contain targetable mutations such as *EGFR* mutations [52]. In contrast, people with a history of smoking might develop either an adenocarcinoma or a squamous cell carcinoma. They are much more likely to benefit from checkpoint inhibitor immunotherapy than a person who has never smoked. This is presumably due to the high number of mutations found in the cancer cells of smokers and ex-smokers, and their visibility to the immune system [53].

Lastly, angiogenesis inhibitors have also proven to be useful treatments for people with lung cancer, with a few caveats: [54]

- Problems with side effects mean that they're less likely to be given to someone with squamous cell lung cancer.

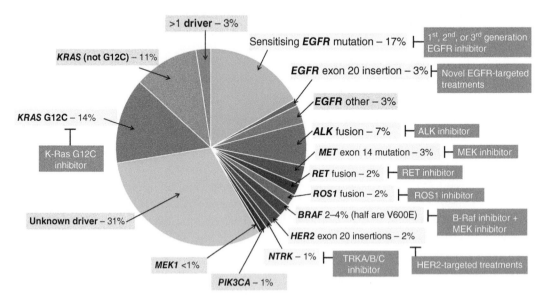

Figure 7.3 Targetable mutations in adenocarcinoma NSCLC. A pie-chart showing some of the mutations found in the cancer cells of people with adenocarcinoma NSCLC and the matching treatment approach for each mutation. Pink text boxes denote mutations for which there is not yet an established tailored treatment approach.

- Their effects tend to be modest, and they're usually combined with other treatments, such as targeted therapy, immunotherapy, and/or chemotherapy.
- As in other cancers, we don't have any biomarkers to help us identify patients

who would derive the greatest benefit from them.

Below, I provide more detail as to the targeted therapies and immunotherapies that are licensed or that look particularly promising as treatments for people with NSCLC.

Table 7.9   A summary of relevant treatment approaches for NSCLC, with or without actionable mutations.[a]

	NSCLC with actionable mutations	NSCLCs without actionable mutations
Targeted therapies matched with mutations and/or protein expression	**Yes:** • **Kinase inhibitors targeting: EGFR, ALK, ROS1, MET, RET, HER2, K-Ras G12C, B-Raf, TRKA/B/C** • **Dual-targeted EGFR and MET antibody**	**No**
Targeted therapy: angiogenesis inhibitors	**Yes: combined with other treatments**	**Yes: combined with other treatments**
Targeted therapy: antibody-drug conjugates	**Yes: targets include HER2, HER3, TROP2, MET, CEACAM5**	
Immunotherapy with immune checkpoint inhibitors	**Immune checkpoint inhibitors are less effective in this group of patients, but they may be helpful if combined with other treatments**	**Yes**

[a] Defined as mutations that can be matched to a specific targeted treatment approach such as an EGFR inhibitor or an ALK inhibitor.

7.4.2 Treatments for NSCLCs <u>with</u> an Actionable Mutation

Table 7.10   Targets and treatments for people with NSCLC with an actionable mutation.

Relevant targets	Treatment approach	Treatment examples	Relevant book sections
EGFR sensitizing mutations, e.g., L858R, ex19del	First, second, or third generation EGFR inhibitors	Erlotinib, gefitinib, afatinib, dacomitinib, osimertinib, lazertinib	Section 3.4.2
	EGFR and MET dual-targeted antibodies	Amivantamab	
EGFR exon 20 insertions	Potent inhibitors of EGFR	Mobocertinib, poziotinib	
	EGFR and MET dual-targeted antibodies	Amivantamab	
ALK fusion proteins	First, second, or third generation ALK inhibitors	Crizotinib, ceritinib, alectinib, brigatinib, lorlatinib, ensartinib	Section 3.6.5
ROS1 fusion proteins	ROS1 inhibitors	Crizotinib, entrectinib	
NTRK gene fusions	TRKA/B/C inhibitors	Entrectinib, larotrectinib, repotrectinib	Section 3.6.6

(Continued)

Table 7.10 (Continued)

Relevant targets	Treatment approach	Treatment examples	Relevant book sections
BRAF V600E mutation	B-Raf inhibitor + MEK inhibitor combinations	Dabrafenib + trametinib	Section 3.7.5
MET exon 14 skipping mutations	MET inhibitors	Capmatinib, tepotinib	Section 3.6.3
RET fusion proteins	RET inhibitors	Pralsetinib, selpercatinib	Section 3.6.4
HER2-altered NSCLCs[a]	HER2-targeted kinase inhibitors	Pyrotinib, poziotinib	Section 3.5
	HER2-targeted ADCs	Trastuzumab deruxtecan	
KRAS G12C mutation	K-Ras G12C inhibitors	Adagrasib, sotorasib	Section 3.7.4
Cell surface protein: HER3	ADCs targeting HER3	Patritumab deruxtecan	Section 3.6.7
Cell surface protein: MET	ADCs targeting MET	Telisotuzumab vedotin	Section 3.6.3

[a] This includes NSCLCs in which the *HER2* gene is mutated or amplified, and/or where the HER2 protein is over-expressed.

7.4.3 Targets and Treatments for NSCLCs <u>Without</u> an Actionable Mutation

Table 7.11 Targets and treatments for people with NSCLC that are not known to contain an actionable mutation.

Relevant targets	Treatment approach	Treatment examples	Relevant book sections
Immune checkpoint proteins on T cells	Immune checkpoint inhibitors targeting PD-1 or PD-L1	Nivolumab, pembrolizumab, durvalumab, atezolizumab, cemiplimab	Chapter 5
	Immune checkpoint inhibitors targeting CTLA-4	Ipilimumab, tremelimumab	
Cell surface protein: TROP2	ADCs targeting TROP2	Datopotamab deruxtecan, sacituzumab govitecan	Section 4.2
Cell surface protein: HER3	ADCs targeting HER3	Patritumab deruxtecan	
Cell surface protein: MET	ADCs targeting MET	Telisotuzumab vedotin	
Cell surface protein: CEACAM5	ADCs targeting CEACAM5	Tusamitamab ravtansine	
Angiogenesis	Angiogenesis inhibitors	Bevacizumab, nintedanib (non-sq only); ramucirumab	Section 4.1

Abbreviations: ADC – antibody-drug conjugate; non-sq – non-squamous NSCLC.

7.4.4 Treatments for Small Cell Lung Cancer

Small-cell lung cancer (SCLC) is an incredibly aggressive disease. Although it generally responds to chemotherapy and radiotherapy, it rapidly becomes resistant, and people often only survive a few months. Because it almost always develops in smokers, the cells of SCLC have one of the highest levels of DNA mutations of any cancer [55].

You might be tempted to think that this high number of mutations would make SCLC highly sensitive to immune checkpoint inhibitor therapy, but you'd be wrong [56]. Granted, checkpoint inhibitors (atezolizumab and durvalumab) combined with chemotherapy are licensed treatments for some people with SCLC. However, many immunotherapy trials have failed to demonstrate any meaningful benefit [56].

In addition, the two most common mutations found in SCLC are not ones that we can effectively target (they are *RB* and *TP53* mutations) [57]. Cell surface proteins that are targetable with ADCs look more promising. The first ADC to enter a Phase 3 trial in SCLC (an ADC called rovalpituzumab tesirine that targets DLL3) was later withdrawn and the trial was stopped due to poor results [58]. However, a second DLL-targeted treatment, a T cell engager targeting DLL3 and CD3 called tarlatamab, was approved by the FDA in May 2024 [59] (for an idea of its structure, look at Figure 6.18d). Other potential cell surface targets include CD56 (the target of lorvotuzumab mertansine) and TROP2, a target being explored in many cancer types [60].

7.4.5 Treatments for Mesothelioma

Mesothelioma is almost always linked to exposure to asbestos, a naturally occurring mineral that comes in various forms. Asbestos fibers irritate and inflame the lining of the lungs as white blood cells attempt, but fail, to destroy them. This unresolved (chronic) inflammation creates an environment that creates, supports, and protects faulty cells. Through a gradual process of mutation and evolution, these cells ultimately cause mesothelioma. The whole process usually takes several decades [61].

Common mutations in mesothelioma include those affecting tumor suppressor genes such as *CDKN2A* and *BAP1* [61]. As I've mentioned before, these aren't the sort of mutations that we can currently target.

In recent years, immune checkpoint inhibitors such as nivolumab and ipilimumab have

become important treatments for people with mesothelioma. Trials such as CheckMate 743 have proven to increase the proportion of long-term survivors [62, 63]. Various trials involving checkpoint inhibitors combined with other treatments, such as chemotherapy and/or angiogenesis inhibitors, are ongoing. Angiogenesis inhibitors are also combined with chemotherapy [64].

7.5 TREATMENTS FOR PROSTATE, TESTICULAR, AND PENILE CANCERS

Although the affected sites are close to one another in location, the treatments that are effective against prostate, testicular, and penile cancers are very different. With prostate cancer, the focus for many decades has been on the creation of more and more potent hormone therapies. In contrast, chemotherapy has been extremely successful in curing most patients with testicular cancer, with just a handful of other treatments in trials. In penile cancer, the current focus is on the potential of immunotherapy with checkpoint inhibitors.

7.5.1 Treatment Targets in Prostate Cancer

As I've just said, the most important target in prostate cancer is the androgen receptor. This receptor protein is found inside the cells of virtually 100% of prostate cancers and is vitally important for their growth and survival [65, 66]. It is normally activated by the circulating hormones testosterone and dihydrotestosterone. In their presence, androgen receptors pair up, move into the cell's nucleus, attach to genes, and force the cell to make a wide range of proteins (they are a type of transcription factor).

Hormone therapies either work by blocking the production of androgens or by blocking the actions of androgen receptors [67].

If prostate cancer becomes resistant to hormone therapies, it's often referred to as being "castration-resistant." Yet, scientists believe that many of these cancers remain dependent on androgen receptors and might yet respond to a more powerful hormone therapy or one that works through a novel mechanism [67].

Because this book is all about targeted therapies and immunotherapies, I'm not going to discuss hormone therapies further, but there's plenty of information online [67, 68]. Another treatment approach that I don't cover in this book, but that is given as a systemic treatment for prostate cancer, is the radioactive isotopes that relieve bone pain and treat bone metastases, which are common metastases in prostate cancer [69]. These treatments include Strontium-89, Samarium-153, Rhenium-186, Rhenium-188, and Radium-223. My reason for not discussing them is that they target the bone rather than directly targeting cancer cells or the cancer microenvironment.

Aside from the strides made with hormone therapies, we've made very little progress in creating effective targeted therapies or immunotherapies for prostate cancer. This is for reasons, such as: [70]

- The most common mutations in prostate cancer are not ones we can currently target,

such as the mutation that creates a fusion between the *TMPRSS2* and *ERG* genes (see Section 1.2.2).
- Prostate cancers tend to contain relatively few mutations and very few T cells, and the microenvironment is generally very immune suppressing. Thus far, immunotherapies tested as treatments for prostate cancer haven't been very helpful.

Despite these problems, there are some promising strategies for hormone therapy-resistant prostate cancer, such as: [70–78]

- PARP inhibitors for prostate cancers with defects in homologous recombination due to a *BRCA* gene defect or other mutation, or given regardless of the presence of a mutation in combination with hormone therapy.
- Radioactively-labeled ligands and antibodies that attach to cell surface proteins such as PSMA (prostate-specific membrane antigen).
- Treatments that can block mutated versions of the androgen receptor found in the cells of hormone therapy-resistant prostate cancer.
- Targeting the PI3K pathway. *PTEN* loss and other mutations that affect this pathway are common in prostate cancer, and AKT inhibitors are in trials.
- Immune checkpoint inhibitors for the 2%–3% that are MSI.

Table 7.12   A summary of treatment approaches relevant to prostate cancer.

	Prostate cancers sensitive to standard hormone therapies	Prostate cancers resistant to standard hormone therapies
Hormone therapy	Yes	Yes: these cancers are often still reliant on their androgen receptors for growth and survival
Targeted therapies matched with mutations and/or protein expression	Not yet	Yes: PARP inhibitors are often matched to *BRCA* gene and other mutations
Targeted therapy: angiogenesis inhibitors	No	No

Table 7.12 (Continued)

Targeted therapy: antibody-drug conjugates	No	None licensed yet. Possible targets include PSMA, TROP2, STEAP1, tissue factor, DLL-3, B7-H3, CD46, and HER2
Targeted therapy: radioactively labeled ligands and antibodies	Possibly	Yes: targeting PSMA
Immunotherapy with checkpoint inhibitors	Seems unlikely	Not in general, but possibly for the fraction that exhibits MSI

In the tables below I have again split the targets and treatments according to their relevance to people with hormone therapy-sensitive or castration-resistant prostate cancer.

However, please do note a couple of things before looking at the tables:

1. What we call "hormone therapy-sensitive" or "castration-resistant" disease changes over time as new hormone therapies come along. For example, prostate cancer that is resistant to an older hormone therapy (and which used to be considered castration-resistant) is likely to still respond to a more potent treatment such as enzalutamide. Cancers that are resistant to enzalutamide (and are now thought of as being castration-resistant) might yet be sensitive to an even newer, and more potent, hormone therapy that doesn't yet exist.

2. Treatments that are currently only pre-scribed if hormone therapy has stopped working might yet be combined with hormone therapy in the future (i.e., given to people with hormone therapy-sensitive cancer) if this is found to be worthwhile in trials.

7.5.2 Treatments for Hormone Therapy-Sensitive Prostate Cancer

Table 7.13 Targets and treatments for hormone-sensitive prostate cancer.

Relevant targets	Treatment approach	Treatment examples	Relevant book sections
Production of androgen by the testes and other tissues	LHRH/GnRH agonists	Goserelin, leuprorelin, buserelin, triptorelin, histrelin	Not covered, see [67, 68]
	LHRH/GnRH antagonists	Degarelix, relugolix	
	CYP17A1 enzyme blockers	Abiraterone	
Activity of androgen receptors	Androgen receptor antagonists & anti-androgens	Bicalutamide, nilutamide, flutamide, cyproterone, enzalutamide, apalutamide, darolutamide	Not covered, see [67, 68]

Abbreviations: GnRH – gonadotropin-releasing hormone; LHRH – luteinizing hormone-releasing hormone.

7.5.3 Treatments for Castration-Resistant Prostate Cancer

Table 7.14 Targets and treatments for castration-resistant prostate cancer.

Relevant targets	Treatment approach	Treatment examples	Relevant book sections
Mutated versions of the androgen receptor found in castration-resistant prostate cancer	Novel hormone therapies targeting the androgen receptor	Masofaniten, AR-V7 antagonists, bavdegalutamide	Not covered, see [76–78]
Homologous recombination deficiency	PARP inhibitors	Olaparib, niraparib, rucaparib, talazoparib	Section 4.3
PSMA (prostate-specific membrane antigen)	Radioactively-labeled ligands for PSMA	^{177}Lu-PSMA-617, ^{225}Ac-PSMA-617, ^{225}Ac-PSMA-I&T	Section 4.2.7
	Radioactively-labeled antibodies that target PSMA	^{177}Lu-DOTA-rosopatamab, ^{225}Ac-pelgifatamab	Section 4.2.7
Cell surface proteins	ADCs	ADCs targeting PSMA, TROP2, STEAP1, tissue factor, DLL-3, B7-H3, CD46, and HER2	Section 4.2 Also see [73, 74]

7.5.4 Treatments for Testicular Cancer

More than 90% of testicular cancers begin in the germ cells – the cells in the testes that produce sperm. Most testicular cancers are highly sensitive to chemotherapy, even when the cancer has spread, and most patients are cured [79]. In chemotherapy-resistant testicular cancer, immunotherapy with checkpoint inhibitors has been tried but doesn't appear to be helpful [80]. Possible cell surface proteins in testicular cancer that can be used as targets for ADCs or novel immunotherapies (such as CAR T cells) include CLDN6 (Claudin 6) and CD30 [79, 81]. Another possible target is PARP [79].

7.5.5 Treatments for Penile Cancer

In contrast to testicular cancer, penile cancer is often resistant to chemotherapy. Penile cancers tend to either be associated with HPV infection or with skin inflammation [82].

Several clinical trials are exploring the usefulness of immune checkpoint inhibitors as treatments for penile cancer [83, 84]. In some of these trials, the checkpoint inhibitor is combined with another treatment such as chemotherapy or a PARP inhibitor.

Some penile cancers express EGFR. EGFR-targeted treatments have only been given to small numbers of patients, so it's difficult to know whether they might be helpful [85]. In addition, in a quarter of cases, there is HER2 on the surface of the patient's cancer cells, and this could be targeted with an ADC such as trastuzumab deruxtecan [86].

7.6 TREATMENTS FOR HEAD AND NECK CANCER

Head and neck cancers include, at least anatomically, cancers of the mouth, nose, lymph nodes, sinuses, salivary glands, throat, and neck, including the thyroid gland. However, different countries and organizations use different criteria as to what to include under this umbrella. I'm just going to look at head and neck squamous cell carcinoma (HNSCC), and thyroid cancer, as these are the most common types of head and neck cancer in the UK [87].

7.6.1 Treatment Targets for Head and Neck Squamous Cell Cancer and Thyroid Cancer

HNSCC develops in the mucosal lining of the mouth, pharynx, or larynx. Exposure to tobacco (through smoking or chewing it), drinking a lot of alcohol, and HPV infection (generally transmitted through sexual contact) are important causes.

As in bowel cancer, the cancer cells of HNSCC often have excessive amounts of unmutated EGFR on their surface. An EGFR-targeted antibody combined with chemotherapy has been a standard treatment approach for over 20 years [88].

More recently, it's been checkpoint inhibitor immunotherapy that has taken over in terms of the number of trials that have been undertaken or that are currently underway [89]. These trials have led to improved survival times when checkpoint inhibitors are combined with chemotherapy for people with advanced disease. However, the results of some trials have been negative, particularly when checkpoint inhibitors have been combined with both chemotherapy and radiotherapy [90].

Other treatment approaches in trials for HNSCC include a wide range of ADCs targeted against cell surface proteins [91].

Thyroid cancer treatments are very different from those of HNSCC. Thyroid cancers commonly contain relatively few mutations overall (especially compared to a genetically complex HNSCC in a person with a history of tobacco use). However, thyroid cancers do often contain powerful driver mutations, some of which are targetable with current treatments [92, 93].

For example, one of the most common types of thyroid cancer, papillary thyroid carcinoma, often contains a *BRAF* mutation or a *RET* gene rearrangement. In addition, *RET* mutations are common in a much rarer form of thyroid cancer, medullary thyroid cancer. *BRAF* mutations also occur in another rare type of thyroid cancer, anaplastic thyroid cancer.

An important class of treatments approved for thyroid cancer is the angiogenesis inhibitors (also called multi-kinase inhibitors) such as lenvatinib, sorafenib, cabozantinib, and vandetanib. All these agents target multiple kinases involved in angiogenesis and other kinases such as RET. Recently, much more selective RET inhibitors (pralsetinib, selpercatinib) have given impressive results in clinical trials [94].

Table 7.15 A summary of treatment approaches relevant to head and neck squamous cell carcinoma and thyroid cancer.

	Head and neck squamous cell carcinoma	Thyroid cancer
Targeted therapies matched with mutations and/or protein expression	Yes: • EGFR-targeted treatments	Yes: • RET-targeted treatments • B-Raf + MEK inhibitors
Targeted therapy: angiogenesis inhibitors	Not yet, but several are in trials	Yes (but some/most of their effects could be due to RET inhibition)
Targeted therapy: antibody-drug conjugates	Not yet, although an EGFR-targeted ADC is approved for use in Japan (cetuximab saratolacan) Other targets include: Nectin-4, HER2 (salivary gland cancer), tissue factor, TROP2	None licensed yet. Possible targets include ICAM1
Immunotherapy with immune checkpoint inhibitors	Yes	Not yet

7.6.2 Treatments for Head and Neck Squamous Cell Carcinoma

Table 7.16   Targets and treatments for people with head and neck squamous cell carcinoma.

Relevant targets	Treatment approach	Treatment examples	Relevant book sections
EGFR	EGFR-targeted antibodies	Cetuximab	Section 3.4.1
Immune checkpoint proteins on T cells	Immune checkpoint inhibitors targeting PD-1 or PD-L1	Nivolumab, pembrolizumab, toripalimab	Chapter 5
Various cell surface proteins	ADCs	ADCs targeting EGFR, TROP2, Integrin-beta6, tissue factor, CD44v6, CD166, CD71, ROR2	Section 4.2

7.6.3 Treatments for Thyroid Cancer

Table 7.17   Targets and treatments for people with thyroid cancer.

Relevant targets	Treatment approach	Treatment examples	Relevant book sections
Angiogenesis (RET?)	Multi-kinase inhibitors	Cabozantinib, vandetanib, lenvatinib, sorafenib	Section 4.1
RET	RET inhibitors	Pralsetinib, selpercatinib	Section 3.6.4
BRAF V600E mutation	B-Raf inhibitor + MEK inhibitor combinations	Dabrafenib + trametinib	Section 3.7.5

7.7 TREATMENTS FOR ESOPHAGEAL, GASTROESOPHAGEAL JUNCTION, AND STOMACH CANCERS

The esophagus, gastroesophageal junction (GEJ), and stomach form a continual tube. It's therefore not surprising that cancers that develop in these locations have overlapping properties. This is particularly true when you look at adenocarcinomas affecting the lower third of the esophagus, the GEJ, and the stomach [95, 96].

In contrast, cancers of the top portion of the esophagus are usually squamous cell carcinomas and have more in common with HNSCC [96].

7.7.1 Treatment Targets in Esophageal, GEJ, and Stomach Cancer

As of Spring 2024, the only targeted therapies approved as treatments for esophageal, GEJ, or stomach (gastric) cancer are HER2-targeted treatments (for patients with HER2-positive cancers) and angiogenesis inhibitors. This is despite many large clinical trials testing out targeted therapies such as cetuximab and panitumumab, both of which are EGFR-targeted antibodies [97]. It is also despite a growing understanding of the distinctions between different types (squamous cell vs. adenocarcinoma) and subtypes of these diseases.

More progress has been made with immunotherapy using immune checkpoint inhibitors, which have become part of the standard treatment approach for all these cancers. A large number of trials are ongoing to test out various timings and combinations, many of which include chemotherapy, radiotherapy, or additional immunotherapies. Scientists are also keen to put into practice the differences they have uncovered between different subtypes of stomach cancer. For example, around 20% of stomach cancers are known to be MSI (this reduces to about 5% in advanced stomach cancer) and are particularly sensitive to immune checkpoint inhibitors [98].

Adenocarcinomas of the GEJ and stomach also have cell surface proteins that are being explored as targets for treatments such as naked antibodies, antibody-drug conjugates, and CAR T cells. These include FGFR2 (a growth factor receptor) and claudin 18.2 (CLDN18.2) [99–101].

As well as adenocarcinoma stomach cancer, there are some rarer stomach cancers such as gastrointestinal stromal tumors (GIST), lymphoma, and neuroendocrine tumors. I'm not going to say anything more about GIST here, but the vast majority of GISTs contain a *PDGFRA* or *KIT* mutation. PDGFR and KIT inhibitors are covered in Section 3.6.1.

Table 7.18 A summary of the treatment approaches relevant to esophageal, gastroesophageal junction, and stomach cancers.

	Esophageal cancer	**GEJ cancer/stomach cancer**
Targeted therapies matched with mutations and/or protein expression	**No**	**Yes, in use:** • **HER2-targeted treatments** **In trials:** • **FGFR2b-targeted treatments**
Targeted therapy: angiogenesis inhibitors	**Not yet**	**Yes**
Targeted therapy: antibody-drug conjugates and other antibody-based treatments	**Not yet: targets include Nectin-4**	**Yes: targeting HER2** **Other targets include: CLDN18.2, TROP-2, HER3, CEACAM5**
Immunotherapy with checkpoint inhibitors	**Yes**	**Yes**

Because there is so much overlap between esophageal, GEJ, and stomach cancers, it's difficult to provide separate tables on relevant treatment approaches. I've therefore chosen to provide a single table of relevant targets and treatments in Table 7.19.

7.7.2 Treatments for Esophageal Cancer, GEJ Cancer, and Stomach Cancer

Table 7.19 Targets and treatments for esophageal cancer, GEJ cancer, or stomach cancer.

Relevant targets	Treatment approach	Treatment examples	Relevant book sections
HER2	Naked antibody therapies	Trastuzumab, pertuzumab, margetuximab	Section 3.5
	ADCs	Trastuzumab emtansine, trastuzumab deruxtecan	Sections 3.5 and 4.2
	HER2-targeted kinase inhibitors	Lapatinib, neratinib, tucatinib	Section 3.5
FGFR2	Naked antibody therapies	Bemarituzumab	Section 3.6.2
	FGFR2-targeted kinase inhibitors	Erdafitinib, pemigatinib	Section 3.6.2

(Continued)

Table 7.19 (Continued)

Relevant targets	Treatment approach	Treatment examples	Relevant book sections
Claudin 18.2	Various antibody-based treatments	Zolbetuximab	Section 2.2.7
Angiogenesis	Angiogenesis inhibitors	Bevacizumab, ramucirumab	Section 4.1
Immune checkpoint proteins on T cells	Immune checkpoint inhibitors targeting PD-1, PD-L1 or CTLA-4	Nivolumab, pembrolizumab, tislelizumab, ipilimumab	Chapter 5

7.8 TREATMENTS FOR PANCREATIC, BILE DUCT, AND PRIMARY LIVER CANCERS

7.8.1 Treatment Targets in Pancreatic, Bile Duct, and Primary Liver Cancer

Pancreatic Cancer

Pancreatic cancer, more than 90% of which are pancreatic ductal adenocarcinomas (PDACs), is one of the most difficult cancers to treat successfully (the other main group of pancreatic cancers are the pancreatic neuroendocrine tumors, which I mention later). I could fill an entire book with all the treatment approaches that have been tried, but that have failed to make a positive difference for people diagnosed with PDAC.

There are various aspects of PDAC that make it incredibly difficult to treat: [102–104]

- It is generally diagnosed after it has started to spread.
- The cancer cells sit in an impenetrable network of fibrous proteins called desmoplasia, hindering drugs' ability to penetrate.
- Cancer cells are protected by other cell types in their environment, such as cancer-associated fibroblasts.
- There are very few blood vessels in pancreatic cancers, and those that do exist are squashed and flattened – again, hindering drugs' penetration.

- The most common mutations (*KRAS*, *TP53*, *SMAD4*, and *CDKN2A*) cannot be usefully matched to existing targeted therapies.
- Cancer cells often spread via nerve bundles, where they are protected from cancer treatments.
- The immune microenvironment is dominated by immune-suppressing and cancer-protecting white blood cells, such as regulatory T cells, myeloid-derived suppressor cells, and tumor-associated macrophages. There is generally little evidence of a useful immune response that could be enhanced by immunotherapy.

A recent (albeit limited) success has come from the use of PARP inhibitors for the small proportion of patients with PDAC who have inherited a *BRCA* gene mutation [105]. In addition, as I mentioned briefly back in Section 3.7.4, scientists are now making progress in creating inhibitors of mutated forms of K-Ras found in pancreatic cancer cells. These include inhibitors of K-Ras G12D, a mutated form of K-Ras found in around 45% of cases. Unlike in lung cancer, where *KRAS* gene mutations seem to be a late event, and therefore only found in a proportion of a person's cancer cells, *KRAS* mutations in PDAC appear to be an initiating event – present in every cancer cell [106]. This makes K-Ras inhibitors a promising treatment approach for *KRAS*-mutated PDAC. Lastly, around 1%–2% of PDAC are MSI and therefore could be sensitive to immune checkpoint inhibitors [107].

Primary Liver Cancer

In contrast to PDAC, we have made significant progress in developing targeted therapies and immunotherapies for people with primary liver cancer (called hepatocellular carcinoma). Various combinations involving checkpoint inhibitors and angiogenesis inhibitors have proven useful. Scientists and doctors are keen to build on this progress and many more combinations are in trials [108].

Bile Duct Cancer (Cholangiocarcinoma)

There's also progress to report in the treatment of people with bile duct cancer

(also called cholangiocarcinoma). Mutations found in the cells of this cancer include those in *IDH1* and *IDH2* (in 10%–23% of patients), *FGFR2* (in 13%–20%), and *BRAF* V600E (in ~5%). Around 15%–20% of cases contain a *HER2* gene amplification and/or overexpress HER2 protein [109]. In addition, a small proportion (roughly 2%) are MSI and have a high likelihood of being sensitive to checkpoint inhibitor immunotherapy [110, 111].

ADCs targeted at various cell surface proteins are in clinical trials for all three cancers [112–114].

Table 7.20 A summary of treatment approaches relevant to pancreatic ductal adenocarcinoma, primary liver cancer, and bile duct cancer.

	Pancreatic cancer (pancreatic ductal adenocarcinoma)	Primary liver cancer (hepatocellular carcinoma)	Bile duct cancer (cholangiocarcinoma)
Targeted therapies matched with mutations and/or protein expression	**Yes:** • **PARP inhibitors matched to *BRCA* gene mutations**	**No**	**Yes:** • **Kinase inhibitors targeting FGFR2** • **IDH1 inhibitors** • **B-Raf inhibitors**
Targeted therapy: angiogenesis inhibitors	**No**	**Yes**	**Not yet**
Targeted therapy: antibody-drug conjugates	**Many are in trials, but tumor penetration is likely to be an issue**	**Not yet; possible targets include GPC3, CD24**	**Not yet; possible targets include HER2, MUC1, GPC1**
Immunotherapy with checkpoint inhibitors	**Not for the vast majority of patients**	**Yes**	**Yes**

7.8.2 Treatments for Pancreatic Cancer

Table 7.21 Targets and treatments for pancreatic ductal adenocarcinoma.

Relevant targets	Treatment approach	Treatment examples	Relevant book sections
EGFR	EGFR-targeted kinase inhibitors	Erlotinib	Section 3.4.2
Inherited defects in *BRCA* genes causing genomic instability	PARP inhibitors	Olaparib	Section 4.3
Mutated K-Ras proteins	Novel K-Ras inhibitors	MRTX1133, TH-Z827, TH-Z835, KD-8	Section 3.7.4
Microsatellite instability (MSI)	Immune checkpoint inhibitors	Nivolumab, pembrolizumab	Chapter 5

7.8.3 Treatments for Primary Liver Cancer

Table 7.22   Targets and treatments for primary liver cancer.

Relevant targets	Treatment approach	Treatment examples	Relevant book sections
Angiogenesis	Angiogenesis inhibitors	Bevacizumab, ramucirumab, cabozantinib, lenvatinib, sorafenib, regorafenib	Section 4.1
Immune checkpoint proteins on T cells	Immune checkpoint inhibitors targeting PD-1 or PD-L1	Nivolumab, pembrolizumab, atezolizumab, durvalumab	Chapter 5
	Immune checkpoint inhibitors targeting CTLA-4	Tremelimumab, ipilimumab	Chapter 5

7.8.4 Treatments for Bile Duct Cancer (Cholangiocarcinoma)

Table 7.23   Targets and treatments for bile duct cancer.

Relevant targets	Treatment approach	Treatment examples	Relevant book sections
FGFR2	FGFR2-targeted kinase inhibitors	Infigratinib, pemigatinib, futibatinib, erdafitinib	Section 3.6.2
IDH1	IDH1 inhibitors	Ivosidinib	Section 4.6
BRAF V600E mutation	B-Raf inhibitors with or without MEK inhibitors	Dabrafenib + trametinib	Section 3.7.5
HER2	HER2-targeted therapies	Trastuzumab, pertuzumab	Section 3.5
Immune checkpoint proteins on T cells	Immune checkpoint inhibitors targeting PD-1 or PD-L1	Pembrolizumab, durvalumab	Chapter 5

7.8.5 Treatments for Pancreatic Neuroendocrine Tumors

Pancreatic neuroendocrine tumors (PNETs) represent around 5%–10% of pancreatic cancers. They are generally less aggressive and slower-growing cancers than PDAC, and they often develop from hormone-producing cells in the pancreas. Targeted treatments licensed for people with PNETs include sunitinib, surufatinib, and belzutifan (angiogenesis inhibitors), and everolimus (an mTOR inhibitor) [115].

Another class of treatment licensed for people with PNETs is the somatostatin analogs. These treatments block the overproduction of various hormones by PNET cells, and they improve symptoms and increase survival times. They include lanreotide, octreotide, pasireotide, and a radioactive somatostatin analogue, Lutetium Lu-177-dotatate [116].

7.8.6 Treatments for Cancers of the Small Intestine

Despite being between 4 and 6 m long, cancers of the small intestine account for only 3% of cancers of the digestive system [117]. Most are adenocarcinomas, neuroendocrine tumors, or GISTs. A proportion are MSI and likely to be sensitive to checkpoint inhibitors [111]. Angiogenesis inhibitors added to chemotherapy have also proven helpful in some people [118].

7.9 TREATMENTS FOR KIDNEY AND BLADDER CANCERS

7.9.1 Treatment Targets in Kidney and Bladder Cancer

Kidney Cancer (Renal Cell Carcinoma)

The most common type of kidney cancer is clear cell renal cell carcinoma (ccRCC). It accounts for around 75% of renal cell carcinomas (RCC).

The most important targetable gene mutations in ccRCC are those affecting the *VHL* gene. These mutations cause cells to lose the VHL tumor suppressor protein, which normally (amongst other things) prevents angiogenesis (see Section 4.1.7 for more about this gene and its role in controlling angiogenesis) [119]. Without VHL to prevent angiogenesis, ccRCCs are usually full of blood vessels and sensitive to angiogenesis inhibitors [120]. The latest iteration of angiogenesis inhibitors is the creation of treatments that target HIF-2α such as belzutifan (Section 4.1.8).

Another important set of treatments for people with ccRCC is the immune checkpoint inhibitors. Surprisingly, given ccRCC's relatively low tumor mutation burden, this cancer appears to be visible to the immune system and sensitive to immune checkpoint inhibitors [121]. People with advanced ccRCC are often prescribed a combination involving both an angiogenesis inhibitor and an immune checkpoint inhibitor, or a combination of two checkpoint inhibitors.

Bladder Cancer (Urothelial Carcinoma)

Immune checkpoint inhibitors have also become part of the standard treatment approach for people with urothelial cancer (the most common form of bladder cancer) [122, 123]. In addition, treatments targeting the growth factor receptor FGFR2 are available to 20% or so of people with bladder cancer whose cancer cells contain an *FGFR2* or *FGFR3* mutation [124].

As in many other cancer types, various ADCs have been explored as treatments for urothelial cancer, and two have been approved: enfortumab vedotin, which targets a cell surface protein called nectin-4, and sacituzumab govitecan, which targets TROP2. ADCs targeting HER2, SLITRK6, and EpCAM are also in trials [125].

There are also two treatment vaccines approved for people with non-muscle invasive bladder cancer (where the cancer is still just in the inner lining of the bladder and hasn't penetrated more deeply). These are the BCG vaccine and nadofaragene firadenovec. Lastly, a novel immunotherapy called nogapendekin alfa inbakicept was approved by the FDA in April 2024. This treatment is designed to activate NK cells and cytotoxic T cells [126].

Table 7.24 A summary of treatment approaches relevant for clear cell renal cell carcinoma and urothelial cancer.

	Clear cell renal cell carcinoma	Urothelial cancer
Targeted therapies matched with mutations and/or protein expression	No	Yes: • Kinase inhibitors targeting FGFR2 or FGFR3
Targeted therapy: angiogenesis inhibitors	Yes: usually a kinase inhibitor rather than bevacizumab	No
Targeted therapy: antibody-drug conjugates	Not yet; possible targets include CD70, ENPP3, CDH6	Yes: targeting nectin-4, TROP2, SLITRK6, HER2, EpCAM
Immunotherapy with checkpoint inhibitors	Yes	Yes
Other immunotherapies	Yes: IL-2	Yes: BCG vaccine, nadofaragene firadenovec, nogapendekin alfa inbakicept

7.9.2 Treatments for Clear Cell Renal Cell Carcinoma

Table 7.25   Targets and treatments for clear cell renal cell carcinoma.

Relevant targets	Treatment approach	Treatment examples	Relevant book sections
Angiogenesis	Naked antibodies targeting VEGF	Bevacizumab	Section 4.1
	Kinase inhibitors targeting VEGFRs, PDGFRs, etc.	Axitinib, cabozantinib, tivozanib, lenvatinib, sorafenib, sunitinib, pazopinib	Section 4.1
	mTOR inhibitors	Everolimus, temsirolimus	Section 4.1
	HIF-2a inhibitors	Belzutifan	Section 4.1
Immune checkpoint proteins on T cells	Immune checkpoint inhibitors targeting PD-1 or PD-L1	Pembrolizumab, nivolumab, avelumab	Chapter 5
	Immune checkpoint inhibitors targeting CTLA-4	Ipilimumab	Chapter 5

7.9.3 Treatments for Urothelial Carcinoma

Table 7.26   Targets and treatments for urothelial carcinoma.

Relevant targets	Treatment approach	Treatment examples	Relevant book sections
FGFR2/3	FGFR2-targeted kinase inhibitors	Infigratinib, pemigatinib, futibatinib, erdafitinib	Section 3.6.2
Cell surface protein: Nectin-4	ADCs	Enfortumab vedotin	Section 4.2
Cell surface protein: TROP2	ADCs	Sacituzumab govitecan	Section 4.2
Immune checkpoint proteins on T cells	Immune checkpoint inhibitors targeting PD-1 or PD-L1	Pembrolizumab, nivolumab, avelumab	Chapter 5
Unknown	Enhance cancer cell recognition by the immune system	BCG vaccine	Section 6.10
Unknown	An adenovirus carrying the gene for Interferon-alpha 2b, which activates and immune response	Nadofaragene firadenovec	Not covered
Interleukin-15 (IL-15)	An IL-15 "superagonist" that activates NK cells and T cells	Nogapendekin alfa inbakicept	Not covered

7.9.4 Treatments for Other Kidney Cancers

Aside from ccRCC, other forms of RCC include papillary RCC and chromophobe RCC. Papillary RCC is generally an aggressive disease, whereas chromophobe RCC is more slow-growing.

Immune checkpoint inhibitors (a PD-1 or PD-L1 antibody alone, combined with a CTLA-4 antibody, or combined with an angiogenesis inhibitor) have been explored as treatments for these cancers. They appear to be helpful for some patients with papillary RCC, but less likely to help people with chromophobe RCC [127].

7.10 TREATMENTS FOR OVARIAN CANCER

7.10.1 Treatment Targets in Ovarian Cancer

Around 80% of newly diagnosed ovarian cancers are high-grade serous ovarian cancers (HGSOC)[3]. Many of the most common mutations in HGSOC are not targetable with current treatments (e.g., *TP53, NF1, RB1, CDK12*) [128].

In recent years, the main focus of clinical research into targeted treatments for people with HGSOC has been on the use of PARP inhibitors (see Section 4.3). These treatments can be effective against HGSOCs that are sensitive to platinum-based chemotherapy, and those in which the cancer cells are unable to perform homologous recombination due to a *BRCA* gene defect or other mechanism [129]. Researchers have been testing out various timings, durations, combinations,

and biomarkers, to get the best out of these treatments. Angiogenesis inhibitors are also an established treatment option.

HGSOC is generally seen as a cold, immune-suppressing cancer. The cancer cells tend to have a low mutation burden and are not MSI. Clinical trials in which immune checkpoint inhibitors have been given to patients with ovarian cancer have generally reported no, or minimal, benefits [130].

ADCs may be more successful as treatments for ovarian cancer. Mirvetuximab soravtansine is an ADC that targets the folate receptor-alpha (FRα). It has been approved for the roughly 35% of patients with HGSOC in whom FRα is found on at least 75% of their cancer cells. Other ADCs in trials for people with HGSOC include those that target NaPi2, HER2, tissue factor, mesothelin, MUC16, protein tyrosine kinase 7, and TROP2 [131].

In contrast to HGSOC, low-grade serous ovarian cancer (LGSOC) tends to be slower growing. Clinical research is focused on the use of hormone therapies, CDK4/6 inhibitors, and treatments that target the MAPK pathway (B-Raf or MEK inhibitors) or PI3K pathway [132, 133].

Table 7.27   A summary of treatment approaches relevant to serous ovarian cancer.

	High-grade serous ovarian cancer	Low-grade serous ovarian cancer
Targeted therapies matched with mutations and/or protein expression	Yes: PARP inhibitors, often matched to homologous recombination deficiency	Not yet
Targeted therapy: angiogenesis inhibitors	Yes	Not yet
Targeted therapy: antibody-drug conjugates	Yes: targeting FRα Other possible targets include NaPi2, tissue factor, mesothelin, MUC16, protein tyrosine kinase 7, TROP2, HER2	No
Immunotherapy with checkpoint inhibitors	No	No

---

[3] As in other parts of this book, I'm using the term "ovarian cancer" to include primary peritoneal and fallopian tube cancer.

7.10.2 Treatments for High-Grade Serous Ovarian Cancer

Table 7.28   Targets and treatments for high-grade serous ovarian cancer.

Relevant targets	Treatment approach	Treatment examples	Relevant book sections
Homologous recombination deficiency and platinum sensitivity	PARP inhibitors	Olaparib, talazoparib, niraparib, rucaparib	Section 4.3
Angiogenesis	Angiogenesis inhibitors	Bevacizumab	Section 4.1
Cell surface protein: FRα	ADCs targeting FRα	Mirvetuximab soravtansine	Section 4.2

7.10.3 Treatments for Low-Grade Serous Ovarian Cancer

Table 7.29   Targets and treatments for low-grade serous ovarian cancer.

Relevant targets	Treatment approach	Treatment examples	Relevant book sections
Estrogen receptors/estrogen production	Hormone therapies blocking estrogen synthesis or targeting estrogen receptors	Tamoxifen, letrozole	Not covered, see [22–24]
Angiogenesis	Angiogenesis inhibitors	Bevacizumab	Section 4.1
Overactive MAPK pathway	MEK inhibitors	Trametinib	Section 3.7.5
Overactive PI3K pathway	mTOR inhibitors	Metformin	Section 3.8

7.11 TREATMENTS FOR OTHER GYNAECOLOGICAL CANCERS

7.11.1 Treatment Targets in Endometrial, Cervical, Vulvar, and Vaginal Cancer

Endometrial (Uterine) Cancer

Endometrial cancers are a varied group of diseases – some highly aggressive, some much less so.

A relatively high proportion (around 30%) of endometrial cancers are MSI and are likely to be sensitive to checkpoint inhibitor immunotherapy. Around 3% of these occur in people with Lynch Syndrome (a condition that occurs in people with an inherited mutation in a mismatch repair gene) [134]. Checkpoint inhibitors have been approved for people with MSI endometrial cancer, and for people whose cancer is not MSI if given as part of a combination [135].

A further 7%–10% of endometrial cancers contain mutations affecting DNA Polymerase epsilon (POLE) and are "ultra-mutated." Theoretically, you'd expect these cancers to be highly sensitive to immunotherapy because of the sheer volume of mutations they contain. But, perhaps because of their inherent visibility to the immune system, POLE-mutated cancers are usually cured with standard treatments [136, 137].

Other potential targets include HER2, the PI3K pathway, and the MAPK pathway. The PI3K pathway is generally overactive due to loss of PTEN, and the MAPK pathway is overactive due to currently untargetable mutations in the KRAS gene. As in ovarian cancer, a proportion are unable to perform homologous recombination and might be sensitive to a PARP inhibitor.

Potential ADC targets in endometrial cancer include HER2, FRα, and TROP2 [138].

Cervical Cancer

Almost all cervical cancers are associated with HPV infection. The presence of this virus is necessary for cervical cancer to develop, but it is insufficient on its own to cause the disease. Perhaps because of the presence of viral proteins in cancer cells, immunotherapy with checkpoint inhibitors is effective for a proportion of patients, particularly if PD-L1 is present. Various other forms of immunotherapy, such as treatment vaccines, TILs (tumor-infiltrating lymphocytes), and CAR T cells, are in trials [139].

An ADC called tisotumab vedotin, which targets a protein called tissue factor, is also an approved treatment approach. A proportion of cervical cancers also express HER2, and

the ADC trastuzumab deruxtecan has given promising results in these patients [140]. Bevacizumab, an angiogenesis inhibitor, is licensed in combination with other treatments [141].

Vulvar and Vaginal Cancer

Approximately 40% of vulvar cancers and most vaginal cancers are associated with HPV infection [142, 143]. These cancers are rare, making clinical trials difficult to perform. Treatment approaches that have been investigated and have shown some signs of effectiveness include EGFR inhibitors, angiogenesis inhibitors, and immune checkpoint inhibitors. A small fraction of vulvar cancers express HER2 and could be sensitive to HER2-targeted therapies [144].

Table 7.30 A summary of treatment approaches relevant to endometrial, cervical, vulvar, and vaginal cancer.

	Endometrial (uterine) cancer	Cervical cancer	Vulvar and vaginal cancer
Targeted therapies matched with mutations and/or protein expression	No	No	Not yet
Targeted therapy: angiogenesis inhibitors	Yes	Yes	Not yet
Targeted therapy: antibody-drug conjugates	Potential targets include HER2, TROP2	Yes: targeting tissue factor

Other potential targets include HER2, TROP2 | No |
| Immunotherapy with checkpoint inhibitors | Yes | Yes | Not yet |
| Other forms of immunotherapy: e.g., treatment vaccines, TILs | No | Not yet | Not yet |

7.11.2 Treatments for Endometrial Cancer

Table 7.31 Targets and treatments for endometrial cancer.

Relevant targets	Treatment approach	Treatment examples	Relevant book sections
Immune checkpoint proteins on T cells	Immune checkpoint inhibitors targeting PD-1 or PD-L1	Pembrolizumab, dostarlimab	Chapter 5
Angiogenesis	Angiogenesis inhibitors	Lenvatinib	Section 4.1
Cell surface proteins	ADCs	Various targets, including HER2, FRα, and TROP2	Section 4.2

7.11.3 Treatments for Cervical Cancer

Table 7.32 Targets and treatments for cervical cancer.

Relevant targets	Treatment approach	Treatment examples	Relevant book sections
Immune checkpoint proteins on T cells	Immune checkpoint inhibitors targeting PD-1 or PD-L1	Pembrolizumab	Chapter 5
Cell surface protein: TROP2	ADCs targeting TROP2	Tisotumab vedotin	Section 4.2
Angiogenesis	Angiogenesis inhibitors	Bevacizumab	Section 4.1

7.12 TREATMENTS FOR BRAIN AND CNS CANCERS

There are over 130 different types of brain and CNS tumors. However, the most common and most aggressive type of brain tumor is glioblastoma (also called glioblastoma multiforme), an aggressive form of glioma. Gliomas are cancers derived from glial cells, the brain's support cells. Other forms of glioma include astrocytomas and oligodendrogliomas.

One of the difficulties in treating brain and CNS cancers with any systemic treatment is that these tissues are protected by the blood–brain barrier (BBB) – the less penetrable lining of blood vessels in these locations. The BBB becomes disrupted and more permeable as a brain tumor forms (it's sometimes referred to as the BTB – the blood-tumor barrier). However, the BTB still represents a barrier to the effectiveness and penetration of most cancer drugs, including small molecules and monoclonal antibodies [145, 146].

7.12.1 Treatment Targets in Brain and CNS Tumors

Glioblastoma

So far, we've made little progress in identifying treatments that are effective against glioblastoma. The only targeted therapy currently in use is bevacizumab, an angiogenesis inhibitor.

Two major obstacles hinder the creation of effective targeted therapies and immunotherapies for glioblastoma:

1. Almost as soon as the first cancer cell appears, it mutates further and multiplies to create a diverse mix of cancer cells. Thus, these cancers display an incredibly high degree of intratumoral heterogeneity [147]. This makes it incredibly difficult to identify targets that can be matched with targeted therapies; any potential target identified is likely to only exist in a subset of the person's cancer cells.

2. The overall number of mutations (the tumor mutation burden – TMB) in glioblastoma cells is normally low and the tumor microenvironment is highly immune-suppressing. More unusual is the fact that patients who have a glioblastoma with an unusually high TMB tend to fare worse with immunotherapy than patients with a low TMB [148, 149].

Current treatment targets being explored:

- Immunotherapy with checkpoint inhibitors has been investigated in several trials. It appears that these treatments can be effective, but they benefit less than 10% of patients [150, 151]. Less than 1% of glioblastomas are MSI [110].

- An enormous number of innovative immunotherapies are being explored, such as CAR T cells, oncolytic viruses, and treatment vaccines [150, 151].

- Targetable gene alterations include *EGFR* (mutated and/or amplified in most patients), *PIK3CA, PDGFRA, KIT, BRAF, NTRK, FGFR,* and *MET* gene mutations [152, 153]. However, all these mutations will only exist in a subset of a person's cancer cells, so any benefit from giving a matching treatment is likely to be short-lived.
- Potential cell surface targets for ADCs include EGFR [154, 155].

Other Brain and CNS Tumors

It's not possible for me to summarize the numerous types of brain and CNS tumors and the many and varied mutations, pathways, and aspects of their microenvironment that might be targetable. Below is just a handful of approaches that are either licensed or looking promising in trials.

- Dabrafenib plus trametinib (a B-Raf inhibitor plus a MEK inhibitor), or novel B-Raf inhibitors such as tovorafenib, for children with *BRAF*-mutated, low-grade glioma [156], or people with other *BRAF*-mutated cancers such as papillary craniopharyngioma [157].
- A HIF2α-targeted therapy (belzutifan) for people with CNS hemangioblastoma linked to Von Hippel-Lindau disease [158].
- An mTOR inhibitor (everolimus) is approved to treat children or adults with a condition called tuberous sclerosis if they have developed a brain tumor called subependymal giant cell astrocytoma [159].
- An IDH inhibitor (vorasidenib) for people with low-grade gliomas that have a mutation in either *IDH1* or *IDH2* [160].

Table 7.33 A summary of treatment approaches relevant to glioblastoma and other brain and CNS cancers.

	Glioblastoma	Other brain and CNS cancers
Targeted therapies matched with mutations and/or protein expression	No	Yes: • B-Raf + MEK inhibitors • IDH inhibitors • mTOR inhibitor
Targeted therapy: angiogenesis inhibitors	Yes	Yes
Targeted therapy: antibody-drug conjugates	Not yet; potential targets include EGFR, HER2, IL13Rα2, CD147, DLL3	Not yet; potential targets include HER2, IL13Rα2
Immunotherapy with checkpoint inhibitors	No	No

7.12.2 Treatments for Glioblastoma

Table 7.34 Targets and treatments for glioblastoma.

Relevant targets	Treatment approach	Treatment examples	Relevant book sections
Angiogenesis	Angiogenesis inhibitors	Bevacizumab	Section 4.1
Various	Novel immunotherapies	Many in development	Chapter 6
EGFR	EGFR-targeted treatments	None proven to work but various in trials, including kinase inhibitors, ADCs, immunotherapies	Section 3.4.1

7.12.3 Treatments for Other Brain and CNS Tumors

Table 7.35 Targets and treatments for non-glioblastoma brain and other CNS tumors.

Relevant targets	Treatment approach	Treatment examples	Relevant book sections
BRAF mutations	B-Raf inhibitor + MEK inhibitor combinations, novel B-Raf inhibitors	Dabrafenib + trametinib, tovorafenib	Section 3.7.5
Overactive mTOR	mTOR inhibitors	Everolimus	Section 3.8
Angiogenesis	HIF2α inhibitors	Belzutifan	Section 4.1
IDH gene mutations	IDH inhibitors	Vorasidenib	Section 4.6

7.13 TREATMENTS FOR SKIN CANCER

7.13.1 Treatment Targets in Skin Cancers

The many layers of our skin contain a range of cell types. Melanocytes are relatively rare skin cells, but they lead to the most aggressive and lethal form of skin cancer – melanoma. Squamous cells and basal cells are far more numerous than melanocytes, but the cancers they cause – squamous cell carcinoma (SCC) and basal cell carcinoma (BCC) – are far less likely to invade and spread. Merkel cell carcinoma is a rare, aggressive form of skin cancer linked to UV exposure (usually from sunlight), immune suppression, and infection with the Merkel cell polyomavirus [161].

Because they're often caused by the DNA-mutating effects of UV light (from the sun or sunbeds), the cells of most skin cancers have a very high tumor mutation burden (TMB). This high TMB makes the cells visible to white blood cells and presumably explains why these cancers are often sensitive to immunotherapy.

Immunotherapy with checkpoint inhibitors has become an important treatment option for people with both melanoma and non-melanoma skin cancer in recent years.

Melanoma Skin Cancer

Until 2011, the main treatment options for people with cutaneous melanoma were surgery and a chemotherapy called dacarbazine. This changed dramatically in 2011 with the approval of vemurafenib, a B-Raf inhibitor, and ipilimumab, a checkpoint inhibitor.

Since that time, immune checkpoint inhibitors targeting PD-1, PD-L1, CTLA-4, and LAG-3 have all become licensed treatments for people with melanoma skin cancer. These treatments have had a dramatic impact on the survival of many people. For example, in a study called CheckMate 067, roughly half of the people with advanced melanoma given a combination of a PD-1 antibody and CTLA-4 antibody were alive 6.5 years later [162]. This compares to a median overall survival time prior to 2011 of around 6 months [163]. Checkpoint inhibitors have also improved cure rates for people with operable disease at risk of relapse [163].

Other immunotherapies licensed for people with melanoma skin cancer include tumor-infiltrating lymphocytes (TILs) and an oncolytic virus.

Another approach to the treatment of melanoma skin cancer is to target the faulty B-Raf protein found in the cancer cells of roughly half of patients. 90% of the time, this faulty B-Raf is the V600E version (or, less commonly, V600K) that can be blocked by B-Raf inhibitors. Rarer mutated forms of B-Raf (the remaining 10%) affect various parts of the B-Raf protein. Some of them are sensitive to current B-Raf inhibitors, and some of them are not [164].

There's much more about B-Raf inhibitors in Section 3.7.5, in which I also explain why

B-Raf inhibitors are usually given in combination with an MEK inhibitor.

V600E (and V600K) B-Raf are most common in melanoma skin cancers that develop [165, 166]:

- In patients who are relatively young (under 40 years old).
- On skin that has been intermittently (rather than chronically) exposed to UV light, such as the torso, upper legs, and upper arms.[4]

Melanomas that occur on the hands or face – parts of the body that are exposed to sunlight most of the time – only rarely contain a *BRAF* mutation.

In recent years, researchers have tried to answer the question as to which treatment option should be offered first to someone with a *BRAF*-mutated melanoma, i.e., is it better to give checkpoint inhibitors first, or is it best to prescribe a B-Raf/MEK inhibitor combination and to only follow up with checkpoint inhibitors when the person's cancer progresses? This question has been answered by studies such as SECOMBIT and DREAMseq. The results of these trials have proven that for most people checkpoint inhibitor immunotherapy is the best first treatment [167]. The two approaches have also been combined (e.g., pembrolizumab + dabrafenib + trametinib), but this doesn't seem to provide worthwhile benefits [167, 168].

Non-melanoma Skin Cancer

BCCs very rarely spread and are almost always curable. If they do spread, Hedgehog pathway inhibitors and checkpoint inhibitors are both licensed treatment approaches [169].

SCCs spread in about 3%–7% of people [170]. As with BCCs, there is a strong link between UV light and SCCs, but SCC is also linked to immune suppression, such as in people who have received an organ transplant. Checkpoint inhibitors have become an important treatment for people with advanced SCC.

Merkel cell carcinomas are rare but very aggressive, making them the second most common cause of death due to skin cancer after melanoma [171]. The Merkel cell polyomavirus has been linked to around 80% of cases. Merkel cell carcinomas that don't contain traces of the virus have a much higher number of DNA mutations. Whether the cancer has been caused by the polyomavirus or is a consequence of the accumulation of thousands of mutations due to UV light, you would expect the resulting cancer to be very visible to the person's white blood cells. It therefore seems logical that this cancer would be sensitive to immunotherapy, which it does seem to be. Several different checkpoint inhibitors have been licensed as treatments for people with advanced Merkel cell carcinoma in recent years and many other forms of immunotherapy are in trials [171].

Table 7.36   A summary of treatment approaches relevant to melanoma and non-melanoma skin cancer.

	Melanoma skin cancer	Non-melanoma skin cancer
Targeted therapies matched with mutations and/or protein expression	Yes: *BRAF* V600E or V600K mutation matched with a combination of a B-Raf inhibitor and a MEK inhibitor	Yes: Hedgehog pathway inhibitors for basal cell carcinoma
Targeted therapy: angiogenesis inhibitors	No	No

(Continued)

---

[4] In other words, think of someone who sometimes goes on holiday to somewhere sunny and then wears clothes that expose more of their arms, legs, and/or torso than they usually have bare.

Table 7.36 (Continued)

	Melanoma skin cancer	Non-melanoma skin cancer
Targeted therapy: antibody-drug conjugates	**Not yet, but potential targets include gp100, gpNMB, PMEL17, HER3, GD3** [172]	**No**
Immunotherapy with checkpoint inhibitors	**Yes**	**Yes: for squamous cell carcinoma, basal cell carcinoma, and Merkel cell carcinoma**
Other immunotherapies	**Yes: IL-2, TILs, oncolytic viruses, treatment vaccines, T cell engagers**	**Yes: imiquimod for basal cell carcinoma; various others in trials**

[a] Imiquimod is a compound that activates receptors on macrophages, monocytes, and dendritic cells. It also directly causes the death of cancer cells [173].

7.13.2 Treatments for Melanoma Skin Cancer

Table 7.37 Targets and treatments for melanoma skin cancer.

Relevant targets	Treatment approach	Treatment examples	Relevant book sections
BRAF V600E/K mutation	B-Raf inhibitor + MEK inhibitor combinations	Dabrafenib, vemurafenib, or encorafenib, plus trametinib, cobimetinib, or binimetinib	Section 3.7.5
Immune checkpoint proteins on T cells	Immune checkpoint inhibitors targeting PD-1 or PD-L1	Pembrolizumab, nivolumab, atezolizumab	Chapter 5
	Immune checkpoint inhibitors targeting CTLA-4	Ipilimumab	Chapter 5
	Immune checkpoint inhibitors targeting LAG-3	Relatlimab	Chapter 5
The patient's immune response against their cancer	Boost immune responses	Interleukin-2	Section 6.1
	Use the patient's own T cells from their tumor/s	Tumor-infiltrating lymphocytes (TILs)	Section 6.5
	Oncolytic viruses	T-VEC (talimogene laherparepvec)	Section 6.10.5

7.13.3 Treatments for Non-Melanoma Skin Cancer

Table 7.38 Targets and treatments for non-Melanoma skin cancer.

Relevant targets	Treatment approach	Treatment examples	Relevant book sections
Immune checkpoint proteins on T cells	Immune checkpoint inhibitors targeting PD-1 or PD-L1	Cemiplimab, pembrolizumab, avelumab, retifanlimab	Chapter 5
Hedgehog pathway (basal cell carcinoma)	Smoothened inhibitors	Vismodegib, sonidegib	Section 4.5
Myeloid white blood cells in the immune-microenvironment	Topical application of immune response modifiers [174]	Imiquimod	Not covered

7.14 TREATMENTS FOR B CELL AND T CELL LEUKEMIAS

Back in Section 1.9, I described why most hematological cancers are caused by faulty B cells (you may find it helpful to look back at this information before you continue).

7.14.1 Treatment Targets for B cell and T cell Leukemias

Treatment Targets in B cell ALL

In Figure 1.24, you'll notice that B cell acute lymphoblastic leukemia (B cell ALL) develops if very immature B cells become cancer cells. Two-thirds of cases of ALL are diagnosed in patients who are under 20 years old [175]. The most common age to be diagnosed is as an infant or young child up to 4 years old. Roughly 90% of children with ALL are cured with chemotherapy, whereas the cure rate in adults is less than 50% [176].

There are several targeted therapies and immunotherapies given to some patients with B cell ALL [176, 207]:

- Bcr-Abl inhibitors are appropriate for the 3–4% of children and 25% of adults with ALL whose cancer cells contain the Philadelphia chromosome and hence also the Bcr-Abl fusion protein.
- Various targeted therapies are being investigated as treatments for patients with Philadelphia chromosome-like ALL. These cancers contain a range of mutations that cause them to behave similarly to Bcr-Abl-driven cancers. Some mutations may create sensitivity to Bcr-Abl inhibitors or to JAK2 inhibitors.
- Increasingly, patients whose disease returns following chemotherapy are offered CAR T cell therapy using their own, genetically-modified T cells targeted against the CD19 protein.
- Another CD19-targeted treatment that has made an impact in recent years is the bi-specific T cell engager, blinatumomab.

Treatment Targets in T cell ALL

T cell ALL accounts for around 15% of ALL diagnoses in children and 25% in adults. The cancer cells of T cell ALLs contain a wide range of mutations affecting many different genes. It is theoretically possible to match at least some of these mutations with matching targeted treatments. As of 2024, none are licensed. Developing safe and effective CAR T cell therapies for T cell-derived cancers is also an enormous challenge (see Section 6.6.6 for more detail).

Treatment Targets in CLL

Chronic lymphocytic leukemia (CLL) is usually diagnosed in older age. It develops from mature B cells. If the cancer cells are found mostly in the person's lymph nodes rather than in their blood, then it might be called small lymphocytic lymphoma (SLL) rather than CLL. In 80% of cases, the person's cancer cells contain at least one of the four most common chromosome alterations: a deletion affecting chromosome 13, 11, or 17, or an extra copy of chromosome 12. Deletions in chromosome 17 always chop out the *TP53* gene (the gene for making the p53 tumor suppressor protein).

A range of antibody-based treatments and targeted therapies are available as standard treatment options for people with CLL [177]:

- CD20-targeted antibodies such as rituximab, ofatumumab, and obinutuzumab, have been standard treatments for people with CLL for over 20 years.
- CLL cells rely on the B-cell receptors (BCRs) on their surface for their survival. Treatments that target BCR-controlled signaling pathways include BTK and PI3Kδ inhibitors.
- CLL cells produce high levels of Bcl-2, which protects them from apoptosis. Venetoclax is a potent Bcl-2 inhibitor.
- In early 2024, the first CAR T cell therapy was approved, based on a complete response rate of 20% in a group of 89 patients (see Section 6.6.6 for more on this topic) [178].

Table 7.39 A summary of treatment approaches relevant for B cell ALL and CLL.

	B cell ALL	CLL
Targeted therapies matched with mutations and/or protein expression	**Yes: Bcr-Abl inhibitors**	**Yes: treatments that target B-cell receptor signaling or cell survival (Bcl-2)**
Targeted therapy: antibody-drug conjugates	**Yes: targeting CD22**	**No**
Immunotherapy with checkpoint inhibitors	**No**	**No**
Immunotherapy with a naked antibody	**Yes: targeting CD20**	**Yes: targeting CD20**
Immunotherapy with CAR T cells	**Yes: targeting CD19, CD22**	**Yes: targeting CD19**
Immunotherapy with T cell engagers	**Yes: targeting CD19**	**Yes: targeting CD19**

7.14.2 Treatments for B Cell Acute Lymphoblastic Leukemia

Table 7.40 Targets and treatments for B cell ALL.

Relevant targets	Treatment approach	Treatment examples	Relevant book sections
CD19	T cell engagers	Blinatumomab	Section 6.9
	CAR T cell therapies	Tisagenlecleucel, brexucabtagene autoleucel	Section 6.5
CD20	Naked antibodies	Rituximab	Section 6.2
CD22	ADCs	Inotuzumab ozogamicin	Section 4.2
Bcr-Abl fusion protein	Bcr-Abl inhibitors	Dasatinib, imatinib, ponatinib	Section 3.10

7.14.3 Treatments for Chronic Lymphocytic Leukemia

Table 7.41 Targets and treatments for CLL.

Relevant targets	Treatment approach	Treatment examples	Relevant book sections
CD20	Naked antibodies	Rituximab, ofatumumab, obinutuzumab	Section 6.2
B cell receptor-controlled signaling pathways	BTK inhibitors	Ibrutinib, acalabrutinib, zanubrutinib, pirtobrutinib	Section 4.8
	PI3Kδ inhibitors	Idelalisib, duvelisib	Section 4.8
Apoptosis/cell survival	Bcl-2 inhibitors	Venetoclax	Section 4.7
CD19	CAR T cell therapies	Lisocabtagene maraleucel	Section 6.5

7.15 TREATMENTS FOR NON-HODGKIN LYMPHOMAS

7.15.1 Treatment Targets for Non-Hodgkin Lymphomas

As in CLL, the cancer cells that cause most NHLs are mature B cells (T cell NHLs are also diagnosed, although in a much smaller number of people). There are over 80 different types of B cell NHL, and they're generally split into two groups depending on how aggressively the cancer cells behave [179]:

- "Indolent" (also called low-grade or slow-growing) B cell NHLs include diseases such as follicular lymphoma and marginal zone lymphoma.
- "Aggressive" (also called high-grade or fast-growing) B cell NHLs include diseases such as diffuse large B cell lymphoma (DLBCL) and Burkitt lymphoma.

Again, as with CLL, CD20-targeted antibodies and treatments that target BCR-controlled signaling pathways (such as BTK inhibitors, PI3Kδ inhibitors, and the ADC polatuzumab vedotin) are important treatments for many people with B cell NHL. CAR T cell therapy and an ADC targeting CD19, and T cell engagers targeting CD19 and CD20, have also proven to be effective, particularly for aggressive B cell NHLs [180]. Lenalidomide (an immunomodulator), selinexor (a nuclear transport inhibitor), and tazemetostat (an EZH2 inhibitor) are licensed for specific groups of patients.

The finer details of the person's treatment will depend on:

- What type of B cell NHL the person has been diagnosed with.
- The stage of their disease and its location and/or dissemination through the body.
- The person's age and overall level of fitness.

- Whether their disease is causing symptoms – e.g., for many people diagnosed with follicular lymphoma, their disease develops slowly and initially causes few symptoms. These people might be advised to wait and avoid starting treatment until their disease worsens.
- The details of the person's diagnosis e.g., whether they have ABC (activated B cell-like) or GCB (germinal center B cell-like) DLBCL.
- What previous treatments the person has received, and whether their disease returned after these treatments.
- The presence or absence of high-risk features, such as particular translocations or other mutations.

All the above help the person's medical team to choose between an increasing number of treatment options.

In addition, immune checkpoint inhibitors have been investigated in a variety of trials. They work best when the cancer cells contain a gene amplification affecting the *PD-L1* and *PD-L2* genes on chromosome 9. This amplification is common in primary mediastinal large B cell lymphoma, and in some other rare lymphomas (see Section 5.5.7).

T cell lymphomas are another diverse group of lymphomas that can either be slow- or fast-growing depending on the type. For example, cutaneous T cell lymphomas (which include mycosis fungoides and Sézary syndrome) tend to be indolent, whereas peripheral T cell lymphomas (including anaplastic large cell lymphoma) are usually aggressive [181].

Treatments for T cell lymphomas include [181–183]

- ALK inhibitors (such as crizotinib) for *ALK*-mutated anaplastic large cell lymphoma.
- A CD30-targeted ADC (such as brentuximab vedotin) can be effective against peripheral

and cutaneous T-cell lymphomas if the cancer cells have CD30 on their surface.

- Histone deacetylase (HDAC) inhibitors (such as belinostat and vorinostat) are approved as treatments for peripheral and cutaneous T-cell lymphomas.
- The immunotoxin denileukin diftitox, which targets the IL-2 receptor, has had

a complicated history of approval and withdrawal [183]. In August 2024, it once again received FDA-approval [184].

- A naked antibody, mogamulizumab, targeted against the cytokine receptor CCR4, is approved for some people with cutaneous T cell lymphomas.

Table 7.42 A summary of treatment approaches relevant to NHL.

	B cell NHL	T cell NHL
Targeted therapies matched with mutations and/or protein expression	**Yes: treatments that target B-cell receptor signaling or cell survival; EZH2 inhibitors**	**Yes: ALK inhibitors, HDAC inhibitors**
Targeted therapy: antibody-drug conjugates	**Yes: targeting CD19, CD79B**	**Yes: targeting CD30**
Immunotherapy with checkpoint inhibitors	**Yes: but only for primary mediastinal large B-cell lymphoma**	**No**
Immunotherapy with a naked antibody	**Yes: targeting CD19, CD20**	**Yes: targeting CCR4**
Immunotherapy with CAR T cells	**Yes: targeting CD19**	**No**
Immunotherapy with T cell engagers	**Yes: targeting CD20**	**No**
Other immunotherapies	**Yes: immunomodulators**	**Yes: an immunotoxin targeting the IL-2 receptor**
Anything else?	**Exportin-1 inhibitors; proteasome inhibitors**	

7.15.2 Treatments for B Cell Non-Hodgkin Lymphomas

Table 7.43 Targets and treatments for B cell NHL.

Relevant targets	Treatment approach	Treatment examples	Relevant book sections
CD20	Naked antibodies	Rituximab, obinutuzumab	Section 6.2
	T cell engagers	Glofitamab, epcoritamab, mosunetuzumab	Section 6.9
	Radioactively-labelled antibodies	Ibritumomab tiuxitan	Section 4.2.8
CD19	Naked antibodies	Tafasitamab	Section 6.2
	ADCs	Loncastuximab tesirine	Section 4.2
	CAR T cell therapies	Axicabtagene ciloleucel, brexucabtagene autoleucel, lisocabtagene maraleucel, tisagenlecleucel	Section 6.6

Table 7.43   (Continued)

B-cell receptor-controlled signaling pathways	BTK inhibitors	Ibrutinib, acalabrutinib, zanubrutinib, pirtobrutinib	Section 4.8
	PI3Kδ inhibitors	Idelalisib, duvelisib	Section 4.8
	ADCs targeting CD79B	Polatuzumab vedotin	Sections 4.2 and 4.8
Amplification of *PD-L1* and *PD-L2* genes	PD-1-targeted checkpoint inhibitors	Pembrolizumab	Chapter 5
Proteasomes	Proteasome inhibitors	Bortezomib	Section 4.10
Various aspects of the immune environment	Immuno-modulators	Lenalidomide	Section 6.3
Nuclear transport	Exportin-1 inhibitors	Selinexor	Section 4.9
EZH2 mutations	EZH2 inhibitors	Tazemetostat	Section 4.6

7.15.3 Treatments for T Cell Non-Hodgkin Lymphomas

Table 7.44   Targets and treatments for T cell NHL.

Relevant targets	Treatment approach	Treatment examples	Relevant book sections
CCR4	Naked antibodies	Mogamulizumab	Section 6.2
Epigenetics	HDAC inhibitors	Belinostat, vorinostat, romidepsin	Section 4.6
CD30	ADCs	Brentuximab vedotin	Section 4.2
IL-2 receptors	Immunotoxins	Denileukin diftitox	Section 4.2.8
ALK mutations	ALK inhibitors	Crizotinib	Section 3.6.5

7.16 TREATMENTS FOR HODGKIN LYMPHOMA AND MYELOMA

7.16.1 Treatment Targets in Hodgkin Lymphoma and Myeloma

Hodgkin lymphoma and myeloma are both cancers that develop from faulty B cells (see Figure 1.24).

Hodgkin Lymphoma

Hodgkin lymphoma has one of the strangest age distributions of any cancer. There are two points in life when we're most at risk: as a young adult, and then again in older age [185]. Most people (particularly younger patients) can be cured with a combination of chemotherapy drugs, sometimes with the addition of radiotherapy [186].

The cancer cells that cause classic Hodgkin lymphoma (which accounts for 95% of cases) are called Hodgkin and Reed-Sternberg cells (HRS) cells. HRS cells are thought to be B cells from lymph nodes that have gone through many changes and have lost many of the proteins normally found on B cells (such as CD19, CD20, and the BCR). Instead, they have the CD30 protein, making them sensitive to the ADC brentuximab vedotin [187]. CAR T cell therapies targeting CD30 are also being developed [188].

Another feature of HRS cells is that the segment of chromosome 9 containing the genes for both PD-L1 and PD-L2 is amplified in most cases [189, 190]. This renders classic Hodgkin lymphoma sensitive to checkpoint inhibitors that target PD-1. Some other, much rarer lymphomas have the same amplification (see Section 5.5.7 for more on this).

Myeloma

Myeloma (also referred to as multiple myeloma) develops from long-lived, antibody-producing B cells (called plasma cells) normally found in bone marrow (see Figure 1.25e). It's often preceded by a condition called monoclonal gammopathy of undetermined significance (MGUS), in which mutated plasma cells start outgrowing their healthy counterparts. Myeloma is strongly linked to older age, with most cases occurring in people over 60 years of age [191].

Myeloma cells have many cell surface proteins that are being explored as targets for a wide range of antibody-based treatments, such as naked antibodies, ADCs, CAR T cell therapies, and T cell engagers. Targets include CD38, BCMA, GPRC5D, CD138, CD56, SLAMF7 (also called CS1), CD74, and NKG2D [192–195].

Another important target of myeloma treatments is the relationship between myeloma cells and their noncancer neighbors in the bone marrow. Thalidomide and other cereblon-targeted treatments affect this relationship in a variety of ways (summarized in Table 6.2). The reasons why myeloma cells are sensitive to proteasome inhibitors and exportin-1 inhibitors seem less clear.

Around 15%–20% of myelomas are caused by cells that contain a translocation called t(11;14). Cells with this translocation produce high levels of Bcl-2. Venetoclax, a Bcl-2 inhibitor, is being investigated as a treatment for this group of patients [196].

Table 7.45   A summary of treatment approaches relevant to Hodgkin lymphoma and myeloma.

	Hodgkin lymphoma	Myeloma
Targeted therapies matched with mutations and/or protein expression	No	Not yet
Targeted therapy: antibody-drug conjugates	Yes: targeting CD30 Other possible targets include CD25	Yes: targeting BCMA
Immunotherapy with checkpoint inhibitors	Yes	No
Immunotherapy with a naked antibody	No	Yes: targeting CD38, CS1(SLAMF7)
Immunotherapy with CAR T cells	Not yet: CAR T-cell products targeting CD30 are being developed	Yes: targeting BCMA
Immunotherapy with T cell engagers	No	Yes: targeting BCMA, GPRC5D
Other immunotherapies	No	Yes: immunomodulators/ cereblon modulators
Anything else?	No	Yes: proteasome inhibitors, exportin-1 inhibitors, HDAC inhibitors

7.16.2 Treatments for Hodgkin Lymphoma

Table 7.46 Targets and treatments for Hodgkin lymphoma.

Relevant targets	Treatment approach	Treatment examples	Relevant book sections
CD30	ADCs	Brentuximab vedotin	Section 4.2
Amplification of *PD-L1* and *PD-L2* genes	PD-1-targeted checkpoint inhibitors	Pembrolizumab, nivolumab	Chapter 5

7.16.3 Treatments for Myeloma

Table 7.47 Targets and treatments for myeloma.

Relevant targets	Treatment approach	Treatment examples	Relevant book sections
Proteasomes	Proteasome inhibitors	Bortezomib, carfilzomib, ixazomib	Section 4.10
Various aspects of the immune environment	Immunomodulators and novel cereblon modulators	Thalidomide, lenalidomide, pomalidomide, iberdomide, mezigdomide	Section 6.3
CD38	Naked antibodies	Daratumumab, isatuximab	Section 6.2
CS1/SLAMF7	Naked antibodies	Elotuzumab	Section 6.2
BCMA	CAR T cell therapies	Idecabtagene vicleucel, ciltacabtagene autoleucel	Section 6.6
	T cell engagers	Elranatamab, teclistamab	Section 6.9
	ADCs	Belantamab mafodotin[a]	Section 4.2
GPRC5D	T cell engagers	Talquetamab	Section 6.9
Nuclear transport	Exportin-1 inhibitors	Selinexor	Section 4.9
Epigenetics	Histone deacetylase inhibitors	Panobinostat	Section 4.6

[a] Balantamab mafodotin was approved in 2020 but later withdrawn from use. However, it seems likely that it will be re-approved based on recent trial results.

7.17 TREATMENTS FOR MYELOID CELL CANCERS

7.17.1 Treatment Targets in Myeloid Cell Cancers

Most cancers that develop from myeloid white blood cells are derived from stem cells or very immature myeloid white blood cells in the bone marrow (see Figure 1.24). These cancers include acute myeloid leukemia (AML), various forms of myelodysplastic syndrome (MDS), and myeloproliferative neoplasms (MPNs) – a category that includes chronic myeloid leukemia (CML; sometimes referred to as chronic myelogenous leukemia).

Acute Myeloid Leukemia (AML)

The risk of developing AML increases steadily with age. However, although it's rare in younger age groups, it is also the second most common leukemia diagnosed in children after ALL. Until fairly recently, treatment options were dominated by chemotherapy and stem cell transplantation. As our understanding of AML has increased, this has led to the creation of targeted therapies that benefit some groups of patients. These include: [197–199]

- FLT3 inhibitors for the roughly 30% of patients with AML whose cancer cells are making a mutated and overactive version of the FLT3 protein (see Section 3.6.8 for more detail).
- The Bcl-2 inhibitor venetoclax. AML cells often overproduce Bcl-2, which protects them from apoptosis. Many trials for AML involve venetoclax being combined with a variety of other treatments in a range of patients.
- IDH inhibitors (such as ivosidenib and enasidenib) are approved for patients whose cancer cells contain a mutation in *IDH1* or *IDH2*. These mutations are found in around 5%–15% of patients with newly diagnosed AML. See Section 4.6 for more about IDH inhibitors and hypomethylators such as azacitidine and decitabine.
- Scientists believe that AML is sustained by millions of AML stem cells that can survive chemotherapy [200]. The Hedgehog pathway is important for stem cells, and this may be why AML is sensitive to Hedgehog pathway inhibitors [201] (see Section 4.5).
- The subgroup of patients with AML who have acute promyelocytic leukemia (APL) are given treatments that target the *PML-RARA* fusion gene found in APL cells [202].
- Another group of treatments looking exciting are the menin inhibitors. These could be effective for people with AML whose cancer cells contain KMT2A (also called MLL1) gene rearrangements or NPM1 mutations [208].

An obstacle that stands in the way of the creation of antibody-based treatments and other immunotherapies for patients with AML is that the cancer cells have the same proteins on their surface as healthy stem cells. This makes it enormously difficult to identify safe targets [203]. So far, the only antibody-based treatment for people with AML is an ADC called gemtuzumab ozogamicin, which targets CD33.

Myelodysplastic Syndromes (MDSs)

MDSs are a varied group of cancers that share some properties with AML (in some people, their MDS becomes an AML). As in AML, the cancer cells of some patients contain an *IDH1* or *IDH2* mutation and are sensitive to a matched IDH inhibitor. Other licensed treatment approaches include hypomethylators and lenalidomide [202].

Myeloproliferative Neoplasms (MPNs), Including Chronic Myeloid Leukemia (CML)

MPNs are a group of rare diseases in which the bone marrow produces too many of a particular type of blood cell. CML is the only MPN in which the cancer cells contain the translocation affecting chromosomes 9 and 22 that I described back in Section 1.2.2. This forces the cells to make an overactive kinase called Bcr-Abl. I describe Bcr-Abl inhibitors in detail in Section 3.10.

Polycythemia vera (PV), essential thrombocythemia (ET), and primary myelofibrosis (PMF) are other main types of MPN. All these cancers develop from faulty stem cells and generally develop slowly. However, these diseases can change over time and transform into a much more aggressive disease or turn into acute leukemia. Mutations affecting the JAK-STAT pathway are found in 90% of MPNs [204]. JAK2 inhibitors are important treatments for these conditions, although they improve symptoms and quality of life rather than offering a cure [204–206].

There are also rare cancers classified as "Myeloid/lymphoid neoplasms with eosinophilia and tyrosine kinase gene fusions". As their name might suggest, the cells of these cancers often contain mutated versions of kinases such as PDGFRA or B, FGFR1, JAK2, or FLT3. These overactive kinases can potentially be matched with suitable targeted therapies.

Table 7.48   A summary of treatment approaches relevant to myeloid cell cancers.

	AML and MDS	MPNs (including CML)
Targeted therapies matched with mutations and/or protein expression	**Yes:** • **FLT3 inhibitors** • **IDH1/2 inhibitors** • **Smoothened inhibitors** • **Bcl-2 inhibitors** • **Menin inhibitors**	**Yes:** • **Bcr-Abl inhibitors (for CML)** • **JAK2 inhibitors (for other MPNs)**
Targeted therapy: antibody-drug conjugates	**Yes: targeting CD33**	**No**
Immunotherapy with checkpoint inhibitors	**No**	**No**
Immunotherapy with a naked antibody	**No**	**No**
Immunotherapy with CAR T cells	**Not yet: many targets are being explored**	**No**
Immunotherapy with T cell engagers	**Not yet: many targets are being explored**	**No**
Anything else?	**Yes: hypomethylators, immunomodulators**	**Yes: PEGinterferon-alpha-2a is a treatment for MPNs (excluding CML).**

7.17.2 Treatments for Acute Myeloid Leukemia

Table 7.49   Targets and treatments for AML.

Relevant targets	Treatment approach	Treatment examples	Relevant book sections
CD33	ADCs	Gemtuzumab ozogamicin	Section 4.2
Mutated FLT3	FLT3 inhibitors	Midostaurin, quizartinib, gilteritinib	Section 3.6.8
Epigenetic enzymes	Hypomethylators (DNA methyl transferase inhibitors)	Azacitidine, decitabine	Section 4.6
Mutated versions of IDH1 and IDH2 (epigenetic enzymes)	IDH1 and IDH2 inhibitors	Enasidenib (IDH2 inhibitor); ivosidenib, olutasidenib (IDH1 inhibitors)	Section 4.6
Hedgehog pathway	Smoothened inhibitors	Glasdegib	Section 4.5
Apoptosis/cell survival	Bcl-2 inhibitors	Venetoclax	Section 4.7
Menin	Menin inhibitors	Revumenib	Not covered

7.17.3 Treatments for Myelodysplastic Syndromes

Table 7.50   Targets and treatments for MDS.

Relevant targets	Treatment approach	Treatment examples	Relevant book sections
Epigenetic enzymes	Hypomethylators (DNA methyl transferase inhibitors)	Azacitidine, decitabine	Section 4.6
Mutated versions of IDH1 and IDH2 (epigenetic enzymes)	IDH1 and IDH2 inhibitors	Enasidenib (IDH2 inhibitor); ivosidenib, olutasidenib (IDH1 inhibitors)	Section 4.6
Various aspects of the immune environment	Immunomodulators and novel cereblon modulators	Lenalidomide	Section 6.3

7.17.4 Treatments for Chronic Myeloid Leukemia

Table 7.51   Targets and treatments for CML.

Relevant targets	Treatment approach	Treatment examples	Relevant book sections
Bcr-Abl fusion protein	ATP-competitive Bcr-Abl inhibitors	Imatinib, dasatinib, nilotinib, bosutinib, ponatinib	Section 3.10
	Allosteric Bcr-Abl inhibitors	Asciminib	Section 3.10

7.17.5 Treatments for Myeloproliferative Neoplasms (Other Than CML)

Table 7.52   Targets and treatments for MPNs (other than CML).

Relevant targets	Treatment approach	Treatment examples	Relevant book sections
JAK2	JAK-2 inhibitors	Ruxolitinib, pacritinib, fedratinib, momelotinib	Section 3.9

7.18 TREATMENTS FOR CHILDHOOD CANCERS

All childhood cancers are rare. The most common cancers affecting children are leukemias, cancers of the brain and spinal cord, lymphomas, soft tissue sarcomas, neuroblastoma, kidney cancers, bone tumors, germ cell tumors, retinoblastoma, and liver tumors [207].

Targeted therapies and immunotherapies are not standard treatment options for most of these cancers. In Table 7.53, I have listed the childhood cancers for which there are licensed treatments mentioned elsewhere in this book.

Table 7.53   Targets and treatments for childhood cancers.

Disease	Treatment approach	Treatment examples	Relevant book sections
Acute lymphoblastic leukemia	Relevant targeted treatments and immunotherapies are described in Section 7.14		
Acute myeloid leukemia	Relevant targeted treatments and immunotherapies are described in Section 7.17		
Alveolar soft part sarcoma	PD-L1-targeted checkpoint inhibitors	Atezolizumab	Chapter 5
Epithelioid sarcoma	EZH2 inhibitors	Tazemetostat	Section 4.6
Giant cell astrocytoma	mTOR inhibitors	Everolimus	Section 3.8
Low-grade glioma	B-Raf + MEK inhibitor combinations, novel B-Raf inhibitors	Dabrafenib + trametinib, tovorafenib	Section 3.7.5
Hodgkin lymphoma	Relevant targeted treatments and immunotherapies are described in Section 7.16		
Juvenile myelomonocytic leukemia	Hypomethylators	Azacitidine	Section 4.6
Neuroblastoma	GD2-targeted antibodies	Dinutuximab, naxitamab	Section 6.2

REFERENCES

1 American Cancer Society. Tumor-agnostic drugs. [Online] Available at: https://www.cancer. org/cancer/managing-cancer/treatment-types/tumor-agnostic-drugs.html [Accessed March 26, 2024].

2 Lu CC *et al*. (2024). Tumor-agnostic approvals: Insights and practical considerations. *Clin Cancer Res* **30**(3): 480–488. doi: 10.1158/1078-0432.CCR-23-1340.

3 AstraZeneca. FDA grants accelerated approval to fam-trastuzumab deruxtecan-nxki for unresectable or metastatic HER2-positive solid tumors. [online] Available at: https://www.fda. gov/drugs/resources-information-approved-drugs/fda-grants-accelerated-approval-fam-trastuzumab-deruxtecan-nxki-unresectable-or-metastatic-her2 [Accessed May 10, 2024].

4 Iqbal N, Iqbal N (2014). Human epidermal growth factor receptor 2 (HER2) in cancers: Overexpression and therapeutic implications. *Mol Biol Int* **2014**: 1–9. doi: 10.1155/2014/852748.

5 Fan Y *et al*. (2021). Clinical features of patients with HER2-positive breast cancer and development of a nomogram for predicting survival. *ESMO Open* **6**(4): 100232. doi: 10.1016/j.esmoop. 2021.100232.

6 National Cancer Institute. Cancer stat facts: Female breast cancer subtypes. [Online] Available at: https://seer.cancer.gov/statfacts/ html/breast-subtypes.html [Accessed March 26, 2024].

7 NCI. Cancer stat facts: Female breast cancer subtypes. National Cancer Institute Surveillance, Epidemiology and End Results Program. [Online] Available at: https://seer. cancer.gov/statfacts/html/breast-subtypes. html [Accessed October 17, 2023].

8 Akshata Desai KA (2012). Triple negative breast cancer – An overview. *Hereditary Genet*. doi: 10.4172/2161-1041.S2-001.

9 Modi S *et al*. (2022). Trastuzumab deruxtecan in previously treated HER2-low advanced breast cancer. *N Engl J Med* **387**(1): 9–20. doi: 10.1056/ NEJMoa2203690.

10 Gampenrieder SP *et al*. (2021). Landscape of HER2-low metastatic breast cancer (MBC): Results from the Austrian AGMT_MBC-Registry. *Breast Cancer Res* **23**(1): 112. doi: 10.1186/s13058-021-01492-x.

11 Derakhshan F, Reis-Filho JS (2022). Pathogenesis of triple-negative breast cancer. *Annu Rev Pathol: Pathol Mech Dis* **17**(1): 181–204. doi: 10.1146/annurev-pathol-042420-093238.

12 Reinhardt K *et al*. (2022). PIK3CA-mutations in breast cancer. *Breast Cancer Res Treat* **196**(3): 483–493. doi: 10.1007/s10549-022-06637-w.

13 Cortesi L, Rugo HS, Jackisch C (2021). An overview of PARP inhibitors for the treatment of breast cancer. *Target Oncol* **16**(3): 255–282. doi: 10.1007/s11523-021-00796-4.

14 Cortes J *et al*. (2022). Pembrolizumab plus chemotherapy in advanced triple-negative breast cancer. *N Engl J Med* **387**(3): 217–226. doi: 10.1056/NEJMoa2202809.

15 Schmid P *et al*. (2018). Atezolizumab and nab-paclitaxel in advanced triple-negative breast cancer. *N Engl J Med* **379**(22): 2108–2121. doi: 10.1056/NEJMoa1809615.

16 Pereira B *et al*. (2016). The somatic mutation profiles of 2,433 breast cancers refine their genomic and transcriptomic landscapes. *Nat Commun* **7**(1): 11479. doi: 10.1038/ncomms11479.

17 Connell CM, Doherty GJ (2017). Activating HER2 mutations as emerging targets in multiple solid cancers. *ESMO Open* **2**(5): e000279. doi: 10.1136/esmoopen-2017-000279.

18 Nunes Filho P *et al*. (2023). Immune checkpoint inhibitors in breast cancer: A narrative review. *Oncol Ther* **11**(2): 171–183. doi: 10.1007/ s40487-023-00224-9.

19 Howard FM *et al*. (2022). The emerging role of immune checkpoint inhibitors for the treatment of breast cancer. *Expert Opin Investig Drugs* **31**(6): 531–548. doi: 10.1080/13543784.2022.1986002.

20 Brett JO *et al*. (2021). ESR1 mutation as an emerging clinical biomarker in metastatic hormone receptor-positive breast cancer. *Breast Cancer Res* **23**(1): 85. doi: 10.1186/s13058-021-01462-3.

21 Hare SH, Harvey AJ (2017). mTOR function and therapeutic targeting in breast cancer. *Am J Cancer Res* **7**(3): 383–404.

22 McAndrew NP, Finn RS (2022). Clinical review on the management of hormone receptor–positive

metastatic breast cancer. *JCO Oncol Pract* **18**(5): 319–327. doi: 10.1200/OP.21.00384.

23 NCI. Hormone therapy for breast cancer. cancer.gov. [Online]. Available at: https://www.cancer.gov/types/breast/breast-hormone-therapy-fact-sheet [Accessed October 17, 2023].

24 Gnant M, Turner NC, Hernando C (2023). Managing a long and winding road: Estrogen receptor–positive breast cancer. *Am Soc Clin Oncol Educ Book* **43**. doi: 10.1200/EDBK_390922.

25 Debien V *et al*. (2023). Immunotherapy in breast cancer: An overview of current strategies and perspectives. *NPJ Breast Cancer* **9**(1): 7. doi: 10.1038/s41523-023-00508-3.

26 Liu ZB *et al*. (2020). Combination strategies of checkpoint immunotherapy in metastatic breast cancer. *Onco Targets Ther* **13**: 2657–2666. doi: 10.2147/OTT.S240655.

27 American Cancer Society. Colorectal cancer risk factors. [Online] Available at: https://www.cancer.org/cancer/types/colon-rectal-cancer/causes-risks-prevention/risk-factors.html [Accessed March 26, 2024].

28 André T, Cohen R, Salem ME (2022). Immune checkpoint blockade therapy in patients with colorectal cancer harboring microsatellite instability/mismatch repair deficiency in 2022. *Am Soc Clin Oncol Educ Book* **42**: 233–241. doi: 10.1200/EDBK_349557.

29 Eng C (2016). POLE mutations in colorectal cancer: A new biomarker? *Lancet Gastroenterol Hepatol* **1**(3): 176–177. doi: 10.1016/S2468-1253(16)30030-9.

30 Wang F *et al*. (2019). Evaluation of POLE and POLD1 mutations as biomarkers for immunotherapy outcomes across multiple cancer types. *JAMA Oncol* **5**(10): 1504. doi: 10.1001/jamaoncol.2019.2963.

31 Angell HK *et al*. (2020). The immunoscore: Colon cancer and beyond. *Clin Cancer Res* **26**(2): 332–339. doi: 10.1158/1078-0432.CCR-18-1851.

32 Ros J *et al*. (2023). Advances in immune checkpoint inhibitor combination strategies for microsatellite stable colorectal cancer. *Front Oncol* **13**. doi: 10.3389/fonc.2023.1112276.

33 Dienstmann R, Salazar R, Tabernero J (2018). Molecular subtypes and the evolution of treatment decisions in metastatic colorectal cancer.

Am Soc Clin Oncol Educ Book **38**: 231–238. doi: 10.1200/EDBK_200929.

34 Randon G *et al*. (2022). Negative ultraselection of patients WITH RAS / BRAF wild-type, microsatellite-stable metastatic colorectal cancer receiving anti–EGFR-based therapy. *JCO Precis Oncol* **6**. doi: 10.1200/PO.22.00037.

35 Morano F *et al*. (2019). Negative hyperselection of patients with RAS and BRAF wild-type metastatic colorectal cancer who received panitumumab-based maintenance therapy. *J Clin Oncol* **37**(33): 3099–3110. doi: 10.1200/JCO.19.01254.

36 Hansen TF, Qvortrup C, Pfeiffer P (2021). Angiogenesis inhibitors for colorectal cancer. A review of the clinical data. *Cancers (Basel)* **13**(5): 1031. doi: 10.3390/cancers13051031.

37 Hua H *et al*. (2023). Genomic and transcriptomic analysis of MSI-H colorectal cancer patients with targetable alterations identifies clinical implications for immunotherapy. *Front Immunol* **13**. doi: 10.3389/fimmu.2022.974793.

38 Dhawan N, Afzal MZ, Amin M (2023). Immunotherapy in anal cancer. *Curr Oncol* **30**(5): 4538–4550. doi: 10.3390/curroncol30050343.

39 Eng C *et al*. (2022). Anal cancer: Emerging standards in a rare disease. *J Clin Oncol* **40**(24): 2774–2788. doi: 10.1200/JCO.21.02566.

40 Zhong J *et al*. (2023). Immune checkpoint blockade therapy for BRAF mutant metastatic colorectal cancer: The efficacy, new strategies, and potential biomarkers. *Discov Oncol* **14**(1): 94. doi: 10.1007/s12672-023-00718-y.

41 Frisch M *et al*. (1997). Sexually transmitted infection as a cause of anal cancer. *N Engl J Med* **337**(19): 1350–1358. doi: 10.1056/NEJM199711063371904.

42 Tashiro H, Brenner MK (2017). Immunotherapy against cancer-related viruses. *Cell Res* **27**(1): 59–73. doi: 10.1038/cr.2016.153.

43 Gao P *et al*. (2019). Immune checkpoint inhibitors in the treatment of virus-associated cancers. *J Hematol Oncol* **12**(1): 58. doi: 10.1186/s13045-019-0743-4.

44 Cancer Research UK. Types of lung cancer. [Online] Available at: https://www.cancerresearchuk.org/about-cancer/lung-cancer/stages-types-grades/types [Accessed October 30, 2023].

45 Herbst RS, Morgensztern D, Boshoff C (2018). The biology and management of non-small cell lung cancer. *Nature* **553**(7689): 446–454. doi: 10.1038/nature25183.

46 Chen R *et al.* (2020). Emerging therapeutic agents for advanced non-small cell lung cancer. *J Hematol Oncol* **13**(1): 58. doi: 10.1186/s13045-020-00881-7.

47 Nassar AH, Adib E, Kwiatkowski DJ (2021). Distribution of KRAS G12C somatic mutations across race, sex, and cancer type. *N Engl J Med* **384**(2): 185–187. doi: 10.1056/NEJMc2030638.

48 Burnett H *et al.* (2021). Epidemiological and clinical burden of EGFR Exon 20 insertion in advanced non-small cell lung cancer: A systematic literature review. *PLoS One* **16**(3): e0247620. doi: 10.1371/journal.pone.0247620.

49 Li T *et al.* (2013). Genotyping and genomic profiling of non–small-cell lung cancer: Implications for current and future therapies. *J Clin Oncol* **31**(8): 1039–1049. doi: 10.1200/JCO.2012.45.3753.

50 Tsao AS *et al.* (2016). Scientific advances in lung cancer 2015. *J Thorac Oncol* **11**(5): 613–638. doi: 10.1016/j.jtho.2016.03.012.

51 Redman MW *et al.* (2020). Biomarker-driven therapies for previously treated squamous non-small-cell lung cancer (Lung-MAP SWOG S1400): A biomarker-driven master protocol. *Lancet Oncol* **21**(12): 1589–1601. doi: 10.1016/S1470-2045(20)30475-7.

52 LoPiccolo J *et al.* (2024). Lung cancer in patients who have never smoked — an emerging disease. *Nat Rev Clin Oncol* **21**(2): 121–146. doi: 10.1038/s41571-023-00844-0.

53 Wang X *et al.* (2021). Smoking history as a potential predictor of immune checkpoint inhibitor efficacy in metastatic non-small cell lung cancer. *JNCI J Natl Cancer Inst* **113**(12): 1761–1769. doi: 10.1093/jnci/djab116.

54 Manzo A *et al.* (2017). Angiogenesis inhibitors in NSCLC. *Int J Mol Sci* **18**(10): 2021. doi: 10.3390/ijms18102021.

55 Paglialunga L *et al.* (2016). Immune checkpoint blockade in small cell lung cancer: Is there a light at the end of the tunnel? *ESMO Open* **1**(4): e000022. doi: 10.1136/esmoopen-2015-000022.

56 Meijer J-J *et al.* (2022). Small cell lung cancer: Novel treatments beyond immunotherapy.

Semin Cancer Biol **86**: 376–385. doi: 10.1016/j.semcancer.2022.05.004.

57 George J *et al.* (2015). Comprehensive genomic profiles of small cell lung cancer. *Nature* **524**(7563): 47–53. doi: 10.1038/nature14664.

58 Uprety D, Remon J, Adjei AA (2021). All that glitters is not gold: The story of rovalpituzumab tesirine in SCLC. *J Thorac Oncol* **16**(9): 1429–1433. doi: 10.1016/j.jtho.2021.07.012.

59 Rudin CM *et al.* (2023). Emerging therapies targeting the delta-like ligand 3 (DLL3) in small cell lung cancer. *J Hematol Oncol* **16**(1): 66. doi: 10.1186/s13045-023-01464-y.

60 Rosner S *et al.* (2023). Antibody-drug conjugates for lung cancer: Payloads and progress. *Am Soc Clin Oncol Educ Book* **no. 43**. doi: 10.1200/EDBK_389968.

61 Gaudino G, Xue J, Yang H (2020). How asbestos and other fibers cause mesothelioma. *Transl Lung Cancer Res* **9**(S1): S39–S46. doi: 10.21037/tlcr.2020.02.01.

62 Fennell DA, Dulloo S, Harber J (2022). Immunotherapy approaches for malignant pleural mesothelioma. *Nat Rev Clin Oncol* **19**(9): 573–584. doi: 10.1038/s41571-022-00649-7.

63 Peters S *et al.* (2021). LBA65 First-line nivolumab (NIVO) plus ipilimumab (IPI) vs chemotherapy (chemo) in patients (pts) with unresectable malignant pleural mesothelioma (MPM): 3-year update from CheckMate 743. *Ann Oncol* **32**: S1341–S1342. doi: 10.1016/j.annonc.2021.08.2146.

64 Popat S *et al.* (2022). Malignant pleural mesothelioma: ESMO Clinical Practice Guidelines for diagnosis, treatment and follow-up☆. *Ann Oncol* **33**(2): 129–142. doi: 10.1016/j.annonc.2021.11.005.

65 Dai C, Heemers H, Sharifi N (2017). Androgen signaling in prostate cancer. *Cold Spring Harb Perspect Med* **7**(9): a030452. doi: 10.1101/cshperspect.a030452.

66 Taplin M-E (2007). Drug Insight: Role of the androgen receptor in the development and progression of prostate cancer. *Nat Clin Pract Oncol* **4**(4): 236–244. doi: 10.1038/ncponc0765.

67 Desai K, McManus JM, Sharifi N (2021). Hormonal therapy for prostate cancer. *Endocr Rev* **42**(3): 354–373. doi: 10.1210/endrev/bnab002.

68 National Cancer Institute. Hormone therapy for prostate cancer. [Online] Available at:

https://www.cancer.gov/types/prostate/prostate-hormone-therapy-fact-sheet [Accessed October 31, 2023].

69 Murray I, Du Y (2021). Systemic radiotherapy of bone metastases with radionuclides. *Clin Oncol* **33**(2): 98–105. doi: 10.1016/j.clon.2020.11.028.

70 Sorrentino C, Di Carlo E (2023). Molecular targeted therapies in metastatic prostate cancer: Recent advances and future challenges. *Cancers (Basel)* **15**(11): 2885. doi: 10.3390/cancers 15112885.

71 Hernando Polo S *et al.* (2021). Changing the history of prostate cancer with new targeted therapies. *Biomedicine* **9**(4): 392. doi: 10.3390/biomedicines9040392.

72 Abida W *et al.* (2019). Analysis of the prevalence of microsatellite instability in prostate cancer and response to immune checkpoint blockade. *JAMA Oncol* **5**(4): 471. doi: 10.1001/jamaoncol.2018.5801.

73 Sardinha M *et al.* (2023). Antibody-drug conjugates in prostate cancer: A systematic review. *Cureus.* doi: 10.7759/cureus.34490.

74 Mjaess G *et al.* (2023). Antibody-drug conjugates in prostate cancer: Where are we? *Clin Genitourin Cancer* **21**(1): 171–174. doi: 10.1016/j.clgc.2022.07.009.

75 Czerwińska M *et al.* (2020). Targeted radionuclide therapy of prostate cancer – From basic research to clinical perspectives. *Molecules* **25**(7): 1743. doi: 10.3390/molecules25071743.

76 Maurice-Dror C *et al.* (2022). A phase 1 study to assess the safety, pharmacokinetics, and antitumor activity of the androgen receptor n-terminal domain inhibitor epi-506 in patients with metastatic castration-resistant prostate cancer. *Investig New Drugs* **40**(2): 322–329. doi: 10.1007/s10637-021-01202-6.

77 Hollasch M. Next-generation aniten masofaniten gains momentum in mCRPC. OncLive. [Online] Available at: https://www.onclive.com/view/next-generation-aniten-masofaniten-gains-momentum-in-mcrpc [Accessed October 31, 2023].

78 Avgeris I *et al.* (2022). Targeting androgen receptor for prostate cancer therapy: From small molecules to PROTACs. *Bioorg Chem* **128**: 106089. doi: 10.1016/j.bioorg.2022.106089.

79 Országhová Z *et al.* (2022). Overcoming chemotherapy resistance in germ cell tumors. *Biomedicine* **10**(5): 972. doi: 10.3390/biomedicines 10050972.

80 Labadie BW, Balar AV, Luke JJ (2021). Immune checkpoint inhibitors for genitourinary cancers: Treatment indications, investigational approaches and biomarkers. *Cancers (Basel)* **13**(21): 5415. doi: 10.3390/cancers13215415.

81 Skowron MA *et al.* (2023). Targeting CLDN6 in germ cell tumors by an antibody-drug-conjugate and studying therapy resistance of yolk-sac tumors to identify and screen specific therapeutic options. *Mol Med* **29**(1): 40. doi: 10.1186/s10020-023-00636-3.

82 Ermakov MS, Kashofer K, Regauer S (2023). Different mutational landscapes in human papillomavirus–induced and human papillomavirus–independent invasive penile squamous cell cancers. *Mod Pathol* **36**(10): 100250. doi: 10.1016/j.modpat.2023.100250.

83 Tang Y *et al.* (2022). Immune landscape and immunotherapy for penile cancer. *Front Immunol* **13**. doi: 10.3389/fimmu.2022.1055235.

84 Vanthoor J, Vos G, Albersen M (2021). Penile cancer: Potential target for immunotherapy? *World J Urol* **39**(5): 1405–1411. doi: 10.1007/s00345-020-03510-7.

85 Carthon BC *et al.* (2014). Epidermal growth factor receptor-targeted therapy in locally advanced or metastatic squamous cell carcinoma of the penis. *BJU Int* **113**(6): 871–877. doi: 10.1111/bju.12450.

86 Tan X *et al.* (2023). The role of Her-2 in penile squamous cell carcinoma progression and cisplatin chemoresistance and potential for antibody-drug conjugate-based therapy. *Eur J Cancer* **194**: 113360. doi: 10.1016/j.ejca.2023.113360.

87 Gormley M *et al.* (2022). Reviewing the epidemiology of head and neck cancer: Definitions, trends and risk factors. *Br Dent J* **233**(9): 780–786. doi: 10.1038/s41415-022-5166-x.

88 Li Q *et al.* (2023). Targeted therapy for head and neck cancer: Signaling pathways and clinical studies. *Signal Transduct Target Ther* **8**(1): 31. doi: 10.1038/s41392-022-01297-0.

89 Fasano M *et al.* (2022). Immunotherapy for head and neck cancer: Present and future. *Crit Rev Oncol Hematol* **174**: 103679. doi: 10.1016/j.critrevonc.2022.103679.

90 Worden F, Mierzwa M. JAVELIN head and neck 100 trial: When failure seems fatal, hope is not lost. The ASCO Post. [Online] Available at: https://ascopost.com/issues/august-10-2021/javelin-head-and-neck-100-trial-when-failure-seems-fatal-hope-is-not-lost/ [Accessed November 28, 2023].

91 Filippini D & Le Tourneau C. (2024). The potential roles of antibody-drug conjugates in head and neck squamous cell carcinoma. *Curr Op Oncology* **36**(3): 147–154. doi: 10.1097/CCO.0000000000001022.

92 Zhang L *et al.* (1878). Molecular basis and targeted therapy in thyroid cancer: Progress and opportunities. *Biochimica et Biophysica Acta (BBA) - Reviews on Cancer* **2023**(4): 188928. doi: 10.1016/j.bbcan.2023.188928.

93 Prete A *et al.* (2020). Update on fundamental mechanisms of thyroid cancer. *Front Endocrinol (Lausanne)* **11**. doi: 10.3389/fendo.2020.00102.

94 Subbiah V *et al.* (2020). State-of-the-art strategies for targeting *RET* -dependent cancers. *J Clin Oncol* **38**(11): 1209–1221. doi: 10.1200/JCO.19.02551.

95 Quante M, Wang TC, Bass AJ (2023). Adenocarcinoma of the oesophagus: Is it gastric cancer? *Gut* **72**(6): 1027–1029. doi: 10.1136/gutjnl-2022-327096.

96 Salem ME *et al.* (2018). Comparative molecular analyses of esophageal squamous cell carcinoma, esophageal adenocarcinoma, and gastric adenocarcinoma. *Oncologist* **23**(11): 1319–1327. doi: 10.1634/theoncologist.2018-0143.

97 Ilson DH (2018). Is there a future for EGFR targeted agents in esophageal cancer? *Ann Oncol* **29**(6): 1343–1344. doi: 10.1093/annonc/mdy135.

98 Rodriquenz MG *et al.* (2020). MSI and EBV positive gastric cancer's subgroups and their link with novel immunotherapy. *J Clin Med* **9**(5): 1427. doi: 10.3390/jcm9051427.

99 Grizzi G *et al.* (2023). Anti-claudin treatments in gastroesophageal adenocarcinoma: Mainstream and upcoming strategies. *J Clin Med* **12**(8): 2973. doi: 10.3390/jcm12082973.

100 Lengyel CG *et al.* (2022). FGFR pathway inhibition in gastric cancer: The golden era of an old target? *Life* **12**(1): 81. doi: 10.3390/life12010081.

101 Körfer J, Lordick F, Hacker UT (2021). Molecular targets for gastric cancer treatment and future perspectives from a clinical and translational point of view. *Cancers (Basel)* **13**(20): 5216. doi: 10.3390/cancers13205216.

102 Jiang S *et al.* (2022). A comprehensive review of pancreatic cancer and its therapeutic challenges. *Aging* **14**(18): 7635–7649. doi: 10.18632/aging.204310.

103 Cannon A *et al.* (2018). Desmoplasia in pancreatic ductal adenocarcinoma: Insight into pathological function and therapeutic potential. *Genes Cancer* **9**(3–4): 78–86. doi: 10.18632/genesandcancer.171.

104 Ren B *et al.* (2018). Tumor microenvironment participates in metastasis of pancreatic cancer. *Mol Cancer* **17**(1): 108. doi: 10.1186/s12943-018-0858-1.

105 Chi J *et al.* (2021). The role of PARP inhibitors in BRCA mutated pancreatic cancer. *Ther Adv Gastroenterol* **14**: 175628482110148. doi: 10.1177/17562848211014818.

106 Bannoura SF, Khan HY, Azmi AS (2022). KRAS G12D targeted therapies for pancreatic cancer: Has the fortress been conquered? *Front Oncol* **12**. doi: 10.3389/fonc.2022.1013902.

107 Luchini C *et al.* (2021). Comprehensive characterisation of pancreatic ductal adenocarcinoma with microsatellite instability: Histology, molecular pathology and clinical implications. *Gut* **70**(1): 148–156. doi: 10.1136/gutjnl-2020-320726.

108 Sangro B *et al.* (2021). Advances in immunotherapy for hepatocellular carcinoma. *Nat Rev Gastroenterol Hepatol* **18**(8): 525–543. doi: 10.1038/s41575-021-00438-0.

109 Zhang Y *et al.* (2022). Newest therapies for cholangiocarcinoma: An updated overview of approved treatments with transplant oncology vision. *Cancers (Basel)* **14**(20): 5074. doi: 10.3390/cancers14205074.

110 Bonneville R *et al.* (2017). Landscape of microsatellite instability across 39 cancer types. *JCO Precis Oncol* **1**: 1–15. doi: 10.1200/PO.17.00073.

111 Marabelle A *et al.* (2020). Efficacy of pembroli-zumab in patients with noncolorectal high microsatellite instability/mismatch repair–deficient cancer: Results from the phase II KEYNOTE-158 study. *J Clin Oncol* **38**(1): 1–10. doi: 10.1200/JCO.19.02105.

112 Wittwer NL *et al.* (2023). Antibody drug conju-gates: Hitting the mark in pancreatic cancer? *J Exp Clin Cancer Res* **42**(1): 280. doi: 10.1186/s13046-023-02868-x.

113 Kuwatani M, Sakamoto N (2023). Promising highly targeted therapies for cholangiocarci-noma: A review and future perspectives. *Cancers (Basel)* **15**(14): 3686. doi: 10.3390/cancers15143686.

114 Dahlgren D, Lennernäs H (2020). Antibody-drug conjugates and targeted treatment strategies for hepatocellular carcinoma: A drug-delivery perspective. *Molecules* **25**(12): 2861. doi: 10.3390/molecules25122861.

115 Li Y-L *et al.* (2022). Advances in medical treatment for pancreatic neuroendocrine neo-plasms. *World J Gastroenterol* **28**(20): 2163–2175. doi: 10.3748/wjg.v28.i20.2163.

116 Gomes-Porras M, Cárdenas-Salas J, Álvarez-Escolá C (2020). Somatostatin analogs in clinical practice: A review. *Int J Mol Sci* **21**(5): 1682. doi: 10.3390/ijms21051682.

117 Symons R *et al.* (2023). Progress in the treat-ment of small intestine cancer. *Curr Treat Options in Oncol* **24**(4): 241–261. doi: 10.1007/s11864-023-01058-3.

118 de Back T *et al.* (2023). Evaluation of systemic treatments of small intestinal adenocarcinomas. *JAMA Netw Open* **6**(2): e230631. doi: 10.1001/jamanetworkopen.2023.0631.

119 Clark PE (2009). The role of VHL in clear-cell renal cell carcinoma and its relation to targeted therapy. *Kidney Int* **76**(9): 939–945. doi: 10.1038/ki.2009.296.

120 Canino C *et al.* (2019). Targeting angiogenesis in metastatic renal cell carcinoma. *Expert Rev Anticancer Ther* **19**(3): 245–257. doi: 10.1080/14737140.2019.1574574.

121 Ross K, Jones RJ (2017). Immune checkpoint inhibitors in renal cell carcinoma. *Clin Sci* **131**(21): 2627–2642. doi: 10.1042/CS20160894.

122 Grande E, Molina-Cerrillo J, Necchi A (2021). Coming of age of immunotherapy of

urothelial cancer. *Target Oncol* **16**(3): 283–294. doi: 10.1007/s11523-021-00804-7.

123 Piombino C *et al.* (2023). Immunotherapy in urothelial cancer: Current status and future directions. *Expert Rev Anticancer Ther* **23**(11): 1141–1155. doi: 10.1080/14737140.2023.2265572.

124 Garje R *et al.* (2020). Fibroblast growth factor receptor (FGFR) inhibitors in urothelial cancer. *Oncologist* **25**(11): e1711–e1719. doi: 10.1634/theoncologist.2020-0334.

125 D'Angelo A *et al.* (2022). An update on antibody–drug conjugates in urothelial carci-noma: State of the art strategies and what comes next. *Cancer Chemother Pharmacol* **90**(3): 191–205. doi: 10.1007/s00280-022-04459-7.

126 Chen W *et al.* (2022). ALT-803 in the treatment of non-muscle-invasive bladder cancer: Preclinical and clinical evidence and transla-tional potential. *Front Immunol* **13**: 1040669. doi: 10.3389/fimmu.2022.1040669.

127 Zarrabi K, Walzer E, Zibelman M (2021). Immune checkpoint inhibition in advanced non-clear cell renal cell carcinoma: Leveraging success from clear cell histology into new opportunities. *Cancers (Basel)* **13**(15): 3652. doi: 10.3390/cancers13153652.

128 The Cancer Genome Atlas Research Network (2011). Integrated genomic analyses of ovar-ian carcinoma. *Nature* **474**(7353): 609–615. doi: 10.1038/nature10166.

129 Konstantinopoulos PA *et al.* (2015). Homologous recombination deficiency: Exploiting the fundamental vulnerability of ovarian cancer. *Cancer Discov* **5**(11): 1137–1154. doi: 10.1158/2159-8290.CD-15-0714.

130 Awada A *et al.* (2022). Immunotherapy in the treatment of platinum-resistant ovarian cancer: Current perspectives. *Onco Targets Ther* **15**: 853–866. doi: 10.2147/OTT.S335936.

131 Garg V, Oza AM (2023). Treatment of ovarian cancer beyond PARP inhibition: Current and future options. *Drugs* **83**(15): 1365–1385. doi: 10.1007/s40265-023-01934-0.

132 Cobb L, Gershenson D (2023). Novel therapeu-tics in low-grade serous ovarian cancer. *Int J Gynecol Cancer* **33**(3): 377–384. doi: 10.1136/ijgc-2022-003677.

133 Zwimpfer TA *et al.* (2023). Low grade serous ovarian cancer – A rare disease with increasing

therapeutic options. *Cancer Treat Rev* **112**: 102497. doi: 10.1016/j.ctrv.2022.102497.

134 Ryan NAJ *et al.* (2020). The proportion of endometrial tumours associated with Lynch syndrome (PETALS): A prospective cross-sectional study. *PLoS Med* **17**(9): e1003263. doi: 10.1371/journal.pmed.1003263.

135 Marín-Jiménez JA *et al.* (2022). Facts and hopes in immunotherapy of endometrial cancer. *Clin Cancer Res* **28**(22): 4849–4860. doi: 10.1158/1078-0432.CCR-21-1564.

136 Yen T-T *et al.* (2020). Molecular classification and emerging targeted therapy in endometrial cancer. *Int J Gynecol Pathol* **39**(1): 26–35. doi: 10.1097/PGP.0000000000000585.

137 van den Heerik ASVM *et al.* (2021). Adjuvant therapy for endometrial cancer in the era of molecular classification: Radiotherapy, chemoradiation and novel targets for therapy. *Int J Gynecol Cancer* **31**(4): 594–604. doi: 10.1136/ijgc-2020-001822.

138 Karpel HC, Powell SS, Pothuri B (2023). Antibody-drug conjugates in gynecologic cancer. *Am Soc Clin Oncol Educ Book* **no. 43**. doi: 10.1200/EDBK_390772.

139 Ferrall L *et al.* (2021). Cervical cancer immunotherapy: Facts and hopes. *Clin Cancer Res* **27**(18): 4953–4973. doi: 10.1158/1078-0432.CCR-20-2833.

140 Meric-Bernstam F *et al.* (2023). Efficacy and safety of trastuzumab deruxtecan (T-DXd) in patients (pts) with HER2-expressing solid tumors: DESTINY-PanTumor02 (DP-02) interim results. *J Clin Oncol* **41**(17_suppl): LBA3000. doi: 10.1200/JCO.2023.41.17_suppl.LBA3000.

141 Gennigens C *et al.* (2022). Recurrent or primary metastatic cervical cancer: Current and future treatments. *ESMO Open* **7**(5): 100579. doi: 10.1016/j.esmoop.2022.100579.

142 Woelber L *et al.* (2020). Targeted therapeutic approaches in vulvar squamous cell cancer (VSCC): Case series and review of the literature. *Oncol Res* **28**(6): 645–659. doi: 10.3727/096504020X16076861118243.

143 Kulkarni A, Dogra N, Zigras T (2022). Innovations in the management of vaginal cancer. *Curr Oncol* **29**(5): 3082–3092. doi: 10.3390/curroncol29050250.

144 Palisoul ML *et al.* (2017). Identification of molecular targets in vulvar cancers. *Gynecol Oncol* **146**(2): 305–313. doi: 10.1016/j.ygyno.2017.05.011.

145 Angeli E *et al.* (2019). How to make anticancer drugs cross the blood–brain barrier to treat brain metastases. *Int J Mol Sci* **21**(1): 22. doi: 10.3390/ijms21010022.

146 Arvanitis CD, Ferraro GB, Jain RK (2020). The blood–brain barrier and blood–tumour barrier in brain tumours and metastases. *Nat Rev Cancer* **20**(1): 26–41. doi: 10.1038/s41568-019-0205-x.

147 Becker A *et al.* (2021). Tumor heterogeneity in glioblastomas: From light microscopy to molecular pathology. *Cancers (Basel)* **13**(4): 761. doi: 10.3390/cancers13040761.

148 Gromeier M *et al.* (2021). Very low mutation burden is a feature of inflamed recurrent glioblastomas responsive to cancer immunotherapy. *Nat Commun* **12**(1): 352. doi: 10.1038/s41467-020-20469-6.

149 Zhao J *et al.* (2019). Immune and genomic correlates of response to anti-PD-1 immunotherapy in glioblastoma. *Nat Med* **25**(3): 462–469. doi: 10.1038/s41591-019-0349-y.

150 Rocha Pinheiro SL *et al.* (2023). Immunotherapy in glioblastoma treatment: Current state and future prospects. *World J Clin Oncol* **14**(4): 138–159. doi: 10.5306/wjco.v14.i4.138.

151 Rong L, Li N, Zhang Z (2022). Emerging therapies for glioblastoma: Current state and future directions. *J Exp Clin Cancer Res* **41**(1): 142. doi: 10.1186/s13046-022-02349-7.

152 Le Rhun E *et al.* (2019). Molecular targeted therapy of glioblastoma. *Cancer Treat Rev* **80**: 101896. doi: 10.1016/j.ctrv.2019.101896.

153 Xu H *et al.* (2017). Epidermal growth factor receptor in glioblastoma. *Oncol Lett* **14**(1): 512–516. doi: 10.3892/ol.2017.6221.

154 Mair MJ *et al.* (2023). Understanding the activity of antibody–drug conjugates in primary and secondary brain tumours. *Nat Rev Clin Oncol* **20**(6): 372–389. doi: 10.1038/s41571-023-00756-z.

155 Ramapriyan R *et al.* (2023). The role of antibody-based therapies in neuro-oncology. *Antibodies* **12**(4): 74. doi: 10.3390/antib12040074.

156 Romero D (2023). Dabrafenib–trametinib is effective in paediatric high-grade glioma.

Nat Rev Clin Oncol **20**(11): 734–734. doi: 10.1038/s41571-023-00820-8.

157   Brastianos PK *et al*. (2023). BRAF–MEK inhibition in newly diagnosed papillary craniopharyngiomas. *N Engl J Med* **389**(2): 118–126. doi: 10.1056/NEJMoa2213329.

158   Deeks ED (2021). Belzutifan: First approval. *Drugs* **81**(16): 1921–1927. doi: 10.1007/s40265-021-01606-x.

159   Sasongko TH *et al*. (2023). Rapamycin and rapalogs for tuberous sclerosis complex. *Cochrane Database Syst Rev* **2023**(7). doi: 10.1002/14651858.CD011272.pub3.

160   Mellinghoff IK *et al*. (2023). Vorasidenib in IDH1- or IDH2-mutant low-grade glioma. *N Engl J Med* **389**(7): 589–601. doi: 10.1056/NEJMoa2304194.

161   Coggshall K *et al*. (2018). Merkel cell carcinoma: An update and review. *J Am Acad Dermatol* **78**(3): 433–442. doi: 10.1016/j.jaad.2017.12.001.

162   Wolchok JD *et al*. (2022). Long-term outcomes with nivolumab plus ipilimumab or nivolumab alone versus ipilimumab in patients with advanced melanoma. *J Clin Oncol* **40**(2): 127–137. doi: 10.1200/JCO.21.02229.

163   Knight A, Karapetyan L, Kirkwood JM (2023). Immunotherapy in melanoma: Recent advances and future directions. *Cancers (Basel)* **15**(4): 1106. doi: 10.3390/cancers15041106.

164   Girod M *et al*. (2022). Non-V600E/K BRAF Mutations in Metastatic Melanoma: Molecular Description, Frequency, and Effectiveness of Targeted Therapy in a Large National Cohort. *JCO Precis Oncol* **6**. doi: 10.1200/PO.22.00075.

165   Davis EJ *et al*. (2018). Melanoma: What do all the mutations mean? *Cancer* **124**(17): 3490–3499. doi: 10.1002/cncr.31345.

166   Curtin JA *et al*. (2005). Distinct sets of genetic alterations in melanoma. *N Engl J Med* **353**(20): 2135–2147. doi: 10.1056/NEJMoa050092.

167   Dummer R, Welti M, Ramelyte E (2023). The role of triple therapy and therapy sequence in treatment of BRAF-mutant metastatic melanoma. *J Transl Med* **21**(1): 529. doi: 10.1186/s12967-023-04391-1.

168   Helwick C. Are triplets necessary for BRAF-mutated melanoma? The ASCO Post. [Online] Available at: https://ascopost.com/issues/september-10-2021/are-triplets-necessary-for-braf-mutated-melanoma/ [Accessed December 11, 2023].

169   Villani A *et al*. (2022). New emerging treatment options for advanced basal cell carcinoma and squamous cell carcinoma. *Adv Ther* **39**(3): 1164–1178. doi: 10.1007/s12325-022-02044-1.

170   Nagarajan P *et al*. (2019). Keratinocyte carcinomas: Current concepts and future research priorities. *Clin Cancer Res* **25**(8): 2379–2391. doi: 10.1158/1078-0432.CCR-18-1122.

171   Zaggana E *et al*. (2022). Merkel cell carcinoma—Update on diagnosis, management and future perspectives. *Cancers (Basel)* **15**(1): 103. doi: 10.3390/cancers15010103.

172   Goodman R, Johnson DB (2022). Antibody-drug conjugates for melanoma and other skin malignancies. *Curr Treat Options in Oncol* **23**(10): 1428–1442. doi: 10.1007/s11864-022-01018-3.

173   Garcia-Mouronte E *et al*. (2023). Imiquimod as local immunotherapy in the management of premalignant cutaneous conditions and skin cancer. *Int J Mol Sci* **24**(13): 10835. doi: 10.3390/ijms241310835.

174   Bubna A (2015). Imiquimod – Its role in the treatment of cutaneous malignancies. *Indian J Pharmacol* **47**(4): 354. doi: 10.4103/0253-7613.161249.

175   Cancer Research UK. Acute lymphoblastic leukaemia (ALL) incidence statistics. [Online] Available at: https://www.cancerresearchuk.org/health-professional/cancer-statistics/statistics-by-cancer-type/leukaemia-all#heading-Zero [Accessed December 12, 2023].

176   Pui C-H (2020). Precision medicine in acute lymphoblastic leukemia. *Front Med* **14**(6): 689–700. doi: 10.1007/s11684-020-0759-8.

177   Hallek M, Al-Sawaf O (2021). Chronic lymphocytic leukemia: 2022 update on diagnostic and therapeutic procedures. *Am J Hematol* **96**(12): 1679–1705. doi: 10.1002/ajh.26367.

178   Bristol Myers Squibb. U.S. FDA approves Bristol Myers Squibb's Breyanzi ® as the first and only CAR T cell therapy for adults with relapsed or refractory chronic lymphocytic leukemia (CLL) or small lymphocytic lymphoma

(SLL). [Online] Available at: https://news.bms.com/news/corporate-financial/2024/U.S.-FDA-Approves-Bristol-Myers-Squibbs-Breyanzi--as-the-First-and-Only-CAR-T-Cell-Therapy-for-Adults-with-Relapsed-or-Refractory-Chronic-Lymphocytic-Leukemia-CLL-or-Small-Lymphocytic-Lymphoma-SLL/default.aspx [Accessed March 22, 2024].

179 National Cancer Institute. Non-Hodgkin lymphoma treatment (PDQ®)–Patient version. NIIH website. [Online] Available at: https://www.cancer.gov/types/lymphoma/patient/adult-nhl-treatment-pdq [Accessed December 12, 2023].

180 Russler-Germain DA, Ghobadi A (2023). T-cell redirecting therapies for B-cell non-Hodgkin lymphoma: Recent progress and future directions. *Front Oncol* **13**. doi: 10.3389/fonc.2023.1168622.

181 Park HS *et al.* (2017). T-cell non-Hodgkin lymphomas: Spectrum of disease and the role of imaging in the management of common subtypes. *Korean J Radiol* **18**(1): 71. doi: 10.3348/kjr.2017.18.1.71.

182 Blackmon AL, Pinter-Brown L (2020). Spotlight on mogamulizumab-Kpkc for use in adults with relapsed or refractory mycosis fungoides or sézary syndrome: Efficacy, safety, and patient selection. *Drug Des Devel Ther* **14**: 3747–3754. doi: 10.2147/DDDT.S185896.

183 Zinzani PL *et al.* (2016). Panoptic clinical review of the current and future treatment of relapsed/refractory T-cell lymphomas: Cutaneous T-cell lymphomas. *Crit Rev Oncol Hematol* **99**: 228–240. doi: 10.1016/j.critrevonc.2015.12.018.

184 OncLive. FDA Approves Denileukin Diftitox for R/R Cutaneous T-Cell Lymphoma. [Online] Available at: https://www.onclive.com/view/fda-approves-denileukin-diftitox-for-r-r-cutaneous-t-cell-lymphoma [Accessed August 16, 2024].

185 Cancer Research UK. Hodgkin lymphoma statistics. [Online] Available at: https://www.cancerresearchuk.org/health-professional/cancer-statistics/statistics-by-cancer-type/hodgkin-lymphoma [Accessed December 14, 2023].

186 Brice P, de Kerviler E, Friedberg JW (2021). Classical Hodgkin lymphoma. *Lancet* **398** (10310): 1518–1527. doi: 10.1016/S0140-6736(20)32207-8.

187 Weniger MA, Küppers R (2021). Molecular biology of Hodgkin lymphoma. *Leukemia* **35**(4): 968–981. doi: 10.1038/s41375-021-01204-6.

188 Andrade-Gonzalez X, Ansell SM (2021). Novel therapies in the treatment of Hodgkin lymphoma. *Curr Treat Options in Oncol* **22**(5): 42. doi: 10.1007/s11864-021-00840-5.

189 Roemer MGM *et al.* (2016). PD-L1 and PD-L2 genetic alterations define classical Hodgkin lymphoma and predict outcome. *J Clin Oncol* **34**(23): 2690–2697. doi: 10.1200/JCO.2016.66.4482.

190 Green MR *et al.* (2010). Integrative analysis reveals selective 9p24.1 amplification, increased PD-1 ligand expression, and further induction via JAK2 in nodular sclerosing Hodgkin lymphoma and primary mediastinal large B-cell lymphoma. *Blood* **116**(17): 3268–3277. doi: 10.1182/blood-2010-05-282780.

191 Cancer Research UK. Myeloma incidence statistics. [Online] Available at: https://www.cancerresearchuk.org/health-professional/cancer-statistics/statistics-by-cancer-type/myeloma [Accessed December 14, 2023].

192 Rodríguez-Lobato LG *et al.* (2020). Why immunotherapy fails in multiple myeloma. *Hematology* **2**(1): 1–42. doi: 10.3390/hemato2010001.

193 Zhou X, Einsele H, Danhof S (2020). Bispecific antibodies: A new era of treatment for multiple myeloma. *J Clin Med* **9**(7): 2166. doi: 10.3390/jcm9072166.

194 Sohail A *et al.* (2018). Emerging immune targets for the treatment of multiple myeloma. *Immunotherapy* **10**(4): 265–282. doi: 10.2217/imt-2017-0136.

195 Sherbenou DW, Mark TM, Forsberg P (2017). Monoclonal antibodies in multiple myeloma: A new wave of the future. *Clin Lymphoma Myeloma Leuk* **17**(9): 545–554. doi: 10.1016/j.clml.2017.06.030.

196 Diamantidis MD, Papadaki S, Hatjiharissi E (2022). Exploring the current molecular landscape and management of multiple myeloma

patients with the t(11;14) translocation. *Front Oncol* **12**. doi: 10.3389/fonc.2022.934008.

197 Carter JL *et al.* (2020). Targeting multiple signaling pathways: The new approach to acute myeloid leukemia therapy. *Signal Transduct Target Ther* **5**(1): 288. doi: 10.1038/s41392-020-00361-x.

198 Liu H (2021). Emerging agents and regimens for AML. *J Hematol Oncol* **14**(1): 49. doi: 10.1186/s13045-021-01062-w.

199 Wei Y *et al.* (2020). Targeting Bcl-2 proteins in acute myeloid leukemia. *Front Oncol* **10**. doi: 10.3389/fonc.2020.584974.

200 Thomas D, Majeti R (2017). Biology and relevance of human acute myeloid leukemia stem cells. *Blood* **129**(12): 1577–1585. doi: 10.1182/blood-2016-10-696054.

201 Lainez-González D, Serrano-López J, Alonso-Domínguez JM (2021). Understanding the Hedgehog signaling pathway in acute myeloid leukemia stem cells: A necessary step toward a cure. *Biology (Basel)* **10**(4): 255. doi: 10.3390/biology10040255.

202 Garcia-Manero G, Chien KS, Montalban-Bravo G (2020). Myelodysplastic syndromes: 2021 update on diagnosis, risk stratification and management. *Am J Hematol* **95**(11): 1399–1420. doi: 10.1002/ajh.25950.

203 Gale RP (2023). Can immune therapy cure acute myeloid leukemia? *Curr Treat Options in Oncol* **24**(5): 381–386. doi: 10.1007/s11864-023-01066-3.

204 Baumeister J *et al.* (2021). Progression of myeloproliferative neoplasms (MPN): Diagnostic and therapeutic perspectives. *Cells* **10**(12): 3551. doi: 10.3390/cells10123551.

205 Spivak JL (2017). Myeloproliferative neoplasms. *N Engl J Med* **376**(22): 2168–2181. doi: 10.1056/NEJMra1406186.

206 Pandey G, Kuykendall AT, Reuther GW (2022). JAK2 inhibitor persistence in MPN: Uncovering a central role of ERK activation. *Blood Cancer J* **12**(1): 13. doi: 10.1038/s41408-022-00609-5.

207 Bernt KM & Hunger SP (2014). Current concepts in pediatric Philadelphia chromosome-positive acute lymphoblastic leukemia. *Front Oncol* **4**: 54. doi: 10.3389/fonc.2014.00054.

208 Kuhn MWM & Ganser A (2024). The Menin story in acute myeloid leukaemia-The road to success. *Br J Haematol*. Online ahead of print. doi: 10.1111/bjh.19508.

Appendix

INFORMATION ON CELLS, DNA, GENES, AND CHROMOSOMES

Stated Clearly
statedclearly.com
- An animation-led US website that explains various scientific concepts.
- Their video *What Is DNA and How Does It Work?* is a fantastic starting point for anyone confused about what DNA is and how it contains the instructions for making living things.
- They also have videos called: *What Exactly Is A Gene?*, *What Is A Molecule?*, and: *What Is A Chromosome?*

Let's Communicate Cancer
e-lfh.org.uk/programmes/
lets-communicate-cancer/
- On the *elearning for healthcare* website from NHS England.
- Let's Communicate Cancer is an educational program for community pharmacists but is available to anyone with an elearning for healthcare login.
- The program includes many videos on cancer biology and treatments, written and presented by me.

Genomics Education Programme
genomicseducation.hee.nhs.uk/education/
- A website from NHS England.
- Contains educational resources and courses on topics such as *What is genomics?* and *What is bioinformatics?*

The National Human Genome Research Institute
genome.gov
- From the National Human Genome Research Institute in the United States.
- Contains some useful fact sheets and other resources.
- For example, their DNA fact sheet is nicely written.

DNA Learning Center
Dnalc.cshl.edu
- From Cold Spring Harbor Laboratory in the United States.
- Includes incredible computer-generated animations showing how DNA is used to make mRNA (transcription) and how mRNA is used to make proteins (translation).
- I would recommend the Transcription and Translation animations found on this page: https://dnalc.cshl.edu/resources/animations/

A Beginner's Guide to Targeted Cancer Treatments and Cancer Immunotherapy, Second Edition. Elaine Vickers.
© 2025 John Wiley & Sons Ltd. Published 2025 by John Wiley & Sons Ltd.

The Khan Academy

khanacademy.org/science/biology

- A US organization offering global online education.
- Contains a wealth of information (mostly overviews and videos) on a huge range of subjects.
- Includes "Structure of a Cell," "Cell Signaling," "DNA as the Genetic Material," "Central Dogma (DNA to RNA to Protein)," and "Gene Regulation."

Scitable

nature.com/scitable/topics

- A free online teaching portal from Nature Education.
- For those of you who want more science!
- Contains detailed but fairly straightforward articles with many illustrations.
- I recommend their e-books, *Cell Biology* and *Essentials of Genetics*.

Armando Hasudungan Biology and Medicine Tutorials

armandoh.org/video/

- An Australian doctor who produces educational videos on a wide range of medical topics.
- His videos on immunology topics are particularly useful.

Glossary of Terms

Acute lymphoblastic leukemia (ALL; acute lymphocytic leukemia) An aggressive form of leukemia that is more common in children than adults. It develops from immature white blood cells called lymphocytes in the bone marrow.

Acute myeloid leukemia (AML) An aggressive form of leukemia that is most common in adults aged over 65. It develops from immature white blood cells (granulocytes or monocytes) in the bone marrow.

ADCC (antibody-dependent cell-mediated cytotoxicity) The process by which a white blood cell (such as a macrophage or natural killer cell) binds to an antibody attached to a protein on the surface of a cell and then kills the cell.

Adenocarcinoma A cancer that develops from cells that produce mucus or other substances. Most cancers of the breast, lung, esophagus, stomach, bowel, rectum, pancreas, prostate, and uterus are adenocarcinomas.

Adoptive cell transfer/adoptive cell therapy A form of immunotherapy in which modified cells are transferred into a patient.

Adjuvant treatment A treatment given together with, or following, another treatment. It commonly refers to giving a patient chemotherapy soon after surgery. It might also refer to a treatment given alongside a vaccine that stimulates the immune system.

Adrenal glands Glands that sit on top of our kidneys and produce a range of hormones.

Advanced therapy medicinal product (ATMP) A medicine that involves the manipulation of genes, tissues, or cells. For example, CAR T cell therapy is an ATMP.

Aerobic glycolysis The fermentation of glucose to create lactate and produce energy in the form of ATP. Cancer cells preferentially use this process to create ATP even when they have sufficient oxygen to perform normal respiration.

Allele Different versions of the same gene are called alleles. We are born with two alleles of each gene in our genome, one from each parent.

Allogeneic Derived from someone else's tissues, cells, or DNA.

Amino acids These are small chemical compounds that are attached to one another by ribosomes to create proteins. There are 20 common amino acids. The number and order of amino acids in a protein determine its shape, function, and other properties.

A Beginner's Guide to Targeted Cancer Treatments and Cancer Immunotherapy, Second Edition. Elaine Vickers.
© 2025 John Wiley & Sons Ltd. Published 2025 by John Wiley & Sons Ltd.

Amplification (of a gene) Describes the fact that a cell has accidentally made extra copies of a gene.

Anaplastic lymphoma kinase (ALK) A growth factor receptor that in humans is encoded by the *ALK* gene.

Androgen receptor Part of a family of intracellular receptors that respond to hormones. Androgen receptors are activated by testosterone and dihydrotestosterone.

Aneuploid A word that is used to describe cells that contain the wrong number of chromosomes. Cancer cells are often aneuploid.

Angiogenesis The development of a new blood vessel from a preexisting blood vessel. In terms of tumors, angiogenesis causes small blood vessels to sprout new side branches that grow to form new blood vessels, enabling blood to reach the tumor's cells and fuel its growth. The main trigger for angiogenesis is a growth factor called VEGF.

Angiogenesis inhibitor A treatment that blocks angiogenesis, usually by interfering with VEGF or VEGF receptors.

Antibody A large, Y-shaped protein produced by B cells in response to an infection – also called an immunoglobulin. Antibodies circulate in the blood and attach precisely to their target, after which they attract complement proteins and white blood cells such as macrophages and natural killer cells. They can also be manufactured by living cells and used as cancer treatments (as monoclonal antibodies).

Antibody-drug conjugate An antibody to which a toxic compound (such as chemotherapy) has been attached. The aim is that the antibody attaches to its target on the surface of a cancer cell and then gets drawn inside the cell and delivers the drug, which kills the cell.

Antigen A protein or other molecule that can trigger an immune response from B cells or T cells. Antigens for B cells are usually intact proteins. Antigens for T cells are tiny protein fragments (peptide antigens) displayed by MHC proteins.

Antigen-presenting cells (APCs) White blood cells that process and present antigens to T cells using their MHC proteins. Examples include dendritic cells, macrophages, and B cells.

Adipocytes Specialized cells that store energy as fat (lipid). Also known as lipocytes or fat cells.

APOBEC enzymes A family of enzymes that protect our cells from viruses by chopping up their DNA. Cancer cells often contain DNA mutations caused by overactive APOBEC enzymes.

Apoptosis Also called "programmed cell death." It is a very orderly and tightly controlled process through which a cell self-destructs.

ATMP See the definition for **Advanced therapy medicinal products**.

Adenosine triphosphate (ATP) A chemical produced from the breakdown of glucose from food. It contains high-energy chemical bonds and is used as the source of energy for every chemical reaction and energy-dependent process in our body.

Autologous Derived from the person's own tissues, cells, or DNA.

Base editing A scientific technique used to make precise changes to the sequence of a piece of DNA.

Basket trial A clinical trial in which patients with different types of cancer are entered into a single trial because their cancers share a common feature, such as the presence of a particular DNA mutation.

Basement membrane A thin, fibrous layer of proteins that lies immediately underneath every sheet of epithelial cells in our body. It provides structural support, limits contact between different cell types, and acts as a sieve. Also called the basal lamina.

B cells (B lymphocytes) Specialized white blood cells made in the bone marrow with B cell receptors (BCRs) on their surface. They may release their BCRs (now called antibodies) into the blood if they recognize an infection. An antibody-producing B cell is called a plasma cell.

B cell receptor (BCR) A protein found on the surface of B cells. BCRs are constructed from immunoglobulin (Ig)/antibody genes, which each B cell rearranges and pieces together to create a unique BCR.

Bcl-2 inhibitor A drug that inhibits Bcl-2 (B cell lymphoma 2), a protein that protects our cells from death by apoptosis. So far, they have successfully been used to treat chronic lymphocytic leukemia and acute myeloid leukemia.

Bcr-Abl A fusion protein made from two proteins called Bcr and Abl. This fusion protein is caused by a translocation between chromosomes 9 and 22, which creates the Philadelphia chromosome. This translocation is found in the cells of people with chronic myeloid leukemia (CML). Similar translocations are sometimes found in acute lymphoblastic leukemia (ALL).

Biological therapy A treatment that is manufactured using living cells, such as a monoclonal antibody therapy. However, organizations and individuals often use this term more widely to refer to all modern cancer treatments or all immunotherapies.

Biomarker Something biological (such as the presence or absence of a particular gene mutation) that can be measured and evaluated to give useful information, such as how aggressive a cancer is or whether a patient is likely to benefit from a particular treatment.

Biopsy A small part of a tumor removed using a needle (a needle biopsy) or during surgery for later analysis.

Biosimilar A treatment that is a copycat version of a protein-based treatment such as a monoclonal antibody. They are called biosimilars rather than generic treatments because they are highly complex molecules and are not biologically identical to the original.

Bispecific antibody An antibody-based protein that is designed to attach to two different targets. Often used to create a physical connection between cancer cells and T cells.

Bispecific T cell engager (BiTE®) A protein constructed from the antigen-binding regions of two different antibodies. Often designed to create a physical connection between cancer cells and T cells.

BiTE® See the definition for **Bispecific T cell engager**.

Blood-brain barrier Refers to the fact that in our brain, the cells lining the blood vessels (called endothelial cells) are slightly different, less permeable, and closer together than in the rest of the body. Thus, the brain is protected from many toxins and drugs that might be present in the blood.

B-Raf inhibitor These drugs are sometimes given to people whose melanoma skin cancer (or other cancer) has a mutation in the *BRAF* gene. B-Raf is made from the *BRAF* gene, and it is a component of the MAP kinase (MAPK) signaling pathway.

BRCA1 and BRCA2 Two proteins made from the *BRCA1* and *BRCA2* genes. These proteins are both involved in a DNA repair process called homologous recombination (HR). Loss or suppression of either gene results in HR deficiency. Inherited mutations in either *BRCA1* or *BRCA2* increase a person's risk of several cancer types, including breast and ovarian cancer.

Bruton's tyrosine kinase (BTK) A kinase that plays a crucial role in B cell development and activation.

Cancer germline antigens See the definition for **Cancer testis antigens**.

Cancer growth blockers/Cancer growth inhibitors Sometimes used to describe treatments that block cell communication pathways.

Cancer-immunity cycle Describes the process through which our immune system recognizes and kills cancer cells.

Cancer stem cell A cancer cell that has some of the properties of a normal stem cell; that is, it can both self-renew and give rise to other cancer cell types.

Cancer testis antigens Proteins that are normally only present in germ cells (egg or sperm) and developing embryos, but that are sometimes also found in cancer cells and can lead to a cancer-fighting immune response. They are a type of tumor-associated antigen.

Chimeric antigen receptor (CAR) A protein made from several different protein parts. It usually comprises an antigen-binding region from an antibody plus several other segments taken from other proteins. T cells that have been engineered to produce a CAR protein are known as CAR T cells.

CAR T cell therapy A treatment that involves modifying millions of a patient's T cells so that they produce a CAR protein.

Carcinogen Anything that causes cancer is called a carcinogen.

Carcinoma A cancer that has developed from faulty epithelial cells.

Catalyst Something that causes the rate of a chemical reaction to increase. Enzymes are specialized proteins that act as catalysts in cells.

Cluster of differentiation (CD) antigen CD antigen is a general name used for the proteins and other molecules found on the surface of cells, particularly white blood cells.

Complement-dependent cytotoxicity (CDC) When the complement protein C1q binds to an antibody attached to a protein on the surface of a cell, further complement proteins attach to C1q, forming a "membrane attack complex" that kills the cell.

Cell cycle The ordered and tightly controlled process a cell goes through each time it divides. A cell cycle involves four phases: G1, S, G2, and mitosis.

Cell cycle checkpoints Times within the cell cycle when a cell halts the cell cycle and checks that everything is progressing properly.

Cell division The process by which a cell grows and then splits into two to create two cells.

Cell signaling The processes through which cells communicate with one another. Often involves receptors on the cell surface that can trigger the activity of cell signaling pathways within the cell.

Cereblon E3 ligase modulatory drugs (CELMoDs) Treatments that work by altering the behavior of the cereblon protein, such as mezigdomide and iberdomide. Less used to describe thalidomide, lenalidomide, and pomalidomide, which were only discovered to affect the cereblon after their successful use as cancer treatments.

Checkpoint proteins A group of proteins found on the surface of white blood cells, such as T cells. Our body uses checkpoint proteins on T cells to control their level of activity. Examples include PD-1 and CTLA-4.

Checkpoint inhibitor See the definition for **Immune checkpoint inhibitor**.

Chemotherapy Generally a term used to describe drugs that kill rapidly multiplying cells. Some of these drugs were developed from diverse sources, such as natural chemicals extracted from plants or bacteria or from mustard gases used in warfare.

Chimeric protein A protein created by joining together the information from two or more genes.

Cholangiocarcinoma A cancer that begins in tubes called bile ducts that carry bile from the liver and gallbladder to the small intestine.

Chromosome A structure made from tightly coiled and packaged DNA, which is wrapped around histone proteins. Chromosomes store the DNA in our cells safely. They must be uncoiled for the DNA to be duplicated or for genes to be transcribed to make proteins.

Chromosomal instability (CIN) When a cell's chromosomes contain lots of large-scale defects such as broken, duplicated, or missing chromosomes.

Chromothripsis When a chromosome sustains many mutations simultaneously in a single catastrophic event.

Chronic lymphocytic leukemia (CLL) A type of blood cancer that develops from mature B lymphocytes. Also referred to as small lymphocytic lymphoma (SLL) if the cancer cells are mostly in the lymph nodes rather than the blood and bone marrow.

Chronic myeloid leukemia (CML; chronic myelogenous leukemia) A rare blood cancer that develops from immature granulocyte white blood cells in the bone marrow. A form of myeloproliferative neoplasm.

Circulating tumor DNA (ctDNA) DNA that has leaked out of cancer cells (often from dying cancer cells) and is circulating freely in a patient's blood; it is also called circulating free DNA. ctDNA can be purified and used to detect DNA mutations in cancer cells or to predict cancer recurrence or resistance to treatment.

Clonal mutation A mutation found in all the cells in a tumor rather than being found in just a subset of cells (a subclonal mutation).

Codon Ribosomes "read" mRNA three bases at a time. Each three-base pair grouping is called a codon. Each codon (e.g., CAA, AUU, or GCU) instructs the ribosome to add a particular amino acid (e.g., glutamine, isoleucine, or alanine) to the protein it is making.

Combination therapy The use of two or more treatments that are given together to people with cancer. Often refers to a combination of two or more chemotherapies.

Complement proteins A complex system of proteins found in our blood that form part of our immune system. They work together to kill invaders and send signals to white blood cells.

Complete response When a person's tumor (or tumors) have completely disappeared, as measured using available tests and scans. It may mean something different with hematological cancer, where more and more sensitive tests to detect residual cancer cells have led to new definitions.

Computerized tomography scan See the definition for **CT scan**.

Conjugated antibody An antibody that has something else linked to it, such as chemotherapy (an antibody-drug conjugate) or a radioactive particle (a radioimmunotherapy or radioimmunoconjugate).

Constant region The back end of an antibody (also called the Fc). It is the part of the antibody that attracts white blood cells that have Fc receptors on their surface, such as macrophages and natural killer cells.

CRISPR/Cas 9 A scientific technique used to make precise changes to the sequence of a piece of DNA.

Cross-talk When a protein or other molecule involved in one signaling pathway also influences the activity of another signaling pathway.

ctDNA See the definition for **Circulating tumor DNA**.

Computerized tomography (CT) scan An image that combines images from many X-rays to create a 3D image of the inside of the body.

Cyclins A set of proteins that are manufactured and destroyed at precise points during the cell cycle and that control cyclin-dependent kinases (CDKs).

Cyclin-dependent kinase (CDK) A set of proteins that regulate the progression of a cell through the cell cycle by phosphorylating a protein called retinoblastoma protein (RB). Their activity is controlled by another set of proteins called cyclins.

Cytokines Small proteins used by white blood cells to communicate with one another. White blood cells use an enormous number of them to coordinate one another's movements, activate one another, and manage immune responses. They include chemokines and interleukins.

Cytokine release syndrome (CRS) A combination of symptoms caused by some immunotherapies. Caused by the rapid release of certain cytokines (such as interleukin-6) by white blood cells such as T cells and dying cancer cells. CRS symptoms include fever, nausea, headache, rash, rapid heartbeat, low blood pressure, and trouble breathing.

Cytoplasm The fluid that fills a cell and is enclosed by the cell membrane. It contains thousands of proteins, along with many different structures and compartments.

Cytotoxic Something that is toxic to living cells.

Cytotoxic T cells These are T cells that can directly kill virus-infected cells and cancer cells. Also called cytotoxic T lymphocytes (CTLs).

Dendritic cell A type of white blood cell. Millions of these cells patrol the body, looking for infections, damage, and other problems. They display on their surface fragments of proteins (called peptide antigens), which they present to T cells using their MHC proteins (they are referred to as antigen-presenting cells). They can also display antigens from cancer proteins and initiate a cancer-fighting immune response. A separate type of dendritic cell, called a follicular dendritic cell, displays antigens to B cells rather than T cells.

Desmoplasia Refers to the accumulation of fibrous proteins within the tumor microenvironment. It can act as a physical barrier that prevents cancer treatments from moving freely within a tumor and is a major cause of treatment resistance in pancreatic cancer in particular.

Diagnostic biomarker A biomarker that can be used to diagnose a particular type or subtype of cancer.

Dimer When two identical (or closely related) proteins pair up, they create a dimer.

Dimerization When two proteins bump into one another and stick together to form a dimer. For example, when two epidermal growth factor (EGF) receptors are bound to EGF, they then dimerize and activate the MAPK pathway.

Deoxy ribonucleic acid (DNA) A long, spiraling molecule made of two strands that wind around one another to create a double helix. The double helix is held together by relatively simple chemicals called DNA bases that pair up in a particular way. The order of the four bases in a DNA strand is called the DNA sequence. DNA is packaged in our cells in structures called chromosomes.

DNA base Relatively simple (but vital) chemicals that hold together the DNA double helix. There are four subtly different DNA bases called A (adenine), C (cytosine), G (guanine), and T (thymine). A always pairs with T; C always pairs with G. The order of bases in DNA is critical as this carries the information for making proteins and for constructing the entire organism.

DNA damage response This term is used to describe how cells respond to and repair DNA damage.

DNA repair deficiency (DRD) A term used to describe cancer cells that are unable to detect or repair some types of DNA damage.

DNA polymerase An enzyme that creates DNA from DNA. Used by our cells to create duplicate sets of chromosomes prior to cell division.

Dose-response relationship Where the effects of a treatment are proportional to the dose the person receives.

Driver mutation A mutation found in a cancer cell that is thought to play an important role in driving the cell's abnormal behavior.

Epidermal growth factor (EGF) A growth factor that stimulates cell growth, proliferation, and differentiation of many cell types by binding to its receptor, the EGF receptor (EGFR).

EGF receptor (EGFR) A growth factor receptor found on the surface of many different cell types. EGFR is part of a family of human EGF receptors that comprise EGFR, HER2, HER3 and HER4.

European Medicines Agency (EMA) The organization responsible for the scientific evaluation, supervision, and safety monitoring of medicines in the European Union and the European Economic Area.

Encode A term often used in relation to genes. Each gene encodes (i.e., contains the instructions to manufacture) one or more proteins.

Endothelial cells Specialized cells that line our body's blood and lymph vessels.

Enhancer A short sequence of DNA to which transcription factors and other proteins can attach and that controls the activity of genes. Unlike promoters, they can be found a long way away from the genes they help to control.

Enzyme A protein that catalyzes a chemical reaction; examples include proteases, kinases, and methylases.

Epigenetics Describes changes to a cell's DNA that impact gene activity but don't involve changes to the sequence of DNA bases. Epigenetics often refers to changes to the backbone of the DNA molecule (e.g., by methylation) or to the histone proteins that DNA is wrapped around (e.g., by acetylation). These changes alter how loosely or tightly the DNA is coiled, affecting its accessibility to transcription factors and influencing whether the gene is transcribed.

Epithelial cell A very common type of cell in the body. Sheets of epithelial cells line the body's cavities, organs, and glands, and cover flat surfaces.

Epithelial-to-mesenchymal transition (EMT) A process through which epithelial cells change to become more like mesenchymal cells, which are more mobile, independent, and robust. Cancer cells that go through the EMT are more likely to cause metastasis and survive treatment.

Epitope The precise location on a protein or other complex molecule that an antibody attaches to.

Estrogen receptor (ER) A receptor often found in breast cancer cells. In the presence of estrogen, these receptors pair up and act as transcription factors that activate the transcription of a wide variety of genes.

Exon A region of a gene that is present in the final mRNA copy of the gene and that is used by the cell to make the corresponding protein. Genes usually contain several exons, separated by introns (regions of genes that don't end up in the final mRNA copy).

Extracellular matrix (ECM) A network of proteins and complicated sugar molecules that surround the cells in our tissues and organs.

Fluorescence-activated cell sorting (FACS) A method of separating and sorting cells according to various characteristics, such as what proteins they have on their surface.

Fc region See the definition for **Constant region**.

US Food and Drug Administration (FDA) The organization that regulates human drugs and medical devices (among other things) in the United States.

Fibroblasts A cell in connective tissue (e.g., bones, cartilage, tendons, ligaments, and fatty tissue), which produces collagen and other fibers. They are the most common type of connective tissue cell in the body.

Fluorescence in situ hybridization (FISH) A laboratory technique used to detect the presence of DNA mutation such as an amplification, translocation, or gene rearrangement.

Fusion protein A protein made from parts taken from two or more different proteins. These are made by cells when the DNA in two genes has broken and been spliced together to create a new, mutated gene. Often caused by translocations.

Fv region See the definition for **Variable region**.

Gastrointestinal stromal tumor (GIST) A rare group of cancers that develop in the digestive system.

Gene A stretch of DNA within a chromosome that contains all the information a cell needs to make one or more proteins.

Gene activity Refers to how often a gene's information is accessed by the cell and used to make a particular protein.

Gene activation When a cell "switches on" a gene and starts using the information it contains to make a protein.

Gene expression When a gene's information is being used by a cell to make a protein, that gene is said to be "expressed," "switched on," or "active."

Gene therapy Refers to treatments in which a gene (DNA) is altered or added to living cells. For example, it includes CAR T cell

therapy, where an extra gene is added to a patient's T cells.

Generic treatments These treatments are exact copies of an existing treatment.

Genome The complete set of genetic material in a cell including all the DNA in a cell's chromosomes and the small amount of DNA found in the mitochondria.

Genomic instability A phenomenon seen in cancer cells. Refers to the fact that cancer cells accumulate DNA damage at a faster rate than other cells, largely due to faulty DNA repair proteins and short telomeres.

Germline mutation A mutation found in an egg or sperm and is consequently present in every cell of an organism. Different from a somatic mutation – one that has occurred during the person's lifetime.

Glioblastoma (also called **glioblastoma multiforme)** A highly aggressive form of brain tumor that develops from support cells called glial cells.

G-protein-coupled receptors A group of over 1,000 receptor proteins found on human cells that respond to stimuli such as light, lipids, sugars, proteins, and peptides. They perform a vast array of different functions.

Graft versus host disease (GVHD) A possible complication that can occur when a patient receives a stem cell or bone marrow transplant. It occurs when some of the transplanted cells attack the patient's body.

Growth factor A small protein that binds to specific receptors on target cells called growth factor receptors. Growth factors often promote cell survival and stimulate cell growth and proliferation.

Growth factor receptor Receptor proteins on our cells that respond to the presence of growth factors. There are 58 different growth factor receptors found on the cells in our body. They are also referred to as receptor tyrosine kinases (RTKs).

Hallmarks of cancer A set of behaviors of cancer cells described by two scientists, Douglas Hanahan and Robert Weinberg.

Hedgehog pathway A signaling pathway active in some cell types, including adult and embryonic stem cells and some cancer cells. Involves a receptor called Patched, to which hedgehog proteins can bind.

Helper T cell A type of T cell that activates other white blood cells and coordinates immune responses.

Hematopoiesis The creation of blood cells (red and white) and platelets by stem cells in the bone marrow.

Hematopoietic stem cell See the definition for **Hematopoiesis**.

HER2 Human EGF receptor-2. A member of the EGF receptor family that comprises EGFR, HER2, HER3, and HER4. Also called ErbB2 or Neu.

Heterodimer A dimer made up of two similar but not identical subunits.

HLA See the definition for **MHC protein** for a description.

Hodgkin lymphoma A hematological (blood) cancer usually driven by faulty mature B cells called Reed Sternberg (RS) cells.

Homodimer A dimer made up of two identical subunits.

Homologous recombination (HR) Our cells' most accurate method for repairing double-strand breaks in DNA.

Homologous recombination deficiency (HRD) Cells that cannot perform homologous recombination are said to exhibit HRD. They are forced to use error-prone methods (such as non-homologous end joining [NHEJ]) to repair double-strand DNA breaks and consequently accumulate DNA mutations rapidly.

Hormone receptor (HR)-positive breast cancer A breast cancer in which the cancer cells contain receptors for estrogen and/or progesterone.

Hormone therapy A group of cancer treatments that either reduce the amount of a hormone in the body or block the actions of a hormone receptor.

Humanized antibody An antibody that contains mostly human protein, but a small amount of mouse (or other) protein remains.

Hypothalamus A region of the brain responsible for making a variety of important hormones.

Immune effector cell–associated neurotoxicity syndrome (ICANS) A set of symptoms caused by the release of cytokines in the brain, which is a possible side effect of some forms of immunotherapy such as CAR T cell therapy and T cell engagers. Symptoms include delirium, seizures, agitation, and problems with written and/or verbal communication.

Immunoglobulin G (IgG) The main type of antibody in the blood and the one most used in the creation of antibody-based cancer treatments.

Immune mobilizing monoclonal TCRs against cancer (ImmTAC®) A type of T cell engager that incorporates the antigen-binding site of a T cell receptor and that of an antibody. Designed to create a physical connection between cancer cells and T cells.

Immune checkpoint inhibitor A treatment that boosts T cells by blocking a checkpoint protein on their surface or by interfering with a checkpoint protein ligand.

Immune editing The process through which the immune system shapes the future development of a population of cancer cells by destroying some cancer cells but being unable to destroy others.

Immunogenicity The ability of cells to provoke a response from the immune system. An immunogenic cancer is one highly likely to provoke a response.

Immunoglobulins B cell receptors (BCRs) that have been released by B cells into the blood (also known as antibodies).

Immunohistochemistry (IHC) A laboratory technique that uses antibodies to detect a particular protein of interest in a sample.

Immunomodulators (IMiDs) Drugs that have the ability to affect (modulate) the patient's immune system. Usually used to refer to thalidomide, lenalidomide, and pomalidomide, all of which affect the behavior of a protein called cereblon.

Immunotherapy Treatments that activate or restore the ability of the immune system to fight cancer.

Immunotoxin A treatment that combines part of an antibody or other protein involved in immune responses (such as a cytokine) with a toxic substance, such as a toxic protein made by a bacterium.

Indel The term for small insertions or deletions in a cell's DNA. Often defined as mutations affecting up to 1,000 base pairs.

Intracellular Within the cell rather than on the cell surface.

Intratumoral heterogenicity Describes the fact that a single tumor (or blood cancer) can contain multiple populations of cancer cells with different properties.

Ki-67 A protein only found in multiplying cells. Its presence is sometimes measured to determine what proportion of cells in a tumor are multiplying at a given moment in time. Tumors with a high proportion of multiplying cells are said to be high-grade; these tumors are generally fast-growing and likely to spread.

Kinase An enzyme that can attach phosphate to one or more targets. These targets are often serine, threonine, or tyrosine amino acids in other proteins. The addition of phosphate might activate or inhibit the target or alter its ability to interact with other proteins or DNA.

Kinase inhibitor A drug that blocks the action of one or more kinases.

Ligand Anything (often a small protein) that can bind to a particular receptor.

Liquid biopsy (fluid biopsy) A sample of a patient's blood from which scientists purify and analyze whole cancer cells or DNA that has leaked out from cancer cells (circulating tumor DNA).

Leukocyte A general name for any white blood cell.

Leukemia A cancer of white blood cells found in the blood and bone marrow.

Locus The specific position on a chromosome where a gene is located.

Lymphatic spread When a cancer spreads via the lymph vessels.

Lymph node Small bean-shaped organs located throughout the body. Millions of white blood cells live inside them, and fluid from the body's tissues drains into them.

Lymphocytes These include B cells, T cells, and natural killer (NK) cells.

Lymphoid cells There are two main groups of white blood cells: (1) myeloid cells, such as macrophages and dendritic cells, and (2) lymphoid cells, such as B cells and T cells.

Lymphoma A cancer of mature lymphocytes in a lymph node. Can be non-Hodgkin lymphoma or Hodgkin lymphoma. Most are derived from B cells rather than T cells.

Macrophage A type of white blood cell that engulfs and digests cellular debris, foreign substances, microbes, and cancer cells. It also has many other functions such as playing a pivotal role in inflammation and controlling the activity of T cells in our tissues.

Magnetic resonance imaging See the definition for **MRI scan**.

Maintenance therapy A treatment that is given to patients following another treatment. It may include treatment with drugs, vaccines, or antibodies that kill cancer cells, and it may be given for a long time.

Malignant disease (malignancy) A disease (cancer) in which abnormal cells multiply out of control and have the potential to invade nearby tissues.

MAPKs Mitogen-activated protein kinases – a family of closely related intracellular protein kinases that includes ERK, JNK, and p38.

MAP kinase pathway (MAPK pathway) A signaling pathway commonly activated when a growth factor such as EGF binds to a growth factor receptor such as EGFR. The term specifically refers to signaling pathways involving ERK or other MAPKs such as JNK and p38. Other components of the pathway include Ras, Raf, and MEK proteins.

Mast cell A type of white blood cell involved in allergic reactions and other immune responses.

MDS See the definition for **Myelodysplastic syndromes**.

Myeloid-derived suppressor cells (MDSCs) Refers to various sets of white blood cells that are derived from myeloid white blood cells. They are often found in tumors, where they suppress T cells and prevent an effective, cancer-fighting immune response.

Melanoma skin cancer A cancer of melanin-producing cells (melanocytes) in the skin. This is the most aggressive and dangerous form of skin cancer. It is also referred to as malignant melanoma. (Uveal melanoma develops from cells that make melanin in the eye.)

Menarche The age at which a girl gets her first menstrual period.

Messenger RNA (mRNA) Similar to DNA but exists as a single strand rather than a double helix. mRNA is manufactured by RNA polymerase, which detects the order of DNA bases in a gene and constructs a corresponding strand of mRNA to match. The mRNA is then transported to ribosomes in the cytoplasm, which use the mRNA to make proteins.

Metastasis A secondary cancer that has developed from breakaway cells from the original tumor that have spread to another part of the body.

Major histocompatibility complex (MHC) protein MHC proteins (also called human leukocyte antigen (HLA)) are found on the surface of all our cells. Our cells use MHC class 1 proteins to display fragments from the proteins they make to white blood cells. Specialized white blood cells such as macrophages and dendritic cells (professional antigen-presenting cells) also have MHC class 2 proteins on their surface, which they use to display fragments of proteins they have picked up from their environment.

Medicines and Healthcare products Regulatory Agency (MHRA) The organization in the United Kingdom that regulates medicines, medical devices, and blood components for use in the United Kingdom.

Microenvironment The immediate small-scale environment of a cell or tumor.

Missense mutation A single nucleotide change in DNA, which alters the amino acid sequence of the encoded protein. A type of point mutation.

Mitochondria These are tiny structures within our cells that create energy for the cell in the form of ATP. In addition, when a cell is damaged, its mitochondria may release cytochrome C, which triggers apoptosis.

Mitosis The stage in the cell cycle in which the cell finally splits into two to create two daughter cells.

Monoclonal antibody All antibody treatments for cancer are monoclonal. That is, the millions of copies of the antibody in the treatment are identical to one another and have been manufactured using a population of genetically identical cells (a clone).

MPNs See the definition for **Myelo-proliferative neoplasms**.

Magnetic resonance imaging (MRI) scan Uses powerful magnets to generate an image of the inside of the body.

mRNA See the definition for **messenger RNA;I**.

Microsatellite instability (MSI) A phenomenon seen in cancers in which the cancer cells contain faults in a type of DNA repair called mismatch repair. Regions of the cell's chromosomes called microsatellites consequently contain thousands of mutations. Also called MSI-High, or dMMR (deficient in mismatch repair).

Multidrug resistance (MDR) protein See the definition for **P-glycoprotein**.

Mutation Any change to the DNA of a cell. Can occur naturally or be caused by exposure to DNA-damaging agents (carcinogens) such as cigarette smoke and UV light.

Myc An important oncogene; a transcription factor.

Myeloid cells There are two main groups of white blood cells: (1) myeloid cells, such as macrophages and dendritic cells and (2) lymphoid cells, such as B cells and T cells.

Myeloid-derived suppressor cells See the definition for **MDSCs**.

Myelodysplastic syndromes (MDS; also called myelodysplasia) A group of rare cancers that occur when too few stem cells in the bone marrow mature properly. This leads to a shortage of healthy red blood cells, white blood cells, or platelets.

Myeloma (multiple myeloma) A hematological cancer that develops from faulty plasma cells. Plasma cells are antibody-producing B cells, which are generally found in the bone marrow.

Myeloproliferative neoplasms (MPNs; also called myeloproliferative disorders) A group of rare cancers caused when faulty stem cells multiply and create too many white blood cells, red blood cells, or platelets. MPNs include chronic myeloid leukemia (also called chronic myelogenous leukemia), polycythemia vera, essential thrombocythemia, primary myelofibrosis, chronic neutrophilic leukemia, and chronic eosinophilic leukemia.

Naked antibody An antibody protein to which nothing has been added or removed.

Natural killer cell (NK cell) A type of lymphocyte white blood cell that plays a major role in identifying and destroying faulty cells, including cancer cells and cells infected by viruses.

Neoadjuvant treatment A treatment given before surgery to kill cancer cells, shrink a tumor, and hopefully make surgery more effective.

Neoantigen A neoantigen is a peptide derived from a mutated protein. Crucially, the peptide includes amino acids that are different from normal because of the mutation.

Neuroblastoma A rare cancer affecting children that develops from embryonic cells of the nervous system.

Neuroendocrine tumors (NETs) A group of rare cancers that can occur in many different locations, and where the cancer cells release hormones.

Neutrophil The most abundant type of white blood cell in the human body. A type of myeloid cell. They are short-lived, very mobile, and quickly enter sites of infection.

Next-generation sequencing A term that refers to various modern techniques to sequence DNA.

NHEJ See the definition for **Non-homologous end joining**.

The National Institute for Health and Care Excellence (NICE) The body that provides national guidance on the treatment of cancer and decides which treatments should be available through the NHS in England and Wales.

Non-Hodgkin lymphoma (NHL) A group of hematological cancers caused by faulty, mature lymphocytes (most are caused by faulty B cells). Some are fast-growing, such as diffuse large B cell lymphoma; others are slow-growing, such as follicular lymphoma.

Non-homologous end joining (NHEJ) A method our cells use to repair broken chromosomes; less accurate compared to homologous recombination.

Nonsense mutation A point mutation in a gene that creates a stop codon part way through the gene and hence instructs the cell to make a shortened (truncated) version of a protein.

Nucleus The membrane-bound compartment within a cell that contains the cell's DNA in the form of chromosomes.

Oligometastases When an initial (primary) tumor has spread and created a small number of metastases.

Oncogene A gene that has the potential to cause cancer. In cancer cells, oncogenes are often mutated in such a way that the protein made from the gene has become over-active or is produced at abnormally high levels. Many oncogenes control cell proliferation and survival.

Oncogene addiction When a cancer cell is dependent on the protein made from an oncogene for its survival.

Oncolytic virus A virus that preferentially infects and kills cancer cells.

Overall survival (median) The time it takes for half the patients in a study to die, while the other half remain alive. For each patient, their survival is often defined as the length of time they live after agreeing to participate in a study or from when they start treatment.

Oxygen free radicals (reactive oxygen species or ROS) These are highly active

oxygen atoms that cause DNA damage. They are produced naturally in our body during various essential chemical reactions. They are also released by white blood cells and are present in cigarette smoke, air pollutants, and industrial chemicals, among other things.

p53 A very important tumor suppressor protein made from the *TP53* gene that is commonly deleted or mutated in cancer cells. It controls the production of DNA repair proteins and triggers cell death if the cell's DNA is badly damaged.

Poly (ADP-ribose) polymerase (PARP) A family of proteins that have various functions, one of which is to detect single-strand breaks in DNA and bring in a team of other proteins to perform repair.

PARP inhibitor A treatment that blocks PARP enzymes. These treatments are particularly effective against cancers that have lost the ability to perform error-free DNA repair through a process called homologous recombination (HR).

Partial response When a person's cancer shrinks by at least 30%, and there are no signs the cancer has grown anywhere else in the body.

Passenger mutation A mutation found in a cancer cell that is adding little or nothing to the cell's abnormal behavior.

Pathogen A disease-causing organism such as a bacterium, virus, or parasite. A pathogenic mutation is a DNA mutation that causes a disease or one that puts someone at high risk of developing a disease.

PD-1 One of many checkpoint proteins found on the surface of T cells and the target of some immune checkpoint inhibitors. When PD-1 is triggered by one of its ligands (PD-L1 or PD-L2) the T cell becomes suppressed.

PD-L1 A protein that connects with, and triggers, PD-1. Found on the surface of some white blood cells and often also found on cancer cells.

Peptide/polypeptide A chain of amino acids not long enough to be called a protein.

Peptide antigen A small protein fragment that can fit inside an MHC protein and be displayed to T cells.

Pericytes Elongated cells that are wrapped around our capillaries (small blood vessels). They can control blood flow and provide structural support and growth factors to the endothelial cells that line the capillaries.

Perineural spread When a cancer spreads by traveling along nerve bundles.

PET scan A detailed image of the inside of the body created using a short-lived radioactive drug called a tracer. PET images are often combined with images from CT or MRI scans, called PET-CT or PET-MRI.

P-glycoprotein (P-gp) A protein often made by cancer cells that causes resistance to a range of different treatments. P-gp, also called multidrug resistance-1 (MDR1), is located on the cell surface and pumps harmful chemicals (such as many types of chemotherapy) out of the cell.

Pharmacodynamics The study of the effects that a drug has on the body.

Pharmacokinetics The study of the movement, absorption, distribution, metabolism, and excretion of a drug from the body.

Philadelphia chromosome An extra-short version of chromosome 22 created by a translocation affecting chromosomes 9 and 22. This translocation forces the cell to make an abnormal protein – a fusion protein called Bcr-Abl.

Phosphate A phosphorous atom surround by oxygen atoms.

Phosphorylation The process of adding a phosphate group to a molecule, such as a protein, sugar, or lipid. The addition of a phosphate group to a protein usually triggers its activity or changes its ability to interact with other proteins or DNA.

PI3K/AKT/mTOR pathway A cell signaling pathway important in controlling cell behavior. The target of some cancer treatments.

Pituitary gland A tiny organ the size of a pea located at the base of the brain. It produces various hormones.

Point mutation The mutation of a single base pair (nucleotide) in DNA.

Positron emission tomography scan See the definition for **PET scan**.

Precision medicine An approach in which the characteristics of a patient's cancer are matched with the treatment most likely to be effective for them.

Predictive biomarker A characteristic of cancer cells that can be measured and that tells you whether a particular treatment is likely to be effective or not.

Professional antigen-presenting cells See the definition for **Antigen-presenting cells (APCs)**.

Prognostic biomarker A characteristic of cancer cells that can be measured and that gives an idea of the likely outcome of the patient independently of what treatment they receive. For example, the presence of a particular mutation might be linked to a shortened survival time.

Progression-free survival (median) The time it takes for half the patients in a study to experience disease progression or to die, while the other half remains alive and progression-free.

Proliferation Rapid reproduction of cells through cell division.

Promoter A region of DNA found immediately before the start of a gene. It is a place where transcription factors can attach to the gene and recruit RNA polymerase in order to initiate gene transcription.

Protein A big molecule made up of small chemical components called amino acids.

Hundreds of thousands of proteins are found in our cells and form the basis of body structures such as skin and hair and of substances such as enzymes, cytokines, and antibodies. The instructions for making proteins are found in our genes.

Protein kinase A protein that can add a chemical group called a phosphate group to other proteins, often resulting in a change in their activity.

Proteasome A complicated, cylindrical structure made up of various different proteins. Our cells use them to break down unwanted proteins into their constituent amino acids.

Proto-oncogene A gene involved in normal cell growth. Mutation of a proto-oncogene may cause it to become an oncogene, which can drive the growth of cancer cells. NB. The distinction between proto-oncogenes and oncogenes isn't always adhered to, and the term *proto-oncogene* seems to be falling into disuse.

Prostaglandin A group of tiny, fatty compounds produced by many cells. They are produced at sites of injury or infection and control inflammation, blood flow, and clot formation.

Pseudoprogression When a tumor appears to be growing but will in fact later stabilize or shrink.

PTEN An important tumor suppressor protein that blocks the PI3K/AKT/mTOR pathway and prevents DNA mutations. The gene for PTEN (*PTEN*) is often suppressed or deleted in cancer cells.

Radioimmunotherapy A term used to describe an antibody that has been linked to a radioactive isotope and used to deliver radiotherapy to cancer cells.

Radiolabeled antibody Same as radioimmunotherapy.

Radioactive isotope (radioisotope) A radioactive version of a chemical element.

Radioligand A cancer treatment that contains both a radioisotope and a component, such as the ligand for a receptor, that will seek out cancer cells.

Radiotherapy A treatment given to many patients with cancer that involves the use of high-energy (ionizing) radiation to kill cancer cells. The radiation may be delivered by a machine called a linear accelerator, which points a beam of radiation at the person's cancer. Some radiotherapies involve the insertion of radioactive seeds or implants close to a tumor (brachytherapy). Or it can involve giving the person a radioactive liquid.

Randomized control trial A clinical trial in which patients are allocated randomly (randomized) into different groups. Each group is given a specific treatment or allocated to be a control group that receives a comparison treatment, a dummy treatment (placebo), or no treatment (observation only).

RAS genes An important set of oncogenes that are mutated in many cancers. There are three versions of the gene (*KRAS*, *NRAS*, and *HRAS*), which encode three main Ras proteins (K-Ras, N-Ras, and H-Ras). Ras proteins are an integral part of the MAPK pathway. They are not kinases and hence cannot be blocked with a kinase inhibitor.

Retinoblastoma protein (RB) An important tumor suppressor protein made from the *RB* gene. RB halts the cell cycle unless phosphorylated by CDKs (cyclin-dependent kinases).

Receptor A protein that binds to specific signals from outside the cell, such as growth factors. Many receptors are on the cell surface, such as growth factor receptors. Other receptors, such as some hormone receptors, are found in the cell cytoplasm and nucleus.

Receptor tyrosine kinase (RTK) A class of receptors found on the surface of our cells.

Many of them are growth factor receptors that respond to the presence of growth factors such as EGF.

Response evaluation criteria in solid tumors (RECIST) A standard set of criteria used to determine whether a new treatment or other intervention is having an effect.

Recombinant DNA technology Describes techniques used by scientists to create DNA sequences that wouldn't normally exist.

Reed Sternberg (RS) cells Large abnormal cells derived from B cells that cause Hodgkin lymphoma.

Response rate The proportion of patients who have a complete or partial response to a treatment.

Ribosome A large structure made from ribosomal RNA and various proteins. It uses the information in messenger RNA (mRNA) to select and attach together tens, hundreds, or thousands of amino acids to construct a protein. Thousands of ribosomes are found in the cytoplasm of each cell.

Ribonucleic acid (RNA) A complex molecule similar to DNA. Made from four bases: A, C, G, and U (uracil). Used in the manufacture of proteins. Comes in many forms with different functions, such as messenger RNA (mRNA), ribosomal RNA (rRNA), transfer RNA (tRNA), micro RNA (miRNA), small nuclear RNA (snRNA).

RNA polymerase An enzyme that travels along a stretch of the DNA double helix and creates a single-stranded copy out of RNA. The RNA copy of a gene is called messenger RNA (mRNA). The cell's ribosomes use the information in mRNAs to make proteins.

RTK See the definition for **Receptor Tyrosine Kinase**.

Sarcoma A cancer that has developed from bone, cartilage, fat, muscle, tendons, blood vessels, or other connective tissues.

Senescence A dormant state in which the cell is no longer able to divide. It can be triggered by short telomeres and DNA damage.

Signaling pathway/signal transduction cascade A chain reaction of events triggered by a signal (such as the binding of a growth factor to its receptor) at the cell surface, which is then transmitted through the cell and into the nucleus, where it causes a change in the cell's behavior.

Scottish Medicines Consortium (SMC) The body in Scotland that reviews medicines licensed by the MHRA and decides whether they should be made available to people in Scotland through NHS Scotland.

Squamous cell carcinoma A cancer that develops from faulty squamous cells – flat cells that are found in the skin, in the lining of various organs, and in the respiratory and digestive tracts.

Stem cell A cell that can both self-renew (i.e., produce more stem cells) and give rise to other cell types. Various types of stem cells are found in the developing embryo and in healthy adult tissues.

Somatic mutation A mutation in a cell's DNA that has occurred during the person's lifetime (as opposed to an inherited, germline mutation).

Stromal cells Cells, such as fibroblasts, endothelial cells, pericytes, and adipocytes, that support a tissue or tumor. In a tumor, stromal cells are all the non-cancer cells residing in the tumor microenvironment.

Subclonal mutation See the definition for **Clonal mutation**.

Synthetic lethality When a combination of mutations and/or the inhibition of two or more proteins leads to cell death, whereas the mutation/inhibition of only one of these proteins does not.

Systemic anticancer therapy (SACT) Any medicine/drug treatment used to control or treat cancer. This can be in the form of a tablet or liquid, an infusion into the blood, or given by injection. SACTs include chemotherapy, hormone therapy, targeted therapy, and immunotherapy.

Targeted treatment/therapy A treatment that has the ability to target a particular protein or faulty process found in cancer cells. Targeted treatments are designed to discriminate between cancer cells and healthy cells better than other treatments such as chemotherapy, but in reality, this isn't always achieved.

T cell engager A treatment that creates a physical connection between cancer cells and T cells. Includes approaches such as BiTEs®, bispecific antibodies, and ImmTACs®.

T cell receptor (TCR) Similar to B cell receptors but found on T cells. T cells use their TCRs to respond to peptide antigens – small protein fragments displayed by cells using their MHC proteins.

T cell (T lymphocyte) A type of lymphocyte (white blood cell) that plays a central role in cell-mediated immunity. T cells can be distinguished from other lymphocytes, such as B cells and natural killer cells, by the presence of T cell receptors on the cell surface.

TCR-engineered T cell therapy A treatment approach in which T cells are taken from a patient's blood and then genetically modified so that they produce a new T cell receptor.

Telomerase An enzyme that lengthens telomeres.

Telomere Stretches of DNA at each end of our chromosomes. They protect our genes and prevent gene breakages and rearrangements. As we get older, our cells' telomeres get shorter.

TIL therapy See the definition for **Tumor-infiltrating lymphocyte therapy**.

Therapeutic window The difference between the dose of a drug that is effective and the dose that causes intolerable side effects.

TKI See the definition for **Tyrosine kinase inhibitor**.

Toxin A poisonous substance (often a protein) produced by living cells.

Transcoelomic spread When cancer spreads via the fluid circulating in the abdomen.

Transcription The process by which an enzyme called RNA polymerase reads the order of DNA bases in a gene and uses this information to make a copy of that gene in the form of messenger RNA (mRNA).

Transcription activator-like effector nucleases (TALEN) A series of enzymes engineered to make specific changes to the sequence of a piece of DNA.

Transcription factor A protein that can attach to DNA at particular locations (called gene promoters and enhancers) and that helps switch on the transcription of one or more genes. Examples of transcription factors important in cancer cells include p53, Myc, and the estrogen and androgen receptors.

Translation The process by which a ribosome uses a piece of mRNA to make a protein.

Translocation A chromosome abnormality caused by the rearrangement of parts of two different chromosomes. A gene fusion may be created when the translocation joins two otherwise separate genes.

Trispecific antibodies Antibody-based proteins that attach to three different targets. Some include the Fc portion of an antibody (to extend their longevity), and some do not.

Tumor antigen/tumor-associated antigen A small fragment (a peptide) of a protein that is displayed by cancer cells to the immune system using their MHC proteins or released into their surroundings. May or may not be exclusive to the person's cancer cells.

Tumor-infiltrating lymphocyte therapy (TIL therapy) A treatment that involves isolating the lymphocytes (usually T cells) from a person's tumor, increasing their number in a laboratory, and then returning them to the patient.

Tumor mutation burden (TMB) The total number of mutations found in a person's cancer cells. Often provided as the number of mutations per one million DNA bases (mutations per megabase or muts/Mb). Cancers with a high TMB are often those that are more immunogenic and likely to respond to immunotherapy.

Tumor-specific antigen A tumor antigen that is exclusively displayed or released by cancer cells and is absent from healthy cells.

Tumor suppressor gene A gene that encodes a protein that helps control and limit cell growth or that is able to trigger cell death. In cancer cells, tumor suppressor genes are often deleted, mutated, or suppressed so that their protective function is lost.

Tyrosine kinase inhibitor (TKI) A drug that blocks a tyrosine kinase – a kinase that exclusively attaches phosphates to tyrosine amino acids. However, this term is sometimes erroneously used to describe all drugs that block kinases.

Umbrella trial A type of clinical trial designed to test the impact of multiple drugs on different populations of patients in a single trial. The patients all have the same type of cancer, but are allocated to specific groups based on properties such as the presence of certain mutations.

Vaccine Something (such as a protein fragment from a virus or other disease-causing microorganism) that, when administered to a person, stimulates their immune system in such a way that it provides long-lasting protection against that organism. Cancer treatment vaccines are used to provoke an immune response against an existing cancer in the patient's body.

Variable region The front end of an antibody (also called Fv). This includes the part of the antibody that attaches to its target – the antigen-binding region.

Vascular spread When a cancer spreads via the bloodstream.

Vascular endothelial growth factor (VEGF) A growth factor that attaches to VEGF receptors on endothelial cells that line blood vessels. This causes blood vessels to grow to create new blood vessels through a process called angiogenesis.

VDJ recombination The process by which T cells and B cells assemble different gene segments – known as variable (V), diversity (D), and joining (J) genes – in order to generate unique receptors (B cell receptor or T cell receptor) that they place on their surface to allow them to recognize invading microbes or cancer cells.

Whole genome sequencing When the DNA is extracted from a single cell or sample of tissue and subjected to DNA sequencing analysis. "Whole genome" refers to the fact that the entire genome is sequenced rather than just the genes, which only take up about 1–5% of the cell's DNA.

Wild type The normal, non-mutated version of a gene or protein.

Index

Note: Page numbers in *italic* refer to figures, page numbers in **bold** refer to tables.

A Beginner's Guide to Targeted Cancer Treatments and Cancer Immunotherapy, Second Edition. Elaine Vickers.
© 2025 John Wiley & Sons Ltd. Published 2025 by John Wiley & Sons Ltd.